BRONCHOLOGY:
RESEARCH, DIAGNOSTIC AND THERAPEUTIC ASPECTS

DEVELOPMENTS IN SURGERY

VOLUME 3

BRONCHOLOGY:
RESEARCH, DIAGNOSTIC, AND
THERAPEUTIC ASPECTS

Proceedings of the Second World Congress for Bronchology,
held at Düsseldorf, FRG, 2-4 June 1980

edited by

JOHN A. NAKHOSTEEN, MD
Chest Physician, Consultant Bronchologist,
Ruhrlandklinik, Essen, FRG

and

WERNER MAASSEN, MD
Professor of Medicine, Medical Director,
Ruhrlandklinik, Essem, FRG
President, 2nd World Congress for Bronchology

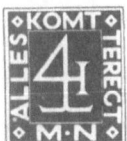 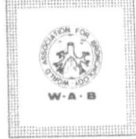

1981

MARTINUS NIJHOFF PUBLISHERS
THE HAGUE / BOSTON / LONDON

Distributors

for the United States and Canada
Kluwer Boston, Inc.
190 Old Derby Street
Hingham, MA 02043
USA

for all other countries
Kluwer Academic Publishers Group
Distribution Center
P.O.Box 322
3300 AH Dordrecht
The Netherlands

This volume is listed in the Library of Congress Cataloging in Publication Data

ISBN-13:978-94-009-8238-3   e-ISBN-13:978-94-009-8236-9
DOI: 10.1007/978-94-009-8236-9

ACKNOWLEDGEMENTS

We would like to express our gratitude to the many colleagues and co-workers who helped make the Second World Congress for Bronchology so successful. Our particular thanks go to the members of the Organizing, Finance, Scientific and Planing Committees. The Technical and Office Staff, which included students, secretaries and other hospital personnel was indispensable in seeing that thousand-and-one details were fulfilled. For the special contribution that each of the following gave, we would like to mention by name Dr. and Mrs. W. Petro, Dr. W. Dams, Mr. M. Leiendecker, Miss I. Angerstein and cand. med. D. Leimenstoll. To Dr. S. Ikeda and the staff of the World Association for Bronchology Head Office in Tokyo we also owe a special thanks for their organizing the far eastern participation and their giving valuable advice.

Generous financial support by Olympus Optical Company, Hamburg and Tokyo, had enabled us to purchase a limited number of copies of BRONCHOLOGY 1980 at a reduced rate and pass this saving on to congress participants placing firm pre-publication orders with us; we would like to thank Olympus for this help.

Mr. Jeffrey Smith of Martinus Nijhoff has readily given valuable advice every time we have had to turn to him, and we appreciate this greatly.

Finally, our unending thanks go to our wives, who, each in her own way, patiently and actively supported us in over two years of work for the Congress and for this book.

J. A. Nakhosteen   W. Maassen

Essen, F.R.G.
August, 1980

TABLE OF CONTENTS

XXII

Chapter I
INTRODUCTION

The papers presented at the Second World Congress for Bronchology, held in Duesseldorf from June 2 to June 4, 1980, have been compiled for this book. The majority of these papers, submitted - as requested - as camera-ready manuscripts for off-set printing, have been reproduced un- altered. A minority which, for one reason or another, did not conform to the detailed instructions for preparing manuscripts, have been subjected to greater or lesser editing, a few papers necessitating major revision. This task, the arrangement of the chapters, and preparation of the various indeces have made up the major part of the editors' contribution.

Because of the topical and socio-economic importance of lung cancer, and the individual suffering this appaling disease causes, Chapter 2 EARLY DIAGNOSIS OF BRONCHOGENIC CARCINOMA, begins with reports by Andersen and Fontana on efforts being undertaken presently at the Mayo Clinic in this field (The Mayo Lung Project), goes on to various diagnostic measures in obtaining material, localizing occult and in-situ neoplasmas, and assessing cytological data. Subtle endoscopic changes are discussed; and in a summary of a film presented on the same subject, one paper shows how diagnostic yield has improved in recent years, in particular with the advent of biplane fluoroscopic guidance in reaching peripheral lesions. Weng's Special Paper on chronic bronchitis in China completes this chapter, because of the great general interest this topic holds.

In Chapter 3 BRONCHOSCOPY AND INTENSIVE CARE MEDICINE, the disad- vantages are discussed of "blind" catheter compared to flexible bron- choscopic suctioning of retained secretions on the intensive care unit, which is yet another reason for the indispensability of the bronchofiber- scope in this context, a point taken up by others. The necessity of trans- bronchial biopsy (TBB) in acute pulmonary failure is emphasized, where the diagnostic yield may justify this procedure in a high-risk group. Finally, the successful use of the bronchofiberscope in treating severe airway burns is reported.

COMPLICATIONS IN BRONCHOLOGIC EXAMINATIONS are discussed in Chapter 4 with most papers dealing with fiberoptic and one with rigid bronchoscopic procedure. Current interest may be more centered on the newer examination, and complications of rigid bronchoscopy are adequately documented in the literature. Nonetheless, in an excellent review, it is pointed out at least two cardiac arrests occurred during rigid bronchoscopic suctioning of retained secretions, and these are situations in which flexible bronchoscopy would definitely be prefered. Various approaches to endobronchial bleeding are also presented, including a new method with instillation of fibrin glue and aprotinin-trans AMCHA combination, and the painstaking approach practiced routinely by Ikeda's group. In general, simple but essential guidelines would, however, seem adequate: is there a bleeding (iatrogenic?) diathesis? Is the patient properly positioned? Is noradrenalin(norepinephrin) 1:10,000 and/or iced physiological saline ready for (prophylactic) intrabronchial instillation? In high-risk cases, is matched blood available for the rare case when it may be needed? Two developements of possible interest in this context are the double-lumen tubes, discussed here. Cardiac rhythm and blood gas disturbances, and various problems in local and general anesthesia round up the chapter.

BRONCHOGRAPHY (Chapter 5) is fast becoming a forgotten skill in certain parts of the globe, but the editors are in complete agreement with Japanese bronchologists, who emphasize its importance in the study of bronchiectasis, lung cancer and other pulmonary disease. Watanabe's and Ikeda's survey of 181,892 bronchographies at 259 Japanese institutes gives an excellent analysis of the present situation there. Using selective bronchography magnified 4 times, bronchographic changes in peripheral adeno and squamous cell carcinoma, as well as tuberculomas are detailed. We feel, however, that a better idea is gained of the topographic situation when the whole left or right side is bronchographed in three planes; although this is possible through flexible bronchoscopic and catheter systems, we generally use Carlens' double-lumen tube in general anesthesia.

The diagnosis of SARCOIDOSIS (Chapter 6) is best obtained by tissue biopsy, but since this is not always possible, great efforts are being made to secure diagnosis by other means. The correlation between raised alveolar T lymphocytes and sarcoidosis and also that between T lymphocytes and serum angiotensin converting enzyme (SACE) is discussed.The ease with which

Kveim test can be carried out - both for patient and doctor - would make it an ideal diagnostic tool, were it not for the difficulty of obtaining properly validated Kveim reagens and for the very high rate(up to 30%) of false positives reported on the European continent. Hence the survey of the results of Kveim tests with 2 sequential lots issued from Colindale, England, between 1971 and 1977 becomes all the more important - in particular, because the rate of false positives(only 4 patients out of 440 eventually found to have another disease) illustrates the very high selectivity of these materials. Bioptic material is nonetheless prefered, and in one specialist European hospital, the introduction of mediastinoscopy in 1961 led to a 99% positive diagnostic rate. Further papers deal with biopsies of mucosa and TBB, and an essential point must be stressed here: multiple biopsies (6 to 8) give better results. The results of per-bronchial biopsies are discussed in Chapter 9.

The four papers in Chapter 7 discuss various aspects of the question, RIGID OR FLEXIBLE BRONCHOSCOPY? During the symposium on this subject - chaired admirably by Penfield Faber - one Japanese panelist reported that in the past seven years, he had not once needed to use the open-tube bronchoscope, a position taken by many colleagues in Japan and America. The opposite view, emphasizing the importance of individual training and available apparatus, was also presented. Between the situations in which the flexible instrument is definitely indicated(i.e., on the intensive care unit) or the open-tube(i.e., in life-threatening hemorrhage) there is a large field in which either instrument, depending on the operator's experience, may be used. The editors certainly agree with the position that the good bronchoscopist must be expert at both methods.

Beginning with the study of pre- and post-operative functional evaluation of tracheal stenoses, Chapter 8 presents four further papers on functional aspects of tracheal disease, going on to tracheoscopy findings after prolonged intubation with a special tracheostomy tube. This paper provides a transition to a series of 10 studies on various aspects of conservative and surgical therapy of tracheal stenoses. The chapter continues with some interesting observations of the bronchi during cough following tracheobronchoplasty, in which the essential collapse of the membranous wall during cough is reported to be virtually absent if denervation has occurred.

The use of the bronchofiberscope in post-operative treatment and evaluation of patients following bronchoplastic surgery concludes this chapter.

Not surprisingly, most contributions on the subject of PER-BRONCHIAL FINE NEEDLE ASPIRATION(Chapter 9 are from the European continent. Hence a report on a vast experience ranging over 30 years in this diagnostic technique is given, and followed up with the cytological evaluation of material thus obtained. The use of flexible needle aspiration through the flexible bronchoscope is then discussed. But although the possibilities of needle aspiration through flexible instruments should be further investigated, it would seem difficult to perforate the bronchial wall with a needle attached to a flexible guide because of the lack of a counter force to overcome resistance offered by the bronchial wall. At present most per-bronchial needle aspirations are performed through the rigid tube, as the rest of the papers on this subject confirm. The chapter concludes with suggestions for applying CT-scan of the mediastinum as an indication for either flexible(when no nodes are involved) or rigid(when lymphadenopathy exists, necessitating per-bronchial aspiration) bronchoscopy.

Transbronchial biopsies(TBB) are discussed in 10 papers given in Chapter 10 Diagnostic rates of 66% in diffuse bilateral parenchymal disease, 80% in sarcoidosis, 40% in fibrosing alveolitis and 63% in peripheral carcinomas, reported from the Brompton Hospital group, reflect, generally, results obtained in most specialist western centers. We have much to learn from our Japanese colleagues here, who, with previous bronchography and under fluroscopic guidance, report positive cytological diagnosis of curettage specimens of 86.0% over-all in peripheral lesions. The interesting combination of TBB with broncho-alveolar lavage ("luobiopsy") completes this chapter.

Under the heading of "FURTHER DIAGNOSTIC PROCEDURE", Chapter 11 begins with an article on endoscopic assay during cytotoxic and radiation therapy of small cell lung cancer and continues with two papers on biochemical assays and bronchogenic carcinoma. Energy-dispersive x-ray microanalysis of fibrotic lung tissue obtained by TBB is an exciting method for finding minute amounts of toxic substances in the lung; the method and some results are presented here. One paper each on pneumediastinography and bronchological regional lung function follows. An excellent detailed analysis of 209 tumors, their topographic relation to bronchial mucosa and histological types is then given. A new diagnostic technique, "lymphoscintigraphy", and the use of the bronchofiberscope for pleuroscopy are discussed.

Beginning with the paper on Immunoglobulins in Bronchial Lavage Fluid, Chapter 12, "PATHOPHYSIOLOGY AND BRONCHOLOGY", initially offers 10 articles on various aspects of the study of the lung pathophysiology by broncho-alveolar lavage (BAL). That many of this studies are done by clinical bronchologists reflects the level to which the field of bronchology has evolved in recent years. These articles are followed by three studies on asthma: endoscopic alterations and microscopic changes reflecting various stages in asthmatic attacks. Earlier reports that long-term inhalation of beclomethasone dipropionate does not cause atrophy of bronchial mucosa are confirmed. Various types of bifurcations seen in normal right and left upper lobes are documentated, based on a series of 300 bronchofiberscopies.

MUCOCILIARY FUNCTION is another theme gaining importance during recent years, and Chapter 13 opens with an article demonstrating in a mathematical model that acute deposition of particles results in a high concentration in the large airways, while continuous exposure leads to a high concentration in the bronchioles, an observation of possible significance in small airways disease. The four major methods available for assessing mucociliary clearance in vivo are then reviewed, and it is postulated that the degree of invasiveness is directly proportional mucociliary rate, and that there may be a causative link there. Modifications of Friedman's roentgenographic-teflon disc method for assessing tracheal clearance are used in assessing the effects of various forms of beta-agonists on clearance and in investigating this function in smokers and non-smokers. A method for measuring ciliary beat frequency in vitro and its use to assess beta-adrenergic effects on cilia are described. This chapter ends with the stimulating scanning electron-microscopic studies on the bronchial mucosa, one on the injurious effects of bronchial brushings, the other on mucosal changes in chronic bronchitis.

Whether bronchological procedures should be allowed as office procedures is discussed in Chapter 14, where a fine summary of the indications and contra-indications for this is given. One word of caution from the editors: because of the danger of tension pneumothorac developing, trans-bronchial biopsies should never be done as an out-patient procedure.

Although PEDIATRIC BRONCHOSCOPY had not been planned as a separate theme, the papers received on this and related topics prompted the editors to group them together in Chapter 15. They range from the use of the bronchofiberscope in small children to indications for bronchological examinations, from case reports to immunological testing in infants.

Commencing with a Special Paper on the use of carbon dioxide laser in laryngeal and bronchial surgery, Chapter 16 continues with four experimental studies on YAG (Yttrium, Argon, Garnet), argon and CO_2 lasers, followed by a clinical study with a YAG laser introduced bronchofiberscopically. Cryo-surgery and electro surgery complete the topics discussed here, in a chapter whose contents are certainly indications of things to come.

The final chapter of this book, Chapter 17, deals with some very interesting case presentations and also reproduces other papers unrelated to the above general themes.

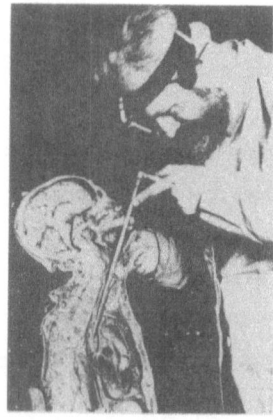

Figure 1.

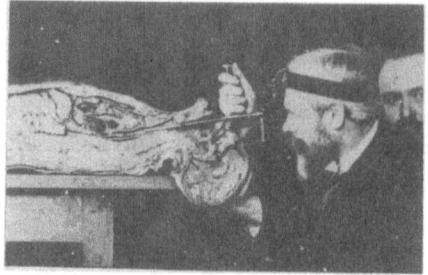

Figure 2.

Finally, in a tribute to the man who started it all, we reprint some rare pictures[*] of Gustav Killian in Freiburg, showing him initially as a younger man in the late 1880's, practicing bronchoscopy on cadavers (Fig. 1 and 2). Figure 3 shows Kilian doing a bronchoscopy in 1897 on a patient in a sitting position, and Fig. 4, using his "floating bronchoscope", which enabled the operator to have both hands free for manipulations. Since those inovativ

[*] The Editors wish to thank Professor H. Killian for his permission to reprint these photographs.

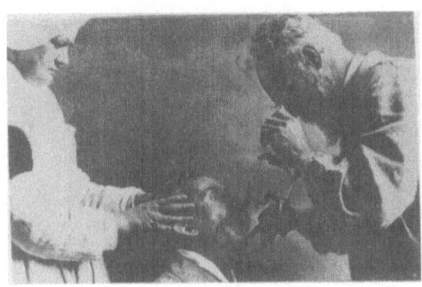

Figure 3.

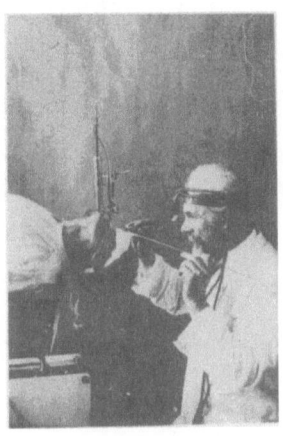

Figure 4.

and primitive beginnings, bronchology has become a medical science in which flexible and open tube bronchoscopes form the basis for optimum diagnosis with least patient discomfort, for elegant therapeutic procedures using bot pharmacological and apparative means, and for research in fundamental proce ses of lung defense and pathological mechanisms. Ikeda's bronchofiberscope has been a milestone in this process; one wonders what the next 80 years will bring.

Chapter II

EARLY DIAGNOSIS BRONCHOGENIC CARCINOMA

II.1.

DIAGNOSIS OF EARLY LUNG CANCER

H. A. ANDERSEN

A cancer of the lung which is not diagnosed until after it causes symptoms
is usually late in the course of the disease and is usually associated with a
poor prognosis. A cancer of the lung diagnosed before the onset of symptoms is
not always early in the course of the disease, but the survival rate is better
when the tumors are small or early. Though it remains to be proved whether the
mortality rate is lower in patients with early lung cancer, it is generally
considered to be a much more desirable situation and considerable effort has been
directed toward this as a goal.

Though it is not the purpose of this presentation to debate the desirabil-
ity of finding lung cancer in its early stages, factors enhancing survival are:

1. Presence of a well differentiated tumor, especially squamous type
2. Slow growth
3. Peripheral location
4. Small size (less than 3 cm in diameter)
5. Normal lung surrounding it
6. Confined to the bronchial wall (in situ or minimally invasive)
7. Lack of spread to lymph nodes or other structures, and
8. Lack of symptoms

Early cancer of the lung is found most easily by chest x-ray and by cytologic examination of sputum. Occult cancer of the lung is detected by the finding
of malignant cells in sputum when the chest x-ray is normal or is similar to
previous x-rays.

EARLY LUNG CANCER

When a new uncalcified lesion is discovered within pulmonary substance and
persists unchanged for four to six weeks, particularly in a person at increased
risk such as a cigarette smoker, the physician is obligated to persist until a
diagnosis is made unless the evidence for benignancy is overwhelming. When that
lesion is 1 cm or less in size, persistence usually means a thoracotomy. Diagnostic procedures such as brushing and biopsy via a bronchoscope or transthoracic
thin needle aspiration using fluoroscopic guidance are poor in obtaining diagnostic material from benign lesions and not sufficiently accurate in obtaining
diagnostic material from malignant lesions of this size to be reliable. It is
possible that some new procedure or refinement of presently known procedures may
change this situation. Currently, for example, studies are under way to determine
whether the x-ray attenuation number (density) on computerized tomographic (CT)
scanning may help in distinguishing between tumors and granulomas.

*J.A. Nakhosteen and W. Maassen (eds.), Bronchology: Research, Diagnostic and
Therapeutic Aspects. All rights reserved.
Copyright 1981. Martinus Nijhoff Publishers bv, The Hague / Boston / London*

OCCULT LUNG CANCER

Occult cancer of the bronchus with a cytologically positive sputum and no roentgenologic evidence of a source of malignant cells presents a different problem. The physician is then obligated to localize the cancer exactly, whether this is in a bronchus or in the upper airway.

Among 75 cases of occult cancer in the Mayo Lung Project 8 have been found in the upper respiratory tract (the larynx or above). Of the remainder only four patients did not have the cancer localized for various reasons. The remainder were localized and 58 were treated. In 31 the lesion was not visible on initial examination but random biopsy was positive in 8. In the remainder repeat examination (two to five times) was necessary in 23.

Localization of occult cancer of the bronchus has been facilitated by use of the flexible fiberbronchoscope. If the initial examination is normal, then one must search diligently with brushing of several segmental bronchi and biopsies of several spurs between segmental bronchi. All specimens are labelled and examined carefully microscopically. The bronchoscopic examination is prolonged and general anesthesia is used for these cases (as opposed to topical anesthesia for the usual bronchoscopic examination at Mayo Clinic). If no evidence of malignancy is found in any of the specimens, repeat examination, including examination of a three-day collection of a pooled specimen of sputum and fiberbronchoscopic examination as described above, is performed.

Recently hematoporphyrin has been helpful in localizing occult cancers of the bronchus. Hematoporphyrin localizes in malignant cells in greater amount than in non-malignant cells causing fluorescence which can be detected by violet light transmitted through the bronchoscope when examination is done 3 to 72 hours later. A technique has been perfected by Drs. Denis Cortese and James Kinsey at Mayo Clinic in which the endoscopist, by use of a rotating disc, can use white light for visualization at the same time that fluorescence can be detected with violet light and transformed to an auditory signal which can provide the endoscopist with exact location of the malignant tissue. This technique has been used in five cases and has provided accurate information concerning not only the presence of malignancy, but also the extent of malignancy. This is very helpful to the surgeon in planning his operation. Otherwise, he must depend on the pathologist for information concerning extent of the lesion after resection because occult bronchial cancers are not palpable. This is important particularly because of emphasis on conservation of as much pulmonary tissue as possible.

Early diagnosis and localization of lung cancer appear to be justified at present. I hope that future determinations of mortality rates vindicates physicians who are trying to help patients inflicted with this terrible disease.

II.2.

SCREENING FOR LUNG CANCER: A PROGRESS REPORT ON THE MAYO LUNG PROJECT

R S FONTANA, D R SANDERSON, W F TAYLOR, M A UHLENHOPP

The high-risk group for lung cancer consists primarily of middle-aged and older men who are chronic excessive cigarette smokers, although the risk is also increasing rapidly among women smokers. In addition, there are significant occupational and environmental risk factors, but these are minor compared to cigarette smoking. It is unfortunate that efforts to reduce smoking have been only partially successful.

Symptomatic lung cancer is usually advanced and incurable. There are only two reliable tests for detecting presymptomatic, localized disease, that is American Joint Committee (AJC) post-surgical stage I cancer. These tests are chest radiography, which is the most sensitive for identifying peripheral tumors, and sputum cytology, which is best for detecting central "hilar-type" squamous cancers that are radiographically occult. The bronchofiberscope has greatly facilitated localization of occult tumors. Therefore, until there are effective preventive measures or effective treatment for symptomatic lung cancer, testing for localized disease by periodic radiography and cytology seems reasonable, especially for those in the high-risk group.

In 1970, in response to concerns expressed by patients known to be at high risk for lung cancer, the Division of Thoracic Diseases of the Mayo Clinic recommended that any man 45 years old or more who smokes one package of cigarettes or more each day should have a sputum cytology test and a chest x-ray film at least once a year. This was and still is, an empiric recommendation without statistical proof.

In 1971 the National Cancer Institute of the United States initiated a randomized controlled study at Mayo with the aim of determining whether lung cancer mortality could be significantly reduced in high-risk patients if chest radiography and sputum cytology were offered every four months rather than simply recommended once a year.

This is the design of the Mayo study, or Mayo Lung Project (MLP): non-volunteer Mayo outpatients who were men over 45 years old and who were chronic excessive cigarette smokers without known lung cancer received chest radiographs and 3-day "pooled" sputum cytology tests. If either test proved positive on this initial screening, the patient became a "prevalence" case. Those with negative initial screens were randomized into two groups. In the screened group the

J.A. Nakhosteen and W. Maassen (eds.), Bronchology: Research, Diagnostic and
Therapeutic Aspects. All rights reserved.
Copyright 1981. Martinus Nijhoff Publishers bv, The Hague / Boston / London

patients were asked (and reminded) to have chest x-ray films and sputum tests at 4-monthly intervals. The comparison (control) group received the standard Mayo recommendation of annual testing and was contacted yearly by letter.

Between November, 1971 and July, 1976, 11,001 candidates were interviewed. The initial screening detected 92 new ("prevalence") lung cancers, nearly half of which were AJC stage I. Most of the cases were detected by radiography, but almost all of those detected cytologically were resectable "for cure". Overall, more than half of the prevalence cases had "curative" resections. The survival rate at 3 years was about 40 percent, much better than that observed in clinical practice at Mayo. About half of the survivors represent cytologically detected cases.

There were 645 patients who either refused or failed to complete the initial screening, and nearly 1,000 more who were excluded from the re-screening (or "incidence") phase of the MLP for other clinical reasons, usually limited life expectancy or pulmonary insufficiency that precluded resection. Thus there were approximately 4,600 patients randomized into each of the two "incidence" populations; the screened group, asked and reminded to have chest radiography and sputum cytology every four months, and the control group, advised to have these tests yearly. Each of these groups has now been observed for 22,000 man-years. Cooperation has been excellent in both groups, and only 73 patients have been lost to follow-up.

A successful screening program should detect more cases, especially more early stage, localized cases, than would be observed if screening were not done. As of January 1, 1980, there had been 108 lung cancers detected in the MLP screened group compared to only 72 in the control group. The difference was composed almost entirely of localized (post-surgical AJC stage I) cancers. However, it was disturbing to observe that nearly 30 percent of the cancers in both groups were of the small cell variety, which has a notoriously poor prognosis.

Two-thirds of the cases in the screened group were actually detected by the 4-monthly screening tests, whereas nearly two-thirds of the control cases presented with symptoms, usually an ominous sign. Almost half of the cancers in the screened group were localized, and more than half were resectable "for cure". In the control group these proportions were much lower.

In the control group, advanced cancers (AJC stages II and III) began to be observed soon after completion of the prevalence screen and have accumulated steadily. The first localized cancer was not observed until 20 months after the prevalence screen, and accumulation of these has been slow. Most of the localized cases have been detected by fortuitous non-study chest radiographs, something that will tend to reduce the contrast between the controls and the study group.

In the 4-monthly screened group both advanced and localized cancers began to be detected shortly after the prevalence screen and have accumulated steadily, in a manner very similar to the accumulation of the advanced cancers in the control group. It is evident that 4-monthly screening is effective in detecting localized, resectable lung cancer. Since the survival of patients with localized lung cancer is much better than the survival of those with advanced cancer, it is not surprising that the survival rate of the 4-monthly screened group has been much better than the survival rate of the control group. One might anticipate that the undetected localized cancers in the control group will eventually progress to advanced cancers and ultimately become symptomatic; but this is speculation.

It must be recalled that the aim of the MLP is to determine whether offering 4-monthly screening with chest radiography and sputum cytology will reduce mortality from lung cancer compared to advising annual screening. Mortality, not survival, is the crucial issue.

On January 1, 1980, there were 50 deaths from lung cancer in the control group and 43 in the 4-monthly screened group. This is not a statistically significant difference. Only recently have the deaths from lung cancer in the control group exceeded those in the study group. If one combines small cell and large cell undifferentiated cancers there appears to be no benefit at all from screening. However, if squamous carcinoma and adenocarcinoma are combined there are 24 lung cancer deaths in the control group and only 13 in the study group. Yet this difference is not statistically significant either. Finally, among those patients who have been in the MLP for 4 years or more the death rate from lung cancer for the controls exceeds that of the study group by a considerable amount, but again this is not statistically significant.

At this time screening for lung cancer seems somewhat promising for squamous cancers and adenocarcinomas, but not for small or large cell undifferentiated cancers, although further observation is needed to clarify this point. There is insufficient evidence now to warrant large-scale screening for lung cancer in the general population of older male smokers, nor is there enough evidence of lack of effectiveness for the physician to deny individual testing to high-risk patients, particularly those seeking a cancer checkup.

II.3.

DIE KATHETERBIOPSIE NACH FRIEDEL BEIM PERIPHEREN BRONCHIALKARZINOM

K. WETZER

EINLEITUNG

Die Katheterbiopsie peripherer Lungenherde wurde 1959 von FRIEDEL mit dem Ziel entwickelt, röntgenologisch suspekte Lungenverschattungen durch bronchologische Materialentnahme einer histologischen Sicherung der Diagnose zuzuführen.

METHODE

Die Katheterbiopsie wird im Rahmen einer Narkosebeatmungsbronchoskopie durchgeführt. Über ein Katheterführungsrohr mit verschieden starken Endkrümmungen, entsprechend den Lappen- und Segmenteingängen, wird ein modifizierter 8 Charr. Herzkatheter unter Röntgenkontrolle in das Herdgebiet vorgeschoben.Dort wird durch wiederholtes kräftiges Einstoßen des Katheters in den pathologischen Prozeß die für eine regelrechte Biopsie erforderliche Traumatisation des Gewebes bewirkt. Das mit starkem Sog aspirierte und anschließend in Alkohol fixierte Material ist fast immer für eine histologische Aufarbeitung ausreichend. Das Herdgebiet wird bis zu viermal in einer Sitzung kathetert, zwischen den Biopsien wird der Katheter jeweils mit Kochsalzlösung durchgesaugt.

ERGEBNISSE

Zur Auswertung gelangten die Katheterbiopsien bei 817 Patienten mit peripheren, rundherdartigen Bronchialkarzinomen im Zeitraum von 1967 bis 1977.

Bei 570 Patienten (69,8%) ergab die histologische Untersuchung des durch Katheterbiopsie gewonnenen Materials die Diagnose des Bronchial karzinom. In den letzten drei Jahren betrug die Trefferquote 75 bis 77%. Der Anteil der mehrfach bronchoskopierten (und kathetertent) Patienten konnte von 79% (1967) auf 7% (1977) reduziert werden.

Die diagnostische Trefferquote zeigte signifikante Abhängigkeit von der Tumorgröße: Sie betrug bei Rundherden bis zu einem Durchmesser von 2,5 cm 38,7%, bei Herden von 2,5 bis 4,5 cm Ø 71,5%, und bei Herden über 4,5 cm Ø

J.A. Nakhosteen and W. Maassen (eds.), Bronchology: Research, Diagnostic and Therapeutic Aspects. All rights reserved.
Copyright 1981. Martinus Nijhoff Publishers bv, The Hague / Boston / London

79,9 %.

An Hand von bronchographischen Untersuchungen konnte festgestellt werden, daß in etwa 15% der peripheren, rundherdartigen Bronchialkarzinome der Biopsiekatheter das Herdgebiet nicht erreichen kann. Bei einem Teil der Fälle geht der befallene Bronchus unter einem so großen Winkel vom Segment- oder Subsegmentbronchus ab, daß der Katheter, der in der Peripherie nur durch Drehung um seine Längsachse in geringem Maße zu steuern ist, diesen Winkel nicht überwinden kann. Bei einem weiteren Teil der Karzinome ist der sondierte Bronchus durch den Tumor nur komprimiert, nicht jedoch infiltriert, und in einigen Fällen ist die Einengung des Bronchus durch das Karzinomgewebe nur gering, so daß der Katheter ohne Widerstand zu finden, d.h. ohne Materialaspiration, diese Stenose passiert.

Neben diesen objektiven Ursachen führen auch untersucherabhängige Fehler bei der Durchführung der Katheterbiopsie zu falsch-negativen Ergebnissen, z.B. die unzureichende Traumatisierung des Herdgebietes oder die Sondierung eines falschen Segment- oder Subsegmentbronchus.

Die Komplikationen der Katheterbiopsie sind gering. Es treten zwar unmittelbar nach der Katheterung ziemlich regelmäßig geringe endobronchiale Blutungen auf, sie sistieren meist nach einmaliger Absaugung. Stärkere Blutungen, die eine temporäre Bronchustamponade erfordern, kommen in etwa 1% der Fälle vor. Blutungen ins Parenchym, erkennbar an einer unscharfen Herdvergrößerung, kommen häufiger vor, bilden sich jedoch symptomlos ohne Therapie zurück.

Eine Tumorzellimplantation in die Bronchialschleimhaut findet nach unseren Erfahrungen und nach den Literaturberichten nicht statt.

SCHLUSSFOLGERUNGEN

Die hohe Trefferquote der Katheterbiopsie, die geringe Komplikationsrate der Methode und die Möglichkeit der sofortigen Behebung der Komplikationen im Rahmen der Narkosebeatmungsbronchoskopie sind für uns Anlaß, die Katheterbiopsie als primäre morphologisch-diagnostische Methode bei tumorverdächtigen peripheren Rundherden einzusetzen. Es erscheint uns dabei zweckmäßig, vor einer bioptischen Untersuchung eine Bronchographie als Pfadfindermethode durchzuführen.

Läßt sich bei einem peripheren tumorverdächtigen Herd trotz bronchographisch nachgewiesenem bronchialem Zugang die Diagnose durch Katheterbiopsie nicht sichern, oder hat der Prozeß keinen bronchialen Anschluß, so wenden wir zur weiteren morphologischen Abklärung die perthorakale Punktionsbiopsie an.

Die Materialentnahme über das flexible Bronchoskop zur zytologischen Untersuchung haben wir den nicht narkosefähigen, inoperablen Patienten vorbehalten.

II.4.

EARLY DIAGNOSIS OF PERIPHERAL BRONCHOGENIC CARCINOMA BY CYTOLOGICAL EXAMINATION OF CATHETER BIOPSIES

WORCH, R., HAMMESFAHR, R. and ATAY, Z.

1. INTRODUCTION

Without using transthoracic lung punctures, the morphological diagnosis of peripheral lung tumours may be most unsatisfactory. After a single examination of sputum or bronchial secretion, one can usually expect a positive result in only 45% of the cases. For small tumours (Stage I) or peripheral circular foci, the success rate may be reduced to 25% (1, 2)

The introduction of catheter biopsies by Friedel (3) considerably improved the histological diagnosis of peripheral tumours. By this method, however, only isolated cells or very small pieces of tissue are obtained and these are often insufficient to make a definitive histological diagnosis. As Kluge(4) reported in 1965, because there is frequently a lack of stroma, histologists tend to use cytological criteria in order to make their diagnosis. For this reason, we decided to examine catheter biopsies by cytology rather than by histology.

In the following report, we contrast the cytological diagnoses of catheter biopsies with those of bronchial secretion samples and compare these with previously published histological findings.

2. MATERIALS AND METHODS

Between 1971 and 1977, 1594 catheter biopsies and bronchial secretion samples were taken simultaneously from patients at the lung clinic of the Dieckholzen Hospital. Malignant tumours diagnosed morphologically and clinically for 437 of these cases, 223 of which were confirmed by histology.

3. RESULTS

The results of all 1594 cases are shown in Table 1. Of these, 0.18% were diagnosed as unrepresentative material (Pap 0) by examination of both catheter biopsies and bronchial secretion, while 3.5% were unclear (Pap III). Positive findings from catheter biopsies (20.2%) were much

J.A. Nakhosteen and W. Maassen (eds.), Bronchology: Research, Diagnostic and
Therapeutic Aspects. All rights reserved.
Copyright 1981. Martinus Nijhoff Publishers bv, The Hague / Boston / London

higher than from bronchial secretion (12.7%). 120 of 474 carcinomas were diagnosed as such by examination of the catheter biopsies alone. This figure is about one third higher than that for carcinomas diagnosed from bronchial secretion.

Table 2 shows the success rate for detection of primary and metastasising tumours by examination of bronchial secretion and catheter biopsies. The rate of accuracy for primary tumours was 36% by bronchial secretion, 60% by catheter biopsy and 66% by a combination of the two. For metastasising tumours, a combination of the two methods did not increase the percentage of positive findings, which was 11.8% by bronchial secretion and 26.5% by catheter biopsies.

Table 3 presents the relation of positive findings with tumour localisation. Tumours were described as being near the hilum if they were bronchoscopically visible but no sample excision could be taken. Diagnoses of malignancy were made for 43% of such cases after examination bronchial secretion, for 78% after examining catheter biopsies and for 81% by a combination. By examination of bronchial secretion, the accuracy rate was very low both for the right upper lobe (36%) and for the left upper lobe (25%); by catheter biopsy on the other hand, it was slightly lower for the right upper lobe only (52%).

The positive results for peripheral circular foci are greatgy dependent upon the size of the tumour. For tumours up to 3 cm in size, the accuracy rate was 9% by bronchial secretion and 20% by catheter biopsy; for tumours up to 6 cm, this was 32% by the former and 58% by the latter; for circular foci over 6 cm, it was 64% and 55% (Table 4).

The tumours were divided according to TNM stage by means of the older method of classification. As can be seen from Table 5, the positive findings from bronchial secretion and catheter biopsies depend on the stage of the tumour. For T_1 tumours, the accuracy rate was 13% by bronchial secretion and 20% by catheter biopsies, while for T_2 tumours it was 44% by the former and 70% by the latter. There are too few cases for the other stages to make a valid assessment of the accuracy rates. The percentages of positive findings for surgical tumour stage II are high by examination of both bronchial secretion (42.5%) catheter biopsies (70%).

The rate of accuracy also appears to depend on histogenetic tumour type. Findings were positive for 80% of the squamous cell carcinomas, 67.4% of the large cell carcinomas, 58% of the small cell carcinomas and 49% of the adenocarcinomas.

As can be seen from Table 6, specimens from 38 carcinoma cases were examined both histologically and cytologically. A definite diagnosis of malignancy was made by cytology for 60.5% of these cases and by histology for 42%. A diagnosis of suspected malignancy was made both by cytology and histology for 10.5% of these cases. The accuracy rate of cytology is therefore about 19% higher than that of histology.

In Table 7, we compared results obtained after the cytological specimens were reexamined and the histological material was prepared as sections. In this way, the percentage of positive findings by cytology was increased to 72.1% and by histology to 60.5%.

4. DISCUSSION

Our comparative findings for peripheral malignant lung processes show that the success rate of catheterbiopsies (72%) is much higher than that of bronchial secretion (36%).

There are no publications with present findings from cytological examinations of catheter biopsies, but for bronchial secretion the reported accuracy rates range between 13% and 59%.

An essential advantage of the catheter biopsy is that it contains a good deal more cells than does bronchial secretion. It is thus easier to discover tumour cells and diagnose malignancy.

As shown by Table 8, at 72.1%, our cytological findings are far higher than published histological results wich range between 32.2% and 53%.

Table 9 compares our false positive results with those wich have been published previously. Kluge made 2 false positive diagnoses from 600 cases and Maaßen made 1 false positive diagnosis from 1200 cases (4,5). Amongst our specimens, there was only one case which could not be confirmed during surgery. This indicates that the false positive rate for cytology is comparable with or even lower than that for histology.

TABLE 1. Comparison of cytological findings from bronchial secretion and catheter biopsies of 1594 cases: The positive results from catheter biopsies (20.2 %) were much higher than those from bronchial secretion (12.7 %).

MATERIAL	CLASSIFICATION ACCORDING PAPANICOLAOU									
	0	I	II	III	IV	+	V		=positive
bronchial secretion	3	891	440	58	57	+	145	=	202
	0.18%	56.0%	27.6%	3.6%	3.6%	+	9.1%	=	12.7%
catheter biopsy	3	815	398	56	68	+	254	=	322
	0.18%	51.1%	25.0%	3.5%	4.3%	+	15.9%	=	20.2%
combination	0	594	457	69	87	+	387	=	474
	–	37.3%	29.0%	4.3%	5.5%	+	24.2%	=	29.7%

TABLE 2. Accuracy rates from bronchial secretion and catheter biopsies for primary and metastasising lung tumours: Positive findings were made for 11.8 % of the metastasising tumours by bronchial secretion and for 26.5% by catheter biopsy. For primary tumours the accuracy rate was 36 % by bronchial secretion and 60 % by catheter biopsy.

TUMOUR TYPE		CYTOLOGY POSITIVE						
		BRONCHIAL SECRETION		CATHETER BIOPSY		COMBINATION		
	n	n	%	n	%	n	%	
primary	398	144	36.0	240	60.0	261	66.0	
metasta.	34	4	11.8	9	26.5	9	26.5	
Total	437	148	33.9	249	57.0	270	61.8	

TABLE 3. Cytological results from bronchial secretion and catheter biopsies and their dependence on tumour localisation: A combination of the two examinations produced positive results for 81% of tumours near the hilus and for 63% of peripheral tumours. The accuracy rate from bronchial secretion is considerably lower for the right and left upper lobes, while that from catheter biopsies is similarly high for all localisations.

LOCALISATION	n	BRONCHIAL SECRETION	CATHETER BIOPSY	COMBINATION
near hilum	54	43%	78%	81%
peripheral	344	35%	58%	63%
right UL	130	36%	59%	63%
right ML	18	44%	61%	72%
right LL	60	47%	52%	60%
left UL	123	25%	60%	63%
lingula	9	56%	67%	89%
left LL	30	43%	60%	67%
some lobes	28	43%	82%	86%

UL = upper lobe; ML = middle lobe; LL = lower lobe;

TABLE 4. Accuracy rates for bronchial secretion and catheter biopsies and their dependence on tumour size: Positive results were obtained by a combination of the two methods for only 23% of the tumours up to 3 cm. As tumour size increases, so too do the accuracy rates to 64% and 73%.

TUMOUR SIZE	n	BRONCHIAL SECRETION		CATHETER BIOPSY		COMBINATION	
		n	%	n	%	n	%
smaller than 3 cm	75	7	9	15	20	17	23
3 cm – 6 cm	74	24	32	43	58	47	64
bigger than 6 cm	11	7	64	6	55	8	73
Total	160	38	24	64	40	72	45

Table 5. Results in connection with tumour stage according to the TNM system: For T1 and surgical tumour stage I, the accuracy rate is only 33% and 34% respectively, and for T2 and stage II positive results increase to 75% and 76% respectively.

TUMOUR-STAGE	n	BRONCHIAL SECRETION	CATHETER BIOPSY	COMBINATION
T_1	87	13.0%	29.0%	33.0%
T_2	261	44.0%	70.0%	75.0%
T_3	14	36.0%	71.0%	79.0%
T_4	6	17.0%	83.0%	83.0%
T_5	8	40.0%	60.0%	66.0%
st. I	50	20.0%	26.0%	34.0%
st. II	127	42.5%	70.9%	76.4%
st. III	97	36.1%	61.9%	63.9%
st. IV	124	36.3%	62.1%	68.5%

TABLE 6. Comparative results of smears and sections from 38 tumour patients: The success rate for cytology (71%) is clearly higher than for histology (52%). A combination of the two methods produced positive results for 73.6% of the cases.

| | n | POSITIVE CASES | | |
		definite	suspected	total
CYTOLOGY	38	23 (60.5%)	4 (10.5%)	27 (71.0%)
HISTOLOGY	38	15 (39.2%)	4 (10.5%)	19 (52.5%)
COMBINATION	38	27 (71.0%)	1 (2.6%)	28 (73.6%)

TABLE 7. Improvement of results after re-checking by experienced cytologists and after second examination of step sections: Positive findings could be increased cytologically by 12% and histologically by 8%.

	n	1st EXAMINATION	2nd EXAMINATION
CYTOLOGY	398	60.3%	72.1%
HISTOLOGY	38	49.7%	57.8%

TABLE 8. Review of published results of histological and cytological evaluations of catheter biopsies from peripheral lung tumours: At 68.9% and 72%, the rate of accuracy for cytology is approximately 20% higher than that for histology.

AUTHOR	n	DEFINITE POSITIVE CASES	
Friedel, 1964	189	47.6%	
Kirsch a. Mucke, 1966	337	53.0%	
Maaßen, 1968	136	48.0%	histology
Menne, 1970	295	32.2%	
+ own	398	72.1%	
++ own	344	68.9%	cytology

+ Total number of peripheral tumours
++ Peripheral tumours which could not be seen bronchoscopical.

TABLE 9. Review of published positive results from catheter biopsies: At 0.06%, the false positive rate by cytology is lower than that by histology.

AUTHOR	NUMBER OF BIOPSIES	FALSE POSITIVE DIAGNOSIS			
		DEFINITE		SUSPECTED	
		TUMOUR CASES		TUMOUR CASES	
		n	%	n	%
Kluge	600	2	0.3	6	1.0
Maaßen	1300	1	0.08	1	0.08
own	1594	1	0.06	5	0.3

II.5.

COMPARATIVE STUDY BETWEEN THE MACROSCOPIC PATHOLOGICAL FINDINGS AND BRONCHOSCOPICAL
FINDINGS AND DIFFICULTIES IN DETECTION OF THE SITES OF EARLY-STAGE LUNG CANCER

RYOSUKE ONO, M.D. AND SHIGETO IKEDA, M.D.

The recent rapid increase in cases of lung cancer has necessitated the early
detection and correct diagnosis of incipient lung cancer in the hilar region of
the lung. Bronchial fiberscopy is very valuable for definitive diagnosis, in
particular for the diagnosis of the site of the cancer in so-called occult lung
cancer cases. Therefore, the authors carried out clinical and pathological studies
in our 16 cases of early lung cancer at the hilum region of the lung.

Macroscopic findings of early stage lung cancer in the hilum region of the
lung are classified into the Polypoid type, Nodular infiltrating type, Superficial
infiltrating type, and Mixed type. The polypoid and superficial infiltrating
types are characterized by little infiltration to deeper sites; therefore, these
cancers may possibly remain for a relatively long period of time. This can also
be deduced from the fact that dilatation change was noted in the peripheral bronchus
in the 3 cases of polypoid cancer. On the other hand, the nodular infiltrating type
is characterized by rapid progression to deeper sites and can be regarded as a
prototype of progressive cancers in the hilum of the lung.

Endoscopic findings of these types of cancers are described on the right end.
In the superficial infiltrating type with longitudinal involvement along the
bronchial wall, it is easy to determine the range of tumor infiltration by endoscopy,
but macroscopic differentiation from the normal mucosa is sometimes impossible
at sites showing intra-epithelial infiltration, and it is often difficult to
identify tumor infiltration at the sites with inflammatory changes or severe
metaplastic changes. Early stage lung cancer at the hilum of the lung has marked
clinical and pathological characteristics. The characteristics of 16 cases were
analyzed and shown in the slide. The findings shown in this slide are consistent
with those of many cases reported in Europe and the United States, making it easy
to establish the high-risk group of this type of cancer.

All the findings were noted predominantly in males and age distribution was
higher than that of general lung cancer. Coughing and blood-tinged sputum appeared
frequently and most of the patients were heavy smokers. The positive rate of cytodiagnosis of the sputum was high, and detection and localization by bronchofiberscopy

J.A. Nakhosteen and W. Maassen (eds.), Bronchology: Research, Diagnostic and
Therapeutic Aspects. All rights reserved.
Copyright 1981. Martinus Nijhoff Publishers bv, The Hague / Boston / London

were possible in almost all cases. The incidence of squamous cell cancer was high and it developed predominantly in the segmental bronchus. In the 11 cases where obstructive pneumonia or segmental apneumatosis was revealed by X-ray examination of the chest, tumors were easy to localize and were observed endoscopically as the polypoid type or nodular infiltrating type cancers.

Diagnostic technique for radiographically occult lung cancer is described below in our 2 cases.

This subject, a 54-year-old male, was a heavy smoker. The cytodiagnosis of the sputum revealed squamous cell cancer, and X-ray findings were normal. Since the location of the site of the lesion was impossible in the first endoscopic examination, the right and left bronchi were examined separately by washing cytodiagnosis, resulting in the detection of tumor cells in the specimen obtained from the right bronchus. The second endoscopy was carried out principally for the right bronchus, but the site of the lesion could not be located. Therefore, the upper, middle, and lower bronchi were examined separately by washing cytodiagnosis, resulting in the detection of tumor cells in the specimen obtained from the right-lower-lobe bronchus. Accordingly, selective bronchography of the right-lower-lobe bronchus was carried out. The image of irregular stenosis was produced in the segmental bronchus at right B7. Following this result, the endoscope was inserted to B7 in the third endoscopy. The bronchus at B7a was obstructed with pus-like secretions, and the membrane from the site of obstruction to the upper margine showed loss of color and luster, appearing pale white. The mucous membrane was finely rugged and the folds of the membrane were obscure, showing hypertrophy and fragmentation. The biopsy on this site revealed squamous cell cancer of the moderately differentiated type. Finally, the resection of the right lower lobe was performed. When the B7 bronchus was opened, the superficial infiltrating and moderately differentiated type squamous cell cancer, which did not infiltrate beyond the tunica muscularis, was noted as indicated by the endoscopic findings. It is considered that diagnosis was difficult in this case because the tumor existed at B7 where we had experienced lesions less often; moreover, the site of tumor was slightly difficult to see. The next case, a 64-year-old male, was also a heavy smoker. Cytodiagnosis of the sputum disclosed squamous cell cancer, and the X-ray findings concerning the chest were normal. Since the first endoscopy failed to locate the site of lesion, the right and left bronchi were examined separately by washing cytodiagnosis, resulting in the detection of tumor cells in the specimen obtained from the right bronchus. Since the site of the lesion also could not be located by the second endoscopy carried out principally for the right bronchus, the upper, middle, and lower bronchi were examined separately by washing cytodiagnosis, resulting in the detection of tumor cells in the specimen from the right-upper-lobe bronchus.

Since the third endoscopy also failed to locate the site of the lesion, the brush was inserted separately into B1, B2, and B3 in the right-upper-lobe bronchus, and the spur was taken from the bronchus of each segment and subsegment and examined separately by biopsy. The spur from B3a and B3b showed no malignant findings, but the cytodiagnosis of the spur from B3 showed tumor cells. Following these results, the resection of the right upper lobe was performed.

A single layer of tumor cells was noted along the peripheral bronchus at B3b and squamous cell cancer was detected with almost no infiltration to deeper sites.

This case was considered not as early lung cancer in the hilum of the lung, but as cancer which had developed along the wall of the peripheral Bullae.

The diagnostic procedure for radiographically occult lung cancer is described below.

At first, local anesthesia is induced in the mouth and upper trachea with 2% xylocaine solution using the apparatus for anesthesia of the larynx. At this point the larynx should be inspected carefully in heavy smokers with a history of cancer of the mouth or the upper trachea, because it is said that such people tend to contract cancer repeatedly.

Then the bronchofiberscope is inserted through a flexible tracheal tube, because it is necessary to secure the respiratory tract against the possible occurrence of complications during bronchofiberscopy, and the fiberscope must be inserted or removed repeatedly.

Then the tip of the fiberscope is inserted into all the segmental bronchi of the right and left bronchi and a careful inspection is carried out. A small T.V. camera is connected to the bronchofiberscope for videotape recording. In addition, fluorescent bronchofiberscopy is carried out with a fluorescein sodium solution and a videotape recording is made using of an ultra-sensitivity T.V. camera.

Then the right and left bronchi are examined by separate washing cytodiagnosis.

When tumor cells are detected, for example, in the right bronchus by the cytodiagnosis, a careful inspection should be made by inserting the tip of the bronchofiberscope into all the segmental bronchi of the right bronchus. Videotape recording is carried out by connecting a small T.V. camera to the bronchofiberscope.

Then the right upper, middle, and lower lobe bronchi are examined by separate washing cytodiagnosis. Inspection and documentation are carried out as described above for the cytodiagnosis-positive lobe bronchi. Finally, separative brushings and biopsies of the spur from each segmental and subsegmental bronchus are performed.

Among 16 cases of early lung cancer in the hilum of the lung, 5 chest-X-ray-negative cases were studied. All the 5 cases underwent bronchofiberscopy, and the site of lesion was located by the first, second, and third bronchoscopy in 3, 2, and 1 cases, respectively. The tumor locations of the 5 cases were the supra-segmental bronchus in 1 and segmental bronchus in 4. Macroscopically, 3 cases were classified as the superficial infiltrating type and 2 cases as the nodular infiltrating type. As endoscopic findings, fine granule-like rugged surfaces of the membrane were noted in 3 cases and nodule-like tumors in 2 cases, but polypoid tumors were not observed in any of them.

In the superficial infiltrating type of cancer with longitudinal involvement along the bronchial wall, determination of the tumor infiltration range by endoscopy is very important to determine the range of resection and to recognize the endoscopic findings of intra-epithelial cancer. Accordingly, the authors made detailed endoscopic observations on the color, luster and roughness of the surface of the membrane and the quality of the mucous folds in the 6 superficial infiltrating cases and compared them with the pathological depth of infiltration.

At the sites where tumors showed intra-epithelial infiltration, the surface of the membrane was not lustrous, changing into the fine granule-like form, but the mucous folds remained unchanged or showed slight coadunation. At the sites where tumors had infiltrated into the region under the mucosa or into the tunica mascularis, the surface was pale white in color and not lustrous, and longitudinal and circular folds were obscure or displayed fragmentation. When a tumor had infiltrated into the cartilage or even into the adventitial coat, the surface was very rugged, with complete disappearance of mucous folds. It was, of course, sometimes impossible to macroscopically distinguish these from normal mucous membranes when the tumor showed intra-epithelial infiltration. It was also sometimes difficult to identify tumor infiltration when inflammatory or severe metaplastic changes existed. Therefore, the authors consider that it is necessary to perform biopsy and cytodiagnosis using a biopsy needle projecting from the bronchofiberscope for the location of the tumor, and the range of resection should be determined prior to resection by means of fresh specimens obtained during the operation.

II.6.

FLUORESCENT BRONCHOSCOPY: A NEW TECHNIQUE AND FURTHER RESULTS

D. HURZELER

1. EINLEITUNG

Seit Okt. 1975 arbeite ich mit der Fluoreszenzbronchoskopie. Im Gegensatz zu der intravenösen Färbemethode mit Haematoporphyrinderivaten, wie sie die Mayo-Klinik, Dr. Doiron und andere verwenden, wählte ich eine Oberflächenmarkierung mit inhalierter Fluoreszeinlösung. Die Fluoreszenz wurde in den ersten 35 Fällen mit einer UV-Lichtquelle induziert.

2. NEUE METHODE

2.1 Voraussetzung

Die Tatsache, dass die Fluoreszeinfluoreszenz auch im sichtbaren Licht induziert werden kann, ermöglicht eine Vereinfachung der apparativen Einrichtung. Wie aus Tabelle I ersichtlich ist, hat das Fluoreszein 3 Erregerfrequenzen (↓), 2 im UV-Bereich und eine im Blaubereich. Die induzierte Fluoreszenz (↑) liegt im Grüngelb-Bereich. Wenn bei einer üblichen Lichtquelle ein Zeiss-Erregerfilter 500 zwischen Lampe und Fiberlichtleiter geschaltet wird, tritt nur das doppelt schraffierte Blaulicht, welches das Fluoreszein zum Leuchten bringt, in den Bronchialbaum ein. Schalten wir vor das Okular der Betrachteroptik das Zeiss-Sperrfilter 520, welches nur das einfach schraffierte Licht durchlässt, wird das gesamte Blaulicht ausgefiltert, und nur das induzierte grüngelbe Fluoreszenzlicht bleibt sichtbar. Somit reduziert sich der apparative Aufwand auf den Gebrauch dieser beiden Filter. Es kann mit einer Standardlichtquelle und einer Routinebronchoskopieeinrichtung gearbeitet werden. Mit dieser Methode wurden weitere 65 Fälle untersucht.

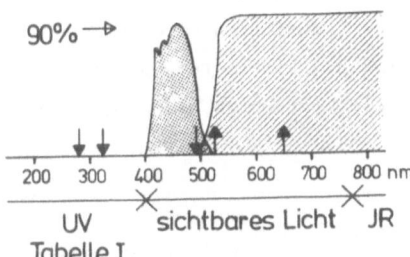

90% →

| 200 | 300 | 400 | 500 | 600 | 700 | 800 nm |

UV   sichtbares Licht   JR

Tabelle I

J.A. Nakhosteen and W. Maassen (eds.), Bronchology: Research, Diagnostic and Therapeutic Aspects. All rights reserved.
Copyright 1981. Martinus Nijhoff Publishers bv, The Hague / Boston / London

2.2 Vorversuche

Anhand von Vorversuchen konnte festgestellt werden, dass 1-2 Std. nach Ueberdruck-
inhalation von 5 ml einer sterilen, wässerigen, 5 %igen Fluoreszeinlösung mit einigen Tropfen eines β_2-Stimulators die cilientragenden Epithelschichten im Bronchialbaum wieder gereinigt sind und cilienlose Partien wie Metaplasien, Tumoren,
neoplastisch veränderte Schleimhaut sowie Schleimhaut mit einer massiven Ansammlung von Schleimdrüsen meist noch mit Fluoreszein markiert sind und demzufolge
fluoreszieren.

2.3 Bemerkungen zur neuen Methode

Die neue Methode erlaubt, eine grosse Energiemenge von Induktionslicht in den
Bronchialbaum zu bringen, was mit einer UV-Lichtquelle schwierig war. Es ist möglich,
dass selbst 2 Stunden nach der Inhalation der normale Bronchialbaum und im besonde-
ren der Bronchialbaum bei entzündlichen Veränderungen noch nicht völlig vom fluoreszierenden Sekret gereinigt ist. Dieses massiv fluoreszierende Sekret, das sich
meist in Streifenform darstellt, kann die Beurteilung erheblich stören. Es muss
deshalb sorgfältig abgesaugt werden, wenn nötig unter Optiksicht mit einem Katheter
und der lenkbaren Instrumentenführung nach Maassen oder mit einer vorsichtigen
Spülung. Es ist darauf zu achten, dass keine Blutung auftritt, da das Maximum der
Lichtabsorption des Haemoglobins genau im Bereiche des induzierten Fluoreszenz-
lichtes liegt und eine Blutung jede Fluoreszenz auslöscht. Eine zarte, flächen-
hafte, netz- oder punktförmige Fluoreszenz entspricht einer echten Wandfluoreszenz.

3. RESULTATE UND AUSWERTUNG

3.1 Schlussdiagnosen

Die Auswertung der erwähnten 100 Fälle ergibt folgende Verhältnisse: Die Schluss-
diagnose lautete bei 27 Patienten auf ein zentrales Bronchuskarzinom. 24 Fälle
zeigten periphere Bronchuskarzinome, bei 7 Fällen handelte es sich um Lungenmeta-
stasen bei Fremdtumoren, und 42 Patienten wiesen übrige, meist entzündliche broncho-
pulmonale Krankheiten auf.

3.2 Sichtbare Tumoren

Von den 28 sichtbaren Tumoren (zu den 27 zentralen Karzinomen gesellte sich noch
ein zentraler Tumordurchbruch bei einem Metastasenfall) fluoreszierten 22. 2 Tumoren
fluoreszierten nicht, trotzdem sie eindeutig makroskopisch als solche zu erkennen
waren. Weitere 4 waren blutbedeckt, weshalb die Fluoreszenz nicht gesehen werden
konnte. Auch fand sich unter den 42 Nichttumorfällen eine Metaplasie der Bronchial-

schleimhaut, die nicht fluoreszierte. Gesmathaft fanden sich also 3 falsch negative Resultate und 4 infolge Blutung nicht beurteilbare Fälle. 39 Schleimhautstellen zeigten die bei Fluoreszenz erwarteten Veränderungen (10 Metaplasien, 29 Tumorinfiltrationen).

3.3 Makroskopisch unveränderte Schleimhaut

Von makroskopisch unveränderten Schleimhautpartien zentral eines Tumors, bei peripheren Tumoren oder Metastasen sowie bei den übrigen bronchopulmonalen Krankheiten fanden sich 30 fluoreszierende Schleimhautpartien. Normal oder entzündlich verändert waren 13. In diesen Fällen wurde eine fluoreszierende Schleimhautauflagerung als echte Schleimhautfluoreszenz beurteilt. Diese 13 Fälle sind als falsch positive Resultate zu werten. Sie hatten aber insofern für den Patienten keine nachteiligen Folgen, als durch die gezielte Biopsie eine ernsthafte Erkrankung ausgeschlossen werden konnte. 10 Stellen zeigten Metaplasien, 7 eine Neoplasie im Sinne einer Lymphangiosis carcinomatosa oder einer Schleimhautkarzinose. Diese waren makroskopisch nicht erkennbar und konnten einzig mit der Fluoreszenz gefunden werden. 35 Routinebiopsien nicht fluoreszierender Schleimhautstellen bestätigten histologisch eine normale oder lediglich entzündlich veränderte Schleimhaut.

4. SCHLUSSFOLGERUNG

Zusammenfassend kann gesagt werden, dass die neue Methode der Fluoreszenzbronchoskopie den apparativen Aufwand wesentlich vereinfacht. Es genügen zu einer Standardbronchoskopie-Ausrüstung ein Erreger- und ein Sperrfilter, die Zeissfilter 500 und 520. Bei der Fluoreszeinmethode handelt es sich um eine Oberflächenmarkierung. Normale oder histologisch nur entzündlich veränderte Schleimhaut, die durch die Cilientätigkeit gereinigt wird, fluoresziert ca. 2 Std. nach der Inhalation in der Regel nicht mehr. Allerdings fanden sich bei 100 Patienten 13 falsch positive Resultate unter den 52 fluoreszierenden Schleimhautstellen (nicht 14 von 53 wie in der veröffentlichten Zusammenfassung erwähnt). Sichtbare Tumoren, Metaplasien, Ansammlung von Schleimdrüsen im Epithel und neoplastisch veränderte Schleimhaut fluoreszieren. Die histologischen Befunde von 39 solcher Schleimhautstellen stimmten mit diesen Diagnosen überein. Nur 3 falsch negative Resultate waren zu beobachten. Es ist vor allem die Tatsache hervorzuheben, dass von den 58 Karzinomfällen 7 neoplastisch veränderte Schleimhautpartien, die makroskopisch weder von blossem Auge noch mit der Hopkinsoptik erkennbar waren, allein mit der Fluoreszenz gefunden werden konnten.

II.7.

THE RELIABILITY OF CYTODIAGNOSIS IN DETERMINING MALIGNANCY AND
 HISTOGENETIC TUMOUR TYPE

Z. ATAY

1. INTRODUCTION
    The morphological determination of peripheral lung tumours is de-
pendent in the majority of cases upon a cytological diagnosis. Here
arises a basic question: Should the attending doctor undertake extensive therapy on the grounds of a positive cytological finding, but
without histological confirmation? An affirmative answer to this
question presupposes two conditions: The degree of certainty in the
diagnosis of malignancy must be as high for cytology as it is for
histology , and the cytologist must define the histogenetic tumour
type as precisely as the histologist does.

2. MATERIAL AND METHOD
    To determine whether cytodiagnosis is as efficient as histology,
the material used for histological and cytological diagnosis must be
identical and should be examined simultaneously. For this purpose, a
subcutaneous cytological examination of imprints from sample excisions
would appear to offer the best possibilities and, since 1966, has been
used extensively by our working group (1, 5).
    To answer the above question, I evaluated 938 sample excisions from
the Heckeshorn Lung Clinic (1966 - 1967) and 6921 cases from the Institute of Pathology of the Medizinische Hochschule Hannover (1970 -
1979), which could be divided as follows: 5679 sample excisions from
the bronchus, 1197 from the pleura and lung, 286 transbronchial lung
biopsies, 619 mediastinoscopies and 150 samples removed during surgery.
    To avoid variations in terminology, I have evaluated only those
cases for wich the histology was carried out in our own Institute of
Pathology. The total number amounted to 3811 cases, 2405 of which involved a benign process and 1406 a malignant process.

J.A. Nakhosteen and W. Maassen (eds.), Bronchology: Research, Diagnostic and
Therapeutic Aspects. All rights reserved.
Copyright 1981. Martinus Nijhoff Publishers bv, The Hague / Boston / London

3. RESULTS AND DISCUSSION

3.1. Diagnosis of malignancy

The distribution of histological and cytological diagnosis from
the same material is summarised in Table 1. Malignancy was histologically diagnosed in 31.5% of the cases, and cytologically in 35.9%. By
cytological examination, a further 128 cases of malignant tumours
could be established.After a second examination of the cytological
material, we were able to raise the rate of malignant diagnoses to
36.1%, because the preparations require longer scrutinisation and because sparse tumour cells could easily be overlooked during routine
examination or by an inexperienced cytologist.

Although a Ca in situ was histologically diagnosed in 13 cases,
cytologically we found no Ca in situ.

In Table 2, I have listed the cytological findings which deviate
from bioptical histology. Of the 2596 cases in which no malignancy
was detected by histology, the cytological findings corresponded for
92%. The concurrence of histological and cytological findings for
dysplasia and for benign tumours amounted to only 49%. In all cases
which were histologically determined as Ca in situ, by cytology we
found tumour cells indicating an invasive carcinoma. 17% of the cases
found to be suspected malignomas by histology were diagnosed likewise
by cytology. For 95% of those cases in which malignancy was histologically certain, the same diagnosis was made by cytology.

The degree of certainty and the validity of the cytological results
can be seen in Table 3. With the exception of one, all 1294 cases
found to be Pap. V, 653 of which were diagnosed by cytology only, were
later confirmed. This means the accuracy rate is 99.9%. In one case
only, a degenerate haemartoma was discovered during surgery which had
been diagnosed histologically as a benign haemartoma.For benign cases,
there is a false positive rate of 0.04%. 97.6% of the Pap IV cases
involved a malignant process. Here the false positive rate is 0.008%.
In 1.1% of the cases for which no definite malignancy could be found
by cytology, a malignant process was in fact present.

I should now explain why, despite identical material, the cytologist tends to discover malignant processes more often than does the
histologist. Firstly, although insufficient for histology, a scanty

amount of material may be optimal for cytology. Decisive criteria for malignancy may be observed in one single tumour cell. In extreme cases, this means that malignancy can be cytologically detected in just one tumour cell. Such diagnoses are easily made for hornified squamous cell carcinomas and anaplastic carninomas.

Particularly in the case of small cell tumours, better results may be achieved by cytology than by histology. By means of step sections and re-examination, histological results can be improved upon by 4.3%, as our group was able to show (5).

In 24 of 27 cytologically false negative cases, we found no tumour cells upon re-examination. These cases predominantly involved lymphangiosis carcinomatosa and fibrotic carcinomas. In two mesotheliomas and one bronchiolo alveolar cell carcinoma, we found plentiful tumour cells which were so highly differentiated that a diagnosis of malignancy could not be made.

It is not possible for me to provide a review of comparable evaluations of combined histological and cytological studies. Only Roglić reports that malignancy was histologically diagnosed in 88% of the sample excisions examined, and cytologically in 98.5% (4).

As early as 1966, our group together with Brandt was able to present our first comparative results from a combined histological and cytological study. Cytology had an accuracy rate of 92.5% and histology 78.4% (3).

With Preußler, we recorded that of the findings for 921 malignant processes, 88.5% were positive for histology and 97.9% for cytology (1).

Here our rate of false positive results is 0.04%. This low percentage indicates the reliability of cytodiagnosis and is far below the false positive rates for histology recorded in other studies; for example, Becker and Knothe reported 3 false positive findings amongst 443 intraoperative thoracotomies (2).

3.2. Definition of histogenetic tumour type

The histogenetic tumour type was cytologically and histologically defined for 1126 cases. Between 1966 and 1969, definitions made by cytology and histology were the same for 88.7% of these cases and between 1970 and 1979, for 92.1% (Table 4).

The highest rate of accuracy was achieved for carcinoid with 100%, followed by malignant lymphomas with 94% and adenocarcinomas with 93.9%. The rate for large-cell carcinomas was only 63%. In intraoperative cytology, the accuracy rate for primary lung carcinomas was 88.9%.

Cytology is more accurate than histology because it can produce a diagnosis of type from very scanty material, in extreme cases with just one tumour cell.

4. SUMMARY

a) In defining malignancy and histogenetic tumour type, cytological diagnoses of smear excisions are of equal value and, in some cases, superior to those made by histology.

b) By combining the method of examination for routine diagnosis, the accuracy rate of histology in determining malignancy, particularly in the case of malignant lymphoma and small-cell carcinomas may be increased by about 15%.

c) Cytology can establish whether a Ca in situ diagnosed by bioptic histology involves offshoots of an invasive carcinoma.

d) Real false negative findings must be reckoned with for bronchiolo-alveolar cell carcinomas and mesotheliomas.

REFERENCES

1. Atay, Z. and Preußler, H.: Ergebnisse der vergleichenden Zytologie und Histologie von 921 malignen Tumoren aus 2500 Biopsien im Thorax. Verh.Dtsch.Ges.Path. 57: 360-362 ,1973.

2. Becker, W.H. and Knothe, W.: Intraoperative Fehldiagnosen: Bronchialcarcinom. Thoraxchirurgie 6: 235-242,1959.

3. Brandt, H.-J. and Atay, Z.: Vergleich von cytologischer und histologischer Diagnostik bei intrathorakalen Erkrankungen. 12. Tagung Dtsch.Ges.Hämatol.,Berlin 1966.

4. Roglić, M.: Cytological examination of forceps - Biopsy materials obtained at bronchoscopy. 6th Congress European Federation of Cytology Societies, Weimar 1976.

5. Siegismund, G. and Atay, Z.: Vergleichende Auswertung der histologischen und cytologischen Präparate vom Bronchus. Schweiz., Öster. u. Dtsch. Ges. für klin. Cytol., Wengen/Schweiz, 1975.

TABLE 1. Distribution of histological and cytological findings according to malignancy: The accuracy rate was 5% higher by cytology than by histology. After a second examination, cytological findings could be improved by 1%.

			CYTOLOGY			
DIAGNOSES	HISTOLOGY		1st examination		2nd examination	
	n	%	n	%	n	%
Pap. 0 - II without atypia	2513	66.0	2395	63.0	2354	61.8
Pap. III unclear	83	2.2	86	2.3	78	2.0
Pap. IV a Ca in situ	13	0.3	-	-	-	-
Pap. IV b suspected malignoma	58	1.5	87	2.3	85	2.2
Pap. V malignoma	1144	30.0	1243	32.6	1294	33.9
Total IV b and V	1202	31.5	1330	34.9	1379	36.1

TABLE 2. Correlation of histological and cytological diagnoses of bioptical material: Cytology correlated with histology for 92% of the benign cases and for 95% of the cases of malignancy, while for Ca in situ no correlation was found.

DIAGNOSES	HISTOLOGY	CYTOLOGY				
		O-II	III	IVa	IVb	V
0 - II	2513	2310 92%	34	-	35	134
III	83	20	41 49%	-	3	19
IVa	13	-	-	-	2	11
IVb	58	7	-		10 17%	41
V	1144	17	3	-	35	1089 95%
Total	3811	2354	78	-	85	1294

TABLE 3. Validity of cytological findings: 99.9 % of the cytological diagnoses of malignancy (Pap V) and 97.6 % of the Pap IV cases were confirmed. 98.9 % of the cases cytologically diagnosed as benign were also found to be correct.

CLASSIFICATION ACCORDING PAPANICOLAOU	CYTOLOGICAL RESULTS	ONLY CYTOLOGY	FINAL DIAGNOSIS MALIGNANT		BENIGN	
	n	n	n	%	n	%
+ V	1294	(153)	1293	99.9	1	0.1
++ IV	85	(38)	83	97.6	2	2.4
0 - III	2432	(164)	27	1.1	2405	98.9

+ false positive: 1/2405 benign cases = 0.04 %
++ false positive: 2/2405 benign cases = 0.08 %

TABLE 4. Cytological definition of histogenetic tumour type: Correct cytological diagnoses were made for 88.7 & of the total number of cases. The accuracy rate was 84.5 % from 1966 to 1969 and 92.1 % from 1970 to 1979.

BIOPTICAL HISTOLOGY	CORRECT CYTOLOGICAL TUMOUR TYPE					
	1966 - 1969		1970 - 1979		ADDITION	
	n	%	n	%	n	%
squamous-cell ca.	177/205	86.3	307/330	93.0	484/535	90.5
adenocarcinoma	92/99	93.0	47/49	96.0	139/148	93.9
small-cell carcinoma	76/87	87.4	159/172	92.4	235/259	90.7
large-cell carcinoma	38/62	61.3	17/26	65.4	55/88	63.0
carcinoid	6/6	100.0	14/14	100.0	20/20	100.0
mesothelioma	18/22	81.8	9/10	90.0	27/32	84.4
the others	7/9	77.8	1/2	-	8/11	72.7
malignant lymphoma	10/12	83.0	21/21	100.0	31/33	94.0
Total	424/502	84.5	575/623	92.1	990/1126	88.7

II.8.

SPUTUMCYTOLOGIC DIAGNOSIS OF EARLY ROENTGENOLOGICALLY OCCULT BRONCHO-
GENIC CARCINOMA

S.HAGLUND,J.KINNMAN,K.NASIELL,M.NASIELL,L.MALMSTRÖM & V.ROGER

INTRODUCTION

A sputumcytologic screening project aiming at early diagnosis and
study of the pathogenesis of bronchogenic carcinoma has been going on
from 1964 to 1979 inclusive. 1974/1975 the project was reorganized to
study a target population of smokers without known lung disease at
high cancer risk from outpatient clinics and various companies and
organizations.

MATERIAL AND METHODS

Three early morning cough specimens (12 slides) are carefully examined by specially trained cytotechnologists using detailed cytomorpho-
logic criteria for the various epithelial abnormalities. Cytologic
evidence of early epithelial injury, various degrees of atypical metaplasia, evidence of early bronchial malignancy and outspoken cancer are
recorded on the patients charts. In addition the archival material has
been used for retrospective quantitative measurements of DNA and simultaneous cytologic re-evaluation (Nasiell et al.,1978). The routine
clinical procedures during the "prevalence", cytology screening study
are shown in Table 1.. The bronchofiberscopy is performed by the otolaryngologist who also makes a routine ENT-examination to exclude malignancies in the upper respiratory and alimentary passages. The otolaryngologist in addition performs the mediastinoscopy in the case
the patient is a candidate for surgical resection.

The material consists of 2.861 men aged 45 smoking 20 cigarettes
per day for 15 years or more. In addition patients from a routine clinical material with normal chest X-rays were examined.

RESULTS

Among the high risk smokers 27 (0.9%) had positive cytology -
most of these were clinically occult carcinomas (Table 1.).

In the routine material 61 patients with clinically occult lung
cancer were found.

*J.A. Nakhosteen and W. Maassen (eds.), Bronchology: Research, Diagnostic and
Therapeutic Aspects. All rights reserved.*
Copyright 1981. Martinus Nijhoff Publishers bv, The Hague / Boston / London

TABLE 1. Sabbatsberg hospital sputum cytology screening study for early bronchogenic carcinoma in high risk smokers

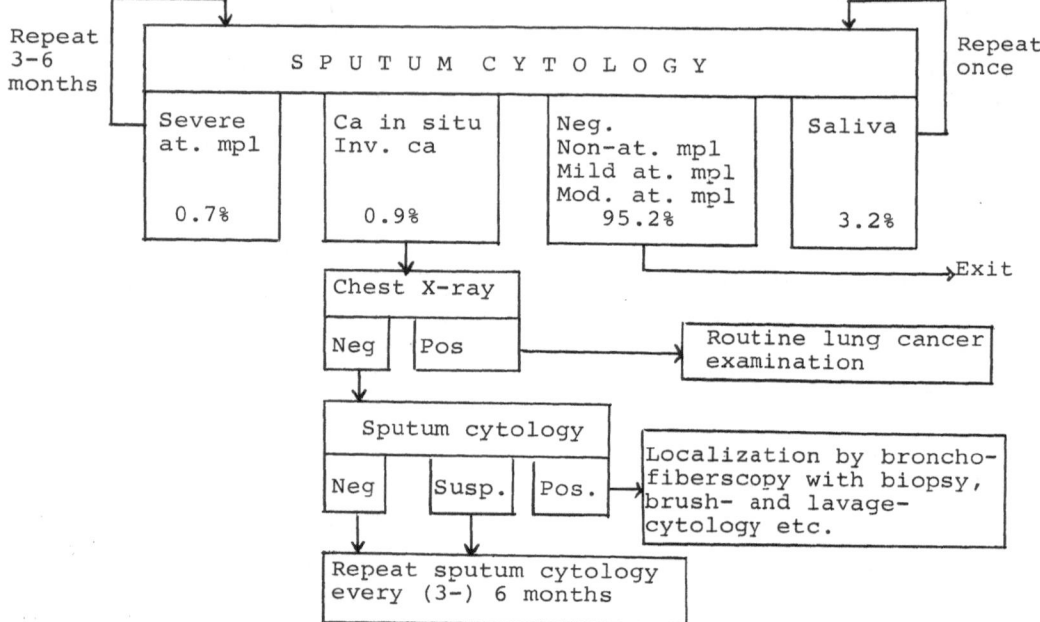

Bronchofiberscopy has been used since 1974/1975, and so far 28 clinically occult bronchogenic carcinomas have been localized - 21 of these underwent surgical resection (Table 2.).

TABLE 2. Resected cases

No sign of recurrence	14[x] (66%)	
Dead from lung cancer	5	
Dead from intercurrent disease	2	
Total	21	

x) Atypia or CIS in resection border: 2

Average age at operation was 61 year (range 48-71) and the average follow-up time 2 years 5 months (range 0-14).
Seventeen of the patients (10 pertaining to the screening project) were operated 1975-1979. During this last period of the project the time lapse from the first positive cytological finding to resection was as an average 3 months (range 1-7).

Among the 67 non-resected patients 20, pertaining to the early part of the series from 1964 to 1974, have died from lung cancer even though the tumor had been diagnosed cytologically before it gave positive radiological changes. Two patients died from hypopharynx cancer, nine from intercurrent diseases. In one patient a larynx cancer was diagnosed (bronchofiberscopy negative at 3 occasions) and after radiotherapy sputum cytology has remained negative.

In 22 cases definite diagnosis is still pending - in 8 of these sputum cytology is definitely indicating cancer, in 14 severe atypic metaplasia or cancer in situ.

The results indicate that, with increasing experiences and more active clinical diagnostic procedures, early bronchogenic carcinoma can be detected and localized by sputum cytology and bronchofiberscopy, which gives hope for a more successful treatment.

Prevalence screening has a tendency to detect cases with relatively long preclinical duration and correspondingly slow growth. The end result will be determined, of course, by total lung cancer deaths. Two main questions remain and will be the subject to further studies:
1) Does early diagnosis influence the natural course of squamous cell bronchogenic carcinoma?
2) How many additional bronchogenic carcinomas (incidense cases) can be expected to develop in the screening material?

REFERENCE
Nasiell,M., Kato,H., Auer,G., Zetterberg,A., Roger,V. & Karlen,L.: Cytomorphological grading and Feulgen DNA-analysis of metaplastic and neoplastic bronchial cells. Cancer 41:1511, 1978.

Reprint requests to Dr. Jan Kinnman, Department of Otolaryngology, Huddinge sjukhus, S-141 86 Huddinge, Sweden.

II.9.

The Diagnosis of Precancerous Lesions and Multifocal Carcinoma of
the Bronchial Epithelium with Fiberoptic Bronchoscopy
F. Klinke, H. Dittrich, R. Achatzy, K. M. Müller, E. Anyanwu,
V. Jelesijevic

Introduction

Bronchoscopy with fiberoptics - as described by Ikeda in 1968 - has
opened up new dimensions in bronchoscopic diagnosis. The bronchoscopy
with an inflexible bronchoscope offers the advantage of stronger
illumination, broader view, and better biopsy possibilities in the
central bronchial area. On the other hand, the fiberoptic bronchoscopy
has the advantage of extending the view into the peripheral bronchial
areas. The duration of the examination using an inflexible bronchoscope is limited by the danger of the patient being hypoventilated in
the open system. The fiberoptic-bronchoscopy on the other hand,
while being carried out under mechanical ventilation using a closed
system, allows examinations lasting for hours, thus making it quite
tolerable to the patients.

Material and methods

For mechanical ventilation, we make use of three different systems:
1.) a short bronchoscope - manufactured by the firm Storz - which we
fit with a cuff, 2.) the bronchoscope of the firm, Olympus, likewise
fitted with a cuff. It has a modified sealing to allow passage of
instruments. Should it not be possible, for any anatomic reason,
to insert an inflexible bronchoscope we use 3.) a shortened portex
tubus fitted with a T-piece, thus allowing the connection of the
respirating system and an air-tight fitting around the fiber bronchoscope.
With the aid of these systems we have carried out a consecutive
bronchoscopy on 345 patients - 309 men and 36 women with an average
age of 58 alternatively 51 years -, who were referred to us with
the tentative diagnosis of a bronchial carcinoma. A mediastinoscopy
was carried out 254 times at the same sitting. 111 patients were
macroscopically carcinoma suspect. Materials won by brushes showed
cancerous cells in 41 cases. 11 patients had already metastasis of

J.A. Nakhosteen and W. Maassen (eds.), Bronchology: Research, Diagnostic and
Therapeutic Aspects. All rights reserved.
Copyright 1981. Martinus Nijhoff Publishers bv, The Hague / Boston / London

bronchial carcinoma in the mediastinal lymph nodes, without our being able to prove the presence of a primary tumor from the histological examination of the material won by fiber optic bronchoscopy. Biopsies confirmed the presence of a tumor in 100 cases. The mediastinoscopy of 107 cases, which were judged to be operable on bronchoscopic examination, revealed metastasis in more than one station of lymph nodes in 69 % of the patients.

Only in 33 cases (21.7 %) was it possible to carry out a curative resection of the lung. The operation was palliative in 5 patients (3. 3 %) and because of the technical inoperability in 12 patients, the operation could not go beyond an explorative thoracotomy.

Of the 152 patients with primary lung cancer 50.7 % or 77 (5 females, 72 males) had squamous cell, 32.2 % or 49 (6 females, 43 males) small cell carcinoma, 3.3 % or 5 (males), oat cell carcinoma, 7.2 % or 11 patients (5 females, 6 males) adenocarcinoma, 3.9 % or 6 (3 females, 3 males) large cell carcinoma, 2 % or 3 (2 females, 1 male) carcinoid with infiltrate growth and finally 1 male had carcinoma-in-situ. Because the pathologists emphasize potentially precancerous lesions (3), we paid particular attention to these lesions and in fact, searched for them.

Incidence of precancerous lesions as found with fiberoptic bronchoscopy in 198 patients with and without lung cancer

Type of lesion	Patients	
	without cancer n = 68	with cancer n = 130
Squamous metaplasia	19, 2 %	18, 5 %
Epithelial dysplasia	15, 8 %	27, 7 %
Micropapillomatosis	2, 9 %	0, 8 %
Dyskariosis	2, 0 %	6, 2 %
Cellular atypia	4, 0	18, 5 %
Chronic inflammation		total 56, 7 %

Table 1

The incidence of these changes, which were found in biopsy materials from suspect bronchial areas and above all, from brush specimens won from the individual lobular and segment bronchi is demonstrated in table 1. In the presence of tumor, different areas of the bronchial system often presented with displasias of a higher grade. Noteworthy is also the histologically proven high incidence of signs of chronic inflammation of the bronchial system (in 56 %). Following the discovery of a tumor macroscopically, we did not restrict the biopsy to the tumor and possible areas of resection, but also all the other areas of the bronchial system were examined systematically. So, we found carcinoma-in-situ in 6 patients (3.9 %) in addition, 5 ipsilaterally and 1 contralaterally.

In 7 patients or 4.6 % (table 2) we discovered a primary multifocal cancer. Excluded from this number are those patients, presenting with cancer in the brush materials and biopsies from the same side at the same time in order to exclude intramural or lymphogenic metastasis.

Multiple primary lung cancers found by fiberoptic bronchoscopy							
Pat.	Age	Sex	Cell type	Location of the greater tumor mass	Other location	Diagnosis of the tumor by Biopsy	Brush
1.	50	Male	Small cell -	r. lower lobe	l. lower lobe	+ +	-
2.	53	Female	Large cell -	r. main stem	l. upper lobe / l. lower lobe	+ - / + -	+
3.	54	Male	Squamous -	r. lower lobe	l. upper lobe / l. lower lobe	+ +	-
4.	55	Male	Squamous -	l. lower lobe	r. upper lobe / r. lower lobe	+ +	-
5.	56	Female	Adenocar.	l. upper lobe / l. lower lobe	middle lobe	+ + / + +	+
6.	65	Male	Squamous -	middle lobe	l. upper lobe / l. lower lobe	+ -	+
7.	50	Male	Squamous -	l. lower lobe	larynx	+ +	-

Table 2

Many cancer patients had severe dysplasia far away from the side of the tumor, or they showed continuous transition from simple to severe displasias, to carcinoma-in-situ and to invasive tumor growth.

Discussion

Our observation of the incidence of potentially precancerous lesions, metaplasia, dysplasia, carcinoma-in-situ and micropapillomatosis has not yet matched their corresponding incidence in the final stages as discovered by the morbid anastomist following post mortem examination or in lung removed at the operation (1, 3). The 4.2 % incidence of multifocal pulmonary cancer in our series stands against 1 % incidence as given in the literature other than pathology (4).

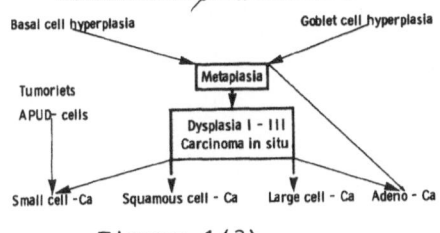

Figure 1(3)

In the light of the fact that today pathology assumes a relation between the precancerous lesions of the bronchial mucous layer and the different histological types of bronchial cancer as shown in figure 1 (3, 5), better results in the treatment of cancer patients can be achieved only be finding the preneoplastic lesions and carcinoma-in-situ and carrying out an early definitive treatment. Bronchoscopy with fiber optics, as described here, presents already today as an instrument for the early diagnosis of the bronchial cancer (2).

References

1. Auerbach, O., Saccomanno, G., Kuschner, M., Brown, R. D., and Garfinkel, L.: Histologic findings in the tracheobronchial tree of uranium miners and non-miners with lung cancer. Cancer 42: 483 - 489, 1978
2. Marsh, B. R., Frost, J. K., Erozan, Y. S., and Cartes, D.: Diagnosis of early bronchiogenic carcinoma. Chest 73: 716 - 717, 1978 (Suppl.)
3. Müller, K.-M.: Krebsvorstadien der Bronchialschleimhaut. Verh. Dtsch. Ges. Pathol. 63: 112 - 131, 1979
4. Martini, N., and Melamed, M. R.: Multiple primary lung cancers. J. Thorac. Cardiovasc. Surg. 70: 606 - 612, 1975
5. Saccomanno, G., Archer, V. E., Auerbach, O., Saunders, R. R., and Brennan, L. M.: Development of carcinoma of the lung as reflected in exfoliated cells. Cancer 33: 256 - 270, 1974

II. 10.

BRONCHOFIBERSCOPIC OBSERVATIONS ON BRONCHIAL **EPITHELIUM** OF
HEAVY SMOKER (Follow-up Data to Preliminary Findings)

H. Iwahashi M.D.   K, Hagiwara M.D.   M, Nogawa M.D.

Histological studies to detect early stage central type pulmonary
carcinoma, and to survey changes in the bronchial epithelium of
heavy smokers were undertaken using the bronchofiberscope. Subjects
were comprised of limited high-risk groups, each of whom satisfied
the following conditions. 1) 40 years of age and over, 2) smoked in
excess of 20 cigarettes per day for more than 20 years. 3) revealed
no abnormal Chest-X-ray findings. The entire bronchial epithelium was
observed by bronchofiberscope. Punch biopsy was carried out at the
site of the **bifurcation** of the right upper bronchus and right intermediate bronchus, even when no abnormal findings were admitted.

The results were as follows: Heavy smokers---goblet cell hyperplasia
34 cases (12.6%), squamous metaplasia 30 cases (11.1%), basal cell
hyperplasia, 60 cases (22.3%). Non-smokers---39 cases (60%) showed no
abnormal findings, only 1 case of goblet cell hyperplasia was admitted.
11 cases (16.9%) of mild basal cell hyperplasia, and 3 cases (4.6%)
    of   squamous metaplasia were found. In heavy smokers, the
percentage of cases with squamous metaplasia findings was 6.5% higher
than that of non-smokers group.

TABLE 1.

Histological Changes of Bronichial Epitherium
in Heavy Smokers and Non-Smokers

	Normal	Inflammatory cell infilt-ration	Goblet cell hyperplasia	Basal cell hyperplasia	Squamous metaplasia	Total
Heavy smokers BI > 400	129 48.1%	16 5.9%	34 12.6%	60 22.3%	30 11.1%	269
Non-smokers	39 60.0%	10 15.3%	1 1.5%	11 16.9%	3 4.6%	64

J.A. Nakhosteen and W. Maassen (eds.), Bronchology: Research, Diagnostic and
Therapeutic Aspects. All rights reserved.
Copyright 1981. Martinus Nijhoff Publishers bv, The Hague / Boston / London

52

FIGURE 1.shows the results of follow-up studies undertaken on
22 of the 30 cases of squamous metaplasia observed. These 22 cases
were classified into 3 groups. 1) squamous metaplasia with atypia,
3 cases. 2) mature squamous metaplasia without atypia, 10 cases.
3) immature squamous metaplasia without atypia, 9 cases. Further,
2 cases of basal cell hyperplasia turning into squamous metaplasia
were also observed during 36 month follow-up period. The 3 cases of
squamous metaplasia with atypia were irreversible. 3 of the 10 cases
all heavy smokers of mature squamous metaplasia without atypia evolved
into atypia after one year. There was tendency for a change back to
normal ɩepithelium if the subject quit smoking.

FIGURE 1.

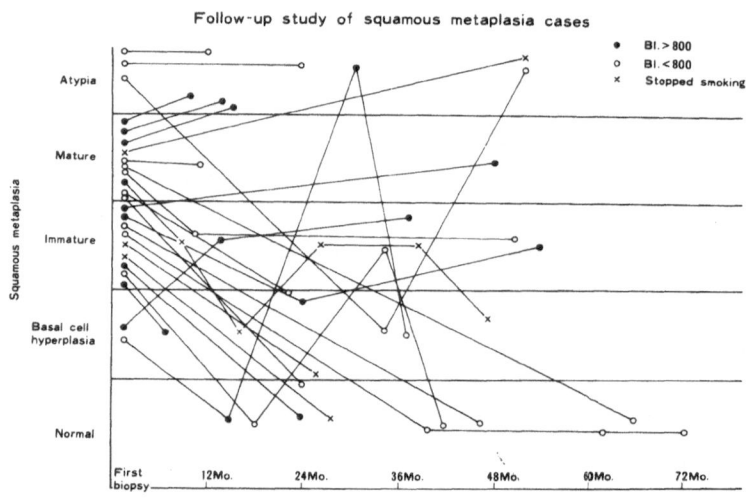

Follow-up study of squamous metaplasia cases

FIGURE 2.

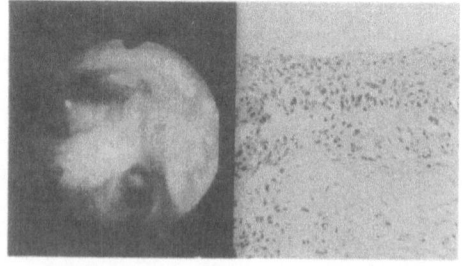

This is the case of 53 year old
male, BI index 700. The left
picture is the left upper bronchial
orifice. The right picture shows
squamous metaplasia with atypia.
The second examination two years
later revealed similar findings.

We are continuing to study the significance of preneonatal
alteration of the bronchial epithelium produced by smoking. No case of
early lung cancer have as yet been detected, however, periodic
observation of squamous metaplasia cases admitted among high-risk groups
will one day verify the evolution of carcinoma in situ and early lung
cancer by providing practical clinical data.

II.11.

FIBEROPTIC BRONCHOSCOPIC FINDINGS IN CASES OF ATYPICAL SQUAMOUS METAPLASIA

Naganobu Hayashi, K. Oho, R. Amemiya, T. Kawauchi, K. Nagai, K. Haya-kawa, I. Iimura, Y. Hayata

Our studies inducing lung cancer in dogs have achieved a high rate of successful induction. In all of our dogs which developed carcinoma of the lung (central type) squamous cell metaplasia preceded the cancer. Although the exact relationship between squamous cell carcinoma and cancer is by no means clear, we feel that it is an important finding in clinical cases. Here we present the fiberoptic bronchoscopic findings of 171 cases of squamous cell metaplasia. All cases presenting at the Department of Surgery, Tokyo Medical Hospital, with respiratory symptoms or abnormal chest X-ray undergo transoral fiberoptic bronchoscopic examination under local anesthesia.

Males predominated over females (136:35) and the average age was 60. Those who responded concerning their smoking habits indicated that 85% of males smoked as compared to about 50% females. Table 1 shows the findings in the 171 cases. Numbers of lung cancer cases and benign cases were roughly equal in number. Even in non-lung cancer cases, a high incidence of cough and bloody sputum. However more than 10% of squamous metaplasia cases showed no symptoms. (Table 2) Typical bronchoscopic findings include thickening and widening of bifurcations and disappearance of mucosal relief. (Fig. 1) Figure 2 shows other typical findings. The mucosa is edematous, irregular and it has lost its transparency. Another finding is redness and vascular engorgement. (Fig. 3) Stenosis (Fig. 4) is another common finding. Rarely, a tumor-like protrusion (Fig. 5) is observed.

We classified the various fiberoptic bronchoscopic findings seen in squamous metaplasia and summarized them in Table 3. The prominent position of squamous metaplasia in the experimental carcinogenetic process in dogs emphasizes the importance of recognizing this finding in clinical cases, and in being able to examine as wide an area of the bronchial tree as possible, for which the fiberoptic bronchoscope is ideally suited.

J.A. Nakhosteen and W. Maassen (eds.), Bronchology: Research, Diagnostic and Therapeutic Aspects. All rights reserved.
Copyright 1981. Martinus Nijhoff Publishers bv, The Hague / Boston / London

54

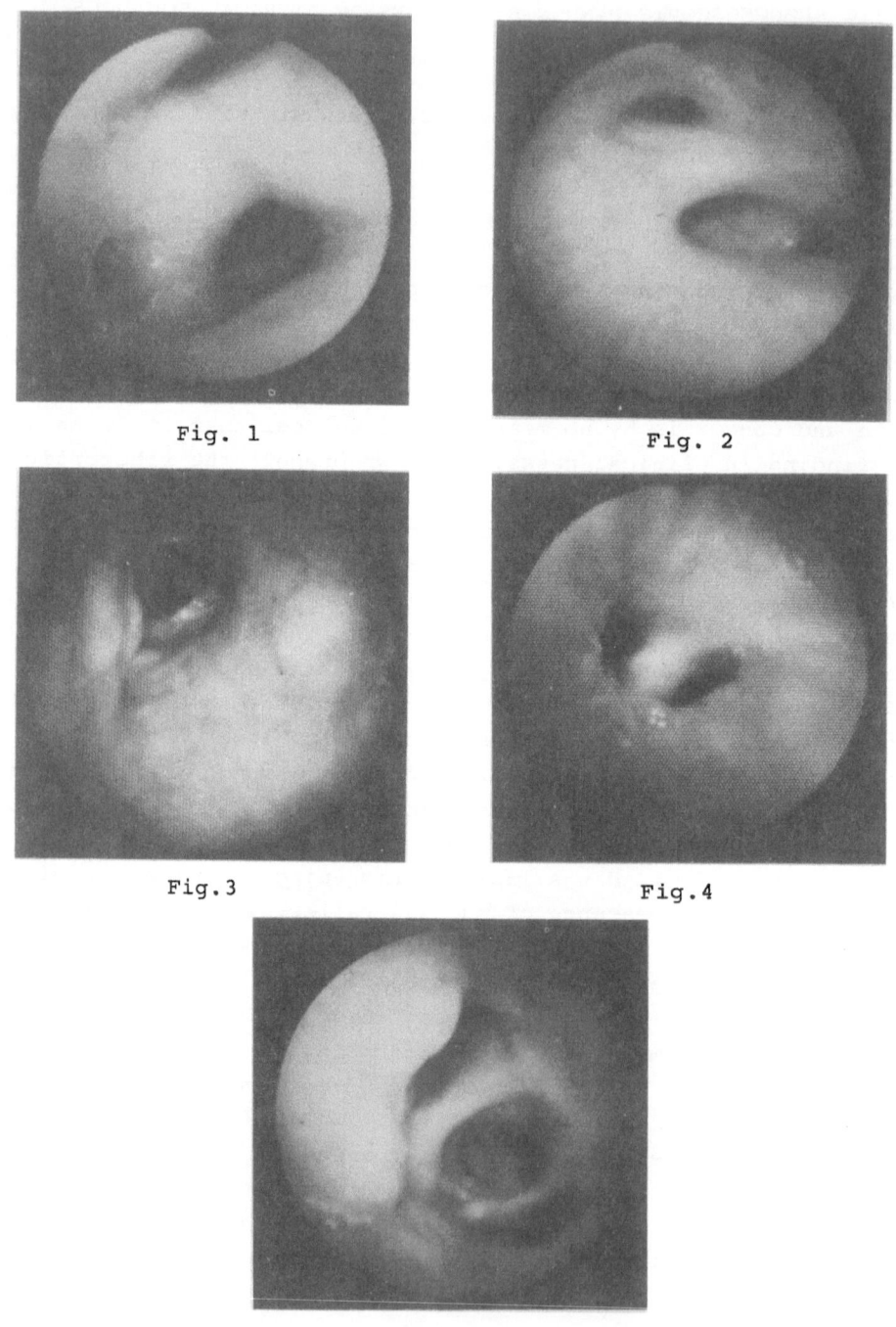

Fig. 1

Fig. 2

Fig.3

Fig.4

Fig. 5

Diseases associated with squamous cell metaplasia
(171 known cases)

	No. of cases	%
Lung cancer	86	50.3
Squamous cell ca	39	22.8
Adeno ca	20	11.7
Small cell ca	14	8.2
Large cell ca	3	1.8
Adenosquamous ca	2	1.2
Other histologic type	8	4.7
Benign diseases	85	49.7
Chronic bronchitis	42	24.6
Pulmonary tuberculosis	12	7.0
Sarcoidosis	12	7.0
Pulmonary fibrosis	4	2.3
Pulmonary suppuration	4	2.3
Bronchiectasis	2	1.2
Pneumonia	2	1.2
Mediastinitis	2	1.2
Others	5	2.9

Table 1

Symptoms associated with squamous cell metaplasia
(85 non-lung cancer cases)

	No. of cases	%
Cough	33	38.8
Bloody sputum	21	24.7
Sputum	8	9.4
Chest pain	5	5.9
Dyspnea	5	5.9
Fever	1	1.2
General fatigue	1	1.2
Another	1	1.2
No symptoms	10	11.8

Table 2

TYPICAL FIBEROPTIC BRONCHOSCOPIC FINDINGS IN SQUAMOUS CELL METAPLASIA

BRONCHIAL WALL
1. Redness
2. Watery edematous swelling
3. Loss of mucosal transparency
4. Mucosal irregularity (Small protrusions)
5. Tumor-like protrusions
6. Thickening and loss of plica
7. Vascular engorgement

LUMEN
1. Stenosis
2. Widened bifurcation

INTRABRONCHIAL MATERIAL
1. Increased secretions
2. Blood

Table 3

VASCULAR PATTERNS OBSERVED VIA THE FIBEROPTIC BRONCHOSCOPE IN CASES OF LUNG CANCER
II.12.
R. Amemiya, K. Oho, M. Aida, N. Hayashi, K. Nagai, N. Takizawa, Y. Hayata

There is no internationally accepted classification of bronchoscopic findings. The classification adopted by the Japanese Lung Cancer Society[1] is shown in Fig. 1, but the only reference to vascular findings in this classification system is the term 'vascular engorgement'. We feel that since cases of lung cancer exhibit a variety of vascular findings which are important in terms of diagnosis and deciding therapeutic strategy. Our purpose was to establish a classification of vascular patterns as observed through the fiberoptic bronchoscope.

It was observed that different histologic types show different tendencies as regards vascular patterns. In the case of squamous cell carcinoma shown in Fig. 2, the vessels are seen to disappear at a site which was demonstrated pathologically to be the border of the lesion. Squamous cell carcinoma tumors exhibiting subepithelial invasion have a tendency to display elevated growth, protruding in the bronchial lumen,[2] as shown in Fig. 3. With deeper invasion, the tumor displays polypoid or nodular protrusion with increased irregularity in the surrounding vascular pattern, and Fig. 4 shows an example of the histology of such a lesion. Viewed through the fiberoptic bronchoscope, the vessels appear irregular. Some appear tortuous and other possible vascular findings include stenosis, engorgement and abruption, (Fig. 5).

Adenocarcinoma and small cell carcinoma exhibit a tendency to proliferate submucosally. Thus, as shown in Fig. 6, blood vessels can be observed extending to the normal mucosa which covers the lesion. However the vessels observed through the transparent mucosa show distention and engorgement, with unequal intervascular distance. Vessels distal to the tumor appear to be nutritive vessels.

Considering the variety of vascular findings which are seen in lung cancer, and since these are related to the various growth patterns of different histologic types of tumors, a detailed classification of their appearance is warranted. Thus we composed the classification of vascular patterns shown in Fig. 7, and use this in clinical evaluation of cases. We realize that it is often difficult to differentiate between neoplastic-like vessels and nonneoplastic-like vessels, but since in clearly distinguishable cases this can be linked to the stage of the case, we feel that this is a valid and important differentiation.

J.A. Nakhosteen and W. Maassen (eds.), Bronchology: Research, Diagnostic and Therapeutic Aspects. All rights reserved.
Copyright 1981. Martinus Nijhoff Publishers bv, The Hague / Boston / London

REFERENCES

1. The Japan Lung Cancer Society: Rules for clinical and pathological records of lung cancer, 41-54, Tokyo, Kanehara-Shuppan, 1978.
2. Oho, K., Amemiya, R.: Practical fiberoptic bronchoscopy, 65-67, Tokyo, Igaku-Shoin, 1980.

Findings in lung cancer cases.

I. Bronchial wall
  1) Tumor
    a. nodular
    b. multinodular
    c. smooth surface
    d. irregular surface
    e. granular surface
    f. necrosis
    g. vascular engorgement
  2) Infiltration
    a. mucosal irregularity
    b. vascular engorgement
    c. loss of luster
    d. necrosis
    e. paleness of mucosa
    f. swelling
    g. redness
    h. indistinct bronchial cartilage
    i. thickened mucosal folds
    j. indistinct mucosal folds

II. Changes in the bronchial lumen
  1) Stenosis
    a. due to tumor
    b. due to infiltration
    c. due to external compression
  2) Obstruction
    a. due to tumor
    b. due to infiltration
    c. due to external compression

Fig. 1

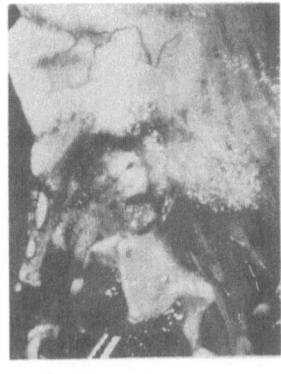

Fig. 2

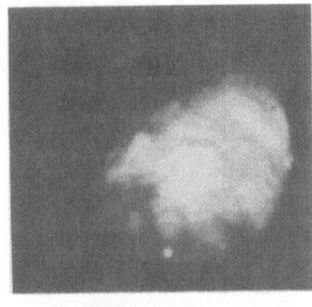

Fig. 3

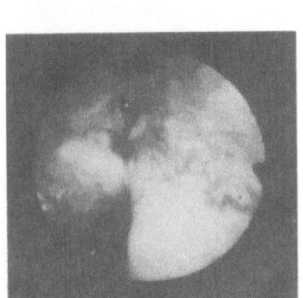

Fig. 5

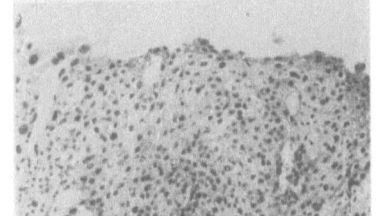

Fig. 4

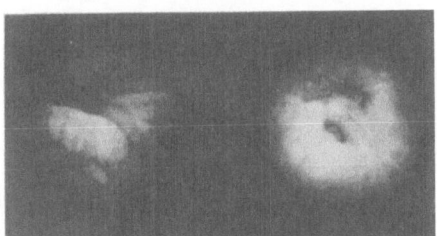

Fig. 6

CLASSIFICATION OF VASCULAR PATTERNS

1. NONNEOPLASTIC-LIKE VESSELS
  1. ENGORGEMENT
  2. DISAPPEARANCE

2. NEOPLASTIC-LIKE VESSELS
  1. ENGORGEMENT
  2. STENOSIS
  3. ABRUPTION
  4. NOT VISIBLE

3. DISTRIBUTION PATTERN
  1. TREE-LIKE BRANCHING
  2. IRREGULAR NETWORK
  3. CORKSCREW-LIKE
  4. NUMEROUS FINE PARALLEL TRACKS

Fig. 7

II.13.
EARLY DETECTION OF HILAR TYPE OF BRONCHOGENIC CARCINOMA

H. MIKAMI, Y.OHSAKI, S. ABE, K. KIMURA, I. TSUNETA AND M. MURAO

Lung cancer among chromate workers has been recognized as one of the occupational lung cancers based on cumulative reports since 1911. We have been
doing health check-ups of chromate workers for detection of bronchogenic carcinoma since 1973. The subjects were 284 chromate workers who were employed
more than one year at a chromate factory in Hokkaido. Of the workers, 266
were men and 18 were women. The methods of check-up were chest roentgenogram,
sputum cytology twice a year and bronchoscopic examination annually. We found
eight cases of bronchogenic carcinoma among chromate workers by health check-
up 1973-1979. All were men. Ages ranged from 45 to 73 years. The period of
exposure to chromate dust or mist ranged from 6 to 36 years. The histology was
squamous cell carcinoma in five, small cell carcinoma in two and poor differentiated adenocarcinoma in one. As to the primary site, seven cases were hilar
and only one was peripheral type. All six cases which were found by chest
roentgenogram were late stage bronchogenic carcinoma. Two cases of early stage
hilar type of bronchogenic carcinoma were found by sputum cytology and bronchoscopic examination. These cases are as follows.

CASE PRESENTAION
Case No. 1.
    The patient was fifty-nine year-old male with no symptoms. He had been
employed at a chromate factory for twenty eight years. He had nasal perforation at health check-up. His smoking index was 600. Laboratory studies were
within normal limits. Chest roentgenogram was negative except small calcifi-
cation in the right middle lung field. The histology of sputum revealed severe
squamous metaplasia. Bronchoscopic examination showed a very small tumor formation in the anterior aspect of the left upper lobe bronchus. The lesion revealed a slight elevation of reddish bronchial mucosa with irregular surface,
whitish coating and slight bleeding. The brushing cytology performed under
bronchoscopic examination revealed squamous cell carcinoma. Left upper lobectomy was done. The size of the tumor was 0.8 X 1.0 cm and its pathology revealed squamous cell carcinoma confined within the mucus membrane of the bronchial wall, namely carcinoma in situ.

J.A. Nakhosteen and W. Maassen (eds.), Bronchology: Research, Diagnostic and
Therapeutic Aspects. All rights reserved.
Copyright 1981. Martinus Nijhoff Publishers bv, The Hague / Boston / London

Case No. 2.

The patient was forty-five year-old male with no symptoms. He had been employed at a chrome factory for twenty six years, and had nasal perforation. His smoking index was 500. Physical examination and laboratory studies were within normal limits. Chest roentgenogram revealed no abnormal findings. Suspecting malignant process based on squamous metaplasia by sputum examination done in 1976, bronchoscopic examination was performed, but it showed no findings. One year later, bronchoscopic examination showed a very small tumor formation with bleeding and whitish coating at the septum of apic-posterior and anterior segmental bronchi of the left upper lobe bronchus. The brushing cytology performed under bronchoscopic examination revealed squamous cell carcinoma. Left upper lobectomy was done. The resected tumor was very small, 0.6 X 0.8 cm in size and its pathology showed early stage squamous cell carcinoma.

CONCLUSION:

1) Chest roentgenogram was not an effective method for detection of hilar type of bronchogenic carcinoma.

2) Final diagnosis should be made with bronchoscopic examination and this is the essential method for detection of early hilar type of bronchogenic carcinoma.

3) Bronchoscopic examination is, however, not applicable for a large number of the subjects, from an economical and time-consuming point of view. So that, it is our policy to select candidates for bronchoscopic examination based on the results of sputum cytology.

II.14.

TUMOROUS DISEASES OF THE TRACHEA AND BRONCHI GIVING NO X-RAY SHADOW

E.BÁNHIDI

Nowadays lung cancer is the most common tumour in men. The forms of clinical appearance, diagnostic and therapeutic results of the 2nd and 3rd stages
are well-known. It is the occult and early invasive carcinoma which stands
in the limelight today. Recently more and more publications were issued
demonstrating tumorous cells by sputum-cytology, but there was no sign of
tumour to be seen on the chest radiogram. These tumours which can not be
observed nor followed by routine examinations are called "occult" carcinomas.
This term was given by Webster.
In the 50-ies Boucot found chest radiograms made half-yearly necessary for
discovering such occult tumours in men over 45, who were heavy smokers and
exposed to carcinogenic dust.
The observation of so called "high-risk" individuals was included in
"screening programmes" by Paerson in 1967 and Sanderson in 1974.
In these male heavy smokers over 45 years sputum-cytology and chest films
were made on 3 consecutive days every 4 months. Occult tumour was discovered
in 13 cases during 18 months, a considerable advance on Boucot.
"In-situ" or early invasive carcinomas comprise these occult carcinomas.
Cells are atypical, but if the basal membrane is intact then a carcinoma
in situ exists. Cells increase in size, lose their polarity, have an atypical
nucleus, the chromatin content of which increases.
Limited at first to the superficial epithelium, it spreads into gland ducts,
then infiltrates the cartilagenous part of the bronchi through the mucosa.
Some basic problems have to be considered in its diagnosis.
1./ Incidence and duration of an in situ lesion before it turns into the
     invasive stage.
2./ Possibility of diagnosis, when there is an occult alteration on the chest
     radiogram beside the positive cytological finding.
3./ Prognosis of in situ carcinoma following surgical intervention.

*J.A. Nakhosteen and W. Maassen (eds.), Bronchology: Research, Diagnostic and
Therapeutic Aspects. All rights reserved.*
Copyright 1981. Martinus Nijhoff Publishers bv, The Hague / Boston / London

It is a well-known fact that there is a long latent period in the pathogenesis of cancer of other organs, e.g. the uterus, until it turns into
invasive carcinoma, and this may also hold true for lung cancer. It may
last for 5-10 years. Radiologically occult tumours may cause symptoms in a
significant number of cases. Episodic pneumonitis, unusual cough or
transient haemoptysis are always warning signs. On the other hand, if the
sputum is suspect or positive, the lesion must be found.
Though hemoptysis occured only in 15 % of the patients in a chest clinic,
carcinoma was found in 30 % of this group.
Usually a small ulceration develops in the main bronchus and may be the
source of hemoptysis. Bronchology is a very important and obvious link
among the diagnostic means. Occult carcinomas afford a favourable opportunity
to try the bronchologist's skill.
Biopsy must be made at once, even if the lesion is slightly suspect. If there
is no pathological change to be observed in the main bronchus, all the
segmental and subsegmental bronchi must be examined by bronchofiberoscopy.
Sometimes a friable, slightly thickened mucous membrane, on other occasions
reddish unevenness indicates the presence of in situ carcinoma.The examination material obtained by brush biopsy and fiberbronchoscopic biopsy is the
most valuable.Spur biopsies have great importance, because in situ carcinomas
often originate from the corners of the bronchi. In cases where no alteration
of the mucous membrane can be observed even by the most thorough examination,
random excisions of the bronchus is rather rare, but most rewarding, both
for surgeon and patient. Often the tumorous lesion can be demonstrated only
by serial sections.

Our patients

During the past 10 years we treated 15 patients who had no X-ray shadow,
but malignant tumour could be demonstrated by bronchological examination
and subsequent histology. All of them were heavy smokers with the exception
of some women patients.
Hemoptysis was the main symptom, in one case frequent pneumonia led to
examination. Endobronchially lymphogranulomatosis was found in one patient,
while the type of the malignant cells was characteristically epithelial
cancer, in agreement with the literature. Following up our cases we can

say, that only 1 patient has been living more than a year, the others
have died in spite of the properly chosen therapy within 1-2 years.

Discussion

In 1951 Papanicolau and Koprowska reported about the first carcinoma in
situ case.

In cases with cough and hemoptysis giving no X-ray shadow positive
cytological finding serves as the first morphological sign to prove the
presence of carcinoma, hence the importance of cytology in early and
in situ carcinoma. Locating the in situ or invasive carcinoma in patients
discovered in this way is the next problem, necessitating further endoscopic intervention of all the segment and lobar bronchi every six months.
Transient pneumonia and hemoptysis are warning signs making detailed and
thorough X-ray film examination and monitoring necessary. Certainly, we are
in an easier situation if recurrent pneumonia or other decisive signs lead
the examination in a certain direction.

The results of surgical resection, those published in the literature and
the long survival indicate that it is worth dealing with these patients.

II.15. ELECTRONMICROSCOPIC STUDY OF LUNG CANCER SPECIMEN BIOPSIED BY
LARGE CHANNEL BRONCHOFIBERSCOPE

T. KAWAI. T. OGATA. K. KIKUCHI. and K. WATANABE

INTRODUCTION

The large channel fiberoptic bronchoscope made the use of large
biopsy forceps feasible. Although this type of fiberscope is usable
to take a biopsy of the lesion only proximal to the segmental bronchus
, large pieces of specimen incluing mucosal lesions can be taken.
We studied biopsied specimens of the hilar pulmonary cancers electronmicroscopically.

MATERIALS, METHODS and RESULTS

The materials are two cases of polypoid type adenocarcinoma and
two cases of polypoid type small cell carcinoma. These biopsy specimens were taken with large channel fiberscope and were examined
under light and electronmicroscope.

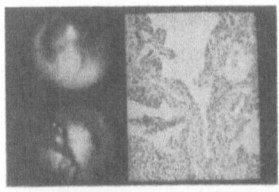

This is a bronchoscopic finding of the hemorrhagic polypoid tumor of the rt.intermediate
bronchus of 32 yrs. old female. Light microscopic
picture shows well differentiated adenocarcinoma
composed of papillary structure of high columnar
cells.

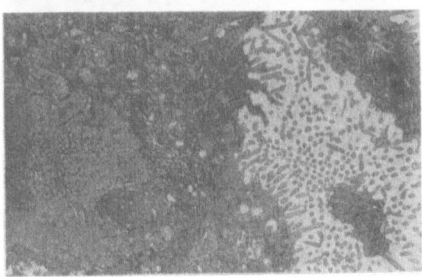 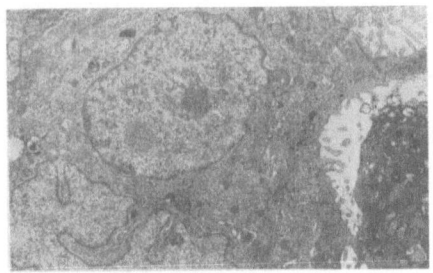

This electronmicroscopic picture indicates a part of papillary
structure. Microvilli and tight junctions near the free edge are
identified and also ample amount of Golgi apparatus and mitochondria
adjacent to nucleus are visualized. Right picture indicates lots of
Golgi vesicle, rough surfaced endoplasmic reticulm (RER) and free

J.A. Nakhosteen and W. Maassen (eds.), Bronchology: Research, Diagnostic and
Therapeutic Aspects. All rights reserved.
Copyright 1981. Martinus Nijhoff Publishers bv, The Hague / Boston / London

ribosome. There are pseudoinclusion in the nucleus. Also a few high density granules are visualized which are suspected to be lysosomal granules, not secretory granules. From these findings, the adenocarcinoma can not be originated in a type II pneumocyte, Clara cell or bronchial gland cell, but bronchial surface cell.

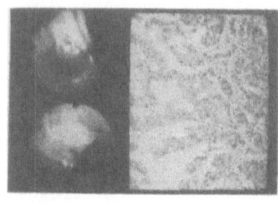

This is the bronchoscopic finding of 48 yrs. old male. Multicentric polypoid tumors coverd with mucosal membrane are identified at the orifices of rt.lower lobe bronchus and lt.lingular bronchus. Light microscopic finding shows geographic pattern of tumor cells composed of non-atypical round nuclei and eosinophilic cytoplasm. Tumor cells appear to be floating in the mucoid substance that is strongly positive to Alcian blue and PAS stain. From these findings, it can be suspected that this tumor originates in bronchial gland cell like a mucoepidermoid carcinoma.

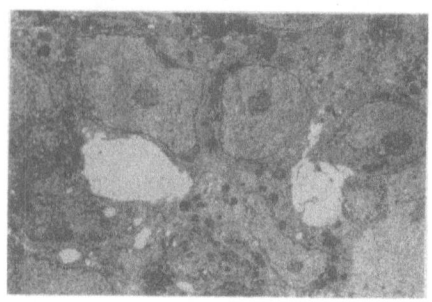

Under the electronmicroscope we can also identify plenty RER, many sized mitochondria and Golgi apparatus. Characteristics of the picture is the visualization of multiple space filled with granular substance lacking in limiting membrane and microvilli inside and outside of the tumor cells. These spaces outside of tumor cells could be a stroma consisted of mucoid substance identified by light microscope. This finding of the stroma suspects the matrix degeneration of tumor cells rather than the secreting figure.

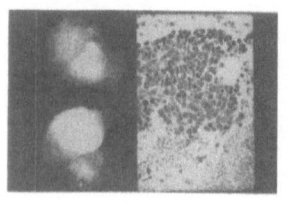

The third patient is a 65 yrs. old male. A polypoid tumor protrudes at the B^3 orifice. A spur between upper and lower bronchus is obtuse and submucosal invasion is evident. Tumor cells are small and have hyperchromatic nuclei without cytoplasm. And there is no specific mode of proliferation. From these finding, this tumor is considered to be small cell anaplastic carcinoma-oat cell type. Electronmicroscopically, a nucleus is a complicated pattern of chromatin agglutination and the irregularity of nuclear outline is evident. Cytoplasm is scarce and simple.Although Golgy apparatus

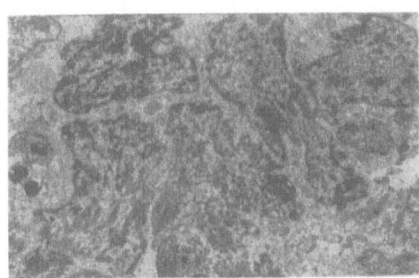

and neurosecretory granules were
not identified. We considered this
oat cell anaplastic carcinoma.

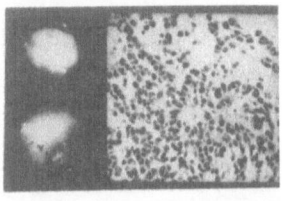

A last case is a 50 yrs. old female. Bronchoscopic findings reveales a large polypoid tumor
arising from lt.main bronchus and extending to
the tracheal bifurcation. Light microscopically,
enough cytoplasm is visualized, even though
N/C ratio is great. With these finding, this
tumor is considered to be small cell carcinoma-intermediate cell type.

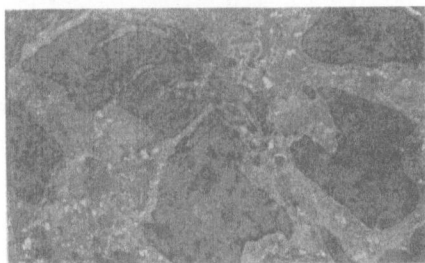 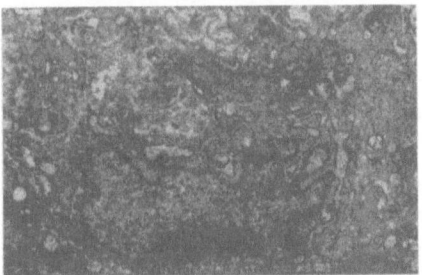

Nuclei of tumor cells show the mosaic pattern of euchromatin and
heterochromatin. The combination of ample mitochondria and scarce
other organella is characteristic of anaplastic type. In addition,
there are many tonofilament bundles are identified everywhere.

Rt.picture is taken from the Epon block of other part of biopsy
material and well developed Golgi apparatus are identified. There
is no microvilli, glandlar space or desmosome. In conclusion, this
tumor could probably originate in basal cell of bronchial epithelium
and epidermoid nature is predominant. Adenocomponent, however, also
noted. Therefore, we considered this tumor small cell carcinoma-intermediate type presenting bidirectional transition.

Biopsied specimens taken by a large channel fiberscope were intact
enough to be examined with an electronmicroscope. Especially subtype
classification of adeno and small cell carcinoma can be done more
efficiently and cell origin was discussed in favorable fashion.
REFERENCE
1) Y. Kimula. : Amer, J. Surg. Pathol., 2, 253-264, 1978.

II.16.

FORCEPS-BIOPSY MATERIAL - A SAMPLE FOR HISTOLOGIC AND CYTOLOGIC
EXAMINATION

M. Roglić

Forceps biopsy was primarily applied to obtain material for
histologic examination. In our hospital forceps-biopsy material
has been analyzed, for more than twenty five years, cytologically
as well as histologically. In this way diagnostic accuracy is
considerably higher.

Materials and methods
Materials obtained by 600 consecutive forceps biopsies during
the last four years, were examined cytologically and histologically.
Cytologic specimens were obtained by imprint method and stained
by the May-Grünwald-Giemsa technique. Hematoxilin and eosin stain
was used for histologic sections.

Results
Results of cytologic and histologic examination as well as the
correlation between cytologic and histologic diagnoses or findings
are presented on the table 1.

TABLE 1. Cytology versus histology of 600 materials

	Carcinoma	Suspicious	Metaplasia	Granuloma	Negative
Carcinoma	296	15	2	1	81
Suspicious	1	2	1	-	6
Metaplasia	1	1	-	-	-
Granuloma	1	-	1	4	5
Negative	3	3	7	6	163

Carcinoma was proved cytologically in 395 materials. Of these, carcinoma was proved by histology in 296, suspicious in 15; further two showed metaplastic and one granulomatous changes. In 81 materials histologic diagnosis was negative.

Out of lo cases which were cytologically suspicious of cancer histology has given following results: one positive, two suspicious, one metaplasia, and six negative.

Metaplasia was found in two cytologic smears, while histology was positive in one and suspicious in the other material. Cytology detected granulomatous changes in 11 cases. Histology correlated with cytology in four cases, proved carcinoma in one, metaplasia in one, and was negative in five.

Out of 182 cases being cytologically negative histology proved carcinoma only in three. Further three findings were suspicious. Metaplasia was found in seven materials and granuloma in six. 163 cases were both negative histologically as well as cytologically.

Correlation rate between cytologic and histologic diagnoses comes to 77.5%.

Out of the total number of 401 carcinomas diagnosed from forceps-biopsy materials, 296 were verified cytologically and histologically, while 99 cytologically and 6 histologically only. Thus 395 carcinomas or 98.5% were proved by cytology, while 302 or 75.3% by histology.

The results of type classification of 296 carcinomas diagnosed by both methods are shown on the table 2.

TABLE 2. Cytologic versus histologic typing of carcinoma

	Carcinoma epidermoides	Carcinoma anaplasticum	Adeno-carcinoma	Carcinoides	Carcinoma
Carcinoma epidermoides	180	1	1	–	1
Carcinoma anaplasticum	3	68	–	–	4
Adeno-carcinoma	–	–	3	–	–
Carcinoides	–	1	–	1	1
Carcinoma	4	–	–	–	28

Cytologic and histologic typing has confirmed the congruity in: 180 epidermoid carcinomas, 68 small-cell anaplastic carcinomas, 3 adenocarcinomas, 1 carcinoid, and 28 carcinomas without distinct type differentiation.

Congruity rate amounts to 94.6%, i.e. in 280 out of 296 cases.

The use of transmural fine needle aspiration biopsy proved carcinoma in 23, and granulomatous changes in 22 out of 163 above mentioned cases, where cytologic and histologic diagnosis was negative.

This was subjoined in order to demonstrate the efficiency of application of other biopsy techniques during the same bronchoscopic procedure to provide better results.

Conclusion

It is obvious how useful it is to examine forceps-biopsy material not only histologically but also cytologically using the imprint method.

The results obtained indicate the advantage of such simultaneous examination. In this way the percentage of positive diagnoses is higher, especially if there is a scanty amount of tumour tissue in the forceps-biopsy material.

II.17.

DIAGNOSTIC FLEXIBLE FIBEROPTIC BRONCHOSCOPY: ANALYSIS OF RESULTS OF BIOPSY AND BRUSH IN 105 PATIENTS

YUAN-CHING HSIEH, C.H. CHIANG, C.Y. SHEN, C.C. YANG

INTRODUCTION

The flexible bronchoscope has achieved wide acceptance as diagnostic and therapeutic tool in various pulmonary disorders. This report involves 105 consecutive cases of bronchial biopsy and brush including both clinical and radiological evidence of bronchopulmonary diseases, the flexible fiberoptic bronchoscope offers increased diagnostic capabilities and a low complication rate. The purpose of this paper is to evaluate the diagnostic accuracy of bronchial forcep biopsy compared to bronchial nylon brushing in diagnosis of suspected bronchopulmonary disease.

MATERIAL AND METHODS

105 consecutive patients, 84 men and 21 women, ages 19 to 84 years at Tri-Service General Hospital in Taipei, underwent Olympus 5.3 mm flexible fiberoptic bronchoscopy, preparation of the patient and premedication were described as Ikeda. All patients received both forceps and a nylon brush passing through the channel of the instrument by introduction of oral route. The brush materials were studied for both cytology and acid-fast stain.

RESULTS

All patients received fiberoptic bronchoscopy and obtained an adequate specimen of bronchial tissue for biopsy and brushing materials for cytology and acid-fast stain. The two histological picture most frequently encounter were bronchogenic carcinoma (CA) in 57/105 (54%) patients and chronic inflammation in 48/105 (45%) patients. The etiological diagnosis of 105 patients by histological picture were shown as in Table I. A comparison of result between biopsy and brush cytology and different bronchoscopic findings were shown as listed in Table II. Which indicated that the positive rate of brush cytology was much higher than forcep tissue biopsy, and 3 of 8 patients without bronchoscopic

J.A. Nakhosteen and W. Maassen (eds.), Bronchology: Research, Diagnostic and Therapeutic Aspects. All rights reserved.

findings were also proved by brush cytology but the brush materials for acid-fast stain was only 3 positives, as shown in Table III. Analysis of the histology type of bronchogenic CA in 57 of 105 patients showed that adeno CA was higher than epidermoid CA in this series. In addition, 3 patients with positive acid-fast stain and graunloma were found, only 5 cases with brisk bleeding and low grade fever for 1-2 days and one patient had psychic reaction with laughing and crying which lasted for half one hour.

DISCUSSION

This report describes using the technique of bronchial forcep biopsy, and brushing materials for cytology and acid-fast stain, through the fiberoptic bronchoscope in manuever similar to that used by Ikeda's oral introduction of the fiberoscope. Emphasis in our analysis was placed on the relative merits of forcep biopsy and brushing in establishing the diagnosis, no attempt was made to compare other established methods of diagnosis in this group of patients. A major advantage of our used method is the combination of oral introduction of fiberoscope, with forceps biopsy and brush studied in a single procedure. The instrument is easier to manipulate, and can be rapidly and atrumatically withdrawn, and repeatedly reinserted for multiple biopsies, and brush or clearing the distal lens. Diagnostic accuracy of endoscopically direct and indirect findings for malignamy, by above mentioned method in this series was only 65% and 79% (Table II), which was relatively lower to compare with Ikeda's 95% and Zavala's 89%, because we had no fluroscopic control, and therefore can not do the transbronchial biopsy for bronchoscopic indirect or negative lesion, but the positive rate on endoscopic visible lesion, including tumor mass, obstruction and mucosa destruction was 80 to 100%, by both forcep biopsy and cytology studies (Table II). However, there was a low positive rate on acid-fast stain although pulmonary tuberculosis among the percentage of chronic inflammation was 16/48 (38%) in this series. This was partly due to the majority of tuberculous lesion were located at peripheral region in this series and another possible reason was all patients had treated with chemotherapy for some times, before they received bronchoscopy to rule out the possibility of malignancy in order to do both cytological study and acid-fast stain.

It was condluded that flexible fiberoptic bronchoscopy with bronchial forcep biopsy and brush were an excellent procedure and provides highly accurate diagnostic information for the diagnosis of bronchopulmonary disease. The examination can be quickly and easily performed with minimal risk or discomfort to the patient.

Table I. Etiological Diagnosis of 105 Patients by Histological Picture

Histological picture and etiological diagnosis		No. of patient
Bronchogenic Carcinoma		57
Chronic inflammation		48
Pulmonary tuberculosis	16	
Bronchiectasis	11	
Bacterial pneumonia	5	
Chronic bronchitis	4	
Lung abscess	2	
Diffuse interstitial fibrosis	3	
Pneumoconiosis	2	
Undeterminated	6	
Total		105

Table II. Comparison of Result between Biopsy and Brush in Different Broncho-scopic Findings of 57 Patients with Bronchogenic Carcinoma

Bronchoscopic finding	No. of patient	Forcep biopsy positive		Nylon brush positive	
		No. of patient	%	No. of patient	%
I.Direct finding					
1. tumor mass	16	14	87	15	94
2. obstruction	10	8	80	8	80
3. mucosa destruction	9	9	100	9	100
II. Indirect finding					
(Narrowing, compression	14	6	43	10	71
swelling, redness)					
III. Negative	8	0	0	3	38
Total	57	37	65	45	79

Table III. Analysis of the Histology Type of Bronchogenic Carcinoma in 57 of 105 Patients

Histology type	No. of patient	%
Adeno Carcinoma	31	54
Epidermoid Carcinoma	18	32
Poorly Differential Carcinoma	4	7
Oat Cell	1	1.8
Large Cell	1	1.8
Anaplastic Carcinoma	1	1.8
Trachea Carcinoma	1	1.8
Total	57	100

II.18.

A Multimodal Diagnostic Approach To Lung Cancer [*]

S.Horie, K.Shimada, K. Matsumura and Y. Seki

1. INTRODUCTION

During the recent 25 years, we have made strenuous efforts to establish the diagnostic methods to carry out preoperative assessment of patients with lung cancer. Bronchoscopic examination is a vital part of diagnosis of lung cancer but some limitations have been pointed out in some occasions since its introduction. To overcome these limitations and to get better diagnostic yields, a multimodal diagnostic approach to lung cancer has been newly introduced in our department.

2. SUBJECTS

All patients except few autopsied cases who entered into this study underwent thoracotomy and all surgical or autopsy specimens were histologically proven. Preoperative histological or cytological diagnosis was all re-evaluated from histological examination of surgical specimens or autopsied specimens.

3. DIAGNOSTIC PROCEDURES

3.1. Bronchoscopy under general anesthesia. Bronchoscopy was routinely performed under general anesthesia with a use of muscle relaxants and inhalation anesthetic gases. A ventilating rigid open tube bronchoscope with a rubber cuff was used. A rigid broncho-telescope was used for endoscopic observation of the trachea and major bronchi with bright illumination. Endoscopic magnification was also possible. Bronchoscopic therapeutic manuvers were also successfully performed with an introduction of a modified bronchotelescope. Flexible bronchofiberscopy was usually done via the rigid open tube bronchoscope under general anesthesia after detailed observation of the trachea and major bronchi.

3.2. Flexible bronchofiberscope. A new type of a flexible bronchofiberscope was introduced. One of the principal features of it is a horizontal movement of the tip of the bronchoscope. The light source apparatus available currently has each different mode

of light guide sockets which are limited in use. A new device can
hook up with any types of light guide sockets.

3.3. Simultaneous use of fluoroscopy. Biplane simultaneous
fluoroscopic apparatus was introduced to confirm a tip of a cytology
brush which is introduced via a bronchofiberscope.

3.4. Bronchoscopy theater. Our bronchoscopy theater is equipped
with an anesthetic apparatus, monitoring television sets, a monitoring
cardiograph, a defibrilator, a cytology display scope in addition to
usual bronchoscopy instruments.

3.5. A cytology display scope with computerized parts was
introduced to observe cytological features obtained in the theater.
A rapid stain according to Shorr was used and cellular features were
possibly evaluated immediately after diagnostic procedure was
completed in the theater. Specialists other than bronchoscopists
joined to determine the character of the specimens. The introduction
of this system into the bronchoscopy theater significantly avoided
the repeated examination that took time.

3.6. Description of bronchoscopic findings. To document
bronchoscopie findings briefly but significantly, two categories
were used to classify the findings related to the presence of the
cancer. One of them was directly tumor-related findings and the
other was indirectly tumor-related findings. These two categories
were justified to use from detailed evaluation of surgical specimens.

4. RESULT

4.1. Figure 1 shows a trend of positive results obtained by
various diagnostic methods. From year to year, the diagnostic yields
become higher especially when the introduction of biplane fluoroscopy
was done. The result was made by means of various diagnostic methods
available currently. The most recent rate has reached 100%.

5. DISCUSSION

Introduction of a flexible bronchofiberscope is definitely a
breakthrough to overcome the limited visibility of a rigid bronchoscope, however, it is not possible to observe all bronchi by a
flexible bronchofiberscope if its size of diameter be so small.
To get a higher result, it was urged to develop many apparatus such
as biplane fluoroscopy and simultaneous use of general anesthesia.
A cytology diaplay scope can make it us possible to observe cellular
features obtained during the diagnostic procedure.

General anesthesia must be mandatory if detailed examination be needed regardless of the location of the tumor in the lung. Modern anesthesiology has widened the indication without any hazards.

REFERENCES
1. Shohei Horie: Bronchoscopic diagnosis of lung cancer, Dokkyo J. Med. Sci., 2: 87 -91, 1975.

---

*The authors presented a film on this subject at the 2d World Congress for Bronchology. Ed.

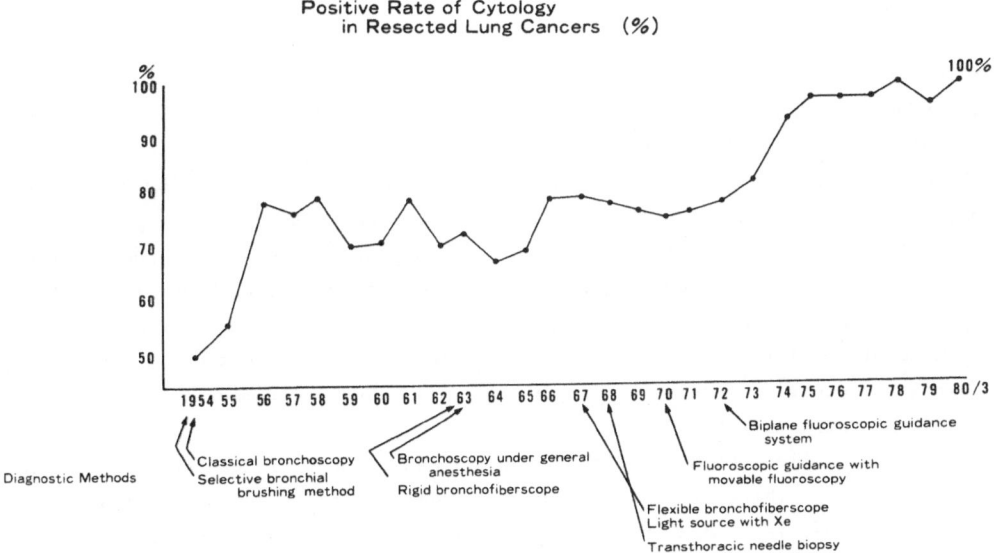

Figure 1

II.19.

Some Aspects of the Research Work on Chronic Bronchitis in China

In the past nine years, a lot of research work had been carried out in our country on chronic bronchitis, here are some related aspects in brief summary.

I. Epidemiology

Nation-wide surveys of 78,920,000 people conducted since 1971, showed an average morbidity of 4.0% (2.5-9.0%), while morbidity in the age group above 50 was as high as 13%. Certain features were noted: incidence higher in the north than in the south; higher in mountaineous areas than in plains; higher in rural areas than in urban areas. This suggests that, the pathogenesis of chronic bronchitis in our country is closely related to meterological factors and Socio-economical status of the people.

II. Etiology

1. Infections: more than ten kinds of viruses have been found which contribute to the pathogenesis of chronic bronchitis. Among them, Influenzae virus and Rhinovirus are the chief agents responsible for the colds. Coronavirus has also been identified in some cases, Viruses were isolated in 16.5% of the patients of chronic bronchitis in its acute stage. Bacterial infections were secondary in most cases, and A type streptococcus and Neisseria were found to be the chief agents, with bacillus influenzae or diplococcus pneumonia ranking next.

2. Meterological factors: The fluctuations of patients' condition in chronic bronchitis are closely correlated with average and, absolute temperature, the daily range and the daily variation of temperature.

3. Physico-chemical stimuli: High incidence was found with heavy air pollution and among smokers. There were about four times more patients in smokers than in nonsmokers. Higher incidence in rural areas may be partly due to the use of firewood for cooking which produces more smoke, and poor heating system and dwelling condition.

Besides hypersensitivity and allergy, senility, consumptive diseases, lack of physical activities, decrease in body resistance, and hypertonia of parasympathetic nervous system are all contributing factors.

J.A. Nakhosteen and W. Maassen (eds.), Bronchology: Research, Diagnostic and Therapeutic Aspects. All rights reserved.
Copyright 1981. Martinus Nijhoff Publishers bv, The Hague / Boston / London

III. Results and outcome of persistent systematic treatment of chronic bronchitis.

In our Hospital, satisfactory therapeutic results were obtained after 9 years of persistent systematic treatment of chronic bronchitls. Remarkable improvement in clinical sysmptoms and progress in varying degrees of physical signs were noted in most cases. In 39 cases (old housewives in urban areas) after 8 year treatment, those with remarkable symptomatic relief or clinical cure made up 33.3%; those with improvement, 53.8%; only 10.9% showed no improvement or even got worse. Another 5 year observation of 94 cases in rural areas showed 2 cases of clinical cure (2.3%), 83 of improvement (88.3%), and only 9 cases showed no effect (9.6%). Works carried out by other hospitals showed similar results.

Parameters of objective observations, however, showed alterations in varying degrees as follows:

1. Dynamic changes in X-ray films of the chest: In a follow-up study of 68 rural patients in our Hospital, incidence of emphysema increased from 33 cases in 1975 to 42 cases in 1979; pulmonary fibrosis was getting more and more severe too. In another report of a 8 year observation of 39 cases of senile chronic bronchitis, those with aggravated reticular streaks and aggravated nodular shadows make up 67.6%; those with widened transverse diameter of right lower pulmonary artery increased from 3 cases in 1972 to 14 cases in 1979; those with right ventricular dilatation from 4 cases to 7 cases.

2. Electrophysiological examination of the heart: Just as in X-ray examination, in spite of remarkable improvement in clinical symptoms, signs of pulmonary hypertension and increase of right ventricular load proceeded steadily. For example, in a report of 41 cases in rural areas from our hospital, 3 year dynamic ECG observations showed considerable changes in frontal axis deviation in QRS and P amplitude and IPIvl in P axis, a 3-5 year dynamic VCG observation on 36 cases in urban areas displayed an increase in incidence of emphysema from 11 cases in 1974 to 15 cases in 1979, and of corpulmonale from 7 cases in 1974 to 11 cases in 1979. In a two year dynamic echocardiographic studies in 18 cases, of 5 cases show with normal findings in 1977, two showed manifestations of pulmonary hypertension one showed manifestation of both pulmonary hypertension and coronary insufficiency, and two showed signs of both cor-pulmonale and coronary insufficiency in 1979.

3. Dynamic examinations of pulmonary functions: In a report from the 1st Military Medical College, a seven year continuous observation on pulmonary ventilation (MMEF and FEV_1) showed a steady drop with time. In a 2-5 year dynamic observation on 62 cases in Amoy (MVV in terms of % of estimated value and FEV_1), overall evaluation of the results point out a definite decline in pulmonary ventilation. It would seem fit to point out that, our pulmonary function tests depend to certain extent on the patients' cooperation and manipulative technics, so that they are not very reliable objective parameters.

4. Bronchofiberscopic examination: In 18 cases under continuous treatment for 7 years in 1st Military Medical College, a check every 3 years displayed a trend towards increase in incidence of mucosal thickening and narrowing of lumen of the bronchi. A self-control biopsy study of 10 cases showed local improvement in 4 cases, aggravation in 5 cases, and indistinct change in 1 case. In their opinion, the submucosal fibrosis which might hinder the improvement in pulmonary function may be the reason why the function tests worsened in spite of symptomatic improvement.

According to the data of Hunan Medical College fewer patients with cor-pulmonale developed from the simple bronchitis than from the asthmatic types; after 7 year treatment, 14.5% were found in the former, while 54.2% were noted in the latter.

The above materials showed that, vigorous measures with the integrative use of both traditional and western medicine cannot put an end to the progress of chronic bronchitis in the later stages of the disease, though the course may be delayed to a certain extent by early treatment. However, Report of Hunan Medical College indicates the remarkable difference of prognosis between the group under persistent systematic treatment (cor-pulmonale in 13%) and the group with interrupted treatment (cor-pulmonale in 26%). Therefore, "persistent treatment and follow-up the patients to the end" will always be the guiding principle in our work for the prevention and treatment of chronic bronchitis. The contradiction between clinical improvement and deterioration of objective parameters needs further investigation. Clinical amelioration and functional improvement are not necessarily correlated with morphological changes. A common experience in clinical practice shows that functions may be improved through excercises. Thus, we enthusiastically recommend the "persistent treatment and follow-up the patients to the end" principle, which may not only alleviate symptoms, preserving or even improving the ability of work, but also retard the progress of disease, prolonging the life span.

IV. Treatment of chronic bronchitis with Chinese traditional medicine

Over 300 Chinese herbs have been explored and studied; over 80 of them are now popularized; chemical structures of the effective components of 180 have been elucidated, and 23 have already been synthesized. Rhododendron simsii (杜鹃), Vitex negundo (牡荆) and some herbs with anticholinergic effects like Radix physochlainae (热参) and Flos daturae (洋金花) were well studied. Among the so-called "rectification drugs", Gonoderma lucidum (灵芝), Acanthopanax senticosus (刺五加), Astragalus membranaceus (黄芪) and some set prescriptions manifest definite therapeutic effects in clinical use.

Chapter III

BRONCHOSCOPY
AND INTENSIVE CARE MEDICINE

III.1.

BRONCHIAL SUCTIONING WITH THE FLEXIBLE BRONCHOSCOPE

BENGT G OLLMAN, CARL-ERIC LINDHOLM, ULF NORDIN

A common problem in postoperative management and in the care of
critically ill patients is the development of pulmonary atelectasis.
The traditional treatment of this condition is physiotherpy, drainage
posture, medication with mucolytic agents and suctioning of the airway with different kinds of catheters.

All manipulations in the airway are apt to cause trauma to the
mucociliary transport system. Great care must therefore be taken as
to the technique used. Lesions of the mucosa will cause retardation
of the mucociliary escalator and new plugs of mucous will form. A.
vicious circle could be created where more suctioning harms more
than it helps.
    A number of catheters of different shape are available on the
market, with special features for effectiveness. By intrabronchial
film-recording in animals and in clinical cases we have studied the
action of some of these catheters and of the flexible bronchoscope,
and how they affect the bronchus and the mucosa.

One catheter has a blunt end and 2 or 3 sideholes. This condition
makes the catheter suitable for suctioning in the trachea and in
larger bronchi, where both holes could be free. In a small bronchus
however occlusion of one hole will cause the other hole to grip the
mucosa and to tear away pieces. Bleeding and scarring will result.
    Another catheter has a curved tip, so that it could be directed
in various directions. If this is done blindly, as it always has
to be, groves and scars are produced in the mucosa. Retardation of
the mucous transport system will result, and mucous plugs will form
in the lesions.
    A third catheter has a protective ring round the open tip. In
spite of this, mucosa will be gripped in the sideholes when the
catheter is introduced in small bronchi. If a tight seal occurs

*J.A. Nakhosteen and W. Maassen (eds.), Bronchology: Research, Diagnostic and
Therapeutic Aspects. All rights reserved.
Copyright 1981. Martinus Nijhoff Publishers bv, The Hague / Boston / London*

when the catheter is introduced in a small bronchus, suctioning
will produce a negative pressure with collaps of the periferal
bronchus. This could lead to formation of a new atelectasis, more
shunting and deterioration of the blood-gas balance.

All catheters have in common that suctioning must be performed
blindly, which means a lot of trial and error when fumbling in the
bronchial tree. The damage will always be widely distributed.

All catheters have in common, that suctioning in the bronchial
tree creates a negative intrabronchial pressure, with the risk of
bronchial collapse and negative effects on respiration.

The Flexible Bronchoscope has the unique ability to guide the
examiner by the eye through the airway directly to the point of
interest, without undue damage to the bronchial wall.

In bronchoscopic treatment of atelectasis, selective suctioning
could be performed in two ways, i.e. either directly through the
instrument channel, or by means of thin catheters introduced under
supervision of the eye through the bronchoscope channel.

With the patient in a respirator a closed system is established
by introducing the bronchoscope through a tight inlet cap. This
creates a Positive End Expiratory Pressure, PEEP, in the region
where the bronchoscope is introduced. This prevents collapse of the
bronchial wall and makes mucous plugs easy to grip with the suction
hole at the end of the bronchoscope. This means effective cleaning
of the bronchus. Periferal, small bronchi should be cleaned with
selective catheters under supervision of the eye, without causing
trauma to the mucosa. These catheters do not grip the mucosa, as
they have no side holes and work under positive pressure.

As long as suctioning through the bronchoscope is performed only
intermittently and only when secretions are presenting in the bronchus
no negative effect on the blood-gas balance has been noted. Resolution
of atelectasis restores PaO_2/$PaCO_2$-balance to normal. X-ray pulmonary
control demonstrates normal aeration of the formerly atelectatic
region.

Summary.

In a comparison between conventional catheters and the flexible
bronchoscope for treatment of pulmonary atelectasis in postoperative
and critically ill patients we have found that using the flexible
bronchoscope is the method of choice.

III.2.

8. THERAPEUTIC BRONCHOSCOPY IN THE OPERATING ROOM AND THE RECOVERY ROOM

J.TAMADA, M.AOKI, Y.SHIMIZU, M.ITO, T.TERAMATSU

Therapeutic bronchofiberscopies have been performed on 56 patients at the department of thoracic surgery of our institute during the last two years. Table 1) gives a breakdown of these bronchofiberscopies. Four of 27 recovery room patients didn't recover, and this was not due to the bronchofiberscopy but their original diseases.

TABLE 1. Therapeutic bronchofiberscopy

(1) In the operating room:total 29 pt.(9.2% of all patients given general anesthesia)
Tracheo-bronchial plasty........................10 pt.
Determining the range of resection.............. 7 pt.
Checking the position of the endotracheal tube.. 4 pt.
Counteracting atelectasis after pneumonectomy... 3 pt.
Checking the bronchi for sputum retainers....... 3 pt.
Aspirating endobronchial blood.................. 1 pt.
Removing a foreign body from a two-year boy...... 1 pt.

(2) In the recovery room:total 27 pt.(9.5% of all recovery room patients)
Counteracting atelectasis............................. 13 pt. (30 times)
Checking sutured lines after tracheo-bronchial plasty.. 5 pt. (7 times)
Aspirating sputa (patients who refused tracheotomy).... 2 pt. (25 times)
Checking the bronchi................................. 2 pt. *(2 times)
*children suspected of having atelectasis
after sterno-turnover for funnel chest

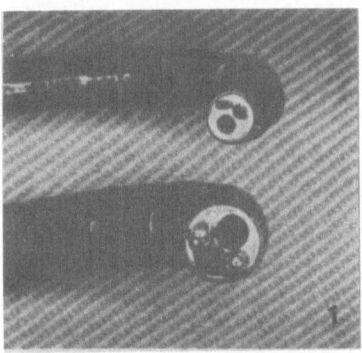
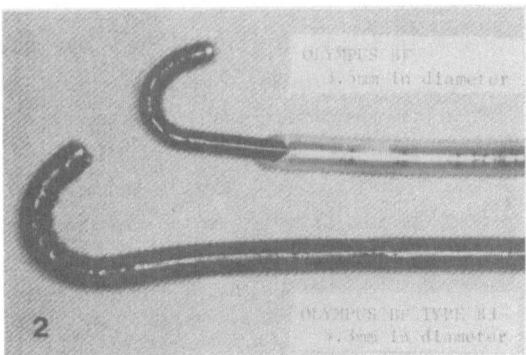

Figure 1) shows the tips of the bronchofiberscopes which we usually use. The lower one is a conventional bronchofiberscope, OLYMPUS BF TYPE B3, whose tip is 5.3mm in diameter. The upper one is a new type of bronchofiberscope, also a product of the OLYMPUS company. It is not on the market as yet. This fiberscope is slender and its tip is 3.5mm in diameter. It has one channel that is open enough to aspirate sputa. And it can be passed through the endotracheal tube which

J.A. Nakhosteen and W. Maassen (eds.), Bronchology: Research, Diagnostic and
Therapeutic Aspects. All rights reserved.
Copyright 1981. Martinus Nijhoff Publishers bv, The Hague / Boston / London

is 4.5mm in inner diameter and mechanical breathing can be done through the space between the scope and the wall of the endotracheal tube. (Figure 2)

In the recovery room, we must often perform bronchofiberscopy alone. In that case we use the attachment shown in Figure 3). It consists of two three-directional cocks and tubes for oxygen supply and wall suction. We can turn the oxygen supply and suction on and off with one hand without interrupting the bronchofiberscope examination. This slender bronchofiberscope is very effective for infants, children and patients who have tracheobronchial stenosis. Even for adult patients without tracheal stenosis, it is advantageous because of the lower resistance of the air way to the bronchofiberscope itself.

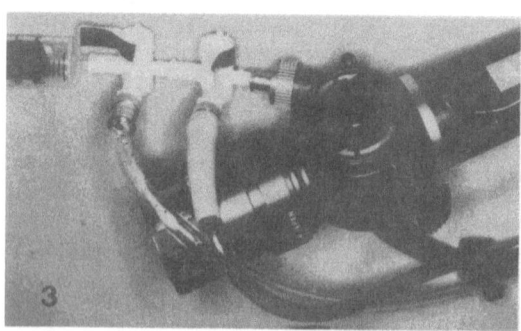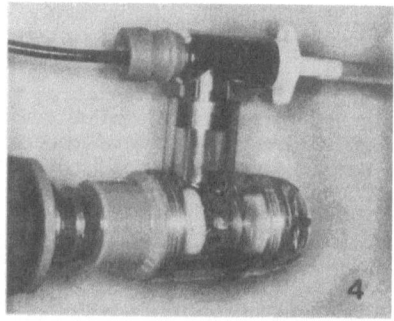

When we perform a bronchoscopy on the patient under mechanical breathing, we use a T-tube not to discontinue breathing. The proximal end of the T-tube is sealed by a rubber cap. (Figure 3)

When performing bronchofiberscopy in the recovery room, direct transnasal insertion of the scope is our first choice, for the following reasons: (1) it is safer and less painful (2) the patient can cough up sputa during the bronchofiberscopy (3) there is no possibility of damage to the fiberscope by biting.

Of cours the direct transnasal insertion of the fiberscope dose result in some bacteria from the surface of the nasal cavity and pharynx being carried into the trachea and bronchi. But the quantities are clinically negligible. Table 2) shows the result of cultures of washings obtained from the surface and the aspiration channel of the bronchofiberscope after direct transnasal insertion.

TABLE 2. Cultures of washings obtained from the surface and the aspiration channel of the bronchofiberscope after direct transnasal insertion

Recovery room patients		Outpatients (diagnostic bronchofiberscopy)	
#1. serratia marcescens	(a few)	#1. klebsiella pneumoniae	(few)
neisseria	(a few)	-hemolytic streptococcus	(few)
klebsiella	(a few)	#2. pseudomonas aeruginosa	(few)
#2. neisseria	(a few)	#3. streptococcus pneumoniae	(few)
escherichia coli	(a few)	#4. klebsiella pneumoniae	(a few)
#3. no growth			

From our experience, bronchofiberscopy is a very useful, easy and safe method to manage the air way of patients in various situations.

III.3.

TRANSBRONCHIAL LUNG BIOPSY FOR DIFFERENTIAL DIAGNOSIS OF ACUTE PULMONARY FAILURE

G. GOECKENJAN, TH. KÖNIGSHAUSEN, W. ELSÄSSER, A. SCHMIDT-GRÄFF

1. INTRODUCTION

Acute pulmonary insufficiency can be caused by numerous lung injuries like different forms of shock, hypoxia, aspiration or toxic agents, and by different inflammatory lung diseases, which often are impossible to differentiate by clinical or radiological examinations. The poor prognosis of these patients may possibly be improved by an early and exact diagnosis followed by an appropriate therapy. During artificial ventilation the application of perthoracic needle biopsy and surgical lung biopsy techniques involves a high risk of complications. Therefore transbronchial lung biopsy could be an alternative in this situation. We report on experiences with the transbronchial lung biopsy in patients who were artificially ventilated.

2. PATIENTS AND METHODS

In 13 adult patients (3 male, 10 female, age 25 to 74 years) suffering from acute respiratory insufficiency and disseminated pulmonary infiltrations a transbronchial lung biopsy was performed as a bedside procedure by means of a fiberoptic bronchoscope. Indication was the diagnosis of pulmonary infiltrations of unknown cause. We used an Olympus BFB2 bronchoscope and a Storz one jaw forceps or an Olympus alligator jaw forceps. Before beginning with the bronchoscopic procedure the inspiratory oxygen concentration was elevated to 100 percent and 0,5 mg Atropine was given intravenously. Fiberoptic bronchoscopy and transbronchial lung biopsy were performed via orotracheal or nasotracheal tube or tracheotomy cannula in an intermittent manner, i.e. artificial ventilation was interrupted for the 15 to 25 second period of bronchoscopy or transbronchial lung biopsy. When necessary local anesthesia was established by endobronchial instillation of 5 to 10 ml of Lidocain 2%. 1 to 3 biopsy specimen were taken under fluoroscopy, in most cases from the periphery of the B8 or B9 segment. 5 - 10 minutes after the end of the procedure a fluoroscopic control was made in order to exclude a pneumothorax. Patients with hemorrhagic diathesis were excluded from transbronchial biopsy.

*J.A. Nakhosteen and W. Maassen (eds.), Bronchology: Research, Diagnostic and
Therapeutic Aspects. All rights reserved.*
Copyright 1981. *Martinus Nijhoff Publishers bv, The Hague / Boston / London*

3. RESULTS AND DISCUSSION

In 11 out of the 13 patients sufficient biopsy material could be obtained in order to establish a diagnosis of the lung disease. In the remaining 2 cases only a bronchial wall was found histologically. In one patient 3 lung biopsies were performed, in the other cases only 1 biopsy. The histological examination disclosed focal pneumonia (n = 2), fibrinous pneumonia (n = 1), interstitial pneumonia (n = 1), slight to moderate alveolar edema (n = 3), alveolar hemorrhage in strongyloidiasis (n = 1), recurrent alveolar hemorrhage probably due to idiopathic pulmonary hemorrhage (n = 1), pulmonary hemorrhage after adrenalectomy for pheochromocytoma (n = 1), interstitial lung fibrosis (n = 1), shock lung with concomitant pneumonia and fibrosis (n = 1). In most cases the biopsy diagnosis contributed to the definite diagnosis. In one patient the lung biopsy revealed only a concomitant interstitial pneumonia in a metastasizing peripheral bronchial carcinoma of the oat cell type as it was subsequently diagnosed. In some cases the histological examination yielded surprising diagnoses. A 29 years old female developed sudden respiratory and circulatory failure 5 weeks after renal transplantation. Because of sanguineous tracheobronchial secretions pulmonary hemorrhage was suspected. The radiograph showed diffuse bilateral pulmonary infiltrations. The histological examination disclosed a pulmonary strongyloidiasis with diffuse pulmonary hemorrhage. The histological section showed a strongyloides stercoralis within the lung tissue. A 38 years old female suffered from respiratory failure subsequent to adrenalectomy for pheochromocytoma. The radiograph disclosed diffuse pulmonary infiltrations. Tentative diagnoses were shock lung or lung edema. Histologically we found an intraalveolar hemorrhage in all biopsy specimen. The pulmonary infiltrations resolved within a few days.

In most cases the histological diagnoses led to therapeutic consequences or were of prognostic value. In a 52 years old male who was admitted because of shock, respiratory failure and renal colic in nephrolithiasis the radiograph showed bilateral pulmonary infiltrations. Lung biopsy disclosed a fibrinous pneumonia and no shock lung which could be suspected considering the patient's history. Additionally Pneumococcus was found in blood culture. The patient responded well to Penicillin G. Especially in respiratory failure due to inflammatory lung changes an early histological determination of the type of pneumonia can be essential for a successful therapy.

In two patients the transbronchial biopsy was followed by a pneumothorax which required pleural drainage for 3 days. A considerable hemorrhage or other complications were not observed. 6 patients have died.

We examined the pulmonary gas exchange before and after the transbronchial biopsy using the ratio of arterial PO_2 to inspiratory oxygen concentration

(P/F ratio). There was no considerable deterioration in this P/F ratio in any case.

4. CONCLUSION

Transbronchial lung biopsy is a useful tool in the diagnosis of dissemina-ted lung processes (1-3). It can also be used in the differentiation of diffuse lung diseases leading to an acute pulmonary insufficiency. It has considerable therapeutic consequences especially in inflammatory lung processes. For exact guidance of the biopsy forceps and early detection of a possible pneumothorax fluoroscopy is necessary. Manifest hemorrhagic diathesis, severely reduced lung compliance and pulmonary hypertension are contraindications of the method. Our preliminary results do not allow a definite assessment of the diagnostic value and the complication risk in this field of indication. Additional experiences are necessary. Because of the possible risks of the method in artificially ventilated patients this procedure should at present be restricted to patients in whom the diagnosis cannot be established otherwise.

REFERENCES
1. Andersen HA, Fontana RS: Transbronchoscopic lung biopsy for diffuse pulmo-nary diseases: Techniques and results in 450 cases. Chest 62:125-128, 1972
2. Levin DC, Wicks AB, Ellis JH Jr: Transbronchial lung biopsy via the fibre-optic bronchoscope. Am Rev Respir Dis 110:4-12, 1974
3. Zavala D: Diagnostic fiberoptic bronchoscopy techniques and results in 600 patients. Chest 68:12-19, 1975

III.4.

DIAGNOSTIC AND THERAPEUTIC VALUE OF THE FIBEROPTIC BRONCHOSCOPIC PROCEDURES
IN THE INTENSIVE CARE UNIT AND THE RECOVERY ROOM

Takayoshi KAHI, M.D. and Shiro HANAWA, M.D.

1. INTRODUCTION

In critically ill patients atelectasis and/or collapse of the lung can be life-
threatening and therefore an early diagnosis and its emergency treatment is often
required. In such circumstances the rigid bronchoscopic procedure is so invasive
for these patients that it is hesitated to perform. The flexible fiberoptic bronch-
scopic procedure is on the other hand much safer to perform even in critically ill
patients with respiratory problems. Since the last year we have tried the fiberoptic bronchoscopy on five critically ill patients over 70 years of age at the
bed-side in our ICU or recovery room with good results and without any significant
complications.

2. MATERIALS AND METHODS

Case 1. A 72 year-old woman was admitted because of deterioration of ischemic
heart disease. She underwent implantation of a cardiac pace-maker because of tri-
fascicular block on July 12, 1979. On the seventh day after implantation a mass
lesion was noticed in the left lower lung field (Fig. 1). With bedside fiberoptic
bronchoscopic procedure a diagnosis of a lung abscess was confirmed.

Case 2. A 78 year-old woman with atrial fibrillation was admitted to our
hospital because of trochanteric fracture of the left femur on July 23, 1979.
She was complaining of productive cough but active postural drainage was difficult
to employ because of traction of the femur. On the sixth day total atelectasis
developed in the left lung (Fig.2). By means of bronchoscopic aspiration of bronchial secretions the atelectasis was significantly improved. Arterial PO_2 improved
rapidly from 72 up to 100 Torr in consequence.

Case 3. An 80 year-old woman with hemoptysis of significant degree was hospitalized to our ICU in poor condition on July 2, 1979. Atelectasis was found in the
upper field of the left lung on the chest x-ray film (Fig. 3). Immediate bronchoscopic procedure at the bed-side disclosed a tumor which obstructed the left upper
lobe bronchus and narrowed the lower bronchus. By a punch biopsy of this tumor
a diagnosis of squamous cell carcinoma was made.

Case 4. An 83 year-old man was admitted to our hospital because of gastric

J.A. Nakhosteen and W. Maassen (eds.), Bronchology: Research, Diagnostic and
Therapeutic Aspects. All rights reserved.
Copyright 1981. Martinus Nijhoff Publishers bv, The Hague / Boston / London

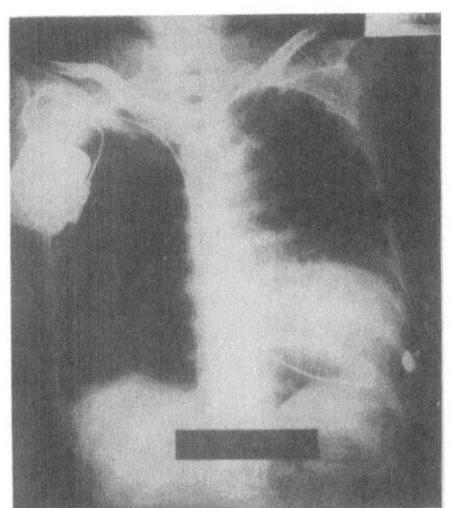

Fig. 1

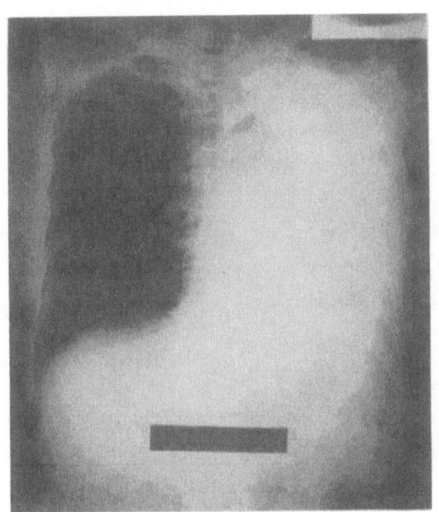

Fig. 2

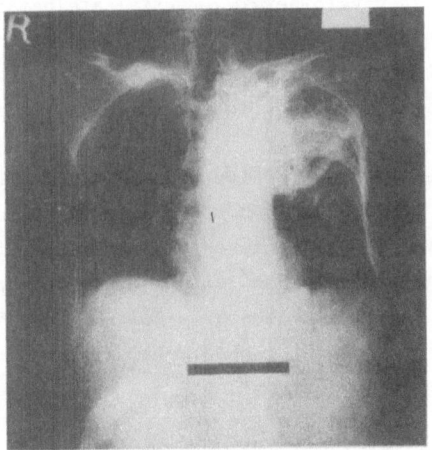
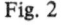

Fig. 3

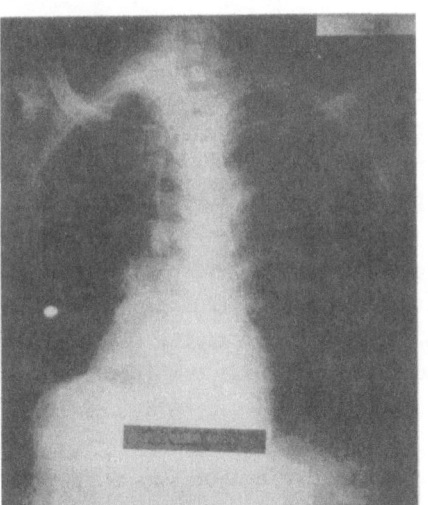

Fig. 4

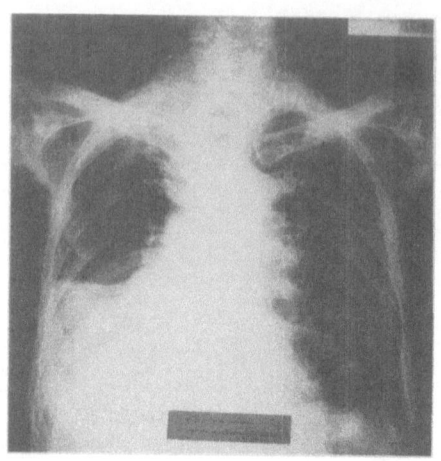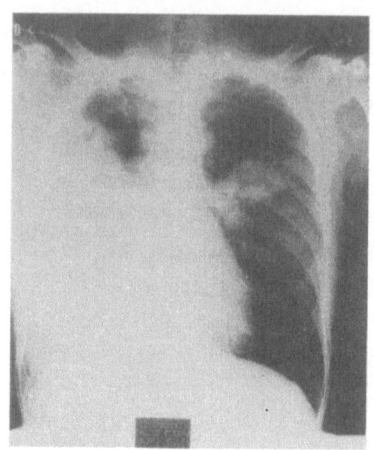

Fig. 5   Fig. 6

bleeding on April 20, 1979. On the third hospital day he underwent an emergency
gastrectomy. In spite of conventional chest physiotherapy, partial atelectasis of
the right lung appeared on the second postoperative day (Fig. 4). The bronchoscopic
drainage in the recovery room allowed satisfactorily the lung to re-expand, although
a band-like atelectasis was remained in the right lower lobe. Arterial PO_2 also
improved from 64 up to 92 Torr.

Case 5. A 95 year-old man was admitted because of dyspnea and difficulty in
expectoration with a temperature of 38 C on July 9, 1979. Atelectasis of the
right middle and lower lobe was superimposed on pneumonia on the third hospital day
(Fig. 5). Vigorous aspiration of tenacious bronchial secretions with fiberoptic
bronchoscope improved the atelectasis efficiently and the arterial PO_2 from 55 up to
70 Torr in consequence. Culture of the secretions disclosed Kebsiella pneumoniae.

Technique of the bedside fiberoptic bronchoscopy. All of the patients are
given oxygen via a nasal catheter before, during and after the procedure. After
premedication with atropine, a four percent solution of lidocaine is sprayed into
the mouth and throat with patients in supine position. The Machida FBS 6TLII fiberoptic bronchoscope is inserted through the mouth into the trachea without the use of
an endotracheal tube. If severe cough was complained of, the same solution is
instilled percutaneously into the trachea prior to insertion of the bronchoscope.
We prefer the transoral approach to the transnasal one, because the nostril of the
Japanese is relatively small. After an initial observation of the tracheobronchial
tree, bronchial secretions and plugs are vigorously aspirated. Repeated lavage of

the involved bronchi with physiologic saline solution is very helpful to aspirate
tenacious secretions. If necessary for diagnosis, bronchial brushings and biopsies
or transbronchial lung biopsies are performed simultaneously. After this methods
we have performed fiberoptic bronchoscopic procedures at the bed-side in the ICU and
recovery room in such critically ill patients over 70 years of age as just presented
and in other ten patients under 70 years of age. Seven of the latter ten patients
underwent bronchoscopic procedures because of postoperative atelectasis and/ or
collapse of the lung and two-because of atelectasis of the lung secondary to pan-
and retroperitonitis with marked improvement in consequence of efficient aspiration
of bronchial secretions. In one patient with hemoptysis and renal failure and with
extensive consolidation of both lungs (Fig. 6), Goodpasture's syndrome was proved
by transbronchial lung biopsy at the bed-side in the ICU. As far as complications
associated with this procedure, we have experienced no significant problems so far.
The duration of each procedure in our series was 15 minutes.

DISCUSSION

The fiberoptic bronchoscope has firmly established itself nowadays in the
field of pulmonary disease not only as a superb diagnostic instument but also as
a therapeutic one. We routinely adopt fiberoptic bronchoscopic procedure in diagnosis and also in treatment of pulmonary disease. Our experience in this series
indicates that the fiberoptic bronchoscopy is such a safe procedure that it can be
performed on and well tolerated by critically ill patients of advanced age in the
ICU and that it is of great value as bedside diagnostic and therapeutic means in
these patients. We have experienced no significant complications yet. However,
cautions and efforts should be directed at minimizing dangers since such major
complications as cardiac and respiratory arrest, myocardial infarction, major
arrhythmias, pulmonary hemorrhage, pneumothorax etc. have been described (1,2,3).
As the fiberoptic bronchoscopic procedure is knwon to cause hypoxemia (4), administration of supplemental oxygen via a nasal catheter and approach without endotracheal
intubation are recommended when patients are seriously ill and/or of advanced age.

REFERENCES

1. Credle WF Jr, Smiddy JF, Elliott RC: Complications of fiberoptic bronchoscopy.
   Am Rev Resp Dis 109: 67,1974
2. Suratt PM, Smiddy JF, Gruber B: Deaths and complications associated with
   Fiberoptic bronchoscopy. Chest 69: 747, 1976
3. Lindhol CE, Ollman B, Snyder JV et al: Cardiorespiratory effects of flexible
   fiberoptic bronchoscopy in critically ill patients. Chest 74: 4, 1978
4. Albertini RE, Harrell JH, Kurihara N, et al: Arterial hypoxemia induced by
   fiberoptic bronchoscopy. JAMA 230: 1666, 1974

A CASE OF SEVERE AIRWAY BURN SUCCESSFULLY TREATED WITH THE FIBEROPTIC
BRONCHOSCOPE
III.5.
Kenkichi Oho, Issei Iimura, Norihiko Kawate

Burns of the airways and lungs were first described in 1943[1]
Despite the high mortality rate, reports on the subject have been few.
Recently we experienced a case of severe airway burn which was diagnos-
ed and successfully treated mainly by fiberoptic bronchoscopy.

The 18 year-old male, who had attempted suicide by igniting inhaled paint thinner, was admitted to Tokyo Medical College Hospital 17
hours after the event. The findings on admission are as shown in Table
1. Fiberoptic bronchoscopy was performed 1 hour after admission, a
diagnosis of airway burn was made, and tracheotomy performed. He was
then placed in a 10 lit/min O_2 tent with a 3 lit/min O2 mask. The
blood gas findings breathing room air are shown in Fig. 1. He was completely weaned from oxygen on day 11.

The fiberoptic bronchoscopy findings on day 2 are shown in Figs 2-
5. Findings varied according to site. Detachment of necrosis and
bleeding was seen on day 3, (Fig.6). Detachment of scabs and viscous
secretions caused respiratory distress and cyanosis, mainly on days 5-6.
Bronchial toilet was performed repeatedly and some large scabs obtained,
(Fig. 12). Gradual healing was seen (Fig. 13) and on day 18 (Fig. 9)
some granulomatous growths were recognized which on day 69 (Fig. 10)
were observed to have developed as pedunculated polyps. They were extirpated by biopsy forceps.

Findings in cases of severe airway burns vary greatly according to
site and post burn period[2] This case showed the importance of the removal of scabs and viscous secretions, especially on days 5-6, and suggests that repeated bronchial toilet performed with the fiberoptic
bronchoscope is the therapeutic method of choice in such cases.

REFERENCES
1. Mallory TB, Brickley WJ: Pathology: With special reference to the
    pulmonary lesions. Ann. Surg., 117: 865, 1943.
2. Oho K, Amemiya R: Practical Fiberoptic Bronchoscopy, Tokyo, Igaku
    Shoin, 1980.

J.A. Nakhosteen and W. Maassen (eds.), Bronchology: Research, Diagnostic and
Therapeutic Aspects. All rights reserved.
Copyright 1981. Martinus Nijhoff Publishers bv, The Hague / Boston / London

96

FINDINGS ON ADMISSION

BURNS : Superficial second degree, face, back of hands, knuckles, fingers
FACE : Charred
EDEMA : Lips, oral and nasal membranes
CONSCIOUSNESS : Clear
RESPIRATION : 40/min
PULSE : 120/min
B.P. : 150/100mm Hg
AUSCULTATION : Wet rales, both lungs, especially upper portions
X-RAY : Slightly infiltrative shadow, extending like branches

Table 1

Changes in blood gas findings in room air.

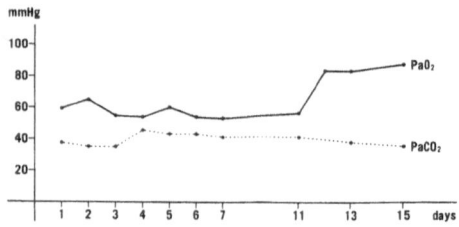

Fig. 1

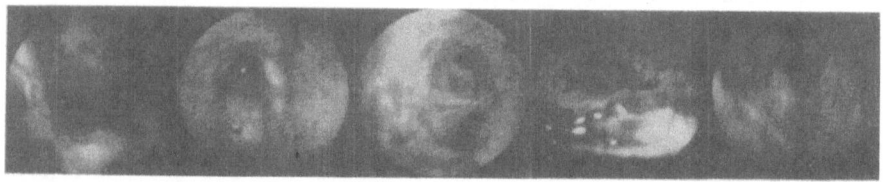

Fig. 2   Fig. 3   Fig. 4   Fig. 5   Fig. 6

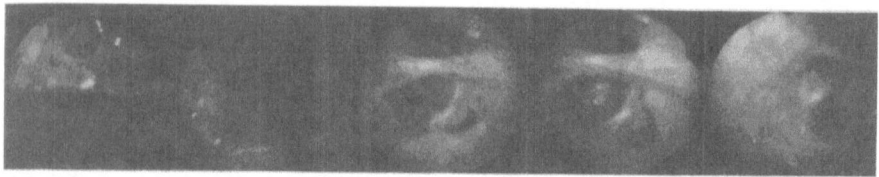

Fig. 7   Fig. 8   Fig. 9   Fig. 10   Fig. 11

Figs. 2-5, Day 2; Fig. 6, Day 3; Figs. 7,8; Fig. 9, Day 18, Fig. 10, Day 69; Fig. 11, 18 months.

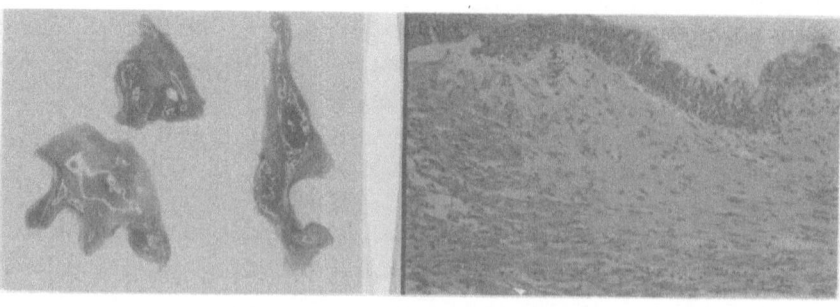

Fig. 12   Bronchial scabs obtained on day 5.

Fig. 13   Histology obtained on day 18.

III.6.

BRONCHOSKOPIE-INTUBATION

R. Schindl, K. Aigner, J. Würz

EINLEITUNG

Die Intubation der Trachea ist zwar nicht unbedingt zwingende Voraus-
setzung für eine Freihaltung der oberen Luftwege und für eine Beatmung, wohl
aber hierfür eine ideale Garantie und gängige Methode. Sie ist aber eine Kon-
dition, wenn eine apparative Beatmung zur Verbesserung bzw. Normalisierung
einer bedrohlich reduzierten alveolären Ventilation indiziert ist. Die spe-
zielle Indikation und Methode der Intubation ist bekannt und vom interdiszi-
plinären Routinebetrieb insbesonders aber aus dem Bereich der Anaesthesie
nicht mehr wegzudenken.

Die zunächst gelegene, weniger frequente Nutzanwendung genießt die Intubation wohl im Bereich der Pneumologie zur Beherrschung einer respirato-
rischen Insuffizienz im Zusammenhang mit einer apparativen Beatmung bedingt
durch bronchiale überwiegend obstruktive, asthmatische- oder parenchymatöse
akute entzündliche Lungenerkrankungen bei entsprechender Vorschädigung oder
einem beacht-lichem Ausmaß.

Es gibt nun Situationen und Gründe, die trotz grundsätzlicher Kenntnis
und einwandfreier Beherrschung der Intubationstechnik über die Möglichkeiten
der blinden oder mehr noch jene mit dem konventionellen Larynxspekulum hinaus,
eine Kombination mit der Bronchoskopie bei folgender Methode nahe legen.

METHODE

Von einem üblichen Trachealtubus wird das Ansatz- bzw. Verbindungsstück
entfernt. Das gesamte Tubuslumen steht nun uneingeengt für die Einführung
eines Kinderbronchoskoprohres mit beschickter Geradeausblickoptik zur Verfügung, begünstigt durch Spray oder Gleitmittel. Gleichermassen ist natürlich
auch ein flexibles Bronchoskop oder eine Geradeausblickoptik alleine, sofern
instrumentell zuträglich, geeignet. Der so mit Rohr und Optik bewehrte Tubus
ermöglicht eine optisch kontrollierte optimale Lagerung mit gleichzeitiger
laufender Exploration.

MOTIVATION

Im nicht anaesthesiologischen Bereich liegt sicher eine weit geringere Routineerfahrung mit der alleinigen Intubation vor. Sie fehlt beispielsweise im pneumologischen Alltag. Aber auch für den Geübten gilt es gelegentlich technisch schwierige, extreme Intubations-Situationen patientenseits. Hierzu kommt vielfach ein Zeitzwang, eine rasche, dringliche Oxygenisierung zu erreichen ohne technische zusätzliche Komplikation. Traumatisch oder neoplastisch, auch degenerativ alterierte Veränderungen der Halswirbelsäule mit behindernder Lagerung, Überstreckung, Anomalien, pathologische Befunde im Bereich der oberen Luftwege, der Stimmbänder, der Verdacht auf derartig zu erwartende Probleme, die eine sorgsame Exploration mit optik-bewehrten Tubus, eine Abweichung von der konvention-llen Vorgangsweise dringlich nahelegen. Die gleiche Vorgangsweise bietet sich aber auch bei bereits liegendem Tubus an zu Klärung der oberen Luftwegsverhältnisse, zur Vermeidung weiterer methodischer Traumatisierung, zur Kontrolle der Bronchialtoilette, isoliert, differenziert, ostiumweise.

ZUSAMMENFASSUNG

Die Erfahrungen der Kombination der Methode der Intubation und der Bronchoskopie in unserem pneumologischen Bereich weisen zwar keine hohen Frequenzen auf. Bei Berücksichtigung der Motivation dieser Vorgangsweise scheinen uns aber die vorhandenen Erfahrungen so günstig, daß sie uns zur Weitergabe als nicht selten sehr konvenierendes konfortables Detail in bedrohlicher Situation und unter Zeitzwang als sinnvolle Vorgangsweise gerechtfertigt erscheint als vereinfachte, optisch gesicherte, insgesamte optimierte Alternative, eine Hilfestellungs-Modifikation.

Chapter IV

COMPLICATIONS IN BRONCHOLOGICAL
INVESTIGATIONS

IV.1. COMPLICATIONS IN BRONCHOLOGICAL INVESTIGATIONS USING A
BRONCHOFIBERSCOPE: RESULTS OF 9,413 PROCEDURES

H.C. KO,   R.P. PERNG,   Y.C. HSIEH,   W.C. HUANG and K.T. LUH

1. INTRODUCTION:

It is an established fact, that the incidence of complication
employing flexible bronchofiberscope is much less than that of the
rigid type. The complications that were encountered before, during
and after bronchofiberscopy were: (1) toxic reaction due to anesthetics, (2) bleeding due to biopsy, (3) laryngospasm and bronchospasm,
(4) fever after examination, (5) pneumothorax caused by transbronchial
biopsy, (6) cardiac arrest, etc.

2. MATERIALS AND METHODS:

From Aug. 1970 to Jan. 1980, a total of 9,413 bronchofiberscopic
examinations were performed in Taipei five major teaching hospitals,
namely: Taipei Municipal Jen-Ai Hospital, Veteran's General Hospital,
National Taiwan University Hospital, Triservice General Hospital and
Mackay Memorial Hospital.

Spray technique using 4% xylocaine is universally used in Taipei,
but 3 different entry routes were employed with or without intratracheal tube via nasal or oral cavity. For premedication atropin sulphate
and meperidin HCl (demerol) were the most common drugs administrated
except National Taiwan University Hospital, which used hyoscine butyl-
bromide (buscopan) only.

3. RESULT:

There were in total 57 complications that were encountered before,
during or after bronchofiberscopic examinations, including four fatal
cases. The most common complication was bleeding caused by biopsy,
which were mostly controlled by continuous suction to keep the air way
patent. The relationship between entry route and complication is shown
in Table. No actual relationship between entry routes, neither from
anesthetic toxic reaction nor bleeding due to biopsy, could be detected.
Actually, drug allergy or over dose was the main cause for anesthetic

J.A. Nakhosteen and W. Maassen (eds.), Bronchology: Research, Diagnostic and
Therapeutic Aspects. All rights reserved.
Copyright 1981. Martinus Nijhoff Publishers bv, The Hague / Boston / London

toxic reaction.

Laryngospasm developed in 2 obese and short neck patients and in a nervous young woman were seen during oral intubation of tracheal tube. Bronchospasm was encountered in a bronchial asthma patient in the direct oral entry technique.

In the intubation group, no remarkable vocal cord injury were reported except for occasional sore throat. Bleeding due to biopsy was controlled easily and safely through intratracheal tube.

Toxic anesthetic reaction symptoms were usually mild, such as tremor, weakness, mental confusion, incoherence of speech, sleepiness and laughing etc. This seems to be due to drug allergy or over dose, the symptoms subsided easily by using oxygen inhalation, keeping the air way patent, injection of diazepan or rest only.

Representative cases of massive bleeding due to biopsy are: 2 cases, died because of massive bleeding after biopsy, were aortic aneurysm which mimicked left hilar cancer by roentgenology, broncho-scopic examination revealed bleeding in the left main bronchus. A uremic pneumonia case required pneumonectomy due to continuous bleed-ing that did not stop for a day after brushing. And a case of foreign body granuloma bleeded profusely for two days after removal of the foreign body. Three cases of protruded intraluminal cancer developed bloody sputum for 2-3 days after biopsy. Those bleeding cases that surgical procedure were not required were put for observation for 10-20 minutes and were treated by suction to keep the air way open. No bleeding tendency were noted in the above cases.

Mild fever were observed in all 6 cases that insertion of fiber-scope was applied by direct oral entry route without tracheal tube, the fever subsided 2-3 days later after antibiotic were administrated.

The other 2 fatal complications were a case of cardiac arrest and pneumothorax respectively. The cardiac arrest case could be avoided if the endoscopist paid more attention to the patient's general condition, comprehended fully his poor lung function and heart condition. It was a case of massive left pleural effusion due to cancer complicated with mild heart failure, his EKG showed myocardial ischemia, the patient died inspite of every measurements taken.

The other was a case of acute myelogenous leukemia with leukemic infiltration in both lungs, pneumothorax developed after transbronchial biopsy, he expired inspite of intercostal drainage that was performed with other resque procedures. This was the result of an over eager or aggressive endoscopist who performed the examination on a poor general condition examinee.

4. CONCLUSION:

A total of 9,413 bronchofiberscopic examinations were performed since Aug. 1970 to Jan. 1980 in Taipei 5 major teaching hospitals. There are various entry routes, however each route has its advantage and disadvantage.

The ways of preventing complications are mapped out as follow: (1) The most common complication was bleeding caused by biopsy, which was controllable by continuous suction to keep the air way free. Here the tracheal tube played an important role for repeated insertion and proved to be more superior than other entry method. (2) Laryngospasm may occur by using intubation of tracheal tube in obese and short neck patient or in nervous young women. So that other entry route methods are more recommendable for such cases. (3) Although fever incidence was low, it could be avoided by careful suctioning of intrabronchial secretion before termination of examination, and here again, the usage of tracheal tube showed its benefit. (4) The causative toxic anesthetic reaction were drug allergy or over dose, hence it is very wise to keep the dosage at the minimal as possible. (5) 2 fatal aortic aneurysm which mimicked left hilar lung cancer roentgenology may be avoided if the patient was well studied before bronchofiberscopic examination. (6) In other respect, we also may avoid serious major complications by strict case selection, well performed and studied lung and cardiac function and patient's general condition before the examination being performed, and lastly, a well equipped endoscopic room including well selected emergency rescue facilities is obligatory.

Table Relationship between Entry Route and Complication

	Oral		Nasal	Total
	Tracheal tube	Direct		
1. Toxic reaction due to anesthetic	1	7	1	9
2. Bleeding due to biopsy				
Controllable	8	13	10	31
Un-controllable	0	3	0	3
3. Laryngospasm, bronchospasm	3	1	0	4
4. Fever investigation	0	6	0	6
5. Pneumothorax due to biopsy	0	1	0	1
6. Cardiac arrest	1	0	0	1
7. Dislocation of jaw	0	2	0	2
Total	13	33	11	57

IV.2.

PREVALENCE AND TREATMENT OF COMPLICATIONS OF 550 FIBERBRONCHOSCOPIES

E. Hershko, N. Reichert and G. L. Baum

In the last 5 years, 550 fiberbronchoscopies have been performed by the Pulmonary Division of the Chaim Sheba Medical Center. The age of the patients ranged between 16 and 85 years. Except for one case, all bronchoscopies were performed transnasally.

The complications observed secondary to the procedure are noted below.

- 12 cases of hemoptysis (2.18%). Of these three were of major importance. Two of them were treated successfully by instillation of epinephrine solution 1/20,000 while one case ended fatally and is described in detail below. The remaining episodes of hemoptysis (9 cases), terminated spontaneously.

- Transbronchial biopsy was complicated by pneumothorax in 3 cases of the 36 cases in which the procedure was performed (8.6%). Only one case required tube drainage.

- Pneumonia occurred post bronchoscopy in 2 cases (0.36%), the causative organism being Pseudomonas aeruginosa. Both cases were successfully treated by appropriate antibiotics. Subsequent to the appearance of these two cases gas sterilization was adopted. Among the 200 bronchoscopies done since the changeover, no post-procedure pneumonia has been observed.

- Bronchospasm developed in two cases of chronic obstructive lung disease imme-diately after the end of the procedure (0.36%). Both cases responded promptly to inhalation of bronchodilator.

- Laryngospasm complicated bronchoscopy in 5 cases (0.9%). One case was treated successfully by steroids intravenously. Another patient was intubated for 24 hours. The rest of the cases recovered spontaneously with continued oxygen therapy transnasally.

- Myocardial ischemia developed in one case (0.18%) associated with transient S-T wave changes in the electrocardiogram. The patient was hospitalized for observation and subsequently had a normal electrocardiogram and no symptoms.

J.A. Nakhosteen and W. Maassen (eds.), Bronchology: Research, Diagnostic and Therapeutic Aspects. All rights reserved.
Copyright 1981. Martinus Nijhoff Publishers bv, The Hague / Boston / London

–   Cardiac arrhythmias were observed in 4 cases (0.73%). Monitoring of cardiac rhythm was done only in patients over 65 years of age and in patients with known cardiac abnormalities. The arrhythmias observed were ventricular premature beats controlled by lidocaine administered intravenously. Sinus tachycardia of 140 to 150 beats per minute developed transiently in 12 cases and disappeared at the end of the procedure.

–   Urinary retention secondary to premedication with morphine and atropine developed in a 75 year old male suffering from prostatic hypertrophy (0.18%). Single catheterization of the urinary bladder resolved the situation.

This experience with complications is essentially similar to that reported in the world literature and the treatment used is standard by comparison to other centers that have reported.

The one fatal case manifested exceptional features. A 54 year old male was first seen with a superior vena cava syndrome associated with pneumonia and a putrid abscess in the right upper lobe. No hemoptysis occurred prior to bronchoscopy. During the procedure a 5 millimeter rose colored tumor protruded into the lumen of the right upper lobe bronchus. Subsequent diagnosis of carcinoma was made. Biopsy and brushing were performed uneventfully and the patient was returned to his ward without any signs of hemoptysis. 3 hours post-bronchoscopy the patient developed slight hemoptysis which progressed into severe bleeding 14 hours post-bronchoscopy. This stopped and the patient remained stable until a massive fatal hemoptysis occurred 36 hours later. Bleeding indices examined prior to the procedure were normal. On post-mortem examination the source of the bleeding could not be identified.

The time interval between the procedure and the development of the hemoptysis indicts the bronchoscopy as the cause of the bleeding. On the other hand, however, all reported cases of fatal hemoptysis that we found in the literature developed during the procedure. Experience in this case suggests that all cases should be observed for 5 to 6 hours after the bronchoscopy and all cases of even slight hemoptysis should be hospitalized for at least 24 hours observation.

In order to minimize the complications of fiberbronchoscopy we suggest the following precautions:

1.   Have a rigid bronchoscope available, especially for bleeding requiring local treatment and have a solution of epinephrine 1/20,000 available at all times.

2. Use an effective sterilization procedure. We prefer gas sterilization. It is imperative to monitor the effectiveness of the sterilization procedures by frequent cultures of the instruments used including all forceps and suction apparatus that enter the patient's upper airways.

3. In older patients, in cases of chronic obstructive lung disease and in asthmatics, give an inhalation of bronchodilator medication immediately prior to the procedure.

4. In severely disabled patients perform bronchoscopies only for clearly indicated reasons... and then think twice!

5. Use effective doses of premedication including atropine.

6. Perform a painstaking topical anesthetic making sure that the vocal cords are well anesthetized. Be careful, however, to use the minimum dose of agent that is compatible. We use a 2.0% solution of esracaine and only for the vocal cords do we use a 4.0% solution.

7. All cases should be given oxygen, by nasal catheter, 4 to 5 liters per minute, during the procedure and for a brief period after.

8. As in all procedures, there should be available equipment and medications to do emergency cardiopulmonary resuscitation.

9. Prepare the patient psychologically by informing him and otherwise allaying his fears as much as possible. This will also give the operator greater likelihood of having a cooperative patient.

10. There should be a recent chest x ray on all patients taken within a day or so before the procedure and a post-operative x ray should be done on all patients who have transbronchial biopsy done. This should be taken within an hour or so after the procedure is completed. Any biopsy procedure after which the patient is uncomfortable or appears uneasy is an indication for a chest x ray.

11. Record preoperative pulse and blood pressure and record the quantity of all medication used including anesthetic.

IV.3.

COMPLICATIONS FOLLOWING FIBEROPTIC BRONCHOSCOPY

Akira KOYAMA and Hiroshi ANNO,

Flexible fiberbronchoscopy has been well evaluated for diagnosis of pulmonary diseases and a few occurrences of complication following the performance is reported. Complications following flexible fiberbronchoscopy in our hospital were reviewed and the treatment and prevention for the complications were studied.

MATERIALS AND METHODS

The kinds and frequencies of complications in 1625 cases on whom flexible fiberbronchoscopy was done during the period of last 5 years were subjected. Among these cases, transbronchial brushing was applied on 117 cases, transbronchial forceps biopsy on 425 cases and both these procedures on 353 cases.

0.5mg/kg of Pentazocin and 0.01mg/kg of atropine sulfate were given half an hour before anesthesia. 5 to 10ml of 4% Lidocain were sprayed for local anesthesia. Flexible fiberbronchoscope is inserted through tracheal tube which was inserted transorally in almost all cases. Several amount of 4% Lidocain is infused for local anesthesia of the bronchus, if necessary. ECG monitoring was applied throughout the examination and transbronchial biopsy was carried out watching biplane X-ray television.

RESULTS

Complications were classified into 4 groups as follows:
1) Complications related to premedication or topical anesthesia.
2) Complications during the bronchoscopic procedure.
3) Complications resulting from transbronchial biopsy.
4) Postbronchoscopic complications.

Complications were classified into two grades. Minor complications were defined as those which was considered to be reversible without resuscitation technique. Major complications were those which was serious and needed special treatment.

Complication related to premedication or topical anesthesia included each one case of hypotension, excitement and wheezing. Symptoms of these 3 cases were mild and bronchoscopic examination could be continued after short time inhalation of oxygen. One case of eruption was also mild and examination was not disturbed.

J.A. Nakhosteen and W. Maassen (eds.), Bronchology: Research, Diagnostic and
Therapeutic Aspects. All rights reserved.
Copyright 1981. Martinus Nijhoff Publishers bv, The Hague / Boston / London

Complications during bronchoscopic procedure were observed in 11 cases. 10 cases out of 11 had minor complication. They included 5 cases of cyanosis, 2 cases of syncope, 2 cases of ST depression with negative T on ECG, and one case of hypotension. One case with major complication was 70 year-old male who had bronchiectasis with hemoptysis. He lost consciousness during bronchoscopic procedure. He recovered after several minutes by assisted respiration.

Complications directly resulting from transbronchial biopsy were hemorrhage and pneumothorax. Small amount of hemorrhage was unavoidable from transbronchial biopsy. Moderate amount of hemorrhage was observed in 31 cases, or 3.6%. Large amount of hemorrhage more than 50ml occurred in 2 cases, or 0.2%. Basic diseases of hemorrhagic cases were consisted of 22 cases of lung cancer, 8 cases of pulmonary tuberculosis and 3 cases of the other pulmonary diseases. Large amount of hemorrhage was occurred in 2 cases with peripheral type of lung cancer. By these cases, rigid type bronchoscope with light guide of glass fiber and with cuff was inserted into the another side of the main bronchus to maintain air way. The bronchoscope was pulled up to trachea after disappearance of cyanosis and suction of the blood was repeated. Bleeding gradually stopped.

Pneumothorax was followed in one case after transbronchial biopsy, but the grade was mild and the lung expanded without drainage.

Cyanosis and hypotension were found respectively in one case as a postbronchoscopic complication. These symptoms get off within a few hours by oxygen inhalation. Though there were a few cases with postbronchoscopic fever, they were mild and transient. No case of postbronchoscopic atelectasis and pneumonia was experienced.

DISCUSSION

Summing up the above presented results (Table 1), complications of flexible fiberbronchoscopy occurred in 51 cases out of 1625 during last 5 years in our hospital. This figure corresponds to around 3.14% of the total performances.

TABLE 1. Complications of flexible fiberbronchoscopy

Complications	Minor	Major	Mortality
1) Premedication or topical anesthesia	4	0	0
2) Bronchoscopic procedure	10	1	0
3) Transbronchial biopsy	32	2	0
4) Postbronchoscopic	2	0	0
Total	48(2.95%)	3(0.18%)	0(0%)
	51(3.14%)		

48 cases, 2.95%, had minor complications and 3 cases, 0.18%, had major complications. We had no mortal case. Complications in 34 cases, around 2/3rd, were related to transbronchial biopsy.

According to the references, major complications had been occurred in 0.08% to 1.5% and mortality were 0.01 to 0.1% of the total performances. Complications due to premedication or topical anesthesia were high in rate and laryngo- or bronchospasm during bronchoscopy were not few in the report collected by Credle. These complications will be avoidable by adequate anesthesia and tracheal intubation before bronchoscopy. Monitoring of ECG, blood pressure and arterial blood gas were very important for aged or pulmonary hypofunction cases because of high appearance rate of hypoventilation or hypoxia. Bronchoscopy under oxygen inhalation is also required in some cases.

Occurrence of hemorrhage related to transbronchial biopsy was around 1 to 9%, pneumothorax 1 to 6% and mortality 0 to 0.2% in the references. Pneumothorax is not a life threatening for the patient, because it is relatively easy to control. Hemorrhage was the most frequent cause of death in the study of Suratt. Our two cases with large amount of hemorrhage were successfully treated by rigid broncho- scope with light guide of glass fiber and with cuff. But transbronchial biopsy for patient with hemorrhagic tendency seems to be contraindication as Zavala reported.

Death case caused by sepsis after transbronchial biopsy was reported by Robbins. In our experiences there were a few cases with postbronchoscopic fever, but they were mild and transient. This might be due to the transoral insertion of broncho- scope through tracheal tube.

CONCLUSION

Diagnostic value of flexible fiberbronchoscopy for pulmonary diseases will be increased when complication related to bronchoscopy is prevented by careful prebron- choscopic examination, adequate premedication and anesthesia, monitoring of general condition and timely oxygen inhalation and other treatment through tracheal tube.

REFERENCES
1. Credle, WF et al: Complications of fiberoptic bronchoscopy. Amer. Rev. Resp. Dis., 109, 67-72, 1974.
2. Pereira, W. et al: A prospective cooperative study of complications following flexible fiberoptic bronchoscopy. Chest, 73, 813-816, 1978.
3. Zavala, DC: Pulmonary hemorrhage in fiberoptic transbronchial biopsy. Chest, 70, 584-588, 1976.
4. Suratt, PM: Deaths and complications associated with transbronchial lung biopsy. Amer. Rev. Resp. Dis., 115, 708-711, 1977.
5. Robbins,H. et al: Failure of a prophylactic antimicrobial drug to prevent sepsis after fiberoptic bronchoscopy. Amer. Rev. Resp. Dis., 116, 325-326, 1977.

IV.4.

A NEW METHOD FOR TREATMENT OF BRONCHIAL AND LUNG BLEEDING

H.SCHLEHE*, H.-M.FRITSCHE**, S.DAUM*

1. INTRODUCTION

Several methods have been described to control endobronchial hemorrhage during bronchoscopic examination and pulmonary hemorrhage after transbronchial lung biopsy. Hemorrhage could be controlled by ice-cold saline (2) or instillation of epinephrine solution. If severe bleeding occurs, the tip of the fiberoptic bronchoscope (4) or a Fogarty balloon catheter inserted through the suction channel of the fiberscope (1) can tamponade the bleeding bronchus.

A modification of the techniques occluding a bronchus is presented here.

2. CASE REPORT

A 47 year old man was admitted to our hospital because of hemoptysis lasting for several weeks. The hematocrit was 27%, the hemoglobin 8,5g%. Two years previously a malignant melanoma was removed from the left axilla. - A radiograph of the chest at the entry in frontal projection disclosed nodular thickening, in lateral projection an area of parenchymal density was suggestive of atelectasis extending over the middle lobe.

Bronchoscopic examination revealed an intrabronchial metastasis of the melanoma with continuous hemorrhage from the tumor in the medial segment bronchus of the middle lobe (fig. 1).

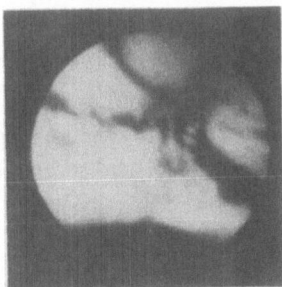

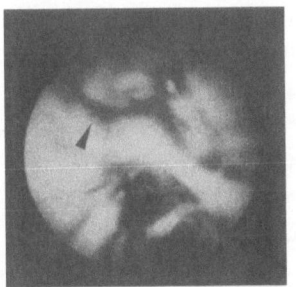

FIGURE 1. View of the bleeding middle lobe bronchus.

FIGURE 2. Fibrin clot occluding the middle lobe bronchus.

J.A. Nakhosteen and W. Maassen (eds.), Bronchology: Research, Diagnostic and Therapeutic Aspects. All rights reserved.
Copyright 1981. Martinus Nijhoff Publishers bv, The Hague / Boston / London

As endobronchial hemorrhage could neither be managed by iced saline solution nor by application of epinephrine solution, three days later a catheter was inserted through the fiberscope channel into the appropiate bronchus in order to perform an occlusion of the bronchus by a fibrin adhesion technique. Fibrin adhesion is prepared with homogenous high concentrated fibrinogen solution, clotted by a fibrinolytic inhibitor containing thrombin solution. After the injection of the fibrin glue, delivered freezed by IMMUNO Comp. Heidelberg, FRG, a solution of aprotinin - trans-AMCHA - $CaCl_2$ - thrombin was added (fig. 3).

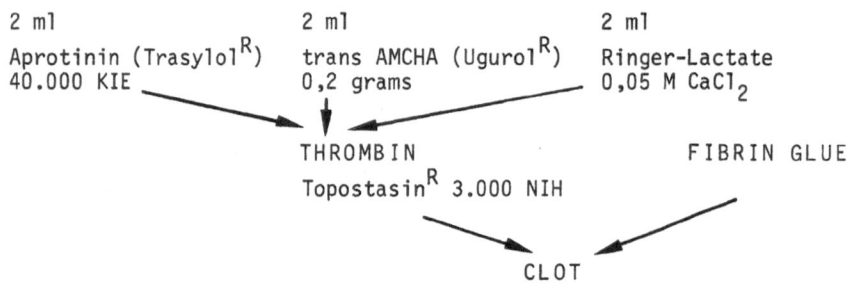

FIGURE 3.   Scheme of fibrin adhesion.

Within a few seconds the clot developed and the middle lobe bronchus was occluded (fig. 2). The bleeding was treated effectively, a third bronchoscopic examination performed two days later showed that there was still evidence of tamponade of the middle lobe bronchus resulting in a complete atelectasis of the middle lobe on X-ray films of the chest.

On the next day the clot was expectorated spontaneously, the patient did no longer suffer from hemoptysis. Another radiograph of the chest, six days later, revealed decrease of atelectasis.

3. DISCUSSION

Fibrin adhesion is a new technique for sealing bleeding areas and adapting tissue (3). It assessed its value in traumatology, vascular surgery, reconstructive surgery, oto-rhino-laryngology, dental medicine and - in our field - in transient occlusion of an airway.

Until now two patients with persistent bleeding from endobronchial tumors and one patient with severe bleeding from segmental pneumonia were successfully treated with this method. The clot was removed by expectoration or by a forceps through fiberoptic bronchoscope.

IV.5.

COMPLICATIONS FOLLOWING FLEXIBLE BRONCHOFIBERSCOPY ─── PREVENTION AND TREATMENT
OF ENDOBRONCHIAL BLEEDING AFTER BIOPSY

M. KANEKO, J. HONDA, K. SOHMA, T. TAKAHASHI, N. YAMAMOTO, H. YOSHIMURA,

T. MATSUBAYASHI, R. ONO, and S. IKEDA, JAPAN

1. INTRODUCTION

Complications subsequent to flexible bronchofiberscopy are as follows:

1. Dyspnea caused by narrowed air passage;

2. Pneumoria caused by an unsanitary flexible bronchofiberscope;

3. Intoxication due to lidocaine;

4. Pulmonary hemorrhage secondary to biopsy, curettage and brushing, and

5. Pneumothorax caused by transbronchial lung biopsy.

Among these complications, pulmonary hemorrhage secondary to biopsy or curettage
is the most frequent. A little bleeding always occurs after intrabronchial or transbronchial biopsies or curettage of peripheral lesions. Controlled minimum hemorrhage
does not interfere with further biopsies, so that many biopsy specimens can be obtained, the examination time is shortened and the patient is more comfortable. On
the other hand, if mild or gross pulmonary hemorrhage occurs, another biopsy cannot
be performed. Thus, it is necessary to prevent these types of hemorrhage following
biopsy.

2. MATERIALS AND RESULTS

Diagnostic flexible bronchofiberscope procedures were performed under local
anesthesia on 5,209 cases at the National Cancer Center Hospital during the period
between January 1968 and December 1979 and on 345 cases at Kitasato University Hospital during the period between June 1977 and December 1979.

Between January 1968 and December 1973, the incidence of mild and gross pulmonary bleeding was 2.9%. Between January 1974 and December 1979, however, this figure
dropped to 1.5%.

3. DISCUSSION

It is believed that this marked lowing of incidence was due to the fact that,
during the former period, after smearing and fixing the collected material, another
bronchofiberscope was introduced through the endotracheal tube in order to ascertain

J.A. Nakhosteen and W. Maassen (eds.), Bronchology: Research, Diagnostic and
Therapeutic Aspects. All rights reserved.
Copyright 1981. Martinus Nijhoff Publishers bv, The Hague / Boston / London

whether hemorrhaging had occurred or not. Thus, during the smearing and fixing process, the patient frequently coughed and spouted a lot of blood through the endotracheal tube.

In the latter period, immediately after the biopsy specimen was taken, another doctor introduced another bronchofiberscope. If a little blood was found, it could be aspirated quickly and quietly until the bleeding stopped, thus preventing the spreading blood from irritating the bronchial mucosa. Even if gross hemorrhage did occur, with the use of this method, the endotracheal tube did not spout any blood.

A little blood flowing into the other side of the bronchus irritates the bronchial mucosa and obstructs the air passage, causing a cough. In turn, the cough results in further bleeding. Thus, a vicious circle is established. In order to prevent gross bleeding, it is necessary to aspirate the initial small quantity of blood completely and not allow the blood to flow into the contralateral side.

We have concluded that the following procedures are mandatory to prevent bleeding after flexible bronchofiberscopic endobronchial biopsy:

1. It must be determined whether the patient has a hemorrhagic diathesis or not;
2. The endotracheal tube must be inserted before the biopsy is undertaken;
3. The mucosal anesthetic agent should be sufficiently administered to the bilateral bronchi just before biopsy;
4. Immediately after the biopsy, another bronchofiberscope must be introduced through the endotracheal tube in order to aspirate blood if endobronchial hemorrhage occurs, and
5. If the hemorrhaging is not terminated quickly by aspiration, it is necessary to put the patient in a lateral decubitus position with the side of the endobronchial hemorrhage down.

REFERENCES

1. Ikeda S: Atlas of flexible bronchofiberscopy, Tokyo, Igaku Shoin, 1974.
2. Pereira W Jr, Kovnat DM, Snider GL: A prospective cooperative study of complications following flexible fiberoptic bronchoscopy. Chest, 74: 813-816, 1978.
3. Zavala DC: Flexible fiberoptic bronchoscopy, A training handbook, Iowa City, Composed at the University of Iowa, 1978.

IV.6.

A SAFETY POSITION IN BRONCHOFIBERSCOPY

DUMON J.F., MD [+]

In general, patients who undergo a fiberscopy are examined either in a sitting position or lying down position. These examination methods have certain incon-
veniences.

- The position of lying down on the back makes the examination of the larynx
difficult, the view of the secretions being prohibited. If the patient is intubated,
the secretions descend along the tube and constrict the bronchial examinations. If
the patient is not intubated, the secretions progress along the fiberscope wich
makes the examination painful for the patient and hinders the endoscopist.

- The sitting position is dangerous in the case of abundant bleeding, because
the blood will flood the entire bronchial branch and is likely to instigate an
asphyxiation. Several deaths have been published in litterature.

This is the reason why we propose a safety position for high risk patients
undergoing a bronchoscopic biopsy.
The patient is examined lying on the side, where the area to be explored is located.
The examiner sits facing the patient, oversees him and explains the operation. The
entrance of the fiberscope is by the mouth or the nose, preferably without intubation. This position makes the examination particularly simple because :

       . there are no secretions from the larynx and the base of the
         tongue does not fall back and block the passage.

       . the patient breathes easily and constantly sees and is in
         contact with the examiner.

       . in the case of a hemmorrhagy the bleeding is easily eliminated
         and in no case the opposite lung is obstructed. This is the
         primary advantage of this position.

+ Médecin des Hôpitaux   Hôpital Salvator
  Chef de Service   13274 MARSEILLE CEDEX 2
  Service Endoscopie thoracique

J.A. Nakhosteen and W. Maassen (eds.), Bronchology: Research, Diagnostic and
Therapeutic Aspects. All rights reserved.
Copyright 1981. Martinus Nijhoff Publishers bv, The Hague / Boston / London

116

The risk of hemorrhagy is slight, but there is
one case out of 1000 fiberscopies of severe
bleeding. In effect, in our statistics, we
reported 6 incidents of severe bleeeding out of
5000 bronchofiberscopies.
(more than 100 cc in which two were more than
200 cc). In one case, a patient with an aneuris-
tic bronchial artery had hemmorrhagy of 500 cc
that was easily controlled by aspiration.
The opposite lung was, at no moment, flooded
with blood.

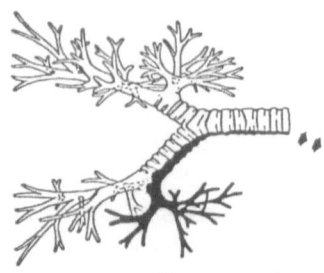

safety position (hemorrhagy)

That position is therefore used for all high
risk patients, that is patients with cardiac
problems (rhythmic anomalies and coronaropathies)
depression of pulmonary fonctions, those with
deficient coagulation and dangerous biopsies
such as transbronchial biopsies.

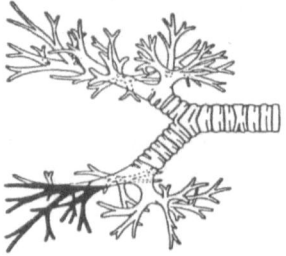

easy position (lung washing)

By analogy, there is also a risk of bronchial
flooding in cases of large lung abcesses or the
presence of a liquid cyst.

    - this lateral position is also practical
for lung washing.

        . according to the same priciple, the
        lung washing is always unilateral.

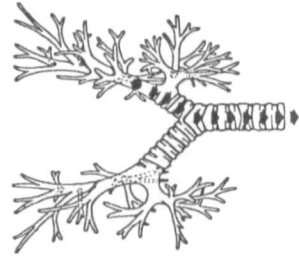

        . the return of the washing liquid from
        the lower lobe is easily accomplished

useful position (foreign body)

        without coughing.

    - Finally, this lateral position is useful for extracting foreign
bodies. The patient is thus placed on the side opposite the location of the
foreign body.
This takes advantage of gravity and facilitates the recuperation.

IV.7.

A NEW DOUBLE LUMEN ENDOTRACHEAL TUBE FOR FIBEROPTIC BRONCHOSCOPY.

H. KRONENBERGER, K.-H. NERGER, M. RUST, M. SCHNEIDER.

Fiberoptic bronchoscopy can be performed transnasally, transorally (with and without tube), through a tracheostoma and through a rigid bronchoscope. For the last several years we preferred the transoral method with an endotracheal tube. We think, it is superior to other methods, as it provides a higher quality of examination and a better management of possible complications. The most important advantage is the possibility to withdraw and to reintroduce easily the bronchoscope during the whole procedure whenever needed without reintubation. Thus for instance the lens of the bronchoscope and the suction channel can be cleaned repeatedly within seconds. In addition it is important that after biopsy the bronchoscope and the forceps can be taken out of the bronchial system as a unit, thus avoiding the loss of diagnostic material during retraction of the forceps through the suction channel. Finally it should be stressed that this method also facilitates removal of foreign bodies.

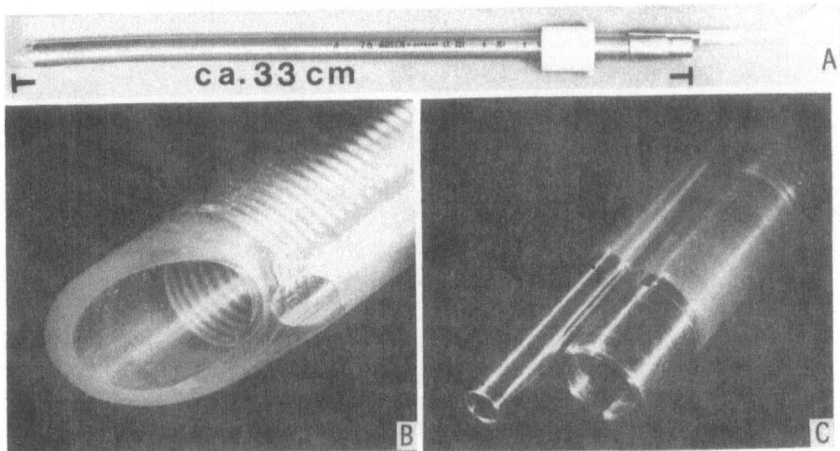

Fig.1: A new double lumen endotracheal tube designed for fiberoptic
bronchoscopy.
A: Total aspect of the new device.
B: Distal tip with two channels, the larger for the bronchoscope,
the smaller for instrumentation.
C: Proximal end of the tube.

J.A. Nakhosteen and W. Maassen (eds.), Bronchology: Research, Diagnostic and
Therapeutic Aspects. All rights reserved.
Copyright 1981. Martinus Nijhoff Publishers bv, The Hague / Boston / London

So far only conventional (single lumen) tubes were available for intubation during fiberoptic bronchoscopy. We present a new flexible endotracheal tube (shown in Fig. 1A) made of PVC with a spiral wire support designed for fiberoptic bronchoscopy. It was manufactured by RUESCH, W.-Germany, according to our specifications. The tube has a lenghts of about 33 cm. Figure 1B shows the distal tip with a larger lumen for the bronchoscope and a smaller one for instrumentation. The large lumen has a diameter of 7.5 mm for the introduction of all common bronchoscopes with an outer diameter up to approximately 6.2 mm. The second smaller channel with a diameter of 3 mm can be used for additional administration of oxygen, the insertion of large diameter suction catheters and instruments. Figure 1C demonstrates a magnification of the proximal end of the double lumen tube. We used this device in more than 300 patients, who all tolerated it well; complications did not occur. Intubation is done according to the method described by IKEDA (1). The tube is guided and advanced into the trachea using the fiberbronchoscope as a stylette which is already positioned in the bronchial tree. This manoevre can be performed within seconds. Three examples shall demonstrate the new options provided by the double lumen tube:

First we want to stress the possibility to insufflate oxygen through the instrumentation channel of the tube in a more comfortable and more effective way. This technique does not interfere with the procedure, nor the operator or the patient. It has been reported that during the whole examination considerable hypoxemia may develop (2). This implies an additional risk for the patients with respiratory failure.

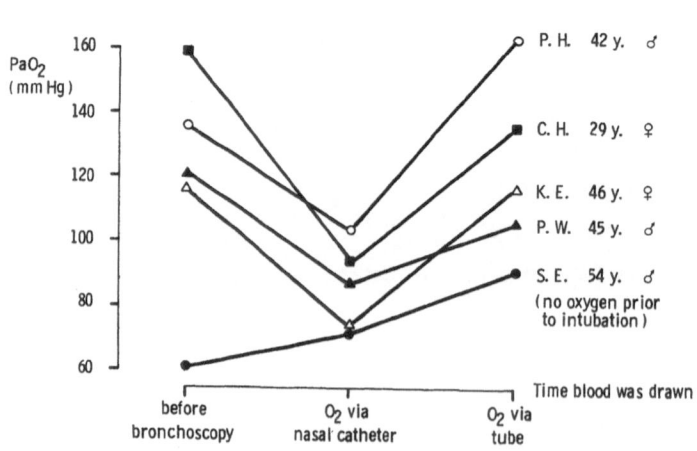

Fig.2: Arterial oxygen tension during different techniques of oxygen administration before and during fiberoptic bronchoscopy.

Figure 2 shows preliminary results of our study on 5 consecutive patients in whom
arterial oxygen tension was measured during the application of 5 liter of oxygen
per minute by nasal catheter before bronchoscopy and 5 minutes after intubation of
the bronchoscope. A significant drop of oxygen tension was observed. After the second blood gas analysis the nasal catheter was withdrawn and oxygen given via tube
at an equal rate resulting in a significant rise of arterial oxygen tension. In another experiment which is not shown, we could demonstrate, that this effect was
not related to the sequence of oxygen administration, as we started with the application via tracheal tube and changed to nasal catheter later on.

As a second example for the use of the double lumen tube we present the feasibi-
lity to insert a larger bipsy forceps made by STORZ, W.-Germany (No. 10358B) through
that second channel. Thus we were able to take larger biopsy specimens from the tracheal bifurcation and from the main stem bronchi.

Figure 3 depicts the histogram of the areas of biopsy particles as estimated by
planimetry. The 5 larger ones were taken by the STORZ forceps the 9 smaller ones
by the OLYMPUS forceps (FB-1c). For the evaluation of the area three random sections
of separately embedded biopsies were used. It is obvious that the areas of the biopsies taken with the STORZ forceps were about ten times larger than the areas obtained by the OLYMPUS forceps. This is an important advantage in early diagnosis

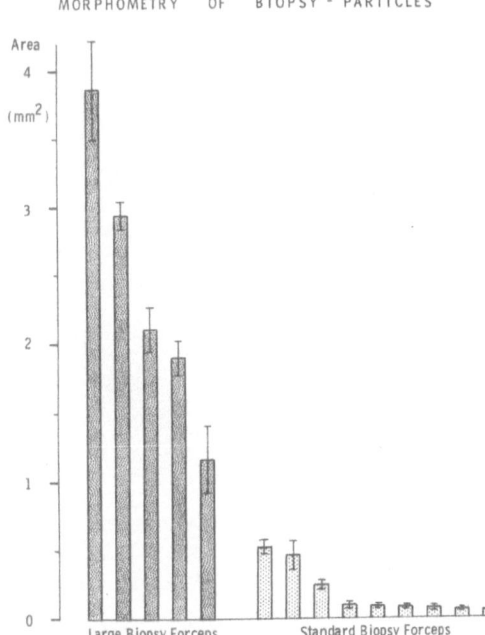

MORPHOMETRY OF BIOPSY - PARTICLES

Fig.3: Areas of biopsy particles estimated by planimetry. The 5 larger
ones were taken by the STORZ forceps the 9 smaller ones by the
OLYMPUS forceps. Three random
sections of all biopsy specimens
were evaluated.

of bronchial carcinoma as the section of the larger biopsy specimens generally re-covered almost the entire lamina muscularis whereas the Standard (OLYMPUS) forceps included only submucosal tissue. At the present time we are trying a curved forceps which may enable us to take larger biopsies also from the carina of the and of the lateral parts of the main stem bronchi.

Further more the tube enables one to perform an intensive bronchial toilet using the double lumen tube in combination with a suction catheter of larger diameter. This is especially helpful during severe bronchial hemorrhage and in case of mucoid impaction with bronchial casts.

In conclusion:
The advantages of the double lumen endotracheal tube are as follows:
1. It has all the capabilities of a single lumen endotracheal tube.
2. It provides more effective and safer oxygen administration even in patients with severe hypoxemia.
3. It enables the introduction of larger instruments that cannot pass through the suction channel of the bronchoscope.
4. It facilitates intensive bronchial toilet while inspecting simultaneously the bronchial tree.

IV.8.

ORO-TRACHEAL INTUBATION USING THE DOUBLE LUMEN TUBE

J H HARRELL II, R G SPRAGG, K M MOSER.

The double lumen tube, first introduced by Carlens in 1949, is used in many clinical conditions where it is necessary to separate the right and left mainstem bronchus. These include massive hemorrhage, manipulation of lung abscesses and differential lavage. Fiberoptiscopes have been used for both naso-tracheal and oro-tracheal intubation with the standard endotracheal tubes. The application of the fiberoptiscope to the double lumen tube was not possible until small fiberoptic bronchoscopes of adequate length and suction channels were developed. The two instruments that fit these criteria are the Machida Pediatric Scope and the Olympus 4 BF2.

Methods: The patient must fit the criteria for Bronchoscopy: 1) PO_2 greater than 50. 2) PCO_2 less than 50. 3) No marked bronchospasm. 4) No serious arrhythmias unless a life threatening situation demands the use of the double lumen tube. The procedure is done in the Operating Room unless emergent conditions, such as hemorrhage, dictate otherwise.

Contra-indications include stenosis or obstruction of the cords, trachea or left mainstem bronchus.

The patient is prepared with 0.5 mg Atropine, topical .45% Tetracaine, and sedation as necessary. Supplemental oxygen is given by nasal canula. The Broncho-cath^{TM}double lumen tube made by National Catheter is used. This tube is indicated for left mainstem intubation and allows selective inflation or deflation of either lung. Before insertion, both balloons of the double lumen tube are inspected, inflated and deflated. The scope and tube are generously lubricated with 2% Xylocaine jelly. The fiberoptiscope is placed through the left arm of the tube.

The scope is passed transorally. The cords are examined. The scope is passed to the carina. Induction of anesthesia can then begin. The double lumen tube is advanced along the fiberoptiscope until it is at the position of the mid trachea. The scope is placed into the left mainstem bronchus

J.A. Nakhosteen and W. Maassen (eds.), Bronchology: Research, Diagnostic and
Therapeutic Aspects. All rights reserved.
Copyright 1981. Martinus Nijhoff Publishers bv, The Hague / Boston / London

at the level of the upper and lower divisions. The tube is passed along over the scope, rotating it to the left. The tip of the tube is placed above the division of the upper lobe and lower lobe on the left.

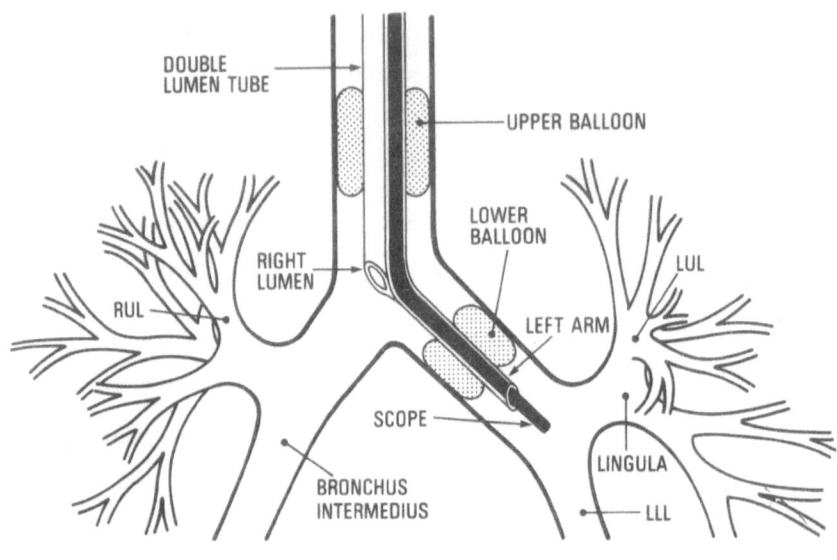

DOUBLE LUMEN TUBE

UPPER BALLOON

LOWER BALLOON

RIGHT LUMEN

LUL

RUL

LEFT ARM

SCOPE

LINGULA

BRONCHUS INTERMEDIUS

LLL

Fig. I

The fiberoptiscope is withdrawn and passed into the right channel. The scope is passed to the right mainstem bronchus orifice, Its patency is insured. The balloon of the left arm is inflated until it is seen to herniate to the level of the carina but not to impinge on the right mainstem bronchus. The tracheal balloon is then inflated. The patient is attached to the anesthesia machine.

The patient is placed in the thoracotomy position. The position of the double lumen tube is again reviewed looking first in the left, and then into the right to insure secure placement of the tube prior to thoracotomy. Therapeutic suctioning in the Operating Room or Recovery Room can be done, e.g., lung abscess and hemorrhage.

Nitrous oxide is known to diffuse through endotracheal tube cuffs, increasing volume; therefore, cuff pressure should be monitored. If lasers are used in this type of PVC tube, HCL gas will be

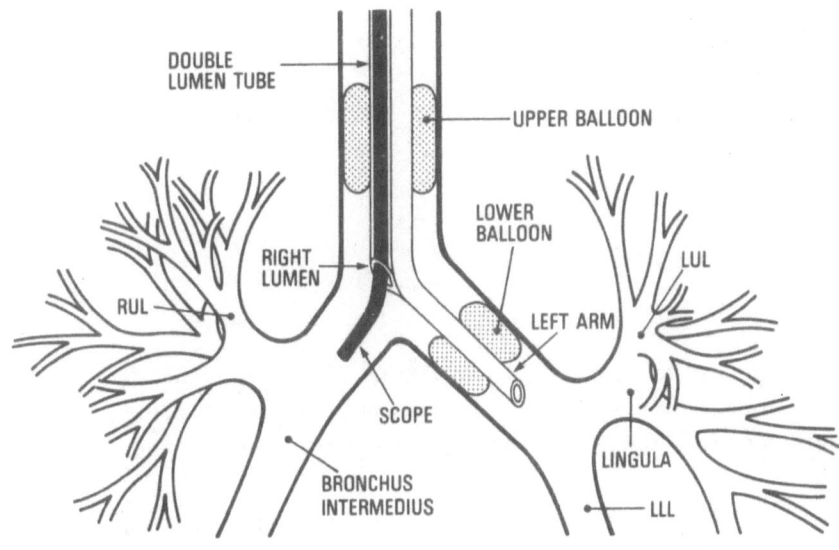

DOUBLE
LUMEN TUBE

UPPER BALLOON

LOWER
BALLOON

RIGHT
LUMEN

LUL

RUL

LEFT ARM

SCOPE

LINGULA

BRONCHUS
INTERMEDIUS

LLL

Fig. 2

released if the tube is touched by the laser beam.

Complications are those of bronchoscopy, cord trauma or tracheal trauma.

Summary: The advent of new small diameter fiberoptic bronchoscopes with large suction channel allows rapid, accurate and secure placement of the double lumen endotracheal tube. This is well tolerated by the patient and results in little or no cord or tracheal trauma. Ease of the procedure allows for repeated examination during surgery and therapeutic intervention if necessary. This type of intubation should only be done by a well trained, experienced bronchoscopist.

IV.9.

CARDIAC ARREST AS COMPLICATION OF BRONCHOLOGIC INVESTIGATION

N. ANTIĆ

Within the period from 1954 to 1979, 5.250 bronchologic procedures have been carried out. Out of this total number 3.136 were bronchoscopies and 2.114 bronchographies due to the following diseases:

neoplasms	2.133	/40%/
tuberculosis	1.461	/28%/
bronchiectasis	991	/19%/
chronic bronchitis	426	/ 8%/
postoperative atelectasis ...	219	/ 4%/
foreign bodies	16	/0,3%/
tracheoesophageal fistula ...	4	/0,07%/

Out of 3.136 bronchoscopies 2.965 /94%/ have been performed un - der local anesthesia and 171 /6%/ under general anesthesia.

Out of 2.114 bronchographies 1.867 /88%/ have been performed under local and 247 /12%/ under general anesthesia.

The age of patients undergone the bronchologic procedures have been from 2 up to 79 years. The distribution to the age group has been following:

2 to 10	106	/ 2%/
11 " 20	314	/ 6%/
21 " 30	842	/16%/
31 " 40	1.207	/23%/
41 " 50	735	/14%/
51 " 60	1.522	/29%/
61 " 70	420	/ 8%/
over 71	104	/ 2%/

At all the patients, except the small children, patients with foreign bodies and therapeutic urgent bronchoscopic aspiration, before the bronchologic procedure, the pulmonary and cardiovascu lar functional sufficiency have been evaluated. Only those pati-

J.A. Nakhosteen and W. Maassen (eds.), Bronchology: Research, Diagnostic and Therapeutic Aspects. All rights reserved.
Copyright 1981. *Martinus Nijhoff Publishers bv, The Hague / Boston / London*

ents, for whom it has been established that they can stand the bronchologic investigation without great risk have been subjected to those procedures.

The bronchologic procedures have been performed in bronchologic laboratory, operating theaters or patient's room by endoscopist and anesthesiologist.

At 26 /0,49%/ the cardiac arrest has occured.

The cardiac arrest took place at 15 patients during the bronchographic procedure, and at 11 cases during bronchoscopy. Out of 15 bronchographic procedures, nine were performed under general and six cases under local anesthesia. Of 11 bronchoscopic procedures, two were performed under general and nine cases without any anesthesia, for the reason that the urgent postoperative aspiration from tracheobronchial tree has been carried out.

The cardiac arrest have suffered patients with following diseases: 5 neoplasms, 8 bronchiectasis, 4 tuberculosis and 9 postoperative atelectasis. The cardiac arrest at bronchiectasis and tuberculosis has occured during the bronchography, at neoplasms it has happend twice during the bronchoscopy and three times during bronchography. All nine cases of cardiac arrest at the postoperative atelectasis have happened during the bronchoscopic aspiration.

Four patients have suffered the cardiac arrest under 10 years of age, one at 26, two at the age between 30 and 40, one at 49, four between 51 and 60, and fourteen have been over 61.

The most probably causes of cardiac arrest at our patients have been following: alveolar hypoventilation provoked by bronchographic contrast material, particularly at children treated under general anethesia, and the deepen of the existing hypoxemia and hypercapnia of bronchoscopic aspiration at older patients with postoperative atelectasis.

Of 26 cardiac arrest cases, three have happened before 1961, what means before the introduction of closed chest cardiac massage, so all of them have been reanimated by thoracotomy and the direct cardiac massage. Two of them died and one survived. All the other have been reanimated by transthoracal cardiac massage, with other measures, as for example: endotracheal intubation, aspiration of contrast material, ventilation with 100% oxygen, defibrillation, cardiotonics and vasopresors, correction of aci-

126

dosis and the postresuscitation care. Of these 23 patients two
have exitated.

Out of four died patients two were children. A six-year child
with bronchiectasis has died due to bronchography in general
anesthesia. The other, seven-year old child with malignant tumor
has suffered the cardiac arrest during the bronchographic procedure, under general anesthesia.

The other two died patients have been older persons. One of them
following the left pneumonectomy due to carcinoma, obtained the
contralateral partial atelectasis due to the impossibility of
expectoration the abundant sputum. At the bronchoscopic aspiration, without anesthesia, the cardiac arrest has followed, which
could not been reanimated with any measures. The other patient,
following thoracoplasty, has not strength to expectorate, and he
fall in hard hypoxemia and hypercapnia. At the bronchoscopic aspiration, without anesthesia, the ventricular fibrillation occured.
Neither the cardiac massage nor the defibrillation could help.

SUMMARY

At 5.250 bronchologic procedures there were 26 /0,49%/ cases of
cardiac arrest, with 4 /0,07%/ lethal results.

Eventhough the cardiac arrest is not such a frequent complication of bronchologic investigation, due to the direct endangere
of patient's life, it is indispensable to do everything in its
prevention and treatment, for it is the only alternative of life.

For that reason, we are of the opinion, that the bronchology
has to be carried out by the qualified team consisted of bronchologist and anesthesiologist-reanimatologist, whitin conditions
which provide the adequate and prompt reanimation.

Rhythmusstörungen bei Bronchoskopien.

IV. 10.

M. Schaefer, V. Rausch

Wir berichten über Rhythmusstörungen bei Bronchoskopien.
Unsere Untersuchungen betreffen 100 Erwachsene, deren Ruhe-EKG keine
Arrhythmien zeigt. In allen Fällen wurden diagnostische Eingriffe mit
dem starren Bronchoskop in Allgemeinnarkose vorgenommen.
Als Praemedikation kamen in aller Regel Atropin, Promethacin und
Pethidin zur Anwendung. Die Halothan-Narkose haben wir mit Hexobarbital
eingeleitet, und die Relaxierung geschah mit Suxamethonium. In allen
Fällen wurde mit reinem Sauerstoff handbeatmet.
Vor und während des Eingriffs haben wir regelmäßig pH, pCO_2 und PO_2
gemessen. Die Herzaktion wurde mit einem EKG-Monitor überwacht. Zur
späteren Auswertung dokumentierten wir die Herzstromkurve mit einem
Ein-Kanal-Schreiber. Die 100 Probanden wurden nach dem Punkte-System
von H. Lutz in Risikogruppen eingeteilt.
In der Tab. I haben wir die Häufigkeit von Rhythmusstörungen für die
einzelnen Risikogruppen aufgeschlüsselt. Die von Lutz angeführte V.
Risikogruppe entfällt hier, weil keiner der von uns untersuchten
Probanden in diese Gruppe des höchsten Risikos zu ordnen war.

Tab. I

Häufigkeit von Rhythmusstörungen bei
Bronchoskopien (n=100)

	Risikogruppe				Σ
	I	II	III	IV	
Anzahl Probanden	34	50	14	2	100
keine Arrhythmien	19	24	5	1	49
Anzahl Arrhythmien	15	26	9	1	51
Prozentzahl Arrhythmien	44%	52%	64%	50%	51%

Wie zu erwarten, nimmt bei schlechtem Allgemeinzustand die prozentuale
Häufigkeit der Rhythmusstörungen zu. Dabei fällt die Risikogruppe IV aus
der Reihe, weil wir nur 2 Probanden dieses Risikofaktors hatten.
Mit dem wachsenden Risiko steigt aber nicht nur die Anzahl der Arrhythmien,
sondern es ändert sich auch deren Qualität. So haben wir - aus der
obigen Tabelle nicht ersichtlich - schwere Rhythmusstörungen, wie
gehäufte ventrikuläre Extrasystolen in der Gruppe I gar nicht gesehen. Unten rechts in der Tab. I ist die
Gesamthäufigkeit von Rhythmusstörungen mit 51 % angegeben. Wir haben
also bei mehr als der Hälfte unserer Bronchoskopien Arrhythmien
festgestellt.

*J.A. Nakhosteen and W. Maassen (eds.), Bronchology: Research, Diagnostic and
Therapeutic Aspects. All rights reserved.
Copyright 1981. Martinus Nijhoff Publishers bv, The Hague / Boston / London*

Die Aufschlüsselung der Arrhythmien in Tab. II zeigt, daß ganz überwiegend supraventrikuläre Rhythmusstörungen auftraten.

Tab. II

Arrhythmien unter
Bronchoskopie (n=100)

Sinustachycardie	38
Sinusbradycardie	2
Sinusarrhythmie	4
Extrasystolen	7
Summe	51

Eine Tachycardie über 100/Min. finden wir in
38 % der Fälle. Sie ist damit die weitaus
häufigste Rhythmusstörung. Sinusbradycardien
erscheinen mit 2 % und Sinusarrhythmien mit
4 %. In 7 Fällen haben wir Extrasystolen
beobachtet. Darunter sind sowohl vereinzelte
ventrikuläre- als auch gehäufte polytope
Extrasystolen. Außerdem sind supraventrikuläre
Extrasystolen sowie Extrasystolen in festem
Zeitverhältnis aufgetreten.

Die häufig beobachtete Sinustachycardie wird gewöhnlich von einem
Blutdruckanstieg begleitet. Diese sympathicotone Kreislaufsituation
entsteht ganz überwiegend bei Einführung des Bronchoskops und ist wohl
auf die Irritation der Atemwege zurückzuführen. Vagale Reaktionen mit
Blutdruck- und Pulsabfall treten dagegen nur selten auf. Letzteres
ist wohl auf die Praemedikation mit dem Parasympatholyticum Atropin
zurückzuführen.
In unseren Untersuchungen haben wir fast regelmäßig eine Hyperkapnie
während des Eingriffs festgestellt. Wie Sechzer et alii beobachteten,
verursacht die Hyperkarbie einen signifikanten Anstieg der Katecholamine
im Serum. Über diesen Mechanismus kann während der Bronchoskopie ein
hohes pCO_2 in ähnlicher Weise sympathikoton und arrhythmogen wirken
wie die mechanische Irritation durch das Instrument.
Aber nicht nur der Eingriff selbst, auch die Narkose und die Adjuvan-
tien der Anästhesie, die wir verwandt haben, sind herzwirksam.
So ist von den Barbituraten eine negativ-inotrope Wirkung bekannt.
Das von uns verwandte Muskelrelaxans vom depolarisierenden Typ
Suxamethonium greift nicht nur an der motorischen Endplatte an, sondern
auch an den parasympathischen Nervenendigungen, wo ebenfalls Acetyl-
cholin Überträgersubstanz ist. Es wirkt deshalb muskarinartig und kann
Bradycardien und Arrhythmien verursachen. Auch die meisten halogenierten
Kohlenwasserstoffe und insbesondere Halothan sind negativ-inotrop und
arrhythmogen. Es ist bekannt, daß Halothan dann besonders arrhythmogen
wirkt, wenn es mit Adrenalin zusammen wirkt. Deshalb kann man nach
W. Hügin die Halothan-Narkose nicht anwenden, wenn bei HNO-ärztlichen
Eingriffen Adrenalin zur lokalen Blutleere der Schleimhäute appliziert

wird.

Da nun bei Bronchoskopien durch Irritation und Hyperkapnie Sympathikus-
reflexe und Adrenalinausschüttung entstehen können, ist wohl auch hier
die Interaktion mit Halothan der Hauptgrund für die beobachteten
Arrhythmien. Wir sind deshalb von der Halothan-Narkose bei Bronchoskopien abgekommen.

Wir verzichten aber nicht gern auf die volatilen Narkosemittel, weil
wir Aufnahme und Ausscheidung der atembaren halogenierten Kohlenwasserstoffe sozusagen in der beatmenden Hand haben, während wir auf das
Schicksal der injizierten Anästhetika im Organismus kaum Einfluß
haben. Wir suchten deshalb ein geeignetes volatiles Narkosemittel für
die Bronchoskopie-Narkose. In diesem Zusammenhang machen die pharmakolo-
gischen Eigenschaften des Ethrane diesen halogenierten Kohlenwasser-
stoff besonders geeignet. Ethrane flutet schneller an und wird schneller
abgeraucht und besitzt damit eine bessere Steuerbarkeit als das Halothan
Auch ist es nicht arrhythmogen. Für die Bronchoskopie-Narkose scheint
uns das Ethrane besonders geeignet, weil nach Johnston und Eger eine
eindeutig geringere Interaktion zwischen Adrenalin und Ethrane als
zwischen Adrenalin und Halothan besteht. Unsere bisherigen Erfahrungen
mit der Ethrane-Narkose für Bronchoskopien sind positiv.

Wir werden darüber zu einem späteren Zeitpunkt berichten.

IV.11.

CARDIAC COMPLICATIONS AND CHANGES OF ARTERIAL BLOOD GAS LEVELS
DURING TRANSBRONCHOSCOPIC LUNG BIOPSY

M. Fukuoka, S. Tamai, M. Takada, N. Okunaka, N. Sakai

We have studied the incidence of cardiac complications
and changes in arterial blood gas levels during and after
transbronchoscopic lung biopsy, hereafter referred to as
TBLB, in an effort to elucidate the influence of TBLB on cardiopulmonary function.

The subjects were 49 patients, i.e., 37 males and 12 females,
whose ages ranged from 19 to 78 years, with a average of 61.6 years.
Their underlying diseases included usual interstitial pneumonitis
in 8 patients, viral pneumonia in 5, lymphangitis carcinomatosa in
5, hypersensitivity pneumonitis in 2, drug induced pneumonitis in 2,
lung cancer in 20, and others in 7.

The patients were given 8mg of oxycodone and 0.3mg of atropine
sulfate intramuscularly 30 minutes prior to the procedure. Local
anesthesia was achieved by spraying of 5ml of 4 % xylocain solution.

In 21 patients TBLB was performed under O_2 inhalation through
a side arm adaptor connected to an endotracheal tube. These patients
are hereafter referred to as the "side-arm-adaptor group". The
remaining 28 patients are referred to as the "no-side-arm-adaptor
group", since TBLB was performed while they breathed ordinary room
air or inhaled transnasally given O_2. Their arterial blood gas was
measured before, during, and after TBLB. In 23 of the 49 patients,
continuous electrocardiograms (Holter Avionics) were recorded for
24 hours before, during and for 24 hours after TBLB. The changes in
average PaO_2 and $PaCO_2$ of the no-side-arm-adaptor group are shown in
Fig. 1. PaO_2 during and after TBLB decreased significantly by 11.5
and 12.5 Torr, respectively, while $PaCO_2$ did not change significantly.
The changes in average PaO_2 and $PaCO_2$ in the side-arm-adaptor group are
shown in Fig. 2. PaO_2 during and after TBLB increased significantly
by 107.4 and 22.1 Torr, respectively, while $PaCO_2$ changed only little.

Major cardiac complications included frequent ventricular premature
contractions (VPC) in 3 patients, a short run of VPC in 2, severe

J.A. Nakhosteen and W. Maassen (eds.), Bronchology: Research, Diagnostic and
Therapeutic Aspects. All rights reserved.

ischemic ST-T changes in 2, and myocardial infarction, atrial fibrillation, and 2nd A-V block, seen in one patient each. The patients with myocardial infarction died 2 hours after completion of TBLB. Minor cardiac complications included sporadic ventricular premature contractions in 5 patients, sporadic supraventricular premature contractions in 4, and sinus bradycardia in 1.

A comparison in incidence of cardiac complications between groups with and without a side arm adaptor are shown in Table 1. The incidence was high in the 14 patients without a side arm adaptor, and was noted in 29 % during TBLB and in 21 % the night after TBLB. On the other hand, no major cardiac complications were noted in the 9 patients with a side arm adaptor.

Conclusions: 1) In the no-side-arm-adaptor group, PaO_2 decreased markedly during and after TBLB. 2) Major cardiac complications associated with TBLB were frequently recorded in the no-side-arm-adaptor group, and were considerd to be due to unavoidable hypoxemia. 3) Increased PaO_2, which occurred during and after TBLB in the side-arm-adaptor group, was considered to contribute to the prevention of cardiac complications.

Table 1. Incidence of cardiac complications
(n=23)

complications	Without side arm adaptor n=14		With side arm adaptor n=9	
	major	minor	major	minor
during TBLB	4 (28.6)	3 (21.4)	0	0
after TBLB	1 (7.1)	4 (28.6)	0	1 (11.1)
night after TBLB	3 (21.4)	3 (21.4)	0	1 (11.1)

( ) %

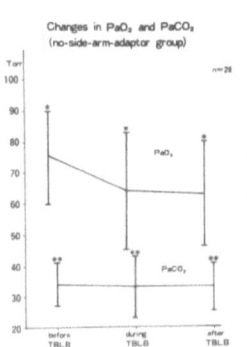

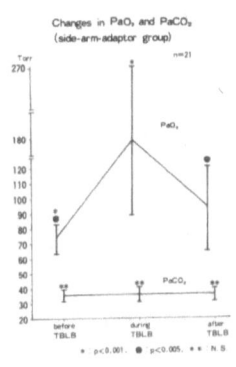

Figure 1.   Figure 2.

REFERENCES

1. Elguindi AS, Harrison GN, Abdulla AM, Chaudhary BA, Vallner JJ, Kolbeck RC, and Speir WA: Cardiac rhythm disturbances during fiberoptic bronchoscopy: A prospective study, The J. Thorac. and Cardiovasc. Surg. 77, 557, 1979.

2. Shrader DL, Lakshminarayan S: The Effect of Fiberoptic Bronchoscopy on Cadiac Rythm. Chest, 73, 6, 821, 1978.

IV.12.

BLOODLESS SO2 MONITORING TO PREVENT COMPLICATIONS IN BRONCHOFIBER-
OPTIC PROCEDURES.

J.M.G. DE VEGA, A. MERIDA, J. MORALES, F. GONZALEZ, J. GUTIERREZ.

INTRODUCTION

The changes produced on saturation by bronchofiberscopy(BF) in
patients with different pathology have been evaluated to prevent
complications stemming from its decrease, and the correlation of
the bloodless method(Oximeter), versus the saturation derived
from gasometry.

MATERIALS AND METHODS

We carried out BF with an Olympus B-3 on 40 patients and arterial gasometry test, before, and inmediately after the conclusion
of the explorations.The patients were monitorized with a saturation
oximeter device, Oximet 1471(Mochida Luketron), and an ECG monitor,
taking saturation values at different airway levels, and upon making the different washing and/or suction maneouvers.The timing
was recorded.

RESULTS

The statistical data obtained are shown in Table 1 and Graphic 1.

TABLE 1. Differences and correlation between bloodless SO2-gasometry.

Absolute differences	$\overline{d}$	Sd
BASAL	3,9	±3,2
FINAL	3,3	±3,2

Correlation	r	
BASAL	0,59	(p < 0,001)
FINAL	0,62	(p < 0,001)
WHOLE	0,60	(p < 0,001)

The values of SO2 at the different airway stretches and basals
and finals, do not undergo any outstanding changes(Graphic 2).The
time consumed has maintained some relation to the desaturation produced at the end of BF.Before any rhythmic alterations were visualized in the ECG monitor, we have already seen important desatura-

J.A. Nakhosteen and W. Maassen (eds.), Bronchology: Research, Diagnostic and
Therapeutic Aspects. All rights reserved.
Copyright 1981. Martinus Nijhoff Publishers bv, The Hague / Boston / London

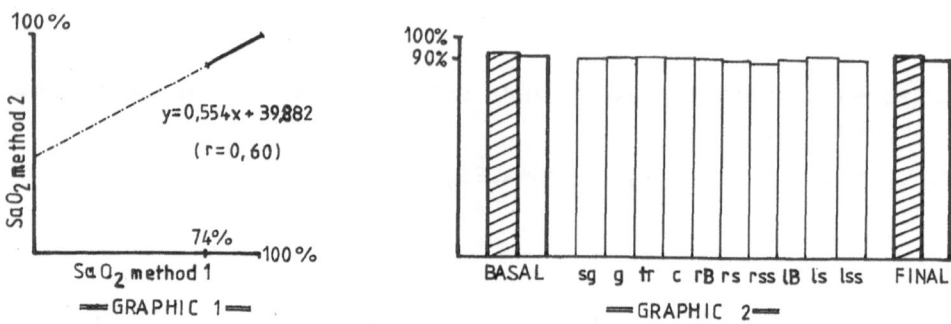

$$y = 0,554x + 39,882$$
$$(r = 0,60)$$

SaO₂ method 2 ... SaO₂ method 1 ... 74% ... 100% ... 100%

═══GRAPHIC 1═══

100% 90% BASAL sg g tr c rB rs rss lB ls lss FINAL

═══GRAPHIC 2═══

tion in the oximeter, which fluctuated between 74 and 60,4 %.

DISCUSSION

The complete absence of any trouble caused to the patient, and the constant gathering of data obtained through the oximeter versus gasometry, has prompted us to judge if the data obtained with the bloodless method are valid.Both methods are not identical and although the correlation may not be the best, it does have an important statistical significance (Tab. 1, Graph. 1).The crossing of the different airway stretches did not show any appreciable change in SO2.However, other authors[1] conclude that P_aO_2 decreases when BF is introduced into a lobe.

The time factor has exerted some influence in the decrease of SO2 at the end of the exploration, as was mentioned before in termes of P_aO_2 by others[2].

When we were alerted by the oximeter, we were able to discontinue temporally the maneouver.The desaturation - cardiac rhythm alteration relation has been previously described,[3,4,5] although they used as a parameter P_aO_2.

Even though the desaturation produced by the washing and/or suction has not been statistical significant, in individual findings, it did take place, for which we do not contradict the finds of Dubrawsky et all.

In conclusion, we believe that the monitorization of the patients by the oximeter is valid, as this method keeps relation with the values of SO2 derived from gasometry, and moreover, it advises us on those cases of desaturation in which serious complications could arise to the patient.

ACKNOWLEDGMENT: M.J. Bolaños from the Biostatistical Section.School of Medicine.University of Granada.

IV.13.

HYPOXEMIA DURING FLEXIBLE FIBERBRONCHOSCOPY

J. Roux, W. Hartmann

INTRODUCTION

Hypoxemia during flexible fiberbronchoscopy has been reported before. The reasons for depression of arterial pO_2 (paO_2) are known only in part and have been discussed in the literature. Whether hypoxemia occurs in all patients is also unclear. And it is also of interest to determine exactly when hypoxemia starts. We investigated these problems by measuring continuously the paO_2 of 20 patients undergoing fiberbronchoscopy. The advantage of continuous registration of arterial pO_2 is the detection even of short periods of hypoxemia.

MATERIALS AND METHODS

The group of 20 patients included 17 males and 3 females, between 33 to 77 years of age. Average age was 58.4 years. Arterial oxygen pressure was measured by a polarographic method. The measurements started about 3 minutes before intubation and terminated 5 minutes following extubation. Mean duration of fiberbronchoscopy was 7 minutes 20 seconds. Thirty minutes before the procedure premedication with atropine, 0.5 mg, and Hydrocodon, 0.2 mg/kg, was given. After local anesthesia transnasal intubation of the bronchofiberscope took place.

RESULTS AND DISCUSSION

An arterial pO_2 below 65 mm Hg was defined as hypoxemia. Seven patients were hypoxemic prior to intubation. During bronchoscopy 13 showed a paO_2 under 65 mm Hg. Two of these 13 reverted to normal blood gas values immediately after extubation, while 11 persisted with hypoxemia.(Figure 1)

The 20 patients were divided into three groups, according to the course of paO_2 during fiberbronchoscopy. Eight showed a decrease of mean paO_2, from 72.4 to 60.4 mm Hg. In a second group of 7, with a mean paO_2 of 60.0 mm Hg, changes in paO_2 during fiberbronchoscopy did not exceed $\pm$ 3 mm Hg. This group showed severe reduction of vital capacity and FEV_1 in pre-bronchoscopy lung function tests. The third group of 5 showed an increase of paO_2 during bronchoscopy. Mean paO_2 increased from 65.0 mm to 75.0 mm Hg. Four of these patients also showed a drop of pCO_2. Because of a severe, purulent bronchitis

J.A. Nakhosteen and W. Maassen (eds.), Bronchology: Research, Diagnostic and Therapeutic Aspects. All rights reserved.
Copyright 1981. Martinus Nijhoff Publishers bv, The Hague / Boston / London

in 3 of these 5 patients, large quantities of sputum had been removed.

Eleven patients showed a sudden decrease of paO_2 three minutes after intubation, nine showed no remarkable change, and none had an increase within the first three minutes. Several mechanisms may be discussed for paO_2 depression: the sudden fall immediately following intubation may be due to reflex mechanisms causing laryngo- or bronchospasm. A further reason may be aspiration of sputum and local anesthetics, which cannot be expectorated and are followed by alteration of ventilation/perfusion ratio.

Nonetheless, hypoxemia is not inevitable during fiberbronchoscopy, in particular (at least in the group of patients here examined) in patients with severe lung disease and low paO_2 before bronchoscopy. Five patients from this group of 20 improved paO_2 during the procedure. This may be due to hyperventilation, evidenced by the drop of $paCO_2$. Finally, removal of purulent sputum may also have led to improved oxygenation.

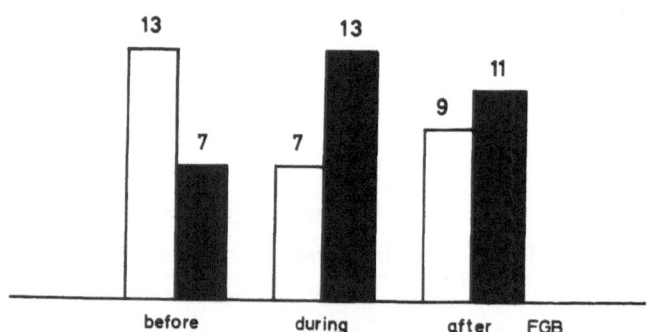

Normal and hypoxemic (black coloured) pO_2 in a group of 20 patients before, during and after FGB

Figure 1

IV.14.

SOME ASPECTS OF COMPLICATIONS ON TRANSBRONCHIAL LUNG BIOPSY

A.KURASHIMA, H.KOMATSU, M.ISHIHARA, R.YONEDA, and T. HAGA

Recently, transbronchial lung biopsy is widely used with the progress of flexible fiberoptic bronchoscopy.

For last three years, from 1977 to 1979, we performed 202 procedures of transbronchial lung biopsy in 177 patients. 106 patients of them had diffuse disseminated lung disease and 71 patients had peripheral pulmonary nodular lesion. In these series, as complications, we encountered one case of acute lung edema, two cases of pneumothorax, and 18 cases of hemorrhage over 50 ml. The acute lung edema occurred in a patient with latent cardiac insufficiency. She had not recﬁeved premedication with atropine-sulfate in error. Immediately after the biopsy in the right lung anterior segment, bilateral lung edema developed rapidly. We think this might have occurred due to vaso-vagal reflex. One of the bleeding cases lead to intra-parenchymal hematoma. This occured after the biopsy for the peripheral coin lesion, chest X-ray film revealed an enlarged round density at the lesion of biopsy. We examined injoured blood vessels in the lung specimens bitten by a biopsy forceps, using a resected human lung whose pulmonary artery was filled with barium-sol. Almost all injoured vesseles belonged to pulmonary circulation. From the histological examination, it revealed that 54 specimens among the 267 specimens (20.2%) had vascular tissues. The frequency distribution of the vascular luminal diameter from the 54 samples indicates that most of the vessels are less than 100 microne of luminal diameter.

For reducing hemorrhage at the procedure of lung parenchymal biopsy, Zavala recommends "Wedge" method.

For purpose to clarify the effect of "Wedge" method, the following clinical experiments were done by ^{99m} Tc perfusion scanning.

J.A. Nakhosteen and W. Maassen (eds.), Bronchology: Research, Diagnostic and
Therapeutic Aspects. All rights reserved.
Copyright 1981. Martinus Nijhoff Publishers bv, The Hague / Boston / London

138

Materials and methods

On the normal human lung, the tip of a flexible fiberoptic bronchoscope was wedged firmely to the selected segmental bronchus, and we
started continuous suction with the negative pressure of 65-70 mmHg.
One minute after the beginning of the suction, ^{99m}Tc-MAA was injected
into the cephric vein, and scanning over the lung was displayed by
the coloured iso-counting method. The result was compared with the
pre-examined control study in the same subject.

Results

Defective region in the wedged segment is apparently shown on the
scintigram. It can be considered as indicating the decrease of regional
pulmonary blood flow caused by "Wedge" method. We examined these radioisotopic experiments in 7 cases and all of them showed the same result.
We approve that "wedge" method is effective to reduce the occurrence
of hemorrhage in the transbronchial lung biopsy.
We usually use "Wedge" method and epinephrine injection into the bronchus just before operation to prevent the hemorrhage.

REFERENCES

1. Zavala, D. C.:Pulmonary Hemorrhage in Transbronchial Biopsy.
   Chest 70:584-591, 1976
2. Nozawa, Y. et al.:Transbronchial Lung Biopsy. The Japanese Journal
   of Thoracic Disease 12:129-136, 1974
3. Moagan, B. C. et al.: Pulmonary Blood Flow and Resistance dualing
   Acute Atelectasis in Intact Dogs. J.Appl.Physiol.28:609-613, 1970
4. Enjeti, Suresh, John T. et al.:Sublobar Atelectasis and Regional
   Pulmonary Blood Flow. J.Appl.Physiol. 47:1245-1250, 1979

IV.15.

TOPICAL ANESTHESIA IN A LARGE NUMBER OF FLEXIBLE BRONCHOSCOPIES

J. ATOCHA

1. INTRODUCTION

Topical anesthesia is the method of choice for a large number of our patients undergoing flexible bronchoscopy because it is simple and almost devoid of significant complications. In a busy thoracic service where flexible bronchoscopies are part of daily diagnostic and therapeutic work, this method fits well and permits normal flow of activities.

2. PROCEDURE

2.1 Materials and methods

From our larger number of flexible bronchoscopies done using a variety of anesthetic drugs and methods, we have selected over two thousand patients for whom lidocaine solution was used. The method of anesthesia consisted of three steps: spraying, swabbing and instillation.

2.1.1 Preparation. The need for premedication is decided primarily by our anesthesiologist after assessing the condition of the patient. Age, cardio-pulmonary status, as well as the general medical condition determine the amount if indicated. In particular cases, no premedication is administered. Diazepan (Valium), hydroxyzine pamoate (Vistaril), atropine and demerol, alone or in combination, are the most commonly used drugs. All elective endoscopies are done on patients who have been fasting at least four hours prior to the procedure. All patients have cardiac monitoring, nasal oxygen by cannula and intravenous fluids. The position of the patient is supine throughout the entire anesthetic and endoscopic procedure.

2.1.2 Site. The operating room is the place of choice, having anesthesia and nursing personnel available. Many emergency bronchoscopies, however, are done in cardiac or respiratory intensive care units or in the emergency suite.

2.1.3 Spraying. We use 4% lidocaine solution directly atomized to the mucosa of the palate, tongue and hypopharynx. Intermittent panting movements help distribute atomized lidocaine throughout the hypopharynx and larynx. The time considered adequate for spraying is about ten minutes. Spraying is completed when the patient states that he has difficulty initiating the swallowing of saliva. When the transnasal route is chosen, both nostrils are also sprayed with the 4% lidocaine solution.

2.1.4 Swabbing. A small cotton ball wrapped around the tip of a right angle Jackson laryngoscopy forceps is soaked in 4% lidocaine solution and used to gently swab the pyriform sinuses and the base of the tongue. On the average, three applications are used to completely abolish the gag reflex.

J.A. Nakhosteen and W. Maassen (eds.), Bronchology: Research, Diagnostic and
Therapeutic Aspects. All rights reserved.
Copyright 1981. Martinus Nijhoff Publishers bv, The Hague / Boston / London

140

2.1.5 Instillation. For this phase of topical anesthesia, we
dilute the lidocaine to 1% and squirt 4 ml. through the vocal cords
two or three times. A blunt-tipped flexible laryngoscopy cannula
is shaped to curve over the posterior tongue and epiglottis and is
attached to a syringe containing 1% lidocaine. The tongue is pulled
outward with a gauze, the cannula is introduced, and the solution is
injected during a deep inspiration. This is repeated one or two
times, as necessary. A sudden cough reflex, mainly on the first
instillation, assures us that the anesthetic entered the trachea.
The induction of anesthesia, we believe, should be a relaxed,
unhurried procedure; the patient being informed, cooperative and
reassured of the benign course of events. Total duration of the
anesthetic procedure from spraying through instillation takes about
15 minutes.

3. BRONCHOSCOPY
    With the patient in the same position, covered with sterile linen,
the flexible bronchoscope is introduced directly into the airway.
The tongue is held outward by the assistant to lift the epiglottis
and expose the vocal cords. The tip of the scope flexed approximately
90 degrees permits rapid visualization of the larynx. In all patients
phonation is observed to evaluate vocal cord function. After the
tip of the scope has passed the larynx the tongue is released. A
systematic observation of the trachea and all visible bronchi is
done. Aspirations of secretions, brushings, washings and biopsies
are done in the routine manner and collected for laboratory evaluation. Additional anesthetic is instilled through the channel of
the scope using about 3 to 4 ml. of lidocaine diluted with lukewarm
saline to make a 1% solution because this produces less cough reflex.
At the completion of the procedure the patient is taken to a recovery
room and kept fasting for one hour.

4. RESULTS
    For the entire group, the process was uncomplicated. Lately,
more and more patients are bronchoscoped as outpatients and released
two hours after the procedure.
    In some bronchitic patients with abundant tracheobronchial
secretions, additional instillation of 2 ml. of the 1% solution of
lidocaine, once or twice, was necessary to complete the procedure.
Laryngospasm was prevented by making sure that the initial spraying
conveyed the mist to the larynx and the subglottic region. Cardiac
arrhythmias and hypoxemia are avoided by proper oxygenation, avoidance of constant aspiration through the suction chamber of the scope
and avoidance of unnecessary delay.

5. CONCLUSION
    The described topical anesthesia with lidocaine solution has
proven safe and practical for flexible bronchoscopy. Multiple
biopsies, brushings and washings were done as necessary, and careful
inspection of all visible orifices was done. In no instance did we
have to change to general anesthesia to complete the procedure. The
gentle manipulation of the fiberscope and careful topical anesthesia
have achieved the goal of many successful bronchoscopies with very
informative results.

REFERENCES
1. Atocha, J. : Available Techniques in Foreign Body Removal.
   Proceedings of the First World Congress on Bronchoscopy, Tokyo,
   Japan, 1978.
2. Ikeda, S.: Atlas of Flexible Bronchofiberscopy.Tokyo, Japan,
   I gaku Shoin Ltd., 1974.

XV.16.

Hemodynamic Effects in Bronchoscopy during Ventilation Bronchoscopy
and Sanders Venturi Ventilation

W. Wrabetz, W. Hartmann

There are two methods available to ventilate patients undergoing bronchoscopy in general anesthesia. One is the ventilation bronchoscopy
which was introduced in 1959. The other was described by Sanders in
1967 using the Venturi effect. We were interested wether both methods
would have different effects on the hemodynamic of the pulmonal circulation if the oxygenation of the arterial blood is comparable.

We examined 15 patients. Lung function tests were carried out before
bronchoscopy was started. 9 of all patients showed either an obstructive
or a restrictive lung disease. Cardiac output (CO) was determined before
and after intubation via a Swan Ganz catheter using the thermodilution
technique. Furthermore we measured the pulmonal arterial pressure (PAP)
blood pressure (BP), heart rate (HR) and arterial blood gases. Arterial
pO_2 was determined continuously by a polarographic electrode. In ventilation bronchoscopy we choose an inspiratory oxygen content of 40 %.
After intubation we first started with ventilation bronchoscopy. When
a steady state of PAP and of art. pO_2 was reached, we switched to Venturi technique. To achieve comparable depth of anesthesia we carried
out our measurements directly before and after change of ventilation
technique.

In 10 patients we measured the art. pO_2 continuously. The control
value showed a reduction of mean art. pO_2 to 68 mm Hg and a reduction
of mean art. pCO_2 to 33 mm Hg. The mean art. pO_2 in Venturi technique
was 219 mm Hg and is above that measured in ventilation bronchoscopy
which was on the avarage 149 mm Hg. The mean art. pCO_2 in Venturi technique was 28 mm Hg showing that hyperventilation took place. In comparison we measured in ventilation bronchoscopy a mean art. pCO_2 of
36 mm Hg. This fact is perhaps explaning the better oxygenation of the
arterial blood using the Venturi technique.

Hemodynamic measurements were carried out in 15 patients. Six of
them already showed elevated PAP before anesthesia. The mean PAP before

142

start of general anesthesia was found to be 20 mm Hg. Mean PAP in ven-.
tilation bronchoscopy was found to be 28 mm Hg. This is significantly
higher than the control value (p < 0.025).

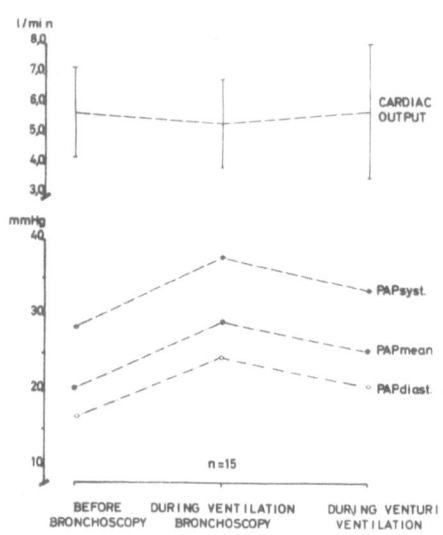

Fig.: Pulmonary arterial pressures and cardiac output before bronchoscopy, during ventilation bronchoscopy and during Venturi ventilation

The other hemodynamic parameters as BP, HR and CO were not significantly altered in comparison to control values. After changing to Venturi
technique we measured a further significant decrease of PAP to 25 mm Hg
(p < 0.025). CO, BP and HR remained unchanged within statistical limits.

Summary

In our opinion the ventilation estimated by the oxygenation of the blood
is in both methods comparable. The arterial pO_2 was higher in Venturi
ventilation probably because of hyperventilation as can be seen in the
lower art. pCO_2 level. The continuously measured art. pO_2 was in both
methods never below 100 mm Hg thus guaranteeing a sufficient oxygenation
of the tissue. The comparison of CO, BP and HR showed no significant
differences. The mean PAP, however, was found to be significantly lower
in Venturi technique. Furthermore it is easier to handle the instruments
as an open system can be used.

IV.17.

INTRAVENOUS ANAESTHESIA TECHNIQUES AS AN ALTERNATIVE TO HALOTHAN
ANAESTHESIA IN BRONCHOSCOPIC PROCEDURES

V.SCHULZ,K.STOSSECK

INTRODUCTION

Routinely bronchoscopic procedures are performed in halothan-oxygen
-inhalation anaesthesia.Anaesthesia induction is done mostly by thio-
pental,succinyl-bischolin is used for muscle relaxation.This procedure is however accompanied by the following disadvantages : halothan concentration as well fresh gas flow is relatively high;there-
fore the halothan exposure to the bronchoscopist and assistants are
considerable.The period of examination is limited with respect to a
maximal dose of succinyl-bischolin.Postnarcotic a high incidence of
cough is observed.At least it should be considered,that halothane in-
terferes with the surfactant metabolism,because it is a lipoid solub-
le agent.Therefore we have proved as an alternative some intravenous
anaesthesia techniques which avoid the discussed disadvantages of the
halothan-oxygen-inhalation anaesthesia.

INTRAVENOUS ANAESTHESIA TECHNIQUES

We proved two techniques.Used medicaments,dosis and form of application during narcosis are developed in the following.

Technique I - premedication : promethazin 1mg/kg BW,pethidin 1mg/kg
BW,atropinum 0,5mg i.m.;introduction of narcosis : atropinum 0,5mg
i.v.,diallylnortoxoferin (alcuronium) 2mg i.v.,following dihydrobenz-
peridol 5mg i.v.,fentanyl 0,2mg i.v.,diazepam 10mg i.v.,after a short
period of ventilation by mask (FIO2 = 1) succinyl-bischolin 100mg i.v.
for intubation by bronchoscop;further managements : 10-15 min. after
intubation renewed application of fentanyl 0,1mg i.v.,Diazepam 5mg
as needed,succinyl-bischolin in single doses to 20-30mg i.v. until to
a total dosis of 400mg;in the postnarcotic state : no antagonists
necessary.

Technique II - premedication : respectively technique I;introduction
of narcosis : atropinum 0,5mg i.v.,diazepam 10mg i.v.,ketamin 100 mg
i.v.,after a short period of ventilation by mask (FIO2 = 1)

J.A. Nakhosteen and W. Maassen (eds.), Bronchology: Research, Diagnostic and
Therapeutic Aspects. All rights reserved.
Copyright 1981. Martinus Nijhoff Publishers bv, The Hague / Boston / London

succinyl-bischolin 100mg i.v. for intubation by bronchoscop;further
managements : 5 min. after intubation 0,07mg/kg BW Org NC45 i.v.,a
new derivate of pancuronium,application of ketamin 50mg i.v. in periods of 10-15 min.,diazepam 5mg i.v. and Org NC45 1mg i.v. as needed;
in the postnarcotic state : physostigmin 5mg i.v. in combination with
atropinum 0,5mg i.v. is used to antagonize Org NC45.

RESULTS

We applied techniqe I to 20 patients.Time of narcosis was 46,5 min.
on average.Arterial blood gases - measured before bronchoscopy and 10
min. after extubation - are comparable and demonstrate normoventilation;therefore postnarcotic spontaneous ventilation of patients was
sufficient,a depression of ventilation due to described technique
could excluded.Postnarcotic a decline of pH was significant,the course of BE showed a developement of a slight metabolic acidosis,possi-
bly a specific effect of this technique.After renewed application of
fentanyl a significant fall of systolic and diastolic systemic arterial pressure and heart rate - evidently the consequence of the anal-
getic effect of fentanyl - to prenarcotic values was noticed.These
values were measured until to the postnarcotic state.All patients were invokeable and took local orientation 10 min. after extubation.
Coughing fits,often observed after halothane-inhalation anaesthesia,
mostly failed to appear.Technique II was proved in 17 patients.Time
of narcosis amounted to 72 min. on average.Arterial blood gases showed
just so 10 min. after extubation a normoventilation pattern.pH and BE
were nor significantly altered.Systolic and diastolic systemic arterial blood pressure arised significantly after intubation;during the
following course of narcosis the values falled again,nevertheless
postnarcotic values were higher than values before bronchoscopy.Heart
rate solely rised significantly after intubation.All patients were
invokeable and took local orientation 10 min. after extubation.In contrast using technique I in this technique a relatively high incidence
of laryngospasm was observed.

CONCLUSIONS

Developed intravenous anaesthesia techniques,especially first descri-
ped modified neurolept analgesia (technique I) can used as an alternative to halothane-inhalation anaesthesia in bronchoscopic procedures,because these techniques avoid the the disadvantages of halothan
-inhalation anaesthesia and permit - as our measurements show - a safe narcosis.

Chapter V

BRONCHOGRAPHY IN THE DIAGNOSIS OF LUNG DISEASE

V.1.

BRONCHOGRAPHY IN PULMONARY DISEASES

K. WATANABE, M.D.* and S. IKEDA, M.D.**

1. INTRODUCTION

Bronchography is used quite extensively now in our hands in the study of various
pulmonary lesions such as cancer, bronchiectasis and diffuse pulmonary diseases.
A 4 times magnified photography of the bronchogram is also taken some times.
Bronchographic images obtained give us valuable clinical informations. There is,
however, difference of opinion as to the value of bronchography among bronchologists
of the world. Japan is a country where this examination is very popular. In the
present study, an inquiry was made as to how often bronchography is performed,
and what kind of a role it is playing in the diagnostic study of pulmonary pathology.

2. PROCEDURE

Inquiries were sent 543 institutes in Japan that had more than 400 beds and
were equipped with thoracic service. They included general hospitals, sanatoriums
and hospitals affiliated with medical schools, but not necessarily exclusively
chest hospitals. 290 institutes (53%) returned their answers, but 31 institutes
were excluded because bronchography was seldom performed.

3. RESULTS

In 74% of the institutes bronchography was
done less than 100 times a year and in 26% of the
institutes more than 100 times a year (Fig. 1).
In 77% of the institutes, aqueous Dionosil is
used (Fig. 1). Metras catheter, Flexible
Bronchial Catheter are most popularly used
(Fig. 1). The Flexible Bronchial Catheter is the
easiest to manipulate, and it is anticipated
that it's use will be expanded in the future.

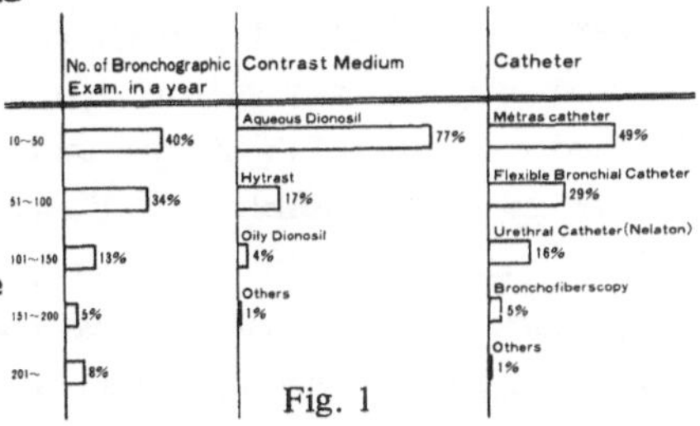

Fig. 1

In 76% of the institutes selective bronchography is performed (Fig. 2). Taking
the discomfort to the patient into consideration, bronchography selective of the
area of the lesion will be adopted more popularly in the future. In 98% of the
institutes, a study is carried out in less than 30 minutes (Fig. 2). In the right

J.A. Nakhosteen and W. Maassen (eds.), Bronchology: Research, Diagnostic and
Therapeutic Aspects. All rights reserved.
Copyright 1981. Martinus Nijhoff Publishers bv, The Hague / Boston / London

graph of Fig. 2, it is shown that in 51% of the
institutes bronchography is done before bronchofiberscopy, whereas in 28% of the institutes
bronchography is performed at the same time or
after bronchofiberscopy. However, these latter
ways of practice are not recommended because the
scar of biopsy and brushing can affect the
bronchogram, and because, in order to make a
definitive diagnosis, it is necessary for the
bronchologist to have a precise localization of
the lesion of the peripheral area, and this is
possible only by performing bronchography before
bronchofiberscopy.

In 30% of the institutes bronchography is
done gradually less frequently either because
other examinations substituted for bronchography
or the patients requiring the study decreased.
In 39% of the institutes the number of the study
per year is unchanged, and in 30% of the
institutes it is increasing either because the
number of patients increased or indications for
bronchography was increased (Fig. 3).

More than 50% of the institutes mentioned
a precise localization of the lesion, diagnosis
of the bronchiectasis, differential diagnosis of
the lesion as the purpose of the bronchography
(Fig. 4). Peripherally located lung cancer,
bronchiectasis and lung cancer in hilum are
mentined as indication of bronchography by more
than 80% of the institutes (Fig. 4).

68% of the institutes responded that
bronchography is very valuable in the properly
selected cases and 21% of the institutes stated
that it is indispensable for diagnosing pulmonary
lesion, thus expressing strong support for the
study (Fig. 5). Although a large number of CT-

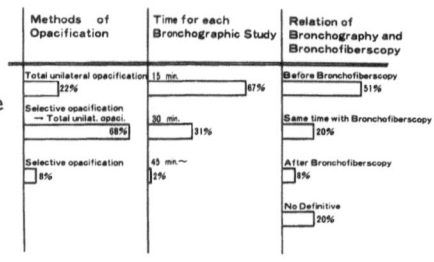

Fig. 2

Recent Trend of Bronchography

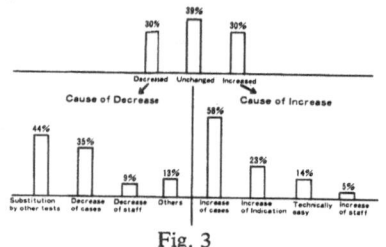

Fig. 3

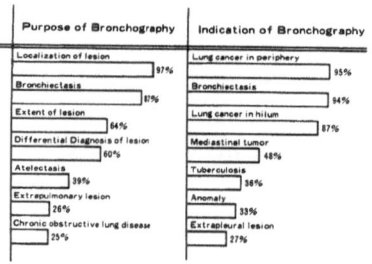

Fig. 4

Opinions about the value of Bronchography

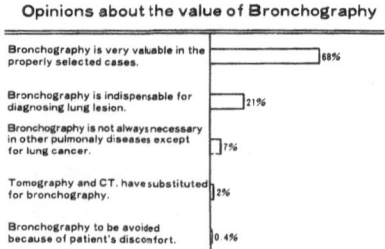

Fig. 5

scanning apparatus are operated in Japan, an opinion in favor of less invasive
CT-scanning or other studies as opposed to bronchography was expressed by only
few institutes.

There were 26 fatal accidents during the study, the incidence being 0.014%,
i.e. 1.4 in 10,000. Respiratory failure, side effects of the local anesthetic was

responsible in 10 and 9 cases respectively. Other non-fatal complications included xylocainisms, pneumonia, aggravation of the lesion, bronchospasm and so on (Fig.6).

Fig. 7 shows the order of the choice of examinations for pulmonary lesion. In the peripheral type, the tomography is mentioned as the first choice. As the second choice bronchography, bronchofiberscopy and CT are mentioned and as the third choice bronchofiberscopy and bronchography are named. In the hilar type, bronchofiberscopy, bronchography and CT are named as the second choice, and as the third choice bronchography and bronchofiberscopy are mentioned. Bronchography occupies different order in choice depending on the location of the lesion, but, in any case it is favored in a large number of institutes.

Complications of Bronchography
in 181,892 exams./259 institutes

Death 26 cases 0.014%(1.4/10.000)

Respiratory failure	10 cases	
Side effects of the local anesthetics	9 cases	
Others	7 cases	

Non-fatal Complications 1440 cases
0.79%(79/10.000)

Xylocainisms	673 cases	0.37%(37 10.000)
Pneumonia	312	0.17 (17 10.000)
Aggravation of the lesion	191	0.11 (11 10.000)
Bronchospasm	164	0.09 (9 10.000)
Hypersensitivity to Iode	36	0.02 (2 10.000)
Others	64	0.04 (4 10.000)

Fig. 6

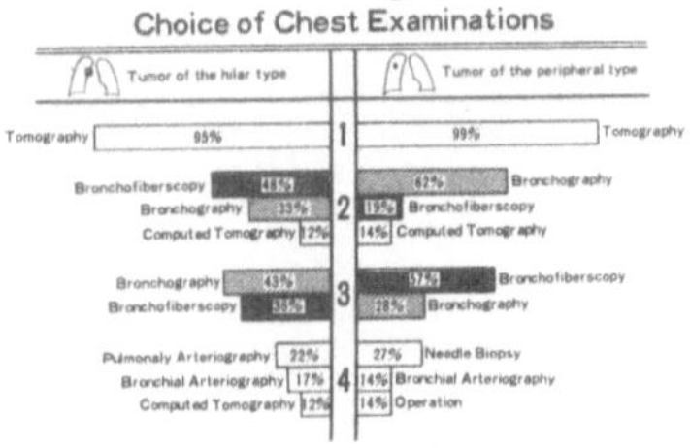

Choice of Chest Examinations

	Tumor of the hilar type	Tumor of the peripheral type	
Tomography	95%	99%	Tomography
	Bronchofiberscopy 44% Bronchography 33% Computed Tomography 22%	47% Bronchography 19% Bronchofiberscopy 14% Computed Tomography	2
	Bronchography 43% Bronchofiberscopy 35%	17% Bronchofiberscopy 17% Bronchography	3
	Pulmonary Arteriography 22% Bronchial Arteriography 17% Computed Tomography	27% Needle Biopsy 14% Bronchial Arteriography 14% Operation	4

Fig. 7

4. CONCLUSION

1. In Japan, bronchography is used mainly in the study of lung cancer and of bronchiectasis. Especially in peripheral lesions, performing bronchography before bronchofiberscopy permits a precise localization of the lesion, and increases accuracy of diagnosis.

2. Bronchography is used for localization of the tumor, examination of the extent and the pathological type of the lesion. In Japan usually a precise preoperative diagnosis of the lesion is requested, and bronchography is carried out for this purpose.

3. The incidence of fatal accidents during the examination is 1.4 in 10,000 studies and that of other non-fatal accidents is 79 in 10,000 examinations. Therefore, it can be stated that bronchography is a safe procedure if a due precaution is observed.

4. In order to minimize the discomfort to the patients, selective bronchography is preferable.

5. In spite of a wide spread use of CT-scanning bronchography remains to be a valuable diagnostic armamentarium except for extrapulmonary lesion such as mediastinal tumor or extrapleural lesion.

REFERENCES
1. Ikeda, S.: Atlas of Flexible Bronchofiberscopy (Igaku Shoin, Tokyo 1974).
2. Ono, R. and Ikeda, S.: Diagnosis of early lung cancer by applying the bronchography. Lung Cancer 15: 319-330 (1975).

V.2.

COURSE OF BRONCHOGRAPHY FROM 1959 TO 1979 IN A DEPARTMENT OF CHEST
DISEASE

J. ENGEL, FRG

From 1959 to 1979, 2414 bronchographies were performed in the Pneumolo-
gical Department of Harburg General Hospital. In relation to the
23,666 bronchoscopies performed during the same period, the percentage
of bronchographies to bronchoscopies decreased rapidly from an initial
94% to a nearly constant final 5%.

Thus, at the beginning of the observation period, bronchographies
were hardly more rarely performed than bronchoscopies. Both operations
were performed at the time in one session under local anesthetic. Apparently bronchography was regarded without much reflection as a more
or less compulsory supplementation to bronchoscopy. The objective was
not only a representation of the bronchial tree extended to the periphery beyond the limitations of what was discernible by bronchoscopy,
which would have been understandable. Rather, records of old examinations show that even the bronchoscopic discovery of central occlusions
of the bronchi was no obstacle to subsequent bronchography. Thus, although the usefulness of the examination to the patient was not always
correctly assessed in our view today, the hazards of anesthesia and/or
contrast media and of impairment in lung function were evidently nonetheless adequately considered. In any case, there was only one serious,
but not fatal contrast medium complication during the entire period;
there were no other complications. A retrospective analysis of the
reasons for the examinations reveals that the detection of cancer was
by far the most frequent, followed by tuberculosis and bronchiectasis.

With the introduction of general anesthesia as standard practice,
the number of bronchoscopies increased at an even rate to twelve times
the initial figure. The number of patients also rose by 61% as compared
to the 1959 figure. An increase in the amount of work with almost the
same labor force is always a reason to review the value of specific
items in the diagnostic procedure. The fact that bronchography lost
ground in favor of other examination procedures, however, is more a
reflection of increasing experience, which led to a restriction to definitive indication, as compared to earlier attempts to apply broncho-

graphy to as many diseases as possible, even those which may have been
less suited to it. Thus the fact was taken into account that direct
inspection, biopsy - including cytology - and bacteriology are usually
of greater significance to the detection of bronchopulmonary ailments
than contrast x-rays of bronchi and drained cavities.

Today we use bronchography routinely for diagnosing supperation
in which we suspect bronchiectasis and for etiologically unclear bleeding which can be located bronchoscopically, the latter with varying
degrees of success. We think that bronchography can nearly always be
dispensed with in diagnosing cancer. We find contrast representation
useful in shrinkage processes under pleural thickening, in post-tuber-
cular syndromes, in alterations after delayed removal of foreign bodies,
in deformations of the bronchial system and occasionally in the detection of major bullae. Finally, it is also useful in confirming the
success of therapeutic cavity fillings, e.g. in the case of inoperable
aspergillom. We have no experience with inhalation bronchography.

Bronchography enthusiasts will surely be able to refine the method further in areas outside of this pragmatic program. In diagnostics
of peripheral bronchial cancer selective bronchography, possibly in
combination with radiological brush biopsy, competes with the usual
bioptic methods of pneumology. As of present, however, we are not
convinced that bronchography shortens the path to the therapeutic objective as compared to endoscopic procedures, perthoracal needle biopsy
and, finally, thoracotomy.

Judging from the number of publications, there has been little
news lately from the field of bronchography. This does not, however,
mean that it is outmoded or old-fashioned. Rather, after initial over-
emphasis it has consolidated on a level on which usefulness, labor
output and possible hazards are in relatively good balance. Its field
of application is most likely found in the gap between bronchoscopy
and tomography. Inhalation bronchography with tantalum is not yet
part of routine diagnostics, to say nothing of that using crypton or
xenon in combination with computer tomography. Only the future will
show how much genuine progress will be made in these areas.

V.3.

SIGNIFICANCE OF PERIPHERAL BRONCHOGRAPHY ON COIN LESION

RYOSUKE ONO, M.D. AND SHIGETO IKEDA, M.D.

The findings peculiar to lung cancer can be obtained by the sufficiently precise and selective bronchography of the peripheral bronchus. These findings are especially important in lung cancer of the lung field type. For this purpose, the authors developed a flexible bronchial catheter.

Since the tip of this catheter is very flexible, it can be inserted easily and certainly, by X-ray fluoroscopy, into the bronchi throughout the region to produce precise images of the peripheral bronchus.

In order to obtain more precise and detail images of the peripheral bronchus, bronchography at 4-fold magnification was carried out using a microfocus of 50 microns. This apparatus was also connected to commonly used X-ray T.V. apparatus to facilitate the transportation of patients and the performance of bronchography. Consequently, it can be used easily even in precise X-ray diagnosis, such as bronchography of the peripheral bronchus; moreover, magnified images can be obtained even in the course of pressurized injection into the lesion bronchus.

In this study, 65 peripheral lung cancer cases which had undergone surgical excision of lung cancer with a tumor diameter of not more than 3 cm (45 adeno-carcinoma cancer cases and 20 squamous cell cancer cases) were studied by this very precise selective bronchography, and comparative studies were made with 30 pulmonary tuberculoma cases, 17 hamartoma cases and 10 sclerosing hemangioma cases. Bronchographic findings were classified according to the Ikeda classification.

In the analysis of bronchographic findings of adenomatous cancer, the lesion bronchus can be detected first as the image of a tapering obstruction, and cases where only one lesion bronchus exists are very rare. Usually several lesion bronchi are noted in the spread of lesions over the segments and subsegments.

Secondly, the lesion bronchi group toward the center of the tumor in a tapering shape to form the image of convergence of peripheral bronchi. Thirdly, the rami in front of the drainage-bronchus are sometimes reproduced in the film, to form so-called peripheral bronchial images.

In the analysis of bronchographic findings of squamous cell cancer, the lesion bronchus can be detected first as the image of a tapering obstruction,

J.A. Nakhosteen and W. Maassen (eds.), Bronchology: Research, Diagnostic and Therapeutic Aspects. All rights reserved.
Copyright 1981. Martinus Nijhoff Publishers bv, The Hague / Boston / London

sharp cut-off obstruction or irregular obstruction. Usually only one lesion bronchus exists when the tumor is less than 2 cm in diameter. Secondly, the tumor shows destructive advancement against the structure of the lung. Reaching the wall of the adjacent bronchus, it infiltrates through the wall to cause tapering or irregular obstruction according to the stage of advancement. Thirdly, since the tumor itself shows active multiplication crowding the surrounding lung parenchyma, the lesion bronchi do not group toward the tumor to produce the image of convergence of peripheral bronchi, and neither deviation nor spreadingout is observed.

In the analysis of bronchographic findings of pulmonary tuberculoma, the tuberculous lesion is often surrounded by the lesions of infiltration in the early stage, which are then encapsulated to form an encapsulated caseous lesion. Shrinkage of the tissue is induced around the tuberculous lesion in most cases, but convergence of peripheral bronchi usually occurs to a slight extent because inflammation spreads to the pleura. In addition, inflammation spreads toward the hilum of the lung, often causing fibrosis and convergence of bronchi in the hilum. The drainage-bronchus dilates and reveals sharp cut-off obstruction with the absence of ramification of bronchi, depending upon the lesion size.

There are many benign lung tumors which should be differentiated from lung cancer. Among such tumors, sclerosing hemangioma and hamartoma are clinically experienced in relatively high numbers. These tumors often develop in the peripheral lung parenchyma near the pluera and are sometimes present with no relation to the bronchus. They occasionally push off the bronchus to a slight extent, but it is rare for the bronchus to undergo tumor invasion. In the bronchographic findings relating to them, smooth stenosis and snaking are noted. In addition, they sometimes exist independently of bronchial images.

In the bronchographic findings of adenomatous cancer obtained at 4-fold magnification, the shape of the lesion bronchus, especially the drainage part, is detected as the image of tapering or irregular obstruction according to the stage of advancement, though it has been so far believed to reveal only tapering obstruction. In the case of tapering obstruction, the tapering part of the tumor shows dilatation. The surrounding bronchioles group toward the tumor in a tapering shape without dilatation.

In the bronchographic findings of squamous cell cancer obtained at 4-fold magnification, the shape of the lesion bronchus appears in the form of irregular obstruction because of the exposed tumor. The surrounding bronchioles are pushed off by the lesion and cause tapering involvement at the margin of the tumor.

In the bronchographic findings concerning pulmonary tuberculoma obtained at 4-fold magnification, the shape of the drainage-bronchus sometimes reveals tapering obstruction depending upon the lesion size, though it has been so far believed to reveal sharp cut-off obstruction with dilatation and absence of ramification of bronchi. The surrounding bronchioles disappear or dilate, showing spreadingout.

In the bronchographic findings relating to benign tumors in the lung obtained at 4-fold magnification, the bronchioles are free from invasion and dilatation, but are pushed off and show stenosis.

CONCLUSION

1) Selective peripheral bronchography was carried out at 4-fold magnification and peripheral mass images were analyzed.

2) In adenomatous cancer, tapering obstruction is noted and the tapering part in the tumor shows the appearance of dilatation. Convergence of peripheral bronchi is not noted toward the tumor. Cases in which only one lesion bronchus exists are very rare, and usually several lesion bronchi are observed. It was also demonstrated that the surrounding bronchioles group toward the tumor in a tapering shape.

3) In squamous cell cancer, the part of drainage does not show the image of dilatation, but shows that of irregular obstruction. The surrounding bronchioles do not show convergence of peripheral bronchi, but are pushed off by the lesion and make tapering involvement.

4) In pulmonary tuberculoma, sharp cut-off obstruction is revealed and there is space between the lesion and the site of obstruction. Dilatation and absence of ramification of bronchi are also observed. The surrounding bronchi show convergence of bronchi in the hilum. The bronchi assume dilatation and absence of ramification of bronchi, and the bronchioles are seen to disappear.

5) In benign tumors in the lung, stenosis due to push-off is noted. The lesion bronchi do not group toward the tumor. The bronchioles appear, showing the appearance of snaking.

V.4.

TRACHEOBRONCHIAL TUBERCULOSIS DIAGNOSED BY BRONCHOSCOPY AND BRONCHOGRAPHY

T. KURASAWA, F. KUZE, M. NAKANISHI, N. MAEKAWA, K. OIDA, T. IWATA AND
Y. ODA

1. INTRODUCTION

Although the number of cases in Japan has been distinctly decreased in
recent years, pulmonary tuberculosis is still a very important bronchopulmonary
infection due to its considerable incidence.

Particularly, the tracheobronchial tuberculosis should be dealt with serious
consideration as to its differentiation from other conditions and also to its
complications during and after treatment.

2. MATERIALS AND RESULTS

For the last six years, twenty seven cases in total, 7 male and 20 female
whose ages were between 21 to 78 years, were diagnosed as tracheobronchial tuberculosis by flexible fiberbronchoscopy (FFB) and bronchography (BG).
Persistent cough, wheezing, dyspnea and chest discomfort were presenting symptoms
in most of the cases.

The main findings of chest roentgenograms on admission showed atelectasis in
15 cases, pulmonary infiltration in 7, cavitary lesion in 3, and no detectable
lesions in P-A chest X-ray in 2 cases.

The main sites of affected lesion on FFB were 1) trachea in 4 cases, 2)
right bronchi in 13 and left bronchi in 10 and   The findings of FFB
were 1) edematous-hyperemic type in 2 cases, 2) infiltrative-proliferative type
in 9, 3) ulcerative-granurative type in 4, 4) fibrostenotic type in 12, according
to Ono's classification reported in 1950.   Additional bronchography was
performed in twenty one cases, which demonstrate total bronchial obstruction in
15 cases, bronchial stenosis in 3 and poststenotic bronchial dilatation in 3.

Thirteen cases among 23 showed positive of smears and/or cultures in their
sputum specimens before FFB and BG procedures, however, in 6 cases tubercle
bacilli were found only in specimens at the time of bronchoscopy and/or in
postbronchoscopy specimens. Six cases among 11 who were submitted to tracheobronchial biopsy, showed histpathological findings compatible with tuberculosis in the histologic section.

3. DISCUSSION

The tracheobronchial tuberculosis has posed still a diagnostic problem here

*J.A. Nakhosteen and W. Maassen (eds.), Bronchology: Research, Diagnostic and
Therapeutic Aspects. All rights reserved.*
Copyright 1981. Martinus Nijhoff Publishers bv, The Hague / Boston / London

in Japan. We are able to recognise it with pulmonary tuberculosis for the most, but the disease is apt to be overlooked mainly due to a rapid increase of bronchogenic carcinoma, which shows rather similar appearance on FFB and BG procedures. P-A chest X-ray shows no detectable changes at times and very often atelectasis is only abnormal findings.

All suspected patients should be submitted to FFB with brushing and biopsy procedures for the confirmation of final diagnosis.

These procedures are the only definitive way which leads us to the correct differential diagnosis of the disease from bronchogenic carcinoma, bronchial asthma and other respiratory diseases.

Tracheobronchial tuberculosis often results in stenosis and obstruction of the affected bronchus due to cicatrization during antituberculous chemotherapy and it gives rise to atelectasis, from which ensues obstructive penumonia, bronchiectasis and so on.

During and after treatment, careful follow up of the patients are mandatory to these complications, surgical intervention should be seriously considered on the bases of carefully performed bronchography and meticulous assessment of pulmonary function as well as general condition.

4. SUMMARY

1) Twenty seven cases of tracheobronchial tuberculosis were discussed. On chest roentgenogram, fifteen cases showed pulmonary atelectasis, which was the most common findings in our cases.

2) FFB is the most useful and indispensable diagnostic technique for tracheobronchial tuberculosis. Careful follow up of the cases during and after treatment with FFB is also necessary.

3) Bronchography is indicated for the assessment of the extent as well as the grade of the intrabronchial disease, particularly in decision as to the indication of surgical treatment and for choosing a surgical procedure.

5. REFERENCES

1) A. Haruhara: Kokenshi 14: 438, 1960
2) S. Awataguchi: J.JPN Bronchoesophagolog. soc. 24: 251, 1973
3) JS. Bower, et al: Amer. Rev. Pulm. Dis. 119: 677, 1979
4) A. Nakashima et al: Jap. Jour. chest Dis. 38: 202, 1979
5) D.J. Pierson et al: CHEST. 64: 537, 1973

V.5.

CLINICAL EXAMINATION OF BRONCHIAL TUBERCULOSIS AS DISTINGUISHED FROM LUNG
CANCER

A. Sato and K. Yoshimura

1. INTRODUCTION

The tubercular lesion of the bronchus has long been studied from various points
of view.[1] With the recent increase of lung cancer, the differential diagnosis of
bronchial tuberculosis from lung cancer has become necessary. We conducted clinical
examinations of bronchial tuberculosis in cases which could not be easily distinguished from lung cancer by chest x-ray.

2. MATERIAL AND METHODS

Examinations involving screening of patients, clinical symptoms, chest roentgenographic findings, bronchographic findings and bronchoscopic findings were performed in 11 cases of bronchial tuberculosis which closely resembled lung cancer on
the chest x-ray findings. Simultaneously, bronchial brushing was performed to
detect bacillus tuberculosis.

3. RESULTS

1) Age and sex: Patients consisted of 11 cases, 2 males and 9 females; their ages
   ranged from 20 to 81.
2) Screening of patients: 2 cases were identified from a mass survey and 9 cases
   from their symptoms.
3) Manifestation of clinical symptoms: 2 cases (12%) asymptomatic, 6 cases (35%)
   of paroxysmal cough, 3 cases (17%) of blood sputum, 2 cases (12%) of chest pain,
   and each 1 case (6%) of dyspnea, fever, sputum and cough.
4) Roentgenographic signs: 8 cases of atelectasis, 1 case of segmental infiltration,
   2 cases of deviation of mediastinum, 2 cases of unilateral hyperlucency, and 1
   case of unilateral change of hilum.
5) Bronchographic findings: The bronchographic findings are shown in Table 1.
   Contraction of the large bronchi and irregular obstruction of the small bronchi
   due to atrophy and stiffening of the lung lesion were different from those of
   lung cancer.
6) Bronchoscopic findings: The bronchoscopic findings are shown in Table 2.
   The direct findings demonstrated mainly scarring stenosis, and also granulomatous

J.A. Nakhosteen and W. Maassen (eds.), Bronchology: Research, Diagnostic and
Therapeutic Aspects. All rights reserved.
Copyright 1981. Martinus Nijhoff Publishers bv, The Hague / Boston / London

stenosis and superficial ulceration were found.

7) Bronchial brushing: 9 cases were positive to bacillus tuberculosis.

8) Prognosis: 10 cases received antituberculosis chemotherapy and 1 case which was negative to bacillus tuberculosis underwent operation. All of them had excellent prognoses.

Table 1   Bronchographic findings

Lesional bronchus	Cases	%
Irregular obstruction	8	45
Irregular stenosis	4	22
Proximal contraction	6	33
		100

Table 2   Bronchoscopic findings

Findings	Cases
Granulation	2
Ulcer	2
Engorgement of blood vessels	3
Irregular mucosa	4
Unclearness of the cartilage	1
Obstruction	2
Stenosis	7
Redness	4

DISCUSSION

The characteristics of bronchial tuberculosis observed by bronchography were proximal contraction of the large bronchi due to atrophy and stiffening caused by lung parenchyma disease and irregular obstruction of the peripheral bronchi instead of the sharp-pointed obstruction which is usually found in lung cancer. Scarring stenosis was the chief bronchoscopic finding. From the finding that the bronchial lesion developed consistently along the inner wall[2] the region of granulomatous ulceration was considered to be widespread. Though bronchography as well as broncho-scopy is useful in diagnosing both diseases, we think it more important to pay attention to the presence of paroxysmal cough and to the detection of bacillus tuberculosis.

References

1. Jones, R.S. and Alley, F.H.: Am. Rev. Tubercul. 63, 381, 1951
2. Macrae, D.M., Hiltz, J.E. and Quinlan, J.J.: Am. Rev. Tubercul. 61, 355, 1950

160

V.6.

Die Möglichkeiten der Bronchographien mit dem Fiberbronchoskop.

R. G. Reimann

1. Einleitung:

Im Anschluß an über 700 flexible transorale oder transnasale
Bronchoskopien in Lokalanaesthesie wurden über 140 Bronchographien durchgeführt. Indikationen waren:
1. Die Feststellung des Schweregrades von Bronchiektasien.
2. Die Lokalisation von Tumoren im Bronchialbaum.
3. Die Darstellung von stenosierenden Bronchialprozesssen.

2. Methode:

Die flexible Bronchoskopie wurde in Lokalanaesthesie mit Nove-
sine 1 %ig ohne eingelegten Trachealtubus bei direkter Sondierung
des Kehlkopfes durchgeführt. Im Anschluß an die Bronchoskopie,
bei der evtl. histologische Proben entnommen wurden, wurde Kontrastmittel, Dianosyl, direkt durch den Instrumentierkanal in den
gewählten Segment bzw. Subsegmentbronchus eingespritzt. Der Patient wurde während des Eingebens des Kontrastmittels aufgefor-
dert, tief ein- und auszuatmen. Dadurch wurde ein gleichmäßiger
Schleimhautbeschlag durch das Kontrastmittel erzeugt. (Abb. 1).
Die Bronchogramme erreichen nahezu Doppeltkontrastqualität und
sind dadurch aussagekräftiger. Auch Volumeneinengung der Bronchien durch stenosierende Bronchialcarcinome sind in der Darstellung des Doppeltkontrast deutlicher festzustellen (Abb. 2).
Da Bronchiektasen schlechter als das übrige Bronchialsystem be-
lüftet sind, erfolgt der Abfluß des Kontrastmittels erschwert.
Sie stellen sich deshalb in aller Regel als Kontrastmitteldepots
(Abb. 3) dar. Die Zuordnung von Tumoren im Thoraxbereich zum
Bronchialsystem ist durch die Bronchographie eindeutig möglich.
Das nachfolgende Bild (Abb. 4) zeigt einen Riesenzelltumor
links thorakal in Verdrängung des Bronchialsystems.

J.A. Nakhosteen and W. Maassen (eds.), Bronchology: Research, Diagnostic and
Therapeutic Aspects. All rights reserved.
Copyright 1981. Martinus Nijhoff Publishers bv, The Hague / Boston / London

Zusammenfassend läßt sich feststellen:

Der Einsatz von Fiberbronchoskopen erweitert nicht nur die Möglichkeit der therapeutischen und diagnostischen Bronchoskopie, sondern er verbessert auch die Möglichkeit der Bronchographie. Die Bronchogramme zeigen bei guter technischer Durchführung nahezu Doppeltkontrastqualität. Bei über 140 Bronchographien wurden Komplikationen von seiten des Patienten ebenso nicht festgestellt wie Beschädigungen des Instrumentes.

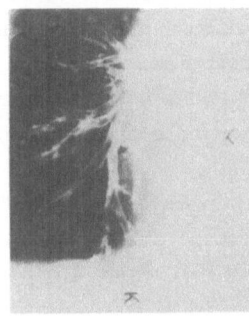 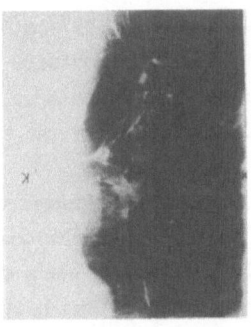

Abb.1.Bronchogramm re. Lunge: Ohne pathologischen

Abb.2. Bronchogramm li. Lunge: Beginnendes stenosierendes Bronchialcarcinom am Abgang des li. Unterlappens.

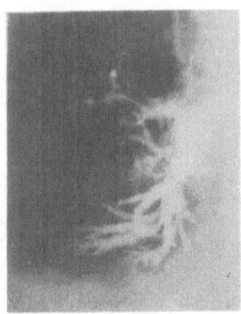 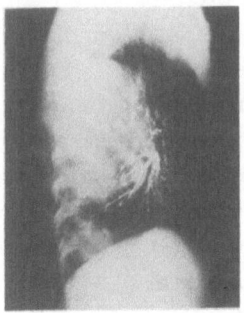

Abb.3.Bronchogramm re. Lunge: Hochgradige zylindrische Bronchiektasien im re. Unterlappen.

Abb.4.Bronchogramm li. Lunge: Aufnahme seitlich, Riesenzelltumor li. thorakal mit Veränderung des Bronchialsystems.

V.7.

SELECTIVE BRONCHOGRAPHY AND TRANSBRONCHIAL BIOPSY

E. Matsui, H. Miyake, S. Yanagawa, M. Shibayama and H. Doi.

The purpose of this paper is to evaluate the diagnostic usefulness of selective bronchography and transbronchial biopsy(TBB). TBB combined with selective broncho-graphy was performed in 1237 patients with localized or diffuse pulmonary diseases.

Metras' catheter was modified for this procedure. We recommend the use of various flexible forceps which were adopted to the Olympus GF and Machida FGS fiberscopes. Under x-ray TV control, TBB was performed immediately after selective bronchography through the same catheter.

Sufficient biopsy specimen was obtained by this method in 690 out of 977 localized lung disease(70.1%) and in 140 out of 164 diffuse lung disease(85.4%). (Table-1).

Bronchographic findings were compaired with the histological examination as the characteristic radiographic findings.

Epidermoid carcinomas presented irregular or cut-off obstructions and irregular margins of the bronchi. A significant features of the adenocarcinomas were tapered obstructions or stenosis of the bronchi and somewhat convergence of the neighbouring bronchi surrounding the foci.

As the distinguished pathologic evidence, small cell carcinoma demonstrated smooth narrowings of the larger bronchi, and large cell carcinoma showed dislocation of the bronchi and loss of arbolization as the characteristic features.

Significant findings of tuberculoma were radish root shaped obstruction and crowded bronchi. Chronic pneumonia presented crowded retracted bronchi and penetration of the bronchi within the radioopacity as the characteristic features.

Table 1. 1237 cases examined by selective bronchography and transbronchial biopsy

Diagnosis		No. of Cases
Localized lesion		977
None or insufficient tissue		32
Positive diagnosis		690(70.6%)
Carcinoma	414	
Non-specific inflammation	160	
Tuberculosis	47	
Metastasis	14	
Lymphoma	3	
Aspergillosis	1	
Thymoma	1	
Others	50	
Negative or incomplete follow-up		255
Diffuse lesion		164
None or insufficient tissue		24
Satisfactory tissue		140(85.4%)
Interstitial pneumonitis	49	
Pneumoconiosis	30	
Sarcoidosis	20	
Normal alveoli	15	
Collagen disease	12	
Berylliosis	5	
Lymphangiosis carcinomatosa	4	
Bronchiolitis	3	
Miliary tuberculosis	2	
COPD		96
Insufficient tissue		14
Satisfactory tissue		71
Normal tissue	11	
Total		1237

J.A. Nakhosteen and W. Maassen (eds.), Bronchology: Research, Diagnostic and Therapeutic Aspects. All rights reserved.
Copyright 1981. Martinus Nijhoff Publishers bv, The Hague / Boston / London

Morphological characteristics of the peripheral bronchi in diffuse pulmonary diseases were clearly demonstrated by the selective bronchography.

As complications of this method, among 1237 patients one death and two brisk hemorrhage were observed. The other complications were minimal. Only one slight pneumothorax was encountered. Selective bronchography made us easy to insert the biopsy forceps deep enough into the focus at the periphery bronchus and to get a safe distance from the visceral pleura. (Table-2).

Case-1; Small peripheral adenocarcinoma, selective bronchography demonstrated tapered obstruction of the left B5a and retraction of the neighbouring peripheral bronchi(left B4b). (Fig. 1-a). Under the guidance of selective bronchography, the biopsy forceps may easily reach to the area of carcinoma. (Fig. 1-b).

Table-2.   Complications

	No. of Cases
Hemoptysis	
Massive(500ml)	2
Moderate(25-100ml)	9
Pneumothorax	1
Death	1
Fever	ca.40% of patients.
Lidocaine reaction	0

Histologically TBB specimen was disclosed as a well differentiated adenocarcinoma with fibrosis.

Case-2; Sarcoidosis. Under the guidance of selective bronchography, the biopsy forceps inserted deeply into the periphery bronchus without any anxiety and may keep a safe distance from the visceral pleura. (Fig-2).

TBB revealed sarcoid nodules among alveoli.

Conclusion

Then, we would like to emphasize that the selective bronchography is quite valuable for the diagnosis of localized and diffuse lung diseases. In addition, selective broncho-graphy is also essential, as a guide of transbronchial biopsy, especially for peripheral localized lesions and diffuse pulmonary diseases.

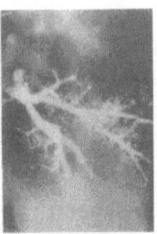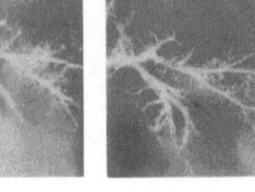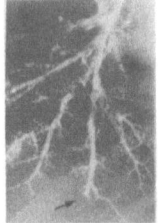

Fig. 1-a   Fig. 1-b   Fig-2

➹ : Biopsy forceps

References

1) Andersen H.A. : Transbronchoscopic Lung Biopsy for Diffuse Pulmonary Diseases. Results in 939 patients. Chest 73 : 734-736, 1978.

2) Matsui E.,Miyake H. et al. : Transbronchial Lung Biopsy via Metra's catheter for Diffuse Pulmonary Disease. Bronchoscopy WCB, Tokyo : 929-32, 1978.

3) Matsui E., Miyake H. et al. : Transbronchial Lung Biopsy. Lung & Heart 25 : 179-190, 1978.

4) Pinet F. et al. : Selective Bronchography and Bronchial Brushing. Springer-Verlag, Berlin, Heidelberg, New York, 1979.

5) Herf S.M. and Suratt P.M. : Complications of Transbronchial Lung Biopsies. Chest 73 : 759-760, 1978.

V.8.

A NEW TECHNIQUE OF BRONCHOGRAPHY & ITS CLINICAL APPLICATION

REURY-PERNG PERNG, CHAO-TO HSING,

1. INTRODUCTION

Conventional technique of bronchography, not only time-consuming, difficult to manipulate but also over-exposure to radiation, caused more discomfort to the patient. For improving these shortcomings of conventional technique we developed a new technique in 1977.

2. TECHNIQUE

The whole procedures are as follows:

Step 1: Preparation of patient and premedication

Step 2: Local anesthesia with Xylocaine

Step 3: Bronchofiberscopy

Step 4: Insertion of bronchocatheter under the guidance of bronchofiberscope and floroscope

Step 5: Injection of contrast medium

Step 6: Taking of X-ray films

3. CLINICAL APPLICATION

From 1977 to 1978 a total of 387 patients were examined by this new technique. It consisted of 91 out-patients and 296 in-patients. The age distribution was from 13 to 79 Y/O. The clinical indications and diagnostic yield from the examination are summarized in Table 1.

TABLE 1: Clinical indications and diagnostic yield

Indications	No.	%	Yield(%)
1. Suspected bronchiectasis	169	43.7	75.7
2. Localization of abnormal shadow	80	20.7	73.7
3. Hemoptysis of unknown causes	54	13.9	38.9
4. Chronic infiltration of lung	36	9.3	41.7
5. Preoperative evaluation	16	4.1	100.0

6. Right middle lobe syndrome	12	3. 1	75. 0
7. Chronic cough of unknown causes	10	2. 6	0. 0
8. Congenital anormaly	1	0. 2	100. 0
9. Others	9	2. 3	22. 2
Total	387	100. 0	64. 9

4. COMPLICATIONS

No major complications occurred in the total examined patients. But 33.8% of the patients developed fever after the examination.

5. DISCUSSION

This new technique has 3 characteristics which are different from conventional technique. a) Flexible bronchocatheter b) Combined with bronchofiberscopy c) Insertion of bronchocatheter is guided by the bronchofiberscope. Because of guidance of bronchofiberscope the insertion of the catheter is very easy. The patient's neck does not need to take any special position. The angulation of the tip of the catheter could be controlled voluntarily. And so selective bronchogram could be taken properly.

We perform bronchofiberscopy prior to the procedure of bronchography. This additional examination could give 3 advantages to the whole procedure. a) Additional anesthesia could be applied b) Clearing of secretions and blood clots c) Recording abnormal changes in the bronchial trees. With a satisfactory anesthesia good films could be obtained. Bronchography combined with bronchofiberscopy could give us more information about the pathological change and got higher diagnostic yield from this examination.

In summary, this new technique has the following advantages:
a) Satisfactory local anesthesia b) Easy insertion of bronchocatheter c) Selective bronchogram can be taken d) Time-saving e) Safe f) Good film can be gotten g) High diagnostic yield h) Reduce patient's discomfort to a minimal.

REFERENCE

1. Perng RP, Tsai CM, Hsing CT: A new technique of bronchography. Chinese J. Radiol. 4:87-94, 1979.
2. Ikeda S, Ono R: Selective bronchography and bronchio-alveolography. Internal Medicine, 37:955-962, 1976.

V.9.

USEFULLNESS OF BRONCHOGRAPHY – WITH SPECIAL EMPHASIS ON DELINEATION OF
MUCOSAL CHANGES OF THE LARGE BRONCHUS –

K. KIMURA, Y. OHSAKI, S. ABE, Y. TSUNETA, H. MIKAMI AND M. MURAO

INTRODUCTION

Bronchography is exculusively utilized for demonstration of distortion of airway anatomy. Usual findings of the bronchography, therefore, are dilated,
stenosed, or obstructed lesions of the bronchial structure.
No attention has been paid until recently to the delineation of mucosal changes
of the large bronchi with usual bronchographic examination.
We tasted and succeeded in demonstating the minute tumor-forming lesions of
the bronchial mucous membrane with our special technique. Furthermore, we
demonstrated its usefulness by model experiment.

METHOD OF BRONCHOGRAPHY

Metras catheter was inserted through the mouth under local anesthesia.
A small amount of contrast media was poured through the catheter, which was
positioned proximally to the lesion. By ordering the patient to take several
deep breaths, the contrast media was expanded on the lesion as this as possible. We called this method light coating bronchography.

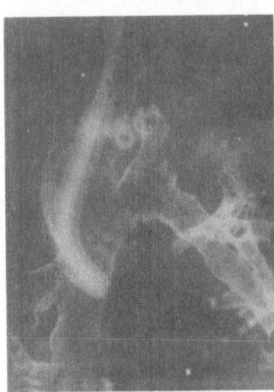

Fig. 1

CASE No. 1

A fifty-nine year old male. Final diagnosis: squamous cell carcinoma.
By our bronchography, the lesion was clearly delineated as a clover-leaf
shaped appearance with irregular margin in enface position. (Fig.1)

J.A. Nakhosteen and W. Maassen (eds.), Bronchology: Research, Diagnostic and
Therapeutic Aspects. All rights reserved.
Copyright 1981. Martinus Nijhoff Publishers bv, The Hague / Boston / London

Bronchoscopy revealed easily hemorrhagic mucosal prominence of the anterior aspect of the left upper lobe bronchus. Contrary to the bronchographic picture, the margin of the tumor is not able to be observed clearly in the broncho-scopic photograph.

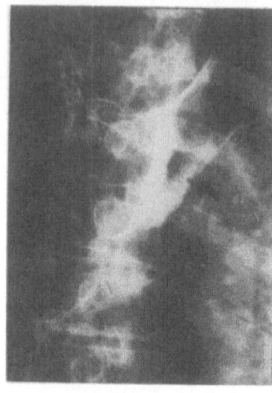

Fig. 2

CASE No. 2

A sixty year old, male. Final diagnosis: inflammatory granuloma of the bron-chial mucous membrane from unknown cause. Bronchoscopic examination revealed a small pin-head polyp-like tumor formation in the lower aspect of the right main bronchus. By bronchographic examination, its prominence was well deline-ated in enface. (Fig. 2)

CASE No. 3

A forty-five year old male. Final diagnosis: squamous cell carcinoma. Bronchoscopic examination revealed easily hemorrhagic small prominence at the base of the apico-anterior of the left upper lobe bronchus. By our broncho-graphy, the lesion was seen as a small defect at the base of the bronchus in profile.

CASE No. 4

A fifty-nine year old male. Chromate worker for 18 years. Final diagnosis: squamous cell carcinoma. Bronchoscopic examination revealed obstruction of the left lower lobe bronchous due to intra-luminal tumor formation. Accidentaly, polypoid tumor formation of the right upper lobe bronchous was detected, indi-cating multiple occurrence of bronchogenic carcinoma. The polypoid tumor was demonstrated as a small defect in profile by bronchography.

MODEL EXPERIMENT

We have done a model experiment to test the usefulness of our method. Small prominence, 0.5 x 0.5 cm in diameter with 0.3 mm prominence, was made in the inner side of a vinyl tube. When the contrast media completely filled the tube, the prominence was only delineated radiographically in profile. On the other hand, when the contrast media coated the inner surface of the tube as thin as possible, the prominence appeared clearly not only in enface but also in profile.

DISCUSSION

Bronchoscopic examination is a very useful method for the detection of bronchial lesion, however, it might be difficult to asses its extent, margin and transition from normal to abnormal mucous membrane changes. By our method, namely light coating bronchographic examination, as we just presented, very tiny mucosal lesions can be clearly delineated either in enface or in profile, so that this procedure can be utilized to examine mucosal changes of the bronchus. We would like to conclude by saying that the indication of bronchography should be expanded not only for demonstration of bronchial anatomy but also for mucosal changes of the bronchi.

Chapter VI
SARCOIDOSIS

VI.1.

BRONCHO-ALVEOLAR LAVAGE(BAL) IN 120 PATIENTS WITH SARCOIDOSIS:CELLU-
LAR DATA AND RELATION WITH SERUM ANGIOTENSIN CONVERTING ENZYME(SACE)

A. ARNOUX, G. STANISLAS-LEGUERN, C. DANEL, J. MARSAC, G. HUCHON,
C. FABRE, R. DUFAT, J. CHRETIEN.

The aim of the present study was to assess the information which
could be drawn from the results of BAL performed on 120 patients
with sarcoidosis, with respect to diagnostic and prognostic.

1.MATERIELS AND METHODS

1.1. Selection of patients.

    The diagnosis of sarcoidosis was established according to the
usual criteria (1). According to their chest X ray abnormalities,
the patients were distributed in 48 Stage I(bilateral hilar lymphadenopathy), 55 Stage II (pulmonary infiltrates with or without hilar lymphadenopathy) and 13 Stage III (mostly fibrosis pattern).23%
were smokers.Nine patients underwent BAL after they had recovered
a normal chest X ray. The results were compared with those obtained
in 16 healthy subjects (8 smokers and 8 non smokers).

1.2. Methods.

    The methods used for BAL and cellular analysis have been pre-
viously published (2).SACE was measured according to Cushman and
Cheung's method (3) modified by Lieberman (4,5).

1.3. Statistical analysis.

    All the results were expressed as a mean ± SEM, mean values were
compared using Student't test analysis.

2. RESULTS

    As it is well known that the smoking habits of subjects (2,6)
play an important role on the cellular results of BAL, the patients
were divided into smokers and non-smokers. When the results of BAL
were compared between controls and sarcoidosis patients, no difference appeared in the recovery of infused fluid (60 ± 4% vs 53 ± 2%
respectively), nor for the total cell yield (40 ± 5 x 10^6 vs 50 ± 3
x 10^6). On table I, the cell recovery was compared between sarcoidosis and controls, a significant increase of cells recovered per

J.A. Nakhosteen and W. Maassen (eds.), Bronchology: Research, Diagnostic and
Therapeutic Aspects. All rights reserved.
Copyright 1981. Martinus Nijhoff Publishers bv, The Hague / Boston / London

ml of fluid was found only in non-smoker patients compared to non
smoker controls.

TABLE I - Cell recovery in BAL fluid of sarcoidosis and control
subjects.

		NON SMOKERS		SMOKERS	
		Controls n=8	Sarcoidosis n=92	Controls n=8	Sarcoidosis n=28
Number of cells (x 10)/ml fluid		143 ± 27	304 ± 20	323 ± 50	448 ± 48
		p < 0.001		N.S.	
Macrophage Recovery	Per cent	82 ± 9	62 ± 2	97 ± 1	75 ± 3
		p < 0.001		p < 0.001	
	10 /ml	130 ± 25	165 ± 9	350 ± 50	360 ± 40
		N.S.		N.S.	
Lymphocyte Recovery	Per cent	10 ± 2	35 ± 2	2 ± 0.5	24 ± 3
		p < 0.001		p < 0.001	
	10 /ml	15 ± 6	120 ± 13	6 ± 2	105 ± 23
		p < 0.001		p < 0.001	

When the recovered cells were expressed in percentage, a significant decrease of macrophages appeared in sarcoidosis,in non smokers as well as in smokers. Consequently, lymphocytes were significantly increased in sarcoid patients. However, when the macrophage
and lymphocyte recovery were expressed in number of cell per ml,the
lymphocyte population,was significantly increased in BAL of sarcoidosis patients. These alveolar lymphocytes were identified as T
lymphocytes by the E rosette test. Compared to their own blood,sar-
coidosis patients had a high level of T lymphocytes in their lung
(66 ± 1% vs 85 ± 1% respectively p < 0.001).

The radiological stage of sarcoidosis did not affect any of
the following BAL parameters: the total cell yield, the cell number
recovered by ml of fluid, the macrophage or lymphocyte recovery
(% or per ml).

When the number of involved organs was correlated with the
lymphocytes (% or per ml), a good relationship was found between
the clinical extrathoracic dissemination of the disease, and the
alveolar lymphocytosis (r = 0.5, n = 100, p < 0.001). A good cor-

relation was also found between alveolar lymphocytosis and SACE particularly in non smoker sarcoidosis patients ($r = 0.5$, $n=84$, $p < 0.001$).

Alveolar lymphocytosis was significantly higher in BAL from patients who had granulomas in bronchial biopsies compared to patients with negative biopsies ($140 \pm 17 \times 10^3$ vs $50 \pm 8 \times 10^3$ Ly/ml $p < 0.001$). One the other hand, SACE was also higher in patients with bronchial granulomas (48 ± 3 u/ml vs 38 ± 2 u/ml, $0.01 < p < 0.02$) compared to patients with negative biopsies.

The data of BAL could be helpful to estimate the evolutivity of the disease, particularly in patients with a radiological fibrosis pattern. Thus, in patients with stage III sarcoidosis, we found a lower cell viability ($86 \pm 5\%$ vs $98 \pm 0.5\%$), significantly less lavage fluid recovered ($42 \pm 6\%$ vs $60 \pm 3\%$) and a significant increase of polymorphonuclear leucocytes ($11.5 \pm 3.7\%$ vs $1.3 \pm 0.2\%$) compared to controls ($p < 0.001$ respectively for each comparison). These results were similar to those obtained in 20 patients with idiopathic pulmonary fibrosis (6). The most striking feature in stage III sarcoidosis was the association of high levels of lymphocytes and polymorphonuclear leukocytes. On the contrary, in idiopathic pulmonary fibrosis, the lymphocyte level was not different from the control group.

BAL was performed in 9 patients after healing. The lymphocyte population showed no difference when compared to the controls.

Sixteen patients underwent two lavages. The second BAL was performed 6 to 18 months after the first. No difference in alveolar lymphocytosis was found in eight patients who had a clinical steady state ($106 \pm 23 \times 10^3$ vs $108 \pm 61 \times 10^3$ Ly/ml). Four patients underwent two BAL before and after healing: whereas the first BAL showed a significant raise in lymphocytosis, the second cell count was within the normal range .

In CONCLUSION, there are much more alveolar lymphocytes and especially T lymphocytes in sarcoidosis. The lymphocytosis is correlated with the clinical dissemination of the disease. A good correlation is found between SACE and alveolar lymphocytosis, that seem to be good criteria both for diagnosis and prognosis in sarcoidosis. For prognosis, it can be useful to repeat BAL in sarcoid patients until the patients recover normal alveolar lymphocytosis. The most important contribution of BAL is perhaps to follow up the patients and particularly to notice an evolution toward pulmonary fibrosis.

VI.2.

THE VALIDATION AND USE OF KVEIM TEST SUSPENSIONS

D.N. MITCHELL, J.R. MIKHAIL, M.W. McNICOL, J.V. COLLINS, D.M. MITCHELL,
M.W. DIGHERO

1. PREPARATION AND VALIDATION OF TEST SUSPENSIONS

Sarcoid spleens removed at operation for valid clinical indications provide the best available source for the provision of continued supplies of potentially satisfactory Kveim test material. Chase-Siltzbach type 1 suspensions (ref. 1) are prepared from deep-frozen splenic tissue either in sequential Lots of approximately 35g each or by processing the whole spleen. The former necessitates the validation of sequential Lots of test material whilst the latter assumes that all parts of the spleen will yield an acceptable test suspension and runs the risk that a portion of the spleen may impair a large volume of a suspension which may otherwise have proved satisfactory. In any event, less than one half of all potentially acceptable sarcoid spleens will provide suspensions which yield the expected proportion of positive reactions among patients at different stages of sarcoidosis and a negligible proportion among patients with other diseases. These acceptable suspensions should comprise fine splenic tissue particles which are evenly dispersible in suspension. The concentration of these tissue particles will usually range between 3.0 mg/ml - 6.0 mg/ml as measured by alcohol precipitable dry weight. The potency and selectivity of test suspensions can be assessed only by validation in man. The reactivity of a suspension is determined by comparison of papule size and histology with that of a simultaneous test using a previously validated suspension in patients with sarcoidosis. The selectivity of a suspension for sarcoidosis is ascertained by comparing the results of identical simultaneous tests in patients with diseases other than sarcoidosis. The histology must be read by an experienced observer who is unaware of the origin of the test suspensions or the nature of the subjects tested. Although test suspensions can usually be kept satisfactorily at $+4^{\circ}$C at least for several years, they should be monitored periodically to ensure that they have not lost either their reactivity or selectivity for sarcoidosis. When a large volume of acceptable test material has been prepared it is therefore usual to ampoule and store at $+4^{\circ}$C; alternatively, it could be freeze dried when it appears to retain its potency for long periods at room temperature (refs. 2,3,4,5,6,7).

J.A. Nakhosteen and W. Maassen (eds.), Bronchology: Research, Diagnostic and Therapeutic Aspects. All rights reserved.
Copyright 1981. Martinus Nijhoff Publishers bv, The Hague / Boston / London

2. USE OF TEST SUSPENSIONS

The results of Kveim tests made with 2 sequential Lots (Lots 19 and 22) of K12 and with 8 sequential Lots (Lots 6-13) of K19 issued from Colindale between 1971 and 1977 (refs. 8,9) are summarized below. Of 644 patients with histologically confirmed or clinically definite sarcoidosis of <2 years' known duration, 439 (68%) had positive tests. By contrast only 66 (47%) of 141 patients with sarcoidosis of >2 years standing yielded positive results. A similar pattern of results was obtained among 1035 patients in whom a diagnosis of sarcoidosis was considered probable (<2 years; 73% positive; >2 years 54% positive). Among 1777 patients in whom a diagnosis of sarcoidosis was considered doubtful 772 (43%) were positive. Overall, of 3597 patients tested 2015 (56%) yielded positive results.

Of 551 patients with Löfgren's syndrome, 464 (84%) had positive tests. Similarly, 71% of 1051 patients with stage I and 70% of 524 patients with stage II sarcoidosis had positive tests. By contrast only 34% of 737 patients with stage III disease, were positive.

There were 776 patients in whom a diagnosis of sarcoidosis was considered highly probable and who presented with extrathoracic lesions only. 28 (20%) of 143 patients presenting with uveitis and 72 (23%) of 319 patients with erythema nodosum had positive tests, whereas of 314 patients who presented with a variety of extrathoracic lesions other than uveitis or erythema nodosum, 109 (31%) were positive.

Of 440 patients who were given Kveim tests during the course of their investigation and in whom a diagnosis other than sarcoidosis was ultimately reached, only 4 had positive Kveim tests: this finding is highly relevant to the selectivity of these Kveim test materials.

3. COMPARISON OF THE RESULTS OF KVEIM TESTS WITH THOSE OF OTHER INVESTIGATIVE PROCEDURES

In a separate but consecutive series of 205 patients with probable sarcoidosis in whom mediastinoscopy was performed (in the absence of accessible tissue for biopsy) and who also had a Kveim test (see table), 167 (80%) had positive lymph node histology; of these, 11 had equivocal and 23 had negative Kveim tests. 133 patients (64%) had both positive lymph node and Kveim test histology. Of 18 patients from whom lymph node tissue was not obtained, 13 showed positive Kveim tests.

Transbronchial and/or bronchial mucosal biopsy and Kveim testing was also undertaken in a further consecutive series of 29 patients in whom a diagnosis of sarcoidosis was ultimately reached. 11 had a positive tissue biopsy (epithelioid and giant cell granulomas) and also had positive Kveim tests whilst 13 had a positive tissue biopsy with a negative (10) or equivocal (3) Kveim test. Of 5 who showed a negative histology following transbronchial and/or bronchial mucosal biopsy, 2 had a positive, 1 an equivocal and 2 a negative Kveim test.

4. SUMMARY AND CONCLUSIONS

The Kveim test using carefully validated test materials is a simple outpatient procedure which in the present context is highly selective for sarcoidosis because other conditions that sometimes yield reactive Kveim tests (refs. 12,13) are un-likely to be confused clinically with sarcoidosis. It has however the disadvantage of a delay of 4 weeks after injection of the test suspension before biopsy can yield meaningful results. Moreover, it is least likely to be of help in patients in whom the disease may have been present for a considerable period eg >2 years, and it is well recognised that such cases not infrequently present with pulmonary mottling only (stage III) and are often a clinical problem in the diagnosis of sarcoidosis.

A negative Kveim test diminishes the likelihood of sarcoidosis but slightly, and where histological support for the diagnosis of sarcoidosis is more urgently required recourse may be made to in-patient procedures such as biopsy of the bronchial mucosa and/or transbronchial biopsy through the fiberoptic bronchoscope, or to mediastinal lymph node biopsy by mediastinsocopy.

Mediastinoscopy should be carried out by an experienced thoracic surgeon. It yields lymph node tissue from which a histological diagnosis can be made in a high proportion (>80%) of cases (ref. 14). Transbronchial biopsy is not entirely without risk but is a simple procedure in experienced hands: although the rate of positive findings is higher among sarcoidosis patients with radiological evidence of pulmonary infiltration, it is also high (>60%) among patients with hilar lymphadenopathy whose chest radiographs show normal lung fields (ref. 15). The pieces obtained may however be unrepresentative or insufficient in size to allow of a satisfactory culture for the detection of acid-fast bacilli whereas mediastinoscopy does permit, additionally, the culture of otherwise inaccessible lymph node tissue for M. tuberculosis. The finding of epithelioid and giant cell granulomas in mediastinal lymph node tissue or in the lung does not necessarily confirm the diagnosis of sarcoidosis since it is recognised that many other conditions including tuberculosis, lymphoma or other malignant diseases, berylliosis, brucellosis, extrinsic allergic alveolitis, histoplasmosis, collagen disorders and antibody deficiency syndromes can produce this type of change (ref. 14).

TABLE. Assessments of mediastinal lymph node and Kveim test biopsies in 205 patients with probable sarcoidosis

		Mediastinoscopy			
		Positive	Negative	Failed	Total
Kveim test	Positive	133(64%)	8	13	154
	Equivocal	11	3	1	15
	Negative	23	9	4	36
	Total	167(80%)	20	18	205

VI.3.

RESULTS OF DIFFERENT BIOPSIES IN SARCOIDOSIS (MEDIASTINOSCOPY, DANIELS'
BIOPSY, BRONCHIAL AND LUNG BIOPSIES)

D. GRESCHUCHNA, W. MAASSEN, CHR. MALCHAU

INTRODUCTION

Diagnosis of sarcoidosis should always be made by biopsy, because even
sarcoid-typical chest films may mask more serious disease. Personal experience and training will influence one to decide whether one or a combination of the following procedures is done: bronchoscopy with biopsy, mediastinoscopy with lymph-node biopsy according to Carlens, needle aspiration,
open lung and pleural biopsy or thoracoscopy. Results of KVEIM tests seem to
us too equivocal and non-specific, and much time can be lost awaiting results. Immunological diagnostic has still to grow out of its infancy.

MATERIAL AND METHODS

In a period of 18 months (1976-1977), a total of 150 patients with sarcoidosis were examined at our hospital. Of these, 127 (85 %) were bronchoscopied. In 36 (28%) bronchoscopy was the only endoscopic procedure. In 108
(72 %) patients mediastinoscopy was performed, this procedure being the
only one done in 17 of these 108 cases. Both bronchoscopy and mediastinoscopy were carried out in 91 (61 %); and in 60 of these (66 %), both procedures were done at one sitting. In 3 patients (2 %), bronchoscopy and a
surgical lung biopsy were performed.

RESULTS AND DISCUSSION

In recent weeks we have analyzed results of open surgical lung and
pleural biopsy in disseminated lung disease, performed in 417 patients between 1971 and 1979. Surprisingly, sarcoidosis was seen fairly rarely in
this group (Table 1). In analyzing this development, we found two stages
in the diagnosis of sarcoidosis in our hospital:

Initially, when we introduced mediastinoscopy here as a routine examination in 1961, we invariably combined it with bronchoscopy; later, with
a Daniels' biopsy; and further on, with muscle biopsy. Our experience until

J.A. Nakhosteen and W. Maassen (eds.), Bronchology: Research, Diagnostic and
Therapeutic Aspects. All rights reserved.
Copyright 1981. Martinus Nijhoff Publishers bv, The Hague / Boston / London

1973 yielded the following results: Out of 472 cases, diagnosis was obtained in 30 % by bronchoscopy, in 69 % by Daniels' biopsy, in 99 % by mediastinoscopy, and, in contrast, only in 6 % by muscle biopsy (Table 2).

TABLE 1. Surgical Lung and Pleural Biopsies in Disseminated Lung Disease from 1971-1979 (n = 417)

Cryptogenic fibrosing alveolitis	171
Fibrosing alveolitis of known etiology	18
Exogenous allergic alveolitis	37
Collagen disease	5
Tuberculosis	6
Sarcoidosis	34
Silicosis	17
Exogenous siderosis	17
Carcinomatosis	23
Histiocytosis X	11
Other	41
Normal findings	20
No diagnosis	17

TABLE 2.

Results of Mediastinoscopy and Other Biopsies in Sarcoidosis

Authors	Bronchusbiopsy		Daniels'Biopsy		Mediastinoscopy		Musclebiopsy	
Friedel et al.	86	11 % +	–		66	98 % +	–	
Löfgren et al.	–		47	32 % +	34	94 % +	–	
Bergh et al.	–		–		33	1oo % +	–	
Palva	–		–		28	96 % +	–	
Carlens	56	2o % +	–		123	96 % +	–	
Jepsen	–		–		43	95 % +	–	
Nielsen and Olsen	–		–		121	95 % +	–	
Maaßen and Greschuchna	472	3o % +	42o	69 % +	534	99 % +	211	6 % +

Subsequently, in a further 763 cases of sarcoidosis, mediastinoscopy led to diagnosis in 99 %, even when different surgeons performed the procedure, whereas other investigations led to poorer results, e.g. Daniels' biopsy was only 66 % positive. As long as all examinations were done by the same surgeon in the initial period, results of Daniels' biopsy were diagnostic in 73 %, and of the muscle biopsy, in 11 % (Fig. 1). Results obtained by mediastinoscopy seemed less likely to be influenced by the operator or the pathologist. In 763 patients with sarcoidosis, who were examined before 1975 and mediastinoscopied and bronchoscopied, 99 % in Stage I and 99 % in Stages II/III gave diagnostic results through mediastinoscopy (Table 3).

FIGURE 1.

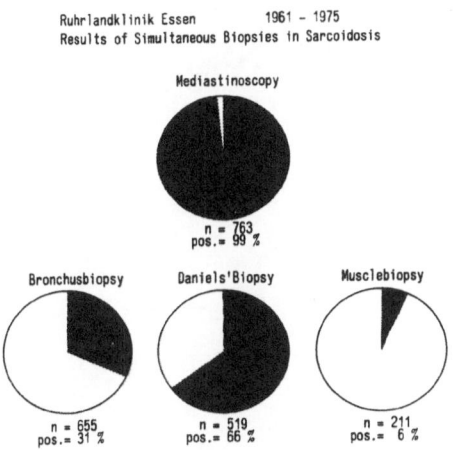

Ruhrlandklinik Essen   1961 - 1975
Results of Simultaneous Biopsies in Sarcoidosis

Mediastinoscopy

n = 763
pos.= 99 %

Bronchusbiopsy   Daniels'Biopsy   Musclebiopsy

n = 655   n = 519   n = 211
pos.= 31 %   pos.= 66 %   pos.= 6 %

In recent years, we have tended more to doing the less invasive procedure of bronchoscopy prior to mediastinoscopy. Figure 2 shows these results in a comparison. Only few (n=7) surgical lung biopsies were carried out; these were limited to cases in which very atypical x-ray presentations led to other diagnoses being considered. Furthermore, mediastinoscopy, with a 99 % diagnostic rate, continued to result in excellent yields, even when different surgeons operated. In bronchial biopsies, a noticeable increase of diagnostic rate was seen, in direct proportion to the number and type of biopsy

FIGURE 2.

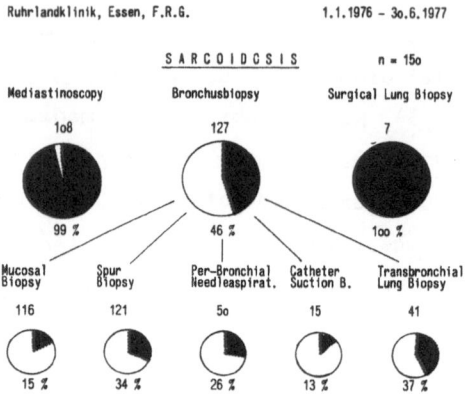

Ruhrlandklinik, Essen, F.R.G.   1.1.1976 – 3o.6.1977

S A R C O I D O S I S   n = 15o

Mediastinoscopy   Bronchusbiopsy   Surgical Lung Biopsy

1o8   127   7

99 %   46 %   1oo %

Mucosal   Spur   Per-Bronchial Catheter   Transbronchial
Biopsy   Biopsy   Needleaspirat. Suction B.   Lung Biopsy

116   121   5o   15   41

15 %   34 %   26 %   13 %   37 %

TABLE 3.

Ruhrlandklinik Essen   1961 – 1975
Results of 763 Mediastinoscopies in Sarcoidosis

		Nr	positive
1	Unknown changes of mediastinal and/or hilar region Sarcoidosis I	44o	438 = 99 %
2	Unknown changes of lung parenchym Sarcoidosis II/III	323	319 = 99 %
		763	757 = 99 %

done. The distribution of various biopsy procedures and their contribution
to diagnosis (bottom row, Fig. 2), leading to total diagnostic rate of 46 %,
was as follows: Mucosal biopsy: 15 %; upper lobe spur:: 36 %; per-bronchial
needle aspiration: 27 %; catheter suction biopsy: 13 %; and trans-bronchial
lung biopsy: 37 %. These results could be improved if increased TBB were performed. Since most of these patients were, however, out-patients, the risk of
pneumothorax developing prevented doing TBB in this group. In contrast, mediastinoscopy can be done on an ambulatory basis in sarcoidosis.

CONCLUSIONS

In the light of the above data, we feel that, as a general rule, bronchoscopy with multiple mucosal biopsies, per-bronchial needle aspiration, and TBB should preceed mediastinoscopy in the diagnosis of sarcoidosis. If diagnosis is not obtained by bronchoscopy, and the slightest doubt remains as to the disease process, mediastinoscopy should be done. Surgical lung biopsy is indicated if another systemic disease is suspected. The last two methods are justified in the diagnosis of sarcoidosis, since their complication rates are not higher than those of bronchoscopy with multiple biopsies and TBB -- provided that the surgeon has mastered the technique of mediastinoscopy.

A Comparison of Fibreoptic Transbronchial Lung Biopsy (TBB) with VI.4.
Other Techniques in the Diagnosis of Sarcoidosis

D.M. Mitchell, D.N. Mitchell, C.J. Emerson, J.V. Collins.

Since the advent of TBB through the fibrescope, the technique
has been used increasingly at Brompton Hospital, London, for the diagnosis of interstitial lung disease and we present here our findings
using this technique and other techniques in the diagnosis of sarcoidosis. We studied a group of 79 patients seen consecutively at Brompton Hospital between January 1977 - December 1978 in whom a diagnosis
of sarcoidosis was made.

Of the 79 patients studied, 40 were male and 39 were female. The
majority were in the 3rd and 4th decades of life, and in the older age
groups there was a slight female predominance. In 55 patients a diagnosis of sarcoidosis was highly probable on clinical grounds. Of
these patients 1 had a normal chest radiograph, 12 had bilateral hilar
lymphadenopathy (BHL), 36 had BHL and pulmonary mottling and 6 had
mottling alone. In a further 8 patients a diagnosis other than sarcoidosis had been made on clinical grounds before investigations were
performed. 3 were thought to have pulmonary tuberculosis, 1 SLE,1
fibrosing alveolitis (UIP), 1 honeycomb lung, 1 budgerigar lung and
1 Hodgkins disease. In the remaining 16 patients, no diagnosis was
made before investigation. Nine had diffuse pulmonary shadows, 2 BHL
and pericarditis, 2 cervical lymph node enlargement and assymetrical
hilar lymphadenopathy, 2 diffuse upper zone shadows and 1 had a pleural effusion.

Histological support for the diagnosis of sarcoidosis was obtained in 73 of the 79 patients. In the remaining 6 no positive histology was obtained. These patients had a negative kveim test or a
negative biopsy but no further invasive diagnostic proceadures were
performed as the diagnosis was highly probable on clinical grounds
alone. Subsequent evolution of the disease in all cases has remained
compatible with the diagnosis of sarcoidosis and no alternative diagnosis have emerged in the follow-up period. Of the 79 patients, FOB
was performed on 50. 42 had TBB performed under fluoroscopic control,
6 - 10 samples being taken in eachcase. In 37 (88%) epitheloid and
giant cell granulomas were seen. Ziehl-Niellsen and Grocott stains
were negative. In 5 normal lung tissue was obtained. 22 patients
had bronchial mucosal biopsy and positive histology was obtained in
17 (77%). Of these 22, 14 also had TBB. 2 patients had positive hist-

J.A. Nakhosteen and W. Maassen (eds.), Bronchology: Research, Diagnostic and
Therapeutic Aspects. All rights reserved.
Copyright 1981. Martinus Nijhoff Publishers bv, The Hague / Boston / London

ology obtained on mediastinal node biopsy. Kveim tests were performed in 44 patients using a suspension of spleen K19. 19 (43%) were positive, 11 equivocal and the remainder negative. The remainder of the patients had extrathoracic manifestations of sarcoidosis, and biopsies were performed as appropriate. Thus 10 had positive histology on cervical lymph node biopsy, 1 had a skin lesion biopsy, 2 had positive liver biopsy and one had positive biopsy of an enlarged parotid gland. TBB or bronchial mucosal biopsy and kveim tests were both performed in 29 patients. Of the 24 patients with positive biopsy histology, 11 had a positive kveim, 3 were equivocal and 10 were negative. On the other hand, of the 5 patients with negative biopsy, 2 had positive kveim, one was equivocal and two were negative.

The patients were grouped according to radiological stage of disease. One patient had a normal chest radiograph. No biopsy was performed but a kveim test was positive. In 12 patients with BHL alone, 2 of 3 who had TBB had positive histology. The presence of granulomas in the lung parenchyma in patients with radiographically normal lung fields is well recognised and has been previously reported both from open biopsy and TBB. The kveim reactivity as might be expected was highest in this group at 58%. In BHL with pulmonary mottling, 12 of 16 patients had positive bronchial mucosa and 19 of 23 (83%) had positive TBB. Kveim reactivity was perhaps lower in this group than one might expect at 36%. This may partly be due to the presence in this group of some patients with known chest radiograph abnormality in excess of 2 years and kveim reactivity is known to decline with time from onset of disease. In patients with pulmonary mottling alone, all patients having mucosal biopsy or TBB were positive as were 3 patients with radiological pulmonary fibrosis. In those patients with radiograph appearances not fitting the usual classification, all those that had biopsy had positive histology.

In summary, in these 79 patients, kveim test provided diagnostic support in 43%, bronchial mucosal biopsy in 77% and TBB in 88%. TBB was particularly useful in patients with diffuse bilateral shadows, pulmonary fibrosis or unusual radiograph appearances. It is in this group of patients where diagnostic problems often occur, and where it is often essential to establish a tissue diagnosis. Overall, TBB provided the highest diagnostic yield in this group. There were no complications from TBB.

VI.5.

TBLB AS A DIAGNOSTIC PROCEDURE FOR SARCOIDOSIS IN JAPAN - A COOPERATIVE STUDY IN TWENTY-FOUR HOSPITALS -

K. HONDA, M. KADO, T. IZUMI, T. OSAKI, Y. HIRAGA, K. IWAI, R. YONEDA, M. WASHIZAKI, H. HOMMA, J. KABE, H. OSADA, H. OKANO, T. FURUIE, H. HOSODA, Y. ITO, K. HIRASAWA, I. MOCHIZUKI, A. SATO, Y. YAMAMOTO, R. AMITANI, R. MIKAMI, N. KURIHARA, T. TACHIBANA, S. HITOMI, N. OCHI, F. KITATANI, J.NAKAI, M. YAMAKIDO, K. SHIMA, S. MIYAGI

1. INTRODUCTION

In recent years, the transbronchial lung biopsy (TBLB) has been introduced as a simple and safe method of diagnosing diffuse pulmonary diseases, especially sarcoidosis. several reports have discribed the usefulness of TBLB (ref. 1). To determine its popularization and clinical significance in Japan, the Japan Sarcoidosis Committee carried out a questionnaire investigation.

2. MATERIALS AND METHODS

Information about sarcoidosis cases in which TBLB were performed at twenty-four hospitals related to the Committee was obtained through a questionnaire.

3. RESULTS

The questionnaire revealed that in 24 hospitals, TBLB were performed for sarcoidosis diagnosis in 207 cases between 1971 and 1979. The frequency of TBLB use has been increasing rapidly, especially in 1979 when TBLB were taken in 104 cases.

TABLE 1. Procedure for sarcoidosis in 207 cases.

TBLB(+)+Mediastinoscopy(+)	13	cases
+Scalene l. n. biopsy(+)	53	"
+Bronchial wall biopsy(+)	10	"
+Kveim test(+)	13	"
+Other biopsy(+)	6	"
TBLB(+) Only	28	cases
TBLB(-)+Mediastinoscopy(+)	5	cases
+Scalene l. n. biopsy(+)	40	"
+Bronchial wall biopsy(+)	3	"
+Open lung biopsy(+)	2	"
+Other biopsy(+)	5	"
TBLB(-)+Clinical finding	29	cases
Total	207	cases

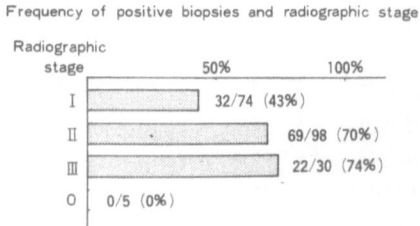

FIGURE 1. Frequency of positive biopsies and radiographic stage.

J.A. Nakhosteen and W. Maassen (eds.), Bronchology: Research, Diagnostic and Therapeutic Aspects. All rights reserved.
Copyright 1981. Martinus Nijhoff Publishers bv, The Hague / Boston / London

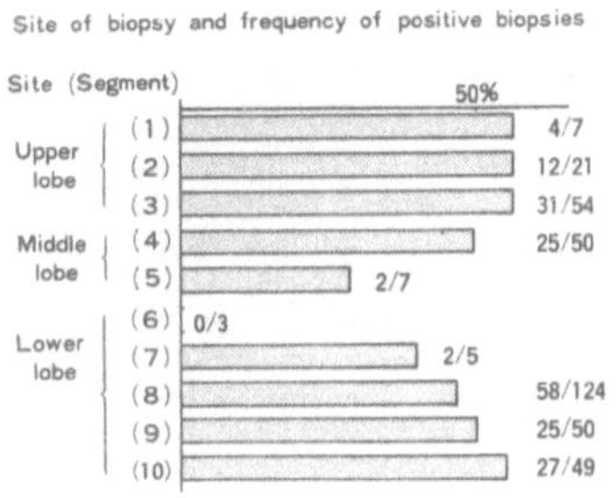

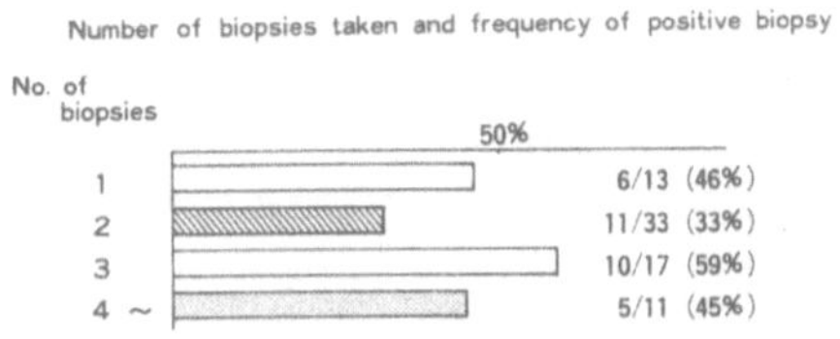

Site of biopsy and frequency of positive biopsies

Site (Segment) 50%

Upper lobe
(1) 4/7
(2) 12/21
(3) 31/54

Middle lobe
(4) 25/50
(5) 2/7

Lower lobe
(6) 0/3
(7) 2/5
(8) 58/124
(9) 25/50
(10) 27/49

Number of biopsies taken and frequency of positive biopsy

No. of biopsies 50%

1 6/13 (46%)
2 11/33 (33%)
3 10/17 (59%)
4 ~ 5/11 (45%)

FIGURE 2. Site of biopsy and frequency of positive biopsies.

FIGURE 3. Number of biopsies taken and frequency of positive biopsies.

These 104 cases were about half of all cases studied. So, this indicates that TBLB may have become a routine method for sarcoidosis diagnosis in 1979 in Japan.

The sex and age distributions of patients examined by TBLB correspond to the sex and age distributions of sarcoidosis.

The procedure for sarcoidosis diagnosis in 207 cases appears in Table 1.

One hundred and twenty-three (59%) of the patients in which TBLB were taken were positive and 84 patients (41%) were negative. Although the percentage of granuloma positive cases were about the same in the second and third radiographic stages (70% and 74% respectively), the percentage was much lower in the first stage (43%). No positive cases were found among stage 0 patients (Fig. 1). No relation was found between extrathoracic lesions and the frequncy of the granuloma positive cases: extrathoracic lesions(-), 64/103(62%), extrathoracic lesions(+), 59/104(57%).

No difference in the frequency of granuloma positive cases was found between the three types of tuberculin status (-, ±, +). Moreover, except for serum gamma-globulin over 2.0 g/dl, serum gammaglobulin groups showed about the same frequency of positive cases.

S3, S4, S8, S9, and S10 were the most frequent biopsy sites. The incidence of positive granuloma was about the same in all of those sites (Fig. 2).

TBLB and mediastinoscopy revealed the same frequencies of positive granuloma in cases in each of the three stages of the diseases. However, TBLB and scalene lymph node biopsies revealed different frequencies among cases of the first stage of the disease (Tab. 2). Therefore, we surmised that taking greater number of TBLB from individual stage I patients would reveal higher frequencies of positive cases. However, this did not prove to be the case (Fig. 3). Therefore, it appears that some sort of other technical problem is involved here.

Complications following TBLB in the 207 cases were few (9%): nine cases exhibited pneumothorax in which 2 cases required chest tubes, 8 cases exhibited bleeding not requiring trans-fusion, and one case experienced severe chest pain for two days.

TABLE 2. Comparison of positive biopsy frequencies between TBLB and other biopsy procedures.

Radiographic stage	TBLB	Med.	TBLB	Scale.
I	10/13	13/13	14/44	30/44
II	2/4	4/4	44/62	51/62
III	1/1	1/1	9/15	11/15

4. DISCUSSION

Our present result that the frequency of positive biopsies in stage I cases was relatively low might reflect the scattered distribution of granulomas and the size of biopsies specimens. Rosen reported that such a low frequency was caused by the fact that biopsy specimens of TBLB were smaller than those of open lung biopsies (ref. 2). So, in order to overcome this handicap, we investigated the relation between the number of biopsies and the frequency of positive cases, but we could not find any significant relation. This might be caused by some sort of technical problem in our cooperative study. Very recently, Roethe reported that by taking ten biopsies, five from both the right-upper and lower lobes in each case, he succeeded in finding granuloma in all stage I cases (ref. 3). This result indicates that TBLB is a reliable diagnostic procedure for sarcoidosis.

5. SUMMARY

The state of TBLB in Japan was investigated by a questionnaire. Results were obtained from 207 patients of 24 hospitals in Japan. TBLB revealed that 59% of the cases were granuloma positive. TBLB also revealed that 43% of the stage I patients were granuloma positive. This confirmed that TBLB has distinct advantages as a sarcoidosis diagnostic technique in Japan.

REFERENCES

1. Koontz CH, Joyner LR, Nelson RA: Transbronchial lung biopsy via the fiberoptic bronchoscope in sarcoidosis. Ann. Intern. Med. 85:64-66, 1976.
2. Rosen Y, Amorosa JK, Moon S, Cohen J, Lyons HA: Occurrence of lung granulomas in patients with stage I sarcoidosis. Am. J. Roentgenol. 129:1083-1085, 1977.
3. Roethe MRA, Fuller LCPB, Byrd CRB, Hafermann LCDR: Transbronchoscopic lung biopsy in sarcoidosis, Optimal number and sites for diagnosis. Chest 77:400-402, 1980.

VI.6.

TRANSBRONCHIAL LUNG BIOPSY IN SARCOIDOSIS

L-G. WIMAN and Y. HÖRNBLAD

INTRODUCTION

In Sweden- like most of the Scandinavian countries - sarcoidosis
is an important medical problem. The prevalence is high, usually
more than 50 cases per 100.000 of the adult population. In the Northern parts of Sweden more than 100 sarcoid patients per 100.000 of
people have been found on mass chest radiography. An increased occurrence of familial sarcoidosis has been reported (Fig. 1).

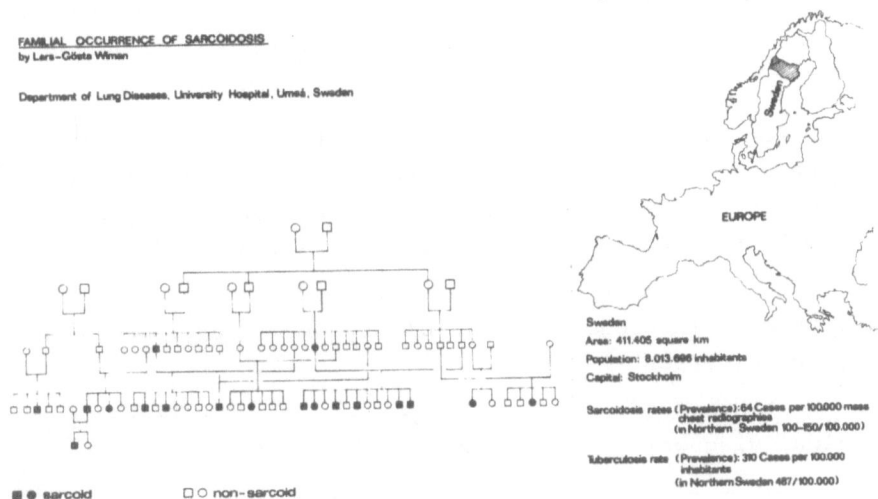

FIGURE 1. Familial occurrence
of sarcoidosis in Northern
Sweden.

PATIENT MATERIAL

One hundred patients presented with disseminated lung lesions
- or with hilar adenopathy only - were examined by fiberoptic bronchoscopy. In 40 patients - 20 males and 21 females between 18-68 years

of age - the clinical diagnosis of sarcoidosis was based upon a history of typical symptoms and signs, and a characteristic appearance of mottling, cloudy shadows or hilar adenopathy in chest radiology.

In a non-sarcoid control group there were 40 patients - 28 males and 12 females between 17-69 years of age.
These patients presented with a great variety of symptoms and signs, and a radiological appearance of irregular and fibrotic lesions. The clinical diagnoses included pulmonary tuberculosis, mycoses, pneumocystis, interstitial pneumonia, asbestoses and many other lesions of known or unknown etiology.

METHOD

All patients were investigated by fiberoptic bronchoscopy in local anesthesia. The instrument was inserted transnasally and via the trachea proceeded to the periphery of the lung, mostly the right lower lobe. Under fluoroscopic guidance the site of biopsy could be precisely determined 1-2 cm from the lung surface. It was important to collect the specimens on the alveolar level to ensure satisfactory material of lung tissue and to avoid excessive bleeding. Biopsy material from the bronchial mucosa was finally secured from the central bronchi.

RESULTS

After transbronchial lung biopsy all patients showing granulomatous tissue were found in the sarcoid group. In some biopsies there were unspecified granulomas, interstitial inflammatory or fibrotic reactions. Normal or insufficient material was obtained in the remaining cases (Table 1).

TABLE 1. Results of transbronchial lung biopsy in 80 patients with disseminated lung diseases.

Histopathological diagnosis	Sarcoid	Non-sarcoid
Epithelioid cell granulomas	16	–
Unspecified granulomas	2	–
Interstitial pneumonitis	4	3
Interstitial fibrosis	3	15
Pneumocystis carinii	–	3
Normal lung tissue	6	15
Insufficient material	9	4
Total	40	40

In light microscopy characteristic granulomas without necroses were found in lung tissue in 40 percent and in bronchial mucosa in 56 percent of the sarcoid patients.

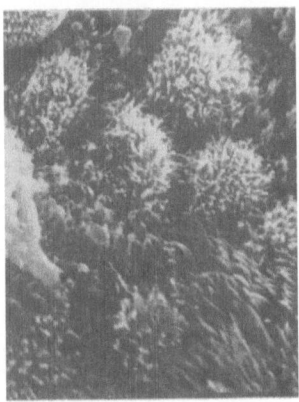 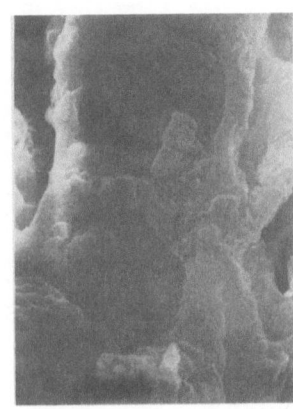 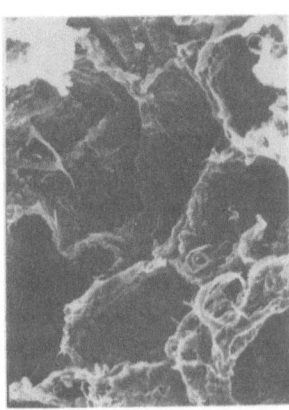

Fig. 2   Fig. 3   Fig. 4

FIGURE 2. Upon scanning electron microscopy the alveolocytes type II are hypertrophied and swollen and the dividing septa are thickened in sarcoidosis.

FIGURE 3. In a normal structure the alveolar surface is smooth and the alveolar septa are sharp.

FIGURE 4. The gross appearance of the bronchial mucosa is usually normal, but microscopically groups of active, abnormal goblet cells are seen in sarcoidosis. Submucosal granulomas were demonstrated in 56 percent of the sarcoid patients using light microscopy.

CONCLUSIONS

Totally, granulomatous tissue was found in 74 percent of biopsies from the lung and bronchi in patients with sarcoidosis. Pneumothorax in three patients were the only complications in this study.

VI.7.

BRONCHOSCOPY IN THE DIAGNOSIS OF SARCOIDOSIS

M. Thunell, R. Lundgren and N. Stjernberg.

In the diagnosis of sarcoidosis histopathological examination of
bronchial mucosa biopsies (Ståhle 1964) and lungbiopsies (Roethe et al,
1980) can be valuable. We have studied the results of bronchoscopy
in the diagnosis of sarcoidosis.

Material and methods

153 patients with clinically and histopathologically established
sarcoidosis were examined by bronchoscopy at our department during
the period July 1974 - December 1979. There were 73 men and 80 women
with ages ranging from 22 to 80 years. Among the patients, 53 had
stage I, 84 stage II and 16 stage III sarcoidosis.

In all patients flexible fiberoptic bronchoscopy (FFB) was performed
under topical anesthesia. Bronchial mucosal changes were noted and
biopsies were taken from different areas of the bronchial mucosa in
all patients. Transbronchial lung biopsies were taken from the right
lower lobe in 55 patients.

Results

Biopsies from the bronchial mucosa showed epitheloid cell granulomas
in 56 of the 153 patients (37%). In stage I, 18% of the biopsies were
positive, in stage II 47% and in stage III 36%. Transbronchial
lung biopsy was positive in 23 of 55 patients (41%). With this method
the highest diagnostic yield was also in stage II and III.
If both bronchial mucosa and lung biopsies were taken, bronchoscopy
gave a histopathological diagnosis in 33 of 55 patients (60%). In
stages II + III, however, the diagnostic yield increased to 75%
(Table 1).

J.A. Nakhosteen and W. Maassen (eds.), Bronchology: Research, Diagnostic and
Therapeutic Aspects. All rights reserved.
Copyright 1981. Martinus Nijhoff Publishers bv, The Hague / Boston / London

TABLE 1. Diagnostic yield from FFB in 153 patients with sarcoidosis (number of patients with positive biopsy/number of patients biopsied).

Chest X-ray stage	Bronchial mucosal biopsy	Trans- bronchial biopsy	Bronchial mucosal and transbronchial biopsy
I (n=53)	10/53 (18%)	4/19 (21%)	6/19 (32%)
II-III (n=100)	46/100 (46%)	19/36 (53%)	27/36 (75%)
All patients	56/153 (37%)	23/55 (41%)	33/55 (60%)

The frequency of positive findings increased with increasing number of biopsies. There were no significant difference in the number of positive biopsies from different areas of the bronchial mucosa. However, when microscopical changes were present in the mucosa, the diagnostic yield increased (Table 2).

TABLE 2. Diagnostic yield with regard to macroscopical findings at bronchoscopy.

Normal mucosa	Unspecific inflammatory	Broncho- stenosis	Yellow-white nodules	Atrophic mucosa
16/81	23/53	8/9	8/11	1/2
19%	43%	88%	72%	50%

Discussion

A number of patients with bronchial sarcoidosis have been reported, as well as bronchostenosis due to sarcoidosis (Olsson et al 1979). Since bronchoscopy is the only way to confirm bronchial involvement in sarcoidosis and transbronchial lung biopsy can be performed at the same time, these methods should be used in the examination of sarcoidosis. In our material, we obtained the highest diagnostic yield in stages II and III, when both bronchial mucosal biopsy and transbronchial lung biopsies were taken.

VI.8.

DIAGNOSIS IN SARCOIDOSIS: HOW MANY BIOPSIES WITH BRONCHOSCOPY?

A. PALOJOKI

Sarcoidosis can produce two principal effects:bronchial distortion because of tracheo-bronchial lymph-node enlargement and mucosal
changes. The mucosa, particularly in the region of the carina and
main bronchi, often shows a vascular engorgement, a sign of inflammation with increased secretion. Small yellowish granulomatous
swellings or plaques are sometimes found, and in later stages of the
disease, scar formation. Normal findings are frequent as well. In
evaluating the patient with suspected sarcoidosis, histological confirmation of the diagnosis is generally desired. The bronchoscopic
biopsy is usually taken from the demonstrable mucosal abnormality,
sometimes with success and sometimes without.

MATERIAL AND METHOD
In order to find the optimal amount of biopsies with bronchoscopy, the number and location of biopsies on 86 patients with sarcoidosis have been retrogradely examined. The subject material (39
men and 47 women) consisted of patients, all of whom had a positive
diagnostic biopsy, and included epitheloid granulomas with giant
cells. Other granulomatous diseases were excluded. Age and sex distribution are shown in table 1.

TABLE 1. Age and sex distribution of 86 patients with sarcoidosis

Age	Male	Female	Total
20-29	10	10	22
30-39	16	9	25
40-49	7	13	20
50-59	6	11	17
60-69	–	4	4
Total	39	47	86

*J.A. Nakhosteen and W. Maassen (eds.), Bronchology: Research, Diagnostic and
Therapeutic Aspects. All rights reserved.*
Copyright 1981. Martinus Nijhoff Publishers bv, The Hague / Boston / London

The roentgenological changes were classified into three stages.
In stage 1 (bilateral hilar adenopathy) were 45 (52.4%), in stage
2 (hilar adenopathy with parenchymal infiltration) were 31 (36%)and
in stage 3 (parenchymal infiltration only) were 10 (11.4%) patients.
The histological confirmation was reached by bronchoscopical biopsy
in 59 cases (68.6%), by mediastinoscopy in 26 cases (30.2%) and
in one case (1.2%) by pleural biopsy, table 2.

TABLE 2. Diagnosis in 86 cases of sarcoidosis

Procedure	Positive	%	
Bronchoscopy			
Mucosal biopsy	54	62.8	
Transbr.lung biopsy	4	4.6	
Transmural needle biopsy	1	1.2	68.6
Pleural biopsy	1		1.2
Mediastinoscopy	26		30.2
Total	86		100.0

RESULTS

One mucosal biopsy produced a positive result in 50 % of the patients, two in 66.7 % and three biopsies produced a positive result
in 64.3 % of the patients, table 3.

TABLE 3. Diagnostic results of biopsies

No. of mucosal biopsies	No. of patients	Positive	%
1	22	11	50
2	45	30	66.7
3	14	9	64.3
4	5	4	80
Total	86	54	62.8
Other bronchoscopic biopsy	5	5	68.6

Transbronchial lung biopsy and transmural needle biopsy increased
the diagnostic yield of 1 - 3 mucosal biopsies to 59 %, 71.1 % and
71.4 % respectively. The diagnostic yield with 4 mucosal biopsies
per patients was 80 %.

In patients who had symptoms of the ailment, bronchoscopic biopsy
brought a positive result slightly more often than it did in patients
without symptoms. The positive result was reached almost as often

in the stage I patients as in the stage II + III patients. Bronchoscopic biopsy brought a positive result in all of the 10 stage III
patients. The bronchoscopy finding was normal in only two patients;
in one the positive result was reached by mediastinoscopy and in the
other by periferic pulmonary lung biopsy.

The main part of the mucosal biopsies were taken from the carina
of the bronchial lobes. As far as the positive results was concerned
there was no difference in the location of the carina biopsy or biopsies from other areas.

DISCUSSION AND CONCLUSIONS

The results imply that, together with bronchoscopy on a patient
suspected of having sarcoidosis, 3 - 4 mucosal biopsies are always
necessary, even if the macroscopic findings would be typical of sarcoidosis. In addition a transmural needle biopsy ought to be done
always, in case enlarged glands are detected. In those with parenchymal involvement, transbronchial biopsies are compulsory; according to one piece of research a minimum of five is necessary. With
these methods the ailment will be recognized in most patients and
too intensive operations, e.g. mediastinoscopy, and open lung biopsy will be avoided.

REFERENCES

1. Dürschmied, H., Stanulla, H., Grollmuss, H. et al.:
   Stand der bioptischen Diagnostik bei intrathorakaler Sarkoidose
   - Erfahrungen von 6 Lungkliniken der DDR. Z. Erkrank.Atm.-Org'
   149:80-83, 1977
2. Roethe, R.A., Fuller, P.B., Byrd, R.B. and Hafermann D.R.:
   Transbronchoscopic Lung Biopsy in Sarcoidosis. Optimal Number
   and Sites for Diagnosis. Chest 77:400-402, 1980.

VI.9.

BRONCHOSCOPIC FINDINGS AND TRANSBRONCHOSCOPIC LUNG BIOPSY IN
SARCOIDOSIS

S. HITOMI, K. MAEZATO[1] AND T. TACHIBANA

We carried out transbronchial lung and bronchial biopsy and endoscopic examination during fiberoptic bronchoscopy in 30 patients with
clinical feature of sarcoidosis. All the cases were in the state before
treatment. As shown in Slide No. 1, of these patients, 20 were male
and 10 were female. The majority (24 cases) of the patients were
twenties of age. The patient of sixties of age was at the stage
III in the course of 18 years. Seven cases (23%) had such subjective
symptoms as coughing, chest-ache, fever, short of breath, and so on.
Twenty-three cases were the symptom-free patients who were discovered
in the mass physical examination. The patients were classified on
the basis of Wurm-Heilmeyer's criteria of chest X-ray examination.
That is to say, 18 cases were placed in the stage I; 11 cases in the
stage II; and 1 case in the stage III. The sites of TBLB were mainly
set at the right S^4 and S^8 in the case of the stage I. In the cases
of the stage II and III, fluoroscopic TBLB was carried out, with a
focus placed around the difuse shadow. The number of biopsy sample
was aimed at three or four per case. As a result, average 2.6 samples per case were obtained.

The Slide No. 2, Table No. 1 shows the results of bronchial and
lung biopsies. Examination was made in 29 cases excluding one case
which was deficient in the lung tissue. The samples obtained through
TBLB were divided into pulmonary lesion and peripheral bronchial lesion. The samples obtained through the direct vision of the bronchus
to the segmental bronchus were regarded as the hilar bronchial lesion.
The histological diagnosis was performed in 18 (62%) of 29 cases.
In terms of the stage, the positive was obtained from 6 (35%) of 17
cases of the stage I of BHL only, and the positive rate of 100% was
obtained from the cases of the stage II and III. The pulmonary lesion (+) was found in 16 of all cases, and the peripheral bronchial
lesion (+) was found in 5 (26%) of 17 cases. The positive of both

*J.A. Nakhosteen and W. Maassen (eds.), Bronchology: Research, Diagnostic and
Therapeutic Aspects. All rights reserved.*

the pulmonary lesion and the peripheral bronchial lesion was found in 3 cases.

TABLE 1. Result of bronchial and lung biopsy in sarcoidosis

X-ray stage	Cases	Positive	Lung lesion	Peripheral bronchial lesion	Central bronchial lesion
I	17	6 (35%)	5/17	2/11	1/11
II	11	11 (100%)	11/11	2/7	0/8
III	1	1 (100%)	0/1	1/1	0/0
Total	29	18 (62%)	16/29	5/17	1/19

Histological diagnosis (lung or bronchial lesion) = $\frac{18}{29}$ (62%)

The third slide shows the histological pictures obtained through TBLB. Granuloma of the epitheloid cells is recognized in the pulmonary tissue in the right slide and in the bronchial submucous tissue in the left slide.

The fourth slide shows the sites where hilar bronchial biopsies were carried out. The biopsy was carried out 24 times in 19 cases. However, the positive was obtained only at the middle lobe bifurcation in 1 case. The positive rate was 5%. TBLB in this case showed the positive both in pulmonary lesion and in peripheral bronchial lesion.

The fifth slide shows the histological picture. The epithelial cell granuloma which consists mainly of Langhans giant cells is recognized at the submucous site.

The sixth slide (Table No. 2) shows the summary of endoscopic findings in 28 cases. Normal findings were obtained in 10 cases (36%); abnormal findings were obtained in 18 cases (64%). In the stage I, normal findings were obtained in 8 cases (47%), while in the stage II, abnormal findings were obtained more than normal findings. In respect to the abnormal findings, the bronchial stenosis and compression were noted in 11 cases; the reddening and edema of the bronchi were noted in 8 cases; mucosal hypervascularity was noted in 5 cases; and yellow plaque was noted in 5 cases.

TABLE 2. Macroscopic findings in bronchi in sarcoidosis (28 cases)

		I	II	III
Normal appearance	10	8	2	0
Abnormal appearance	18	9	8	1
Bronchial stenosis and compression	11	3	6	1
Redness and edema	8	3	5	0
Hypervascularity	5	5	0	0
Yellow plaque	5	2	3	0

The seventh slide shows the endoscopic picture of the left main bronchus. A lot of white-yellow plaques are recognized.

As the complications of TBLB, pneumothorax was noted in 2 (7%) of 30 cases in the present study, bleeding of a large amount was not recognized.

REFERENCES

1) Bennedict, E.B. & Castleman, B.: Sarcoidosis with bronchial involvement. N. Engl. J. Med., 224: 186, 1941.
2) Anderson, H.A.: Transbronchoscopic lung biopsy for diffuse pulmonary diseases: Results in 939 patients. Chest., 73: 734, 1978.
3) Teirstein, A.S., Chuang, M., Miller, A. & Siltzbach, L.E.: Flexible-bronchoscope biopsy of lung and bronchial wall in intrathoracic sarcoidosis. Ann. N. Y. Acad. Sci., 183: 522, 1976.

VI.10.

BRONCHOSCOPY AS A TOOL IN DIAGNOSING SARCOIDOSIS

H.R. Baumann, R. Schwander, M. Winzeler, D. Bernoulli

In order to evaluate the proportion of bronchoscopy in the
diagnosis of endothoracic sarcoidosis, we compared the localisation
of the biopsies and their histological results of the last 54
examined cases. The final diagnosis based upon the radiological
findings of bihilar lymphadenopathy with or without reticulo-
nodulous infiltration of the lungs, histological findings,
compatible clinical symptoms and partly upon positive titers
from circulating anti-bodies against Kveim-antigen.

MATERIALS AND METHODS

The examined group consisted of 20 women with an average age of
35.2 years and 34 men of 33.7 years. All of the endoscopies were
carried out with bronchofiberscopes (1). The rigid bronchoscope
was used, when transbronchial lymph node biopsies or some of the
peripheral transbronchial lung biopsies were planned (2). 49 patients
had several biopsies of the mucosa of large bronchi. In 24 cases
of bihilar lymphadenopathy, where tomographs proved a close relationship of the lymphnodes to the bronchus, transbronchial
aspiration biopsies at the bifurcation carina or the ostium of
the right upper lobe were performed. In a later phase of the series
an average of 3 - 4 peripheral lung biopsies with bronchofiberscopes were carried out on 13 cases with radiologically proved
infiltrations of the parenchyma. The morphological diagnosis was
based only upon the histological examinations; the cytological
findings were not taken into account. 10 patients could be classified
as belonging to stage I, 32 patients to stage II and 12 patients
to stage III. In addition to the 86 biopsies by bronchoscopy,
21 mediastinoscopies and 49 liver biopsies were carried out.

RESULTS

In 24 cases the histological findings of biopsies by bronchoscopy were relevant for the diagnosis of sarcoidosis.
14 diagnosis were determined by liver biopsy and further 14 cases
were determined primarily by mediastinoscopy. 2 diagnosis were
clarified by Daniel's biopsies. In 18 patients the histological
diagnosis was repeatedly reassured, including isolated lymphnode
biopsies, skin biopsies and Kveim-tests. The mediastinoscopy showed
with 20 positive diagnosis from 21 attempts the highest score -
positive resultof 95% - followed by the peripheral parenchyma biopsies
with 69% (9 out of 13), the liver biopsy with 39% (19/49) and
the transbronchial lymphnode biopsy with 38% (9/24). The biopsies
of the mucosa were positive in 27% (13/48). In the whole series
bronchoscopy alone clarified 4 out of 10 cases in stage I, 20 out
of 32 cases in stage II and 7 out of 12 cases in stage III.

CONCLUSIONS

In our experience multiple bronchoscopic biopsy technics are
a valuable method not only in diagnosing interstitial lung diseases
but especially endothoracic sarcoidosis. Our aim tends to reduce the
number of more invasive mediastinoscopies. In our country a more
precise diagnosis of cytologic specimens has to be stressed upon.
According to the latest results in literature (3) the peripheral
transthoracic lung biopsy will in future be undertaken as a routine
method also in bihilar lymphadenopathy without radiologically
identifiable parenchymal infiltration, because stage I sarcoidosis
seems to be characterised in a high percentage by histologically
detectable interstitial lung lesions.

FIBEROPTIC BRONCHOSCOPIC FINDINGS IN SARCOIDOSIS
VI.11.

T. Kawauchi, K. Oho, N. Hayashi, R. Amemiya, M. Aida, Y. Hayata

Sarcoidosis has been described as a systemic disease of unknown etiologycharacterized by the formation of non-caseating epitheloid granuloma, which has a relatively higher incidence in the younger generation, and can occur in all organs except the ovarium and thymus.[1] Although there have been some reports on the findings insarcoidosis,[2,3] classification of the findings as observed through the fiberoptic bronchoscope has not been sufficient, and in this paper the authors attempt to describe and classify the fiberoptic bronchoscopic findings in advanced cases of sarcoidosis.

The case shown in Fig. 1 is a 24 year-old male. Swelling of bilateral lymph nodes was detected in a mass survey. Lung biopsy via the fiberoptic bronchoscope is a relatively simple technique which is being increasingly employed. Even in cases such as this one, in which only bilateral hilar lymphadenopathy could be recognized on X-ray, TBLB (Fig. 2) is an effective method to obtain diagnostic material. As shown in Fig. 3, TBLB obtained granulomatous material composed of epitheloid cells from the periphery of the lung.

Figures 4 through 10 show representative findings of sarcoidosis as observed through the fiberoptic bronchoscope. In the left main bronchus, in Fig. 4, the wall is thickened and irregular due to the thickening and plaque. The bifurcation of the left upper and lower lobe bronchi is thickened (Fig. 5) as is that of the bifurcation of the right upper lobe bronchus and truncus intermedius in Fig. 6, with severe stenosis and vascular engorgement. The reticular vascular pattern resembling crazy paving is another typical indication of sarcoidosis. In the left lower lobe (Fig.7) a remarkably thickened and edematous bifurcation can be seen. Again in the right upper lobe (Fig. 8) remarkable widening, stenosis, plaque and compression can be recognized. Figure 9 shows an unusual case of stenosis of the truncus intermedius with a polyp that appears to bridge the lumen. Much plaque, irregularity and stenosis is seen in the right middle lobe bronchus, (Fig. 10)

As we were not satisfied with existing classifications we developed the classification seen in Fig. 11. Our experience has shown us that sarcoidosis is easily recognized via the fiberoptic bronchoscope,

J.A. Nakhosteen and W. Maassen (eds.), Bronchology: Research, Diagnostic and Therapeutic Aspects. All rights reserved.

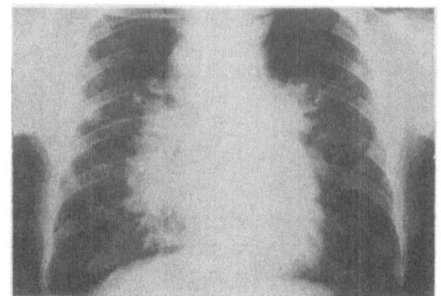

Fig. 1

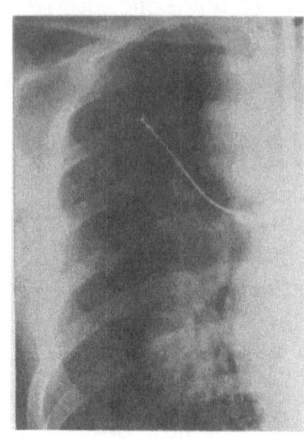

Fig. 2

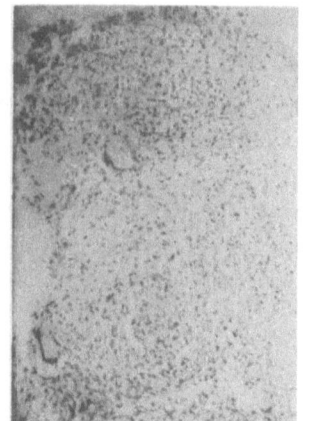

Fig. 3

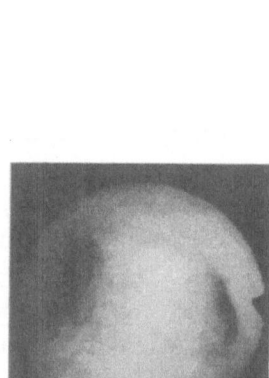

Fig. 4

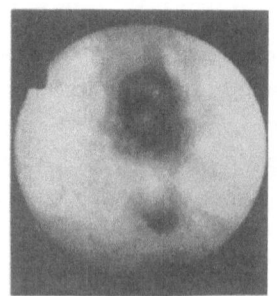

Fig. 5

Fig. 6

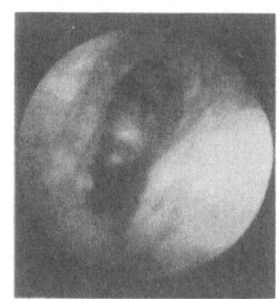

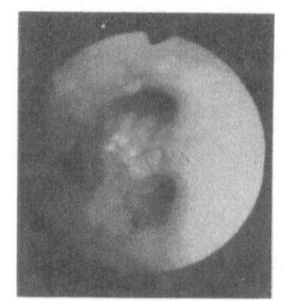

Fig. 7

and that as a diagnostic technique, TBLB through the fiberoptic bronchoscope yields a definitive diagnostic rate of 100%. We feel that vascular findings in sarcoidosis can be of extreme significance, and since they can be observed and biopsied with relative ease via the fiberoptic bronchoscope, their study will provide important information concerning the etiology of the disease.

REFERENCES

1. Kalbian VV: Bronchial involvement in pulmonary sarcoidosis. Proceedings of the Third International Conference on Sarcoidosis, Thorax 12; 18, 1957
2. Roethe RA, Fuller PB, Byrd RE, Haferman DR: Transbronchoscopic lung biopsy in sarcoidosis. Chest, 77: 400-402 March 1980
3. Stahle I: Bronchial involvement in pulmonary sarcoidosis, Acta Med. Scand. Suppl. 425:234, 1964

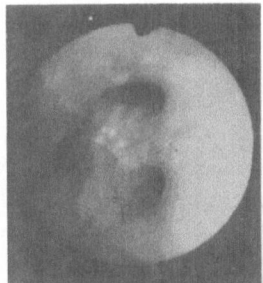 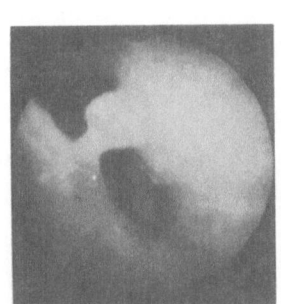 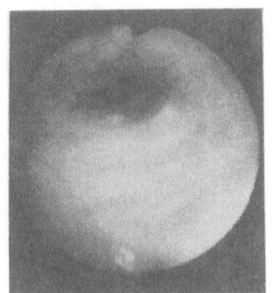

Fig. 8   Fig. 9   Fig. 10

CLASSIFICATION OF FIBEROPTIC BRONCHOSCOPIC FINDINGS IN SARCOIDOSIS

1. Stenosis of bronchi due to external compression
2. Whitish (or yellowish) plaque on mucosal surface
3. Irregular mucosal surface due to plaque
4. Cartilage and longitudinal folds not visible due to thickened edematous mucosa
5. Vascular engorgement (crazy paving-like, reticular)

(Tokyo Medical College Hospital)

Fig. 11

VI.12.

Computed tomography versus conventional tomography of the thorax
in the evaluation of abnormal lymph nodes:
A PROSPECTIVE RADIOLOGIC PATHOLOGIC STUDY.

T.D. TAN, W.J. KÜHLER, W.K. TACONIS, W.K. BRAND, E.L. FRENSDORF,
B.S. ZIENKOWICZ, J.P.M. WAGENAAR, HOLLAND.

INTRODUCTION

Both computed and conventional tomography are useful in evaluating
abnormal hilar lymph nodes (1.2.3.4.). However these reports have
been anecdotal and without consistent pathologic correlation.
The first question to be studied therefore is:
- what is the possible role of C.T. scanning in the evaluation of
  abnormal hilum?
  and if C.T. appears to be useful in this respect, the second
  and third question is:
- is it superior to conventional tomography in the evaluation of
  abnormal hilum? and
- should it replace conventional tomography?

MATERIALS AND METHODS

During a 2-years period from december 1977 to december 1979 we
studied 45 consecutive patients with potentially resectable bronchogenic carcinoma. Two weeks before surgery all patients underwent
C.T. scanning and all but one had postero-anterior conventional
tomograms of the mediastinum, including the hilum. All studies
were done with an EMI 5005 total body scanner. Intravenous infusion
of contrast medium was not used. The conventional tomograms were
made at ½ cm to 1 cm intervals (125 KVP, 29° arc). The hilum was
considered to be abnormal (scored "positive") if a hilar lymph
node larger than 1 cm in diameter was demonstrated on the scan.
The findings were graphically documented in a written standard
report. The results of the standard report were compared with
histological and anatomical findings.

RESULTS

Metastatic hilar lymph nodes.
In 14 out of the 45 cases the hilar lymph nodes showed no

J.A. Nakhosteen and W. Maassen (eds.), Bronchology: Research, Diagnostic and
Therapeutic Aspects. All rights reserved.
Copyright 1981. Martinus Nijhoff Publishers bv, The Hague / Boston / London

abnormalities on the C.T. scans. C.T. showed correctly 3 normal
hilum, which were predicted abnormal by conventional tomography.
In the other 31 cases all but 1 proved to have enlarged lymph nodes
and of those, 22 cases had histologically proven metastases.
There were 2 histologically proven cases in which the conventional
tomography was negative and the C.T. scan was positive. They were
cases with metastatic lymph nodes lying posterior to the pulmonary
artery. C.T. scans demonstrated all abnormalities in which there
were possible metastatic hilar lymph nodes by tomography. In our
patients C.T. had a predictive positive value for hilum metastases
of 0,71 and a predictive negative value of 1,00; on the other hand
for tomography the predictive positive value was 0,72 and the
predictive negative value 0,87.

Enlarged_hilar_lymph_nodes.
In 14 out of 45 cases the hilar lymph nodes showed no abnormalities
on the C.T. scans, all proved to be small lymph nodes at surgery.
C.T. showed correctly 3 normal hilum which were predicted abnormal
by conventional tomography. In the other 31 cases with abnormal
hilum based on C.T. all but one proved to have enlarged lymph
nodes at surgery. In this case the tomography was interpreted as
abnormal also. C.T. detected 5 additional anatomically hilar lymph
nodes which were predicted normal by conventional tomography.
C.T. demonstrated all the abnormalities shown by conventional
tomography. In our patients C.T. had a predictive positive value
of 0,97 and a predictive negative value of 1,00. On the other hand
for conventional tomography the predictive positive value was 0,86
and the predictive negative value was 0,69.

CONCLUSION
1. C.T. scan is useful in the evaluation both of metastatic lymph
   nodes as well as enlarged lymph nodes.
2. C.T. is more accurate than posterior anterior tomography.
3. For metastatic lymph nodes C.T. statistically (two-side
   sign test) cannot replace conventional tomographs (P = 0,72;
   N.S.). On the other hand C.T. can replace conventional
   tomography for enlarged lymph nodes (P = 0,008; S.).

VX.13.

VASCULAR CHANGE IN MAIN BRONCHI OF SARCOIDOSIS

T. Kobayashi, M. Fukushima, K. Ozawa, R. Wada, T. Seki, I. Mochizuki and S. Kusama

In 1978 at the WCB in Tokyo, we reported the bronchial involvement in patients with sarcoidosis and pointed out the profuse, small, engorged vessels, appeared as a network, in bronchoscopic findings and existence of vascular change histologically in biopsied specimens. Now, we report vascular changes in bronchial wall of sarcoidosis in detail.

Table 1   *Bronchoscopic Findings*

No.	age	sex	stage	activity	Branchial distortion Carinal widening	Stenosis	Nodules	Uneven	Vascular engorgement	Rubor
1	22	F	I	—	—	—	╫	+	+	+
2	54	M	I	—	+	—	+	—	╫	+
3	22	M	I	—	+	+	+	+	╫	╫
4	57	F	I	+	+	—	+	+	—	+
5	20	F	I	—	—	—	—	—	+	+
6	37	M	I	+	—	—	+	+	╫	+
7	55	F	I	—	+	—	+	+	+	—
8	21	M	I	+	+	—	—	+	╫	+
9	16	M	I	—	—	╫	—	+	╫	╫
10	27	F	I	+	—	—	—	—	╫	+
11	26	M	I	+	+	+	╫	+	+	+
12	54	F	I	+	╫	+	—	—	+	+
13	44	F	I	—	—	+	—	—	—	—
14	54	F	I	+	—	—	╫	—	+	+
15	28	F	I	—	—	—	—	—	+	—
16	28	F	I	—	—	—	╫	+	+	—
17	30	M	I	—	+	—	+	—	╫	+
18	50	F	I	+	+	—	—	+	+	+
19	57	F	I	—	+	—.	╫	—	╫	+
20	29	F	I	+	╫	+	+	—	╫	╫
21	26	M	I	+	+	—	+	—	╫	╫
22	21	M	I	—	+	—	+	—	+	—
23	14	M	I	—	—	—	+	—	╫	—
24	16	F	I	—	—	—	—	—	—	—
25	54	F	II	+	—	+	+	+	+	+
26	50	F	II	—	+	—	—	—	╫	╫
27	23	F	II	+	+	+	+	╫	╫	+
28	50	F	II	—	—	—	—	+	╫	╫
29	57	F	II	—	—	+	+	+	+	—
30	39	F	II	—	+	+	—	—	—	—
31	19	F	II	—	╫	+	—	+	+	+
32	23	M	II	—	—	—	—	—	—	—
33	53	F	II	+	+	+	+	—	—	—
34	39	F	II	+	—	—	╫	—	╫	+
35	25	M	II	—	—	—	—	—	—	╫

Table 2

Relation between Vascular engorgement and Size of BHL

		Vascular engorgement	
		—	+
Size of BHL	small	1 (14%)	6 (86%)
	middle	3 (19%)	16 (81%)
	large	3 (33%)	6 (67%)

Table 3

Relation between Vascular engorgemenr and Stenosis of main bronchi

		Vascular engorgement	
		—	+
Stenosis of main bronchi	—	4 (21%)	19 (79%)
	+	3 (25%)	9 (75%)

Table 4

Relation between Vascular engorgement and Disease activity in sarcoidosis

	Vascular engorgement	
	—	+
active	2 (15%)	11 (85%)
inactive	6 (26%)	17 (74%)

J.A. Nakhosteen and W. Maassen (eds.), Bronchology: Research, Diagnostic and Therapeutic Aspects. All rights reserved.
Copyright 1981. Martinus Nijhoff Publishers bv, The Hague / Boston / London

Table 5   *Microscopic Findings*

No.	1	2	3	4	5	6	7	8	9	10	11	18	19	20	21	22	25	26	27	28	29
Granuloma	−	−	+	−	−	−	−	−	−	−	−	−	−	−	−	−	−	−	+	−	−
Giant cells	−	−	+	−	−	−	−	−	−	−	−	−	−	−	−	−	−	−	+	−	−
Endothelium swelling	−	−	+	+	+	+	+	+	+	−	+	+	+	+	+	+	+	+	+	−	−
Eosinophils infiltration	−	+	−	−	−	−	+	+	−	+	−	+	+	−	+	−	+	−	+	−	+

Materials and Methods:

We have performed bronchoscopic examination in 35 patients with sarcoidosis
(Table 1). There were 23 women and 12 men. Ages ranged between 14 and 57 years.
Bronchoscopy was performed using standard techniques. Bronchoscopic biopsy was
carried out in the medial wall of the right main bronchi, about 1cm distal from
the tracheal bifurcation.

Results:

The profuse, small, engorged vessels like network-appearance were observed
in trachea, main and segmental bronchi. There was no remarkable difference between
the right and left bronchi. In stage 1, vascular engorgement was observed in 22
out of 24 patients. With regard to the relation between vascular engorgement and
size of BHL, it is difficult to find a certain relation (Table 2). In addition,
vascular engorgement was not related to stenosis the bronchi (Table 3). Therefore,
we think, vascular engorgement was not caused by congestion due to enlargement of
hilar lymphnode, but is characteristic finding of sarcoidosis. It is difficult to
find the relation between the vascular engorgement and disease activity in sarcoidosis (Table 4).

In microscopic findings of biopsied specimens, noncaseating epitheloid cell
granuloma with giant cell were isolated in 2 out of 21, endothelium swelling, 16
out of 21 and eosinophils infiltration around vessel wall, 9 out of 21 (Table 5).

Summary

We suppose vascular engorgement is characteristic finding in sarcoidosis.
Vascular engorgement, as well as white-yellowish nodules, is significant finding
in the bronchoscopic diagnosis on sarcoidosis.

References

1. Bennedict, E.B. and Castleman, B.: Sarcoidosis with bronchial involvement.
   New Eng. J. Med. 224: 186-189, 1941.
2. Huzly, A.: Atlas der Bronchoscopie pp. 24-25. Georg Thieme Verlag. Stuttgart
   1960.

Chapter VII

FLEXIBLE OR RIGID BRONCHOSCOPY?

VII.1.

FLEXIBLE BRONCHOSCOPY IN SCANDINAVIA - A FIVE YEAR SURVEY

BENGT G. OLLMAN, CARL-ERIC LINDHOLM

An increasing interest in environmental questions such as air pollution and the effects of smoking, and also the growth of intensive care medicine as well as a remarkable technical progress in the creation and evolution of the flexible fiberoptic bronchoscope have given us the feeling that bronchoscopy has attached more attention during the last decade than ever before. To investigate whether this feeling is based on a real increase or is just an imaginary transition of proportions we have performed a survey of the bronchoscopic activity in Scandinavia.

This survey is the result of two inquiries, performed with an interval of 5 years. In 1975 an inquiry was sent out to otolaryngologists, anesthesiological departments and pulmonary departments in Sweden, to evaluate the rate and proportion of bronchoscopies performed at that time, and also the technique and type of anesthesia. In spring 1980 a new inquiry was made to the same clinics, and this time also the equivalent clinics in Denmark and Norway were included. The following is therefore a report of bronchoscopic activities in the scandinavian countries, which may also give some hints on the direction of development. The inquiry is supposed to be the base for a similar follow-up study in another 5 years to come.

More than 300 inquiry-forms were sent out to all otolaryngology, anesthesiology and pulmonary departments in Sweden, Norway and Denmark. More than 200 answers returned, but only 194 answers have been included in the survey due to late arrival of the rest. A total of 11.951 bronchoscopies were performed in 1979 in a population of 17 million people. 61 % were performed in Sweden, 21 % in Denmark and 18 % in Norway.

A comparison of bronchoscopy in Sweden between the years 1975 and 1979 (Table I.) demonstrates a numerical rise from 6358 to 7276, which is an increase of 13 %. There is a decrease of rigid bronchoscopies with 1531 and an increase of flexible bronchoscopies with 2442. As can be seen pulmonary physicians perform the equal amount, but have shifted largely from rigid to flexible technique. The otolaryngologists have increased the total number, and mainly added in the amount

J.A. Nakhosteen and W. Maassen (eds.), Bronchology: Research, Diagnostic and Therapeutic Aspects. All rights reserved.
Copyright 1981. Martinus Nijhoff Publishers bv, The Hague / Boston / London

of flexible performances.

TABLE I. Bronchoscopy in Sweden. Comparison 1975 - 1979.

1975	PULM	OTOL + ANEST	TOTAL
RIGID	1265	3382	4647
FLEXIBLE	773	938	1711
	2038	4320	6358
1979			
RIGID	348	2768	3116
FLEXIBLE	1784	2377	4160
	2132	5150	7276

A further analysis of bronchoscopies in Sweden is presented in Table II. From 116 clinics is a reported total of 7276 performances. Only 307 or less than 5 % are performed by the anesthesiologists. The number of flexible instruments is however relatively high by the anesthesiologists. Up to 100 flexible fiberoptic bronchoscopes are in use in Sweden. The missing numbers refers to thoracic surgeons, medical clinics and theoretical institutions.

TABLE II. Bronchoscopy in Sweden 1979.

	FFB	No.Cl	RIGID	%	FLEX	%	TOTAL	%
OTOL	48	49	2592	36	2245	31	4837	67
PULM	19	26	348	5	1784	25	2132	29
ANEST	11	41	176	2	131	1	307	4
	78	116	3116	43	4167	57	7276	100

A similar analysis of bronchoscopies in Denmark 1979 is presented in Table III. Also here the majority is performed by otolaryngologists, but the rigid bronchoscope is here the dominating instrument. The pulmo nay physicians do not seem to so interested in bronchoscopy as their fellow scandinavian doctors.

TABLE III. Bronchoscopy in Denmark 1979.

	FFB	No.Cl	RIGID	%	FLEX	%	TOTAL	%
OTOL	11	19	2042	81	352	14	2394	95
PULM	0	10	17	1	24	1	41	2
ANEST	3	17	59	2	15	1	74	3
	14	46	2118	84	391	16	2509	100

In Norway 2166 bronchoscopies were performed by 32 clinics. The distribution can be seen from Table IV. In contrast to Denmark and Sweden the majority is here performed by the pulmonary physicians.

TABLE IV. Bronchoscopy in Norway 1979.

	FFB	No.Cl	RIGID	%	FLEX	%	TOTAL	%
OTOL	8	15	473	22	121	6	594	28
PULM	17	12	106	5	1436	66	1542	71
ANEST	1	5	16	1	14	1	30	1
	26	32	595	28	1571	72	2166	100

There is a great diversity as to the method of anesthesia both between the rigid and flexible instrument as between the different countries and the different specialities. The rigid bronchoscopies are mainly performed in general anesthesia, with two notable exceptions, viz. pulmonary physicians in Sweden and Norway. Flexible bronchoscopy is generally performed in topical anesthesia, except by anestheiologists in Sweden and otolaryngologists and pulmonary physicians in Denmark.

TABLE V. Anesthesi in Bronchoscopy in Scandinavia 1979.

		% RIGID	%	% FLEX	%
		Gen	Top	Gen	Top
Sweden	OTOL	65	35	35	65
	PULM	1	99	0	100
	ANEST	89	11	67	33
Denmark	OTOL	76	24	81	19
	PULM	75	25	80	20
	ANEST	–	–	–	–
Norway	OTOL	98	2	40	60
	PULM	4	96	2	98
	ANEST	–	–	–	–

A comparison made between anesthesia in otolaryngological clinics in Sweden 1975 and 1979 indicates a trend towards general anesthesia.

TABLE VI. Anesthesia in Otolaryngologic Bronchoscopy 1975 - 1979.

	RIGID				FLEX			
	1975		1979		1975		1979	
	n	%	n	%	n	%	n	%
Topical	2320	50	1279	41	1547	90	3295	79
General	2327	50	1837	59	164	10	866	21
Total:	4647		3116		1711		4161	

As to the method of general anesthesia very few clinics have answered to that question. It seems that intravenous anesthesia with manual ventilation is in high favour, but jet-ventilation and HFPPV is reported in a fair number of cases. Only a few clinics still use the apnoic ventilation method.

For topical anesthesia most instances in Scandinavia use Lidocain-spray. The amount varies between 100 and 800 mg, with a medium value of 220 mg. In Norway ultrasonic nebulisation is reported in a number of places. A few clinics still use Tetracain, Novesin and Cocain.

The method of introduction of the flexible bronchoscope is mainly reported to be the transnasal route. In Denmark 86 % of the procedures in topical anesthesia are made transnasally, in Norway 89 % and in Sweden 89 %. Table VII. shows the change in Sweden during the last 5 years.

TABLE   VII. Introduction method in topical flexible bronchoscopy.

	Trans nasal	Nasal tube	Trans oral	Oral tube
1975 %	38	3	13	46
1979 %	89	1	1	9

Transbronchial lungbiopsy were performed in 221 cases in Norway, 191 cases in Sweden and 123 cases in Denmark during 1979.

Foreign bodies were picked up in 250 cases in Scandinavia during 1979. In 233 cases the rigid method was used. The bronchoscopies were made by otolaryngologists in 227 cases. Pulmonary physicians in Norway reported removal of foreign body with the flexible instrument in 16 cases. Some pulmonary clinics in Sweden reported parttaking in foreign body removal without giving any statistics.

Bronchoscopy in children is reported in 252 cases in Scandinavia during 1979. This is about 2 % of the total amount of bronchoscopies. 230 of these cases were performed with rigid technique. 212 were performed by otolaryngologists.

Complications are rare in bronchoscopy. In 5829 rigid bronchoscopies in Scandinavia in 1979 1 death is reported, 2 cardiac arrests and 3 haemoptysis which needed treatment. In 6122 flexible bronchoscopies 1 death is reported, 3 pneumothorax and 2 haemoptysis which needed treatment.

Thus bronchoscopy, both with the rigid and the flexible instrument seems to be a safe procedure. In 17 million people 2 have died. It would be interesting to know how many have died because they did not have a bronchoscopy performed.

VII.2.

RIGID OR FLEXIBLE BRONCHOSCOPY

E.Th. EDENS, M.D.

In the United States and in Europe there is still a lot of discussion about the question: which instrument shall we use, the rigid
or the flexible bronchoscope ?
In relation to this question I would like to point to a commentary
in the Journal of the American Medical Association (1974) with the
title: "Today's esophagologists autocastrated". If we change the word
esophagus into bronchus the description will fit identical situations
in Holland and perhaps also in Germany.

A passage of this article reads like this: "Since the fiberesopha-
goscope entered the picture, we have raised a generation of esophagologists who are unable to deal with many of the important esophageal
diseases. The ranks of complete esophagologists have thinned alarmingly.
The child with a safety-pin in his esophagus must be sent farther and
farther from home to find a physician capable of getting out it safely.
Perhaps as distressing a tendency as any is the failure of today's
fiberesophagoscopist to appreciate how many important therapeutic
manipulations are possible with the esophagus".
The words of this American editor were quite after my heart. In the
Netherlands it is not uncommon that, especially during the weekend, par-
ents have to drive 200 km. In order to find an endoscopist capable
to extract a foreign body. A bronchotomy to remove an aspirated object
is a testimonium paupertatis for the endoscopist on duty.

Huzly (1977) stated that in his clinic the young surgeon has to
learn the rigid technique in order to get permission to introduce the
flexible fiberscope. In the E.N.T. department of our University Medical
Center where we teach future laryngologists and pneumologists, the
E.N.T. residents get a special training to handle the rigid system
according to practical needs. Especially in childrenbronchoscopy the
rigid scope is the instrument of choice (Sackner, 1975). It is hardly
possible to oxygenate after introducing a 6 mm. fiberscope not men-

*J.A. Nakhosteen and W. Maassen (eds.), Bronchology: Research, Diagnostic and
Therapeutic Aspects. All rights reserved.
Copyright 1981. Martinus Nijhoff Publishers bv, The Hague / Boston / London*

tioning the psychological stress during a procedure in topical anaesthesia. The future Olympus BF-4C3 (with suctionchannel) has a diameter
of 3.4 mm. at the tip and is special designed for endoscopic procedures in children (Oho, 1979). Time and trial will provide sufficient information to make this judgement.

It is difficult to give a survey over the indications for rigid
or flexible bronchoscopy because the choice of instruments is purely
subjective and depends on 25-years experience with rigid technics,
including 12-years work with the flexible bronchoscope. We come to
the conclusion that the rigid bronchoscope is very useful in:

1. Removing foreign bodies
   Recent publications about using the flexible fiberscope in handling
   foreign bodies do not reflect the reality because 92 % of our
   patients with suspected aspiration are children; yet one must not
   condemn the use of the flexible system in adults. Zavala (1980)
   recommends besides the ordinary forceps and baskets the use of Swan-
   Ganz and Fogarty catheters to dislodge foreign bodies. This catheter technic can also be used in the rigid bronchoscope. In children
   under six years of age the open tip bronchoscope is the instrument
   of choice. The use of an optical forceps facilitates the sometimes
   very difficult operation.

2. Intubating acute laryngo-tracheal stenosis
   Well-known are the stridorous episodes in patients (most children)
   with epiglottitis and sub-glottic laryngitis. Severe dyspnea is
   sometimes seen after necksurgery and laryngeal trauma due to edema
   and sub-mucosal bleeding. The rigid bronchoscope is the only instrument that can provide an immediate airway. Katz and Berci
   aware of these problems designed an optical stylet. The stylet is
   in reality a telescope supplied with a stainless steel tube to
   provide support in case of manipulation as well as to prevent break-
   age. In order to get full benefit of this instrument the endoscopist
   (otolaryngologist, anaesthesist, thoracic surgeon or pneumologist)
   must known all the tricks of the rigid intubation technic. With a
   teaching attachment coupled to the stylet the students and residents
   can observe the anatomy of pharynx, larynx and trachea.

3. Dilating tracheastenosis
   All patients with tracheastenosis, mostly of traumatic origin, are
   dilated in our clinic. From 1972-1980 we treated in cooperation
   with the department of thorax-surgery 25 patients with severe
   tracheal stenosis due to high cuff pressure, 5 cases responded

very well to dilation with rigid bronchoscopes and did not need
surgery.

4. Objectivating trachea-esophageal fistulas
The fistulas mostly are of congenital origin. The acquired types
appear sometimes after blunt chest injuries or ingestion of caustic
material. It is nearly impossible to detect a small fistula even
with the help of a telescope. The location of the fistula in the
trachea is seen within seconds after injecting 3-5 cc. methylene
blue in the upper esophagus.

5. Evacuating tough secretions
The diameter of the suction tube in the conventional rigid system
is much larger than the 2 mm. suctionchannel of the widely used
BF-B3. Olympus designed fiberscopes for therapeutic purposes (type
IT and 2T). In comparison to the rigid bronchoscope the price is
extremely high.

6. Coagulation of malignant ingrowth
In cases of palliation electro-coagulation with isolated stainless
steel suction tubes is very helpful. During the time of coagulation
the produced smoke is immediated sucked out of the trachea and
provides an undisturbed vision.

7. Suture excision after tracheal surgery
Suture material in tracheal and bronchial wall often favors the
formation of granulations. This can give rise to very severe stenosis
even of a technically flawless reconstructive procedures with an
anastomosis of initially ample diameter. We designed endobronchial
scissors (Wolf-Knittlingen - W.Germany), to cut the stiches without
any harm to the trachea mucosa. The removal of the suture remnants
with an optical forceps is a matter of seconds (Eygelaar, Edens,
1972).

8. Substantial tumor excision after negative results with the flexible
scope
The cups of a 'rigid' forceps are six times larger than the 'flexible' ones.

9. Punction with 50 cm needles
The punction results of a broad carina or suspected impression of
the bronchial wall are in my opinion superior to those of the existing 'flexible' needles.

10. Objective photodocumentation
The slides produced with the flash generator (Wolf, Storz) are by
far superior in comparison to the results with the flexible fiber
system.

The flexible fiberscope is the first choice for mechanical problems such as trismus, insufficiency of the basilaris artery, torticollis kyphoscoliosis, arthrosis of the temporo-mandibular joints, arthritis and fracture of the cervical spine. The most useful indications for flexible brochofiberscopy are:

1. Intubation problems
   A BF-B3 bronchoscope provided with an endotracheal tube is inserted via the nasopharyngeal airway. Once the distal one third of the scope has been passed through the glottis, the lubricated tube is guided over the bronchoscope into the trachea.
2. Hemoptysis
   More precise localisation of the bleeding site.
3. Peripheral tumors
   Particularly to facilitate placement of a brush or biopsy forceps with or without the help of fluoroscopy.
4. Upper lobe tumors and small hilar lesions
5. Transbronchial biopsy in diffuse pulmonary diseases
6. Negative chest radiograms and positive sputum cytology features
7. Tracheo-bronchial toilet in intensive-care patients
8. Selective collection of secretions for bacteriologic examination
9. Selective bronchography
10. Inspection of partly blocked endobronchial and tracheostomic tubes

There is no doubt that indications for flexible or rigid broncho-scopy will change when smaller diameter flexible fiberscopes enter the market. In the near future the neodyn-yag laser made for flexible bronchoscopes will change the possibilities of pallation in patients with obstructing malignant ingrowth.

Today the flexible and rigid endoscopic systems stand besides each other. The best endoscopist is the doctor who can both handle the rigid and the flexible bronchoscope.

VII.3.

FLEXIBLE OR RIGID BRONCHOSCOPY

I. Pilis

For us who are still employing the rigid bronchoscopic technique
the question may be "to be or not to be". I do not think the question is so serious as, finally, it is not the instrument itself
which determines its futurity but rather the man, bronchologist,
his skill and the results he achieves.

At the beginning I wish to present the advantages and disadvantages of the both techniques, taking Friedel's instrument with the
possibility of performing catheterbiopsy as an example of a rigid
bronchoscope. All that I am going to say is probably already well
known.

Indisputably, the flexible bronchoscope is a great improvement
in bronchology. It is an old endeavour to penetrate visially further into the periphery of the bronchial tree. The above goal is
fulfilled nowadays with the development of the flexible bronchoscope by which 6 - 7 divisions of the subsegmental bronchi can be
explored. Visualization of these minute bronchi is very important
as they harbour small malignant tumours. If no changes are observed and a lesion is located more peripherally, the instrument can
be guided deeper and the specimens taken by the brush or forceps.
Perbronchial lung biopsy is feasible in diffuse and disseminated
lung diseases by the flexible bronchoscope.

Miniaturization of the entire apparatus, particularly its optical instrument has some disadvantages. The optical instruments
diminish and shorten the image, especially the field of visuali-
zations is limited in the central region of the bronchial tree. The
same holds true for the biopsy forceps which is so miniature that
the tissue bits obtained are less suitable for histological examination. The forceps does not satisfy with mucosa biopsy specimens
in sarcoidosis. Frequently indispensable transbronchial puncture
of the nodes or tumours is not feasible by the flexible bronchoscope when external signs of compression on the bronchus are present. Extraction of a foreign body is not feasible with the aid of

*J.A. Nakhosteen and W. Maassen (eds.), Bronchology: Research, Diagnostic and
Therapeutic Aspects. All rights reserved.*
Copyright 1981. Martinus Nijhoff Publishers bv, The Hague / Boston / London

the flexible bronchoscope in adults.

Intubation with the flexible bronchoscope is of minimal discomfort to the patient, less traumatizing and stressful than with the rigid instrument. There are no contraindications for the procedure except for severe heart or respiratory insufficient patients.

Because of miniaturization and high sensitivity, particularly the biopsy forceps and optical instrument, they are liable to frequent defects. The apparatus and its accessories are very expensive and the purchase is time-consuming under our circumstances.

Now I would like to report on Friedel's rigid bronchoscope we have been using in our institution for 15 years. All rigid bronchoscopes are more or less the same and adequate. They may differ only by the quality of their optic instruments. At present all they are very good, particularly Hopkin's optic instruments. They permit visualization only of the lobar and segmental orifice. The optic instruments provide a wide field of visualization and magnify and, hence, the entire bronchial tree can be encompassed. The instrument provides a clear and fine image of the minute details. The tubes are of varying size permitting diversified manipulations such as aspiration, lavage, management of haemorrhage, biopsies with relatively big biopsy forceps and obtaining of adequate material for analysis. The instrument permits a transbronchial puncture of the nodes and tumours and extraction of rather large foreign bodies. Friedel's bronchoscope is used under general anesthesia with relaxation which causes certainly less discomfort for the patient who is asleep throughout the examination so neither intubation nor manipulation within the bronchus causes discomfort that is even less than with flexible bronchoscopy.

Bronchoscopy under local anesthesia with the rigid tube and optical instruments as in flexible bronchoscopy is almost without any contraindications except those mentioned with flexible bronchoscopy. Contrary, bronchoscopy under general anesthesia has more known contraindications. In such circumstances we use the same instrument under local anesthesia.

As far as the periphery is concerned the problem is solved very simply thanks to an exceptional discovery of catheterbiopsy after Friedel. The technical data are well known to all. By skillful manipulation of the guiding wire and the catheter the latter can be guided directly into any subsegmental or more peripheral division controlled by the image intensifuing screen. The material obtainable by catheterbiopsy in majority of cases is a big bit of tissue adequate for the histologic analysis, such as is seen on the presented picture of an epidermoid carcinoma.

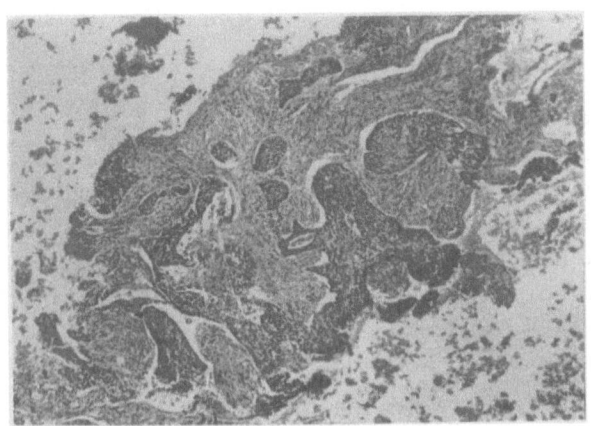

The same catheterbiopsy can be performed under local anesthesia in the cases contraindicated under general anesthesia. In these cases the periphery is not explored visually that is an advantage of flexible bronchoscopy. By any rigid bronchoscope, using Friedel's guiding catheter, perbronchial biopsy of the lung is feasible in diffuse and disseminated diseases. A small flexible bronchoscope forceps is inserted through the canal under the image intensifier reaching any subsegment and further the periphery of the lung area.

Most important are the results obtained. We have been applying Friedel's catheterbiopsy in our institution, since the end of 1966. Thus far we have performed about 3000 catheterbiopsies in different clinical settings. Unfortunately, only the period until July 1975 is analyzed and 1738 catheterbiopsies were performed in that period. The definitive diagnosis was established in 727 malignant tumours, 354 nonspecific inflammatory processes, 278 tuberculoses and 107 other diseases. In all cases the peripheral shadows were concerned. In malignant tumours there were 78.4% positive results and in 92% of cases the diagnosis was established histologically. 1.2% of cases were strongly suspicious for cancer histologically and cytologically indicating that there were 79.6% positive results.

The results obtained by flexible bronchoscopy, according to the literature, range from 51% to 95%. Central carcinoma is included in the above percent. The majority of the results are below 80%. 79.6% positive results of our catheterbiopsies refer exclusively to peripheral carcinoma. The total percentage of the positive fin-

224

dings obtained by the rigid bronchoscope is 88% i.e. an approximate percent as with flexible bronchoscopy.

DISCUSSION

I would repeat the fact that every technique is equally good in the hands of an experienced bronchologist, i.e. it yields approximately the same results. Therefore, I do mean that flexible bronchoscopy and bronchoscopy with the rigid instrument have their "raison d'etre". Either method has its advantages and disadvantages and thus they are complementary to each other. Every bronchologist should actually master the both techniques and have the both instruments. The flexible bronchoscope is certainly a major technical improvement in the development of bronchology. Elegance and ease of its insertion and manipulation makes the examination feasible even in patients with severe debilitating disease and other contraindications in whom the procedure is otherwise impossible with other methods.

The bronchologist has several alternatives at his choice with either bronchoscope:

1) Routine application of the flexible bronchoscope in the combination with the rigid instrument, if necessary, in the particular procedures,

2) Routine use of the rigid bronchoscope with catheterbiopsy in conjunction with the flexible bronchoscope, when necessary, including the cases where general anesthesia is contraindicated and

3) Routine intubation and examination with the rigid bronchoscope under either general or local anesthesia, with the routine peripheral diagnosis by the flexible bronchoscope.

VII.4.
CONTROVERSIES IN FLEXIBLE FIBEROPTIC BRONCHOSCOPY

D.C. Zavala

INTRODUCTION

Since the introduction of the flexible fiberoptic bronchoscope in 1967, most
of the procedural problems have been resolved. However, several important controversies still remain. The author takes a definite position in discussing each of
these topics below.

BRONCHOSCOPY IN CRITICAL CARE MEDICINE

Whereas rigid, open-tube bronchoscopy presents horrendous problems in poor
risk patients on mechanical ventilators, flexible fiberoptic bronchoscopy can be
readily performed through a swivel tracheal tube adapter without interruption of
the ongoing mechanical ventilation. The bronchoscopist should be aware of the
following potential pathophysiologic changes which take place as a result of bronchofiberscopy during mechanical ventilation: (1) Immediately upon insertion of the
fiberoptic bronchoscope a positive end-expiratory effect occurs, accompanied by a
reduction in the patient's exhaled tidal volume; (2) Alterations in the ventilation-
perfusion ratio (V/Q) may develop with a precipitous drop in the PaO_2. This event
is especially likely to happen during vigorous suctioning.

To avoid these potential risks the following recommendations are made: (1)
Use an endotracheal tube which has an internal diameter of at least 8.5 mm; (2)
Increase the FIO_2 to 1.0 (100%); (3) Discontinue PEEP; (4) Monitor the exhaled
tidal volume; (5) Monitor the electrocardiographic pattern, heart rate, and rhythm;
(6) Observe the patient's chest for adequate excursions; (7) Keep the procedure
short; (8) Restrict suction to brief periods; (9) When indicated, monitor the blood
arterial oxygen saturation by ear oximetry; (10) When indicated, obtain a follow-
up chest roentgenogram to rule out pneumothorax and mediastinal emphysema.

PULMONARY HEMORRHAGE

Patients with hemoptysis must be managed according to their clinical condition
and the severity of the bleeding. In mild to moderate bleeding the flexible fiberscope is a super sleuth in tracking down the blood to its source. A meticulous
ENT examination (larynx and nasopharynx) is mandatory. Although bronchitis is
one of the most common causes of blood in the sputum, the reward of a careful examination of the upper and lower airway may be an early laryngeal or bronchogenic
carcinoma. Massive, life-threatening hemoptysis must be handled as an emergency.
The endoscopist has to localize the bleeding site as rapidly as possible and to
control the blood loss by vigorous suction, by application of epinephrine, by pack-
ing with gauze tape, or by inserting a Fogarty balloon catheter. For these maneu-
vers the open-tube, rigid bronchoscope is the preferred instrument without question
since a large amount of blood cannot be removed through the small aspirating channel
of the bronchofiberscope. Also when blood floods the airway, fiberoptic vision is lost

*J.A. Nakhosteen and W. Maassen (eds.), Bronchology: Research, Diagnostic and
Therapeutic Aspects. All rights reserved.
Copyright 1981. Martinus Nijhoff Publishers bv, The Hague / Boston / London*

PEDIATRIC BRONCHOSCOPY

The open-tube ventilating bronchoscope is the instrument of choice in pediatric bronchoscopy; this is primarily because of the small size of the glottis
and trachea. For removal of foreign bodies in infants and children, the rigid,
open-tube bronchoscope is mandatory. Nevertheless, the flexible fiberoptic bronchoscope (small size) plays an important although somewhat limited role in the pediatric age group. One useful function of the fiberscope is to carry out transnasal
laryngoscopy; helpful information may be gained in evaluating a cleft palate, ap-
praising upper airway patency (croup; thermal injury), and in verifying the position of an endotracheal tube. In children as young as two years of age one can
have a brief look at the lower airway using an Olympus BF-3C2 fiberscope. In older
children (usually over 5 to 8 years of age) the new Olympus 4B2 bronchofiberscope
(distal tip 4.9 mm; channel 2 mm) is ideal to visualize the trachea, mainstem and
segmental bronchi. The best route to insert the bronchofiberscope in children
is transnasal, accompanied by supplemental O_2, EKG monitoring, and careful observation of the patient.

FOREIGN BODY REMOVAL

The rigid bronchoscope has been eminently successful in the removal of endobronchial foreign bodies. Even today, large objects in the central airways are
best removed through an open-tube, rigid bronchoscope regardless of the patient's
age. In the pediatric age group where most foreign body aspirations occur in
toddlers and children up to four or five years of age, the rigid bronchoscope remains exclusively the instrument of choice. Until recently, if conventional
methods failed to remove a foreign body in an adult patient, the only other option
was early thoracotomy with transpleural bronchotomy. Currently, however, the
flexible fiberoptic bronchoscope is capable of removing small, peripheral foreign
bodies which lie beyond the reach of the rigid bronchoscope. Recently developed
methods employ new extraction tools (forceps, wire basket, claw, and Fogarty balloon catheter) which are inserted through the biopsy channel of the bronchofiberscope. Proper technique is essential to avoid a number of potential problems.

STAGING FOR LUNG CANCER

In the preoperative assessment of lung cancer for resectability the following
guidelines are important: (1) The presence of tumor within 2 cm of the main carina
indicates inoperability; (2) If a lung cancer is located in either mainstem bronchus
or in the right upper lobe, then forceps biopsies of the main carina (via the
flexible or rigid bronchoscope) produce abnormal results in 10-13% of the cases,
even in the presence of normal appearing mucosa. The finding of malignant cells
in the carinal biopsy specimen decrees that the tumor is unresectable and that
further staging procedures are unnecessary; (3) If a tumor is located in a large
bronchus or a smaller segmental bronchus, routine forceps biopsies of proximal

spurs should be done since spread of carcinoma may be more extensive than is visibly evident; (4) When external compression of the trachea or mainstem bronchus occurs, without thru-and-thru invasion by the extrensic malignancy, a transtracheal or transbronchial needle aspiration biopsy through the bronchoscope (flexible or rigid) may establish the diagnosis.

PERIPHERAL LUNG NODULE

When dealing with a peripheral or subpleural coin lesion there is good evidence to indicate that needle aspiration is the preferred initial procedure rather than bronchofiberscopy. Needle aspiration of outer zone lung lesions has an overall diagnostic yield (sensitivity) of 83% to 90% as compared to a yield of 30% to 70% achieved by flexible fiberoptic bronchoscopy. The exception to these data is the diagnostic success achieved by our Japanese colleagues (Drs. Ikeda and Ono) using a double-hinged curette via the flexible fiberoptic bronchoscope. As yet, the Americans and Europeans have not become proficient in the use of this ingenious biopsy tool.

FLUOROSCOPY

In localized lung disease, endoscopists agree that fluoroscopy is an invaluable aid to accurately position a biopsy tool on a lesion which is located beyond the range of endoscopic vision, but opinions are divided as to the role of the fluoroscope in taking forceps transbronchial biopsies (TBB's) in diffuse lung disease. One subtle factor is that physical limitations at many institutions make the routine use of fluoroscopic techniques difficult, so that TBB's often are carried out without fluoroscopic guidance. And yet, it is much safer and more accurate to perform forceps TBB's under fluoroscopic control. Thus, the operator can make certain that the forceps does not penetrate the visceral pleura and that the jaws of the biopsy tool open properly. Needless to say, it is vital for any physician operating a fluoroscope to be thoroughly trained in its proper usage.

METHODS OF INSERTION: TRANSNASAL VS TRANSORAL

Each method has its advantages and limitations. Thus, one technique should not be used to the total exclusion of the other.

Transnasal insertion is the best route in pediatric bronchoscopy. This technique conveniently provides entrance to the tracheobronchial tree but does not establish an airway. In adult patients, transnasal insertion is preferable in those who are likely to (or attempt to) bite during oral insertion, in those who are unduely apprehensive or refuse to accept oral insertion, and when only an examination of the airway is needed without anticipation of transbronchial biopsy. The potential problems with the transnasal approach are: (1) Forced insertion through a small nasal passageway can produce trauma; (2) There may be considerable loss of biopsy material if the brush is withdrawn through the channel of the fiberscope; (3) The insertion shaft of the bronchoscope may rub the vocal cords sufficiently to cause excessive coughing and thus necessitate the administration of more lidocaine locally.

Transoral insertion of the fiberoptic bronchoscope through an ET tube is especially indicated in transbronchial lung biopsy and in high risk situations. The advantages of carrying out fiberoptic bronchoscopy by this method are: (1) An airway is established for insertion of a large bore sucker to control major hemorrhage or an outpouring of thick pus; (2) Additional O_2 can be given through the ET tube; (3) The fiberoptic bronchoscope can be rapidly withdrawn and reinserted with ease for multiple biopsies, for clearing of the distal lens, or simply to change instruments. Note: An ET tube is contraindicated in pediatric bronchoscopy, in patients with thermal injury, and in subjects with suspected subglottic or upper tracheal lesions.

TRAINING

It is a waste of time, effort, and money to train any physician in fiberoptic bronchoscopy who will not be able to maintain and further develop this art by frequent endoscopy. The best candidates for instruction in pulmonary endoscopy are those in pulmonary medicine, thoracic surgery, and otolaryngology. In addition to these subspecialties, anesthesiologists are using the fiberscope for difficult intubations, and pediatricians are showing interest in miniaturized fiberoptic bronchoscopes. In the training of a competent endoscopist, two important aspects are the education of the hands to maneuver the bronchoscope and the education of the eyes to recognize and correctly interpret the view. Manipulation of the instrument should be natural and spontaneous. All of this takes time and experience, which can be gained only by enlightened, closely supervised training. Although the use of lung models, illustrations, photography, and cinematography is tremendously rewarding, nothing can take the place of the real thing. The ratio of the skilled, dedicated teacher to the committed student must remain one to one. Since each trainee differs in the acquisition of new skills, the operator's performance must be judged on an individual basis.

REFERENCES

1. Zavala DC: Flexible Fiberoptic Bronchoscopy: A Training Handbook. Iowa City, Ia, The University of Iowa Publications Order Department, 1978.
2. Ikeda S: Atlas of Flexible Bronchofiberscopy. Tokyo, Igaku Shoin Ltd, 1974 (also Baltimore and London, University Park Press, 1974).
3. Sackner MA: Bronchofiberscopy: State of the art. Am Rev Respir Dis 111: 62-88, 1975.

Chapter VIII
TRACHEO-BRONCHIAL CORRECTIVE AND PLASTIC SURGERY

Section 1
ENDOSCOPIC AND FUNCTIONAL CRITERIA

RESULTS OF PRE- AND POSTOPERATIVE FUNCTIONAL EVALUATION IN TRACHEAL STENOSIS

W. Petro, W. Maaßen, J.A. Nakhosteen, N. Konietzko

Stenosis of the upper respiratory tract causes complaints by patients especially in cases of severe tracheal stenosis combined with in- and expiratory
stridor.

We investigated 12 patients (8 males and 4 females) suffering from extrathoracic tracheal stenosis causes by long term artificial respiration in 8 and
by benign or malignant tumors in 4 cases.

All of them were cured by trachea sleeve resection and end-to-end-anastomosis.

Preoperative function tests and bronchoscopy take place 2 to 14 days before
operation. The postoperative controls were done within 7 days to three months
after operation. In both tracheal diameter was estimated pre- and postoperatively by endoscopic and roentgenographic methods. Lung mechanics were estimated
by bodyplethysmography (IVC, FEV_1, $FEV_{0.5}$, FIV_1, $FIV_{0.5}$, FRC, TLC, sR_{aw}, sG_{aw}),
flow-volume curve ($\dot{V}_{max\ exp.}$, $\dot{V}_{5o\ exp.}$, $\dot{V}_{max\ in.}$, $\dot{V}_{5o\ in.}$), bronchodilator and
acetylcholin challenge tests (sR_{aw}, sG_{aw}) by application of two puffs of fenoterol
respectively lo breaths of a 2 % acetylcholin solution. Blood gases were also
determined (P_aO_2, P_aCO_2).

Trachea sleeve resection and end-toend anastomosis increase the diameter of
the trachea from 5.9 $\pm$ 2.5 to 11.o $\pm$ 2.9 mm. Similarly the shapes of resistance
loops and flow volume curves change. Resistance loop which is s-shaped in extrathoracic fixed stenosis becomes steeper. The egg-shaped flow-volume-curve changes
into normal form (ref. 3). Resistance parameters were the most sensitive in
describing tracheal obstruction (ref. 1). Hence close correlation was found between pre- and postoperative tracheal diameter changes and changes of specific
conductance (fig. 1) and specific resistance (fig. 2). The same is valid for
conductance (r = o.61). In cases of a tracheal diameter lower than 5 mm one can
find a severe functional distortion and a good improvement by resection. Disturbances and operative effect are only slight in cases of a diameter more than lo mm.

Figure 1 (left)
Correlation between diameter of the trachea and specific conductance (sG_{aw}); values
before (●) and after trachea resection (▲); main regression line – black line;
$y= 22.4 \ x^{0.34}$; r = o.71

Figure 2 (right)
Correlation between diameter of the trachea and specific resistance (sR_{aw})
according figure 1; $y = 22.o \ x^{-0.33}$; r = o.7o

J.A. Nakhosteen and W. Maassen (eds.), Bronchology: Research, Diagnostic and
Therapeutic Aspects. All rights reserved.
Copyright 1981. Martinus Nijhoff Publishers bv, The Hague / Boston / London

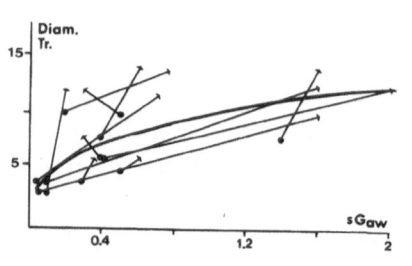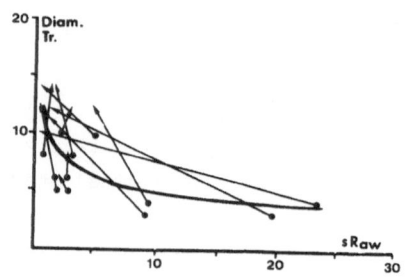

Parameters of flow-volume-curve and forced expiration show a significant correlation to the pre-postoperative tracheal diameter also. One can find correlation coefficients from o.62 ($\dot{V}_{max\ exp.}$), o.48 (FEV_1) and o.48 ($FEV_{o.5}$). There was no close correlation **between** mechanical improvement in FIV_1, $FIV_{o.5}$, $\dot{V}_{max\ in.}$, $\dot{V}_{5o\ in.}$, RV/TLC and blood gases. Reviewing the **functional** effects of increased tracheal diameter (Tab. 1), significant changes were shown by specific resistance and conductance and by further parameters of forced expiration as $\dot{V}_{max\ exp.}$, $\dot{V}_{5o\ exp.}$, FEV_1 and $FEV_{o.5}$.

Table 1: Comparison of pre- and postoperative functional parameters

Parameter	$\bar{x} \pm$ s.d. before		$\bar{x} \pm$ s.d. after resection		t	p
sR_{aw} (kPa s)	6.84	5.49	1.87	1.36	2.26	o.o5
G_{aw} (kPa $1^{-1}s)^{-1}$	1.18	o.68	1.83	1.9	2.72	o.o2
sG_{aw} (kPa s)$^{-1}$	o.37	o.37	o.89	o.63	2.5o	o.o25
$\dot{V}_{max\ exp.}$ (1/s)	2.9	1.6	5.2	2.7	2.48	o.o25
$\dot{V}_{5o\ exp.}$ (1/s)	1.6	o.8	2.8	1.3	2.36	o.o5
FEV_1 (1/s)	1.7	o.7	2.3	o.7	1.8o	o.o5
$FEV_{o.5}$ (1/s)	o.9	o.5	1.3	o.6	2.17	o.o5

Table 2: Preoperative broncholytic effect after 2 puffs of fenoterol

parameter	$\bar{x} \pm$ s.d.		$\bar{x} \pm$ s.d.		t.	p
sR_{aw} (kPa s)	8.33	6.25	6.88	5.61	o.22	n.s.
sG_{aw} (kPa s)$^{-1}$	o.29	o.21	o.42	o.41	o.57	n.s.

Table 3: Postoperative challenge test (1o breaths of 2 % acetylcholin)

parameter	$\bar{x} \pm$ s.d.		$\bar{x} \pm$ s.d.		t.	p
sR_{aw} (kPa s)	1.53	1.06	2.25	1.o8	1.23	n.s.
sG_{aw} (kPa s)$^{-1}$	1.o2	o.68	o.57	o.27	1.65	o.o5

No significant functional effect is demonstrable in lung volumes and capacities like RV/RLC, IVC, blood gases and parameters of forced inspiration. These results lead to the conclusion that forced expiration which is most reduced in tracheal stenosis before resection is most improved following operation.

Fixed extrathoracic stenosis is not influenced by bronchodilator therapy. Specific resistance as well as specific conductance do not show significant changes (tab. 2).

Similarly lung mechanics were not improved by application of bronchodilator substances after surgical intervention. On the contrary a bronchial hyperreactivity is evident after surgical therapy in all patients. Specific resistance as well as specific conductance decreased (tab. 3). This postoperativ hyperreactivity should be treated by bronchodilators and/or corticosteroids.

Summarising these results we find specific functional patterns in extrathoracic stenosis. The most sensitive parameters describing this obstruction are the specific conductance, specific resistance and forced expiratory flow , whereas lung volumes, blood gases and parameters of forced inspiration are not helpful in detection of disturbance. Trachea sleeve resection results in a doubled tracheal diameter followed by significant improvement of resistance parameters and values of forced expiration. Bronchodilator therapy is **ineffective in pre-opera-tive**obstruction. After surgical intervention a bronchial hyperreacitivity is present in all cases.

References
1. Konietzko, N., Querfurt, H.
   Lungenfunktionsanalytische Differenzierung von Stenosen im Bereich der großen Atemwege
   Thoraxchirurgie 26 (1978) 286 - 29o

2. Kummer, F., Oppholzer, R.
   Das typische Funktionsbild der Stenose im Laryngo-Tracheal-Bereich
   Prax. Pneumol. 29 (1975) 3oo - 3o4

3. Maaßen, W., Konietzko, N.
   Ätiologie, Diagnostik und Therapie der Trachealstenosen
   Med. Welt 22 (1977) 3 - 12

VIII.2.
FUNCTIONAL APPRAISAL OF BRONCHOPLASTIC OPERATION

Y. KOTAKE, H. TANABE, Y. ITO, M. MAEDA,

Effect of bronchial surgery on the ventilatory functions and the pathophysiology of the reconstructed pulmonary lobes have not beeen studied well. The purpose of this work is to study the effects with patients receiving bronchial reconstructive surgery.

Fifty three cases receiving bronchial reconstructive surgery consisting of 37 cases of sleeve lobectomy, 4 cases of sleeve resection, 6 cases of wedge resection, and 6 cases of bronchotomy were chosen for the studies, whereas 144 cases of lobectomy, 45 cases of pneumonectomy and 18 cases of open chest surgery were served as controls.

In the first place, 9 cases of sleeve lobectomy were compared with 72 cases of lobectomy during the first week following operation, a period representing post-operative acute phase. Immediately before, and on the 1st, 2nd, 3rd, and 7th days after the operation, A-aDO$_2$ was calculated and variation profiles were prepared for each group. The preoperative A-aDO$_2$ was significantly higher in patients to receive sleeve lobectomy than those to receive lobectomy, possibly due to localized lesion in the former. In patients receiving sleeve lobectomy, A-aDO$_2$ increased post-operatively until the value marked the highest value on the 2nd postoperative day, hten turned off to improvement, and restored the preoperative level on the 7th postoperative day. As for those receiving lobectomy, although the value increased at first, the variation profile revealed a plateau after the 2nd postoperative day. Consequently, even on the 7th postoperative day, the value was somewhat higher than that determined before operation. Little difference could be observed between the value for the sleeve lobectomy group and that for the lobectomy group on the 7th postoperative day. The equalization noted in A-aDO$_2$ may be attributable to the fact that the lesions, which had made A-aDO$_2$ higher in the sleeve lobectomy group than

*J.A. Nakhosteen and W. Maassen (eds.), Bronchology: Research, Diagnostic and
Therapeutic Aspects. All rights reserved.*
Copyright 1981. Martinus Nijhoff Publishers bv, The Hague / Boston / London

in the lobectomy group before operation, was removed so that the A-aDO$_2$ was comparable in the two groups on the 7th postoperative day when the effect of operation per se disappeared. The patients receiving sleeve lobectomy were characterized by the appearance of a peak of A-aDO$_2$ on the 2nd postoperative day. The maximal A-aDO$_2$ value, which is produced by decreased blood oxidation efficiency in the alveoli in the lung reconstructed in association with the bronchial reconstruction, was significantly higher than the control. The finding strongly suggests existence of intrapulmonary shunts and uneveness of ventilation and blood flow.

In the next place, ventilatory functions during a period following postoperative acute phase were studied in patients who received bronchial reconstructive surgery. Percent VC and FEV$_{1.0}$/pred.VC. were chosen as parameter for the evauation. The data obtained were measured at 2 months intervals and compared with those obtained from controls such as patients receiving one lobe lobectomy and those receiving pneumonectomy. Although, before the operation, the %VC in the sleeve lobectomy group was lower than that in the control group, to show the indication of this mode of operation, %VC gains after sleeve lobectomy exceeded those after lobectomy. Subsequently %VC after sleeve lobectomy caught up those after lobectomy in 4 months and were always higher than those after pneumonectomy.

Fev$_{1.0}$/pred.VC., the function index under forced expiration, for the sleeve lobectomy group caught up the counterpart for the lobectomy group at the time somewhat later than the 4th month after the operation, and the value for the two groups were comparable after the 6th month. These results indicate function-preserving effect of the bronchial reconstructive surgery as well as disappearance of influence of the surgery later than the 4th month after the operation.

Conclusions: Upon the basis of examination of postoperative course in patients receiving sleeve lobectomy, function-preserving effect was demonstrated as follws;

1) Although postoperatively increasing A-aDO$_2$ marked the highest on the 2nd postoperative day, the A-aDO$_2$ recovered to a level comparable with that for lobectomy group on the 7th postoperative day. 2) There was practically no difference between the sleeve lobectomy group and lobectomy group in ventilatory function tests (%VC and FEV$_{1.0}$/pred.VC.) later than 4th month after operation.

VIII.3.
DIAGNOSIS AND TREATMENT OF TRACHEOBRONCHOMALACIA WITH ASTHMATIC ATTACK

T.FUNATSU, T.TAKI, Y.MATSUBARA, R.HATAKENAKA, Y.MIYAMOTO, S.KOSABA, K.NINOMIYA AND S.IKEDA,

1.INTRODUCTION

The patients with tracheobronchomalacia are often overlooked and sometimes treated as drug-resistant asthmatics because of their symptomatic similarities. The purpose of this study is to propose a classification for tracheobronchomalacia and a screening criteria for its diagnosis, which are based on a statistical analysis of the tracheal air-column diameter of healthy Japanese.

2.CLASSIFICATION OF TRACHEOBRONCHOMALACIA

The tracheobronchomalacia or tracheomalacia are divided into two categories by the onset of its symptoms, congenital and acquired. We propose that this acquired tracheobronchomalacia should be classified into two groups, primary and secondary. The secondary tracheobronchomalacia is a group caused by tissue destruction of the tracheobronchial wall resulting from endotracheal intubation, tracheostomy and tumor infiltration. The primary tracheobronchomalacia consists of two types according to the deformity of the air-way collapse, a saber sheath-shaped type and a crescent shaped type.

The saber sheath type is the frontal narrowing of tracheobronchial wall during expiration, when the tracheal lumen looks like a saber sheath under fiber bronchoscopy. The cause of this type is suspected to be the softening of tracheal cartilage. The crescent type is the sagittal narrowing of tracheal lumen resulting from hypotonia of the myoelastic elements of the tracheal membranous wall, looking like a crescent moon or C-shaped under fiber bronchoscopy. This crescent type can be observed through the trachea to the bilateral main bronchus. It is more suitable to designate it as tracheobronchomalacia, not tracheomalacia.

  A.congenital
  B.acquired 1.primary.....a)saber sheath type
              b)crescent type
       2.secondary

J.A. Nakhosteen and W. Maassen (eds.), Bronchology: Research, Diagnostic and Therapeutic Aspects. All rights reserved.
Copyright 1981. Martinus Nijhoff Publishers bv, The Hague / Boston / London

[CASE 1] A 57-year-old woman had been treated as a bronchial asthmatic for a long period, and had had 4 episodes of cardiac arrest while she had been undergoing an inhalation therapy with a bronchodilator. The X-ray films of the chest revealed a giant bullous shadow in the right middle lobe. In the postero-anterior view the tracheal air-column was remarkably narrow and its calibre was 9mm. The degree of her saber sheath type tracheobronchomalacia was classified to the fourth degree by Johson's criteria.

A right thoracotomy was performed from the fifth intercostal space and a giant bulla in the middle lobe was resected. The width of the membranous wall of the tracheal, right main bronchus and left main bronchus were 1.2cm, 1.8cm and 1.5cm respectively. The strut plates made from her sixth rib were sutured to the membranous wall of the trachea and the bilateral main bronchus. Her post-operative course was satisfactoty and she did not complain of dyspnea on exertion. Tomography and CT scan revealed the strut plate in the backwall of trachea and it was observed to maintain sufficient air-space under fiber bronchoscopy.

[CASE 2] A 50-year-old woman had been treated as a severe bronchial asthmatic for 10 years. Her symptoms and the shest X-ray findings coincided to our screening criteria of tracheobronchomalacia. After the fiber bronchoscopy and the spot filming, her tracheobronchomalacia was diagnosed to the saber sheath type. A right thoracotomy was performed. The autologous strut made from her rib were sutured onto trachea and the bilateral main bronchus, as described in CASE 1. In post-operative course severe dyspnea disappeared and her slight wheezing was relieved by bronchodilators.

6.CONCLUSION

It is difficult to differentiate tracheobronchomalacia from bronchial asthma and emphysema because of their symptomatic similarities. After a statistical analysis of the trachea air-column diameters of 1680 healthy Japanese, we revealed the correlation between tracheal diameter and height. With this correlative formula and symptoms we propose a screening criteria to diagnose the tracheobronchomalacia. We show here our classification of tracheobronchomalacia, it is divided into 2 categories, congenital and acquired. Further the acquired is classified into primary and secondary, and the primary was also classified into 2 types, saber sheath type and crescent type.

The fiber bronchoscopy and the fluoroscopic motion recording are very valuable in establishing a definitive diagnosis. The two cases with saber sheath type tracheobronchomalacia, were operated with the span plasty by R.Nissen, which originated as a corrective method for the crescent type of tracheomalacia.

3.SCREENING CRITERIA FOR DIAGNOSIS

For outpatients we used the following criteria for screening to differentiate from other air-way obstructive diseases.

1) The diameter of the tracheal air-column in X-ray films of the chest is out of the range for healthy Japanese.

2) In auscultation expiratory wheezes are more closely audible on the upper sternum than other portion. They diminish in inspiration.

3) The chief complaint is usually a feeling of laryngeal blockage.

Dr.Taki, a colleague of our institute, measured the diameters of tracheal air-columns of chest X-ray films of mass health examinations and investigated the correlation between tracheal diameter and height on 1680 healthy Japanese, aged from 6 months to 83 years. The correlation between height and diameter was confirmed and the tracheal diameter was not correlated to sex or age.

The normal range of the tracheal air-column diameter of a healthy Japanese was indicated as the correlative formula and standard deviation as follows. $Y=0.12X-4.596\pm4.12$, where Y is tracheal diameter in mm and X is height in cm.

4.METHODS FOR DEFINITIVE DIAGNOSIS

The fiber bronchoscopy and the fluoroscopic motion recording are very valuable in confirming the definitive diagnosis of tracheobronchomalacia. A fiber broncho-scopy is easy to perform under local anaesthesia and has a high diagnostic value in observing the degree of air-way collapse in deep expiration and coughing.

In our experiences with fiber bronchoscopy, cases of the saber sheath type are observed in the elderly with asthmatoid attack and are localized only in the trachea. In the fluoroscopic motion recording, the spot filming was carried out using 3 exposures per second for 5 seconds with PUCK, while the patient was forced to cough in the antero-posterior position. For some patients the cine-radiography, using 25 exposures per second, was carried out with them lying in the left anterior oblique position. The changes of the tracheal air-column were easily observed by these spot filming without contrast material and correlated to the findings with fiber bronchoscopy.

5.PATIENTS AND TREATMENT

We applied our screening criteria to the patients with asthmatoid attacks and confirmed the diagnosis of tracheobronchomalacia, saber sheath type in 10 patients. In 2 of those cases we performed the strut operation and had good results. The strut operation is the method in which a straight plate made of the patient's own rib is sutured to the membranous wall of the trachea and bilateral main bronchus. This method, the span plasty, was originated by R.Nissen in 1954 and used with the crescent type of tracheomalacia.

VIII.4.

DIAGNOSTIC MEANINGS OF MEFV-CURVE FOR PATIENTS WITH STRICTURE OF
UPPER AIRWAY: VALUE AND LIMITATION OF EMPEY'S INDEX

H. TANABE, Y. KOTAKE, Y. ITO, M. MAEDA,

The purpose of this study is to investigate the diagnostic
significance of Empey's index in the cases of upper airway stenosis.
Materials and methods.

The subjects of investigation consisted of 28 persons with normal
ventilatory function, 30 patients with asthma and 9 patients with
stricture of the upper airway. The patients with asthma were regarded
as the models of lower airway obstructive disease and the diagnosis
of asthma was made according to the definition of American Thoracic
Society. As the cases of upper airway stricture, the patients with
tracheal stricture, were chosen for this study.

The Empey's index was calculated by the equation $FEV_{1.0}/PEFR$
(ml./l./min.). The Fig.1 was a radiogram of a glass tube with stricture
and in order to measure the maximum diameter and the minimum diameter
of it, lines were drawn at 2mm. intervals and measured Is. or stenotic
index assuming the inner space of the glass tube as a circle. In the
experimental group, 20 subjects with normal ventilatory function held
the glass tubes with various degrees of stricture in their mouth and
expired with a maximum effort and then the above mentioned parameters
were calculated.

Results.

Empey's indices of 28 subjects with normal ventilatory function
were 6.74 ± 1.03 on the average. In no case it exceeded 10, the
upper limit value for diagnosis of upper airway stricture stated by

*J.A. Nakhosteen and W. Maassen (eds.), Bronchology: Research, Diagnostic and
Therapeutic Aspects. All rights reserved.*
Copyright 1981. Martinus Nijhoff Publishers bv, The Hague / Boston / London

Empey.

The Empey's indices of 30 patients with asthma were 6.85 $\pm$ 1.32 on the average and in any case it did not exceed 10. The mean of Empey's indices in the patients with stricture of the upper airway was 10.9 $\pm$ 4.48, showing significantly increased value compared to the other two groups, and five out of nine patients showed value over 10. In three out of four patients who had no increase in Empey's index, the degree of the stenosis was slight.

We have operatively reconstructed the trachea in seven patients with upper airway stricture: the mean of Empey's indices decreased significantly from 11.3 $\pm$ 4.9 before operation to 6.7 $\pm$ 1.1 after operation, reaching to the normal range, that is, below 10 in all the patients. The Fig.2 shows the correlation between the Empey's indices and the stenotic indices which were calculated from the radiograms in nine patients with upper airway stenosis. It was noted that Empey's index tended to becoming high, when the stenotic index was high. The Fig.3 shows the stenotic index is plotted as abscissa and Empey's index as ordinate when the Empey's index was measured using various glass tubes. The screen tone indicates a sphere of 2SD of the Empey's indices in 28 subjects with normal ventilatory functions. The correlation of both indices was regarded as exponential, and when the curve of exponential revolution was calculated. A formula $Y = 5.24e^{0.96x}$ ($r^2 = 0.68$) was obtained. The rise from normal range on this curve is coincident with about 0.7 of the stenotic index, and when the stenotic index is below 0.7, imcrease of Empey's index was not observed.

The Fig.4 showed the correlation between the stenotic index and the values of PEFR and $FEV_{1.0}$ when the Empey's index was calculated. When the value of PEFR was plotted as 1/10, being conscious of 10, the PEFR curve and the $FEV_{1.0}$ curve met at the point E, in other

242

words, Empey's index was 10. As can be seen in the figure, the curve
of $FEV_{1.0}$ remained almost constant until the point E and the rise
of Empey's index was due to the decrease in PEFR. After passing the
point E, those curves crossed and the exponential rise of Empey's
index was attributed to this. Empey's index was over 10 when stenotic
index was over 0.85 and when the latter was below 10, it was recognized
only as a rise from the normal range. This point was considered,
therefore, as a limit of Empey's index.

Conclusions:

1) Five out of nine patients with stricture of upper airway showed
Empey's index higher than 10.

2) All of the indices lowered to below 10 in nine patients who
underwent tracheal reconstruction.

3) As a result of expiration test with a stricture tube, a positive
correlation was evidenced between the Empey's index and degree of
stricture.

From the above mentioned results, it was concluded that Empey's
index is useful for making a functional diagnosis of the upper airway
stricture, though there is some limitation.

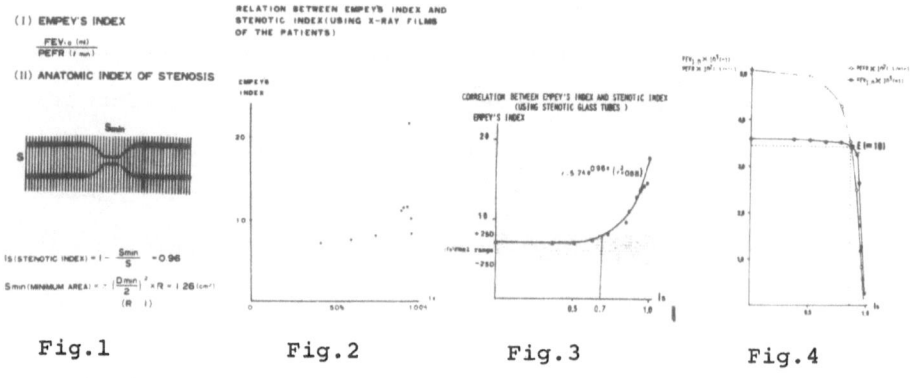

Fig.1   Fig.2   Fig.3   Fig.4

REFERENCE

1. D.W.EMPEY:Assessment of Upper Airways Obstruction;British Medical
Journal,1972,3,503-505

VIII.5.

Endoskopische Befunde bei Trachealstenosen in Beziehung zu funktionell meßbaren Ventilationsstörungen vor und nach Therapie.

H.J.KLIPPE, D.SOMMERWERCK und K.VON WINDHEIM

In der klinischen Arbeit fällt immer wieder auf, daß bei Trachealstenosen eine erhebliche Diskrepanz zwischen der Enge der Stenose und der vom Patienten selbst empfundenen Störung seiner ventilatorischen Funktion besteht. Erst ab einem kritischen Wert von 30-25 % der normalen lichten Weite der Trachea erreicht die Widerstandserhöhung durch Einengung der Strombahn einen kritischen Punkt. Dann jedoch führt der erhebliche, nichtlineare Anstieg des Widerstandes, z.B. durch Wandrauhigkeit, Schleimmembranen und erhöhte Turbulenz zu einer raschen, oft dramatischen Progredienz der Dyspnoe. Hier nun zur Demonstration einige unserer Fälle:

Fall 1: Pat.H.P.,♂,57 J. - 5-tägige Respiratortherapie nach Cardiaresektion, postop. Pleuraempyem links, Restriktion. 3 Monate später Trachealstenose. Keine OP wegen schlechter Atemmechanik (Restriktion, erhebliche Störung der Zwerchfellmotilität li.). Zudem auch keine OP-Willigkeit des Patienten.

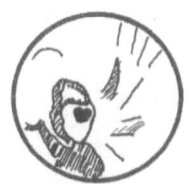

Befund am 9.9.77

Lungenfunktion am 6.9.77

VK = 3100 ml

SekKap exsp = 1330 ml = 41 % der VK

SekKap insp = 1200 ml

R insp = 13,19 cmH$_2$O/l/sec

R exsp = 8,77 cmH$_2$O/l/sec

Bei kombinierter in- und exspiratorischer Störung endoskopisch 2 Granulome subglottisch und fibrös stenosierender Narbenring von 2 mm Ø im unteren Trachealdrittel.

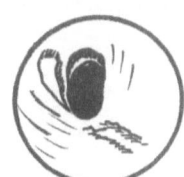

Befund am 16.11.79
nach Bougierung in
18 Einzelsitzungen

Lungenfunktion am 31.8.79

VK = 3100 ml

SekKap exsp = 2500 ml = 80 % der VK

SekKap insp = 2600 ml

R insp = 3,83 cmH$_2$O/l/sec

R exsp = 3,91 cmH$_2$O/l/sec

Fall 2: Pat.Th.W.,♀,58 J. - 21 Tage Respiratortherapie nach SHT, Rippenserienfrakturen rechts, Zwerchfellparese rechts. Nach 1 Monat Trachealstenose von ca. 4 mm Ø in Jugulumhöhe.

J.A. Nakhosteen and W. Maassen (eds.), Bronchology: Research, Diagnostic and Therapeutic Aspects. All rights reserved.
Copyright 1981. Martinus Nijhoff Publishers bv, The Hague / Boston / London

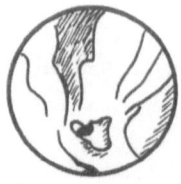

Befund am 28.1.77

Blutgase 26.1.77 unter 2,5 1 O_2

pO_2	81,2 mmHg
pCO_2	42,0 mmHg
pH	7,45
BE	+ 5

10 Tage nach Resektion der Stenose dramatische Luftnot durch Verlegung der Trachea durch Borken, Granulome und Fadenteile. Endoskopische Wiederherstellung der Passage. Danach Wohlbefinden.

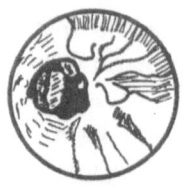

Befund am 10.2.77

Blutgase 10.2.77 unter 4 1 O_2

pO_2	40,0 mmHg
pCO_2	46,2 mmHg
pH	7,38
BE	+ 2

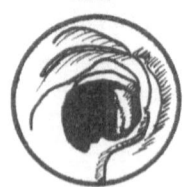

Endzustand postop
am 28.2.77

Blutgase 28.2.77 ohne O_2

pO_2	76,2 mmHg
pCO_2	37,8 mmHg
pH	7,45
BE	+ 2,5

Fall 3: Pat.R.L.,♀,36 J. - Status nach 4-tägiger Respiratortherapie nach Suicidversuch. 3 Monate später tiefsitzende Trachealstenose von ca. 3 mm Ø. Hochgradigste Dyspnoe, Stridor.

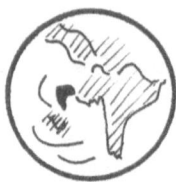

Zustand praeop.

Blutgase 20.3.75 unter 4 1 O_2

pO_2	69 mmHg
pCO_2	49 mmHg
pH	7,36
BE	+ 1,5

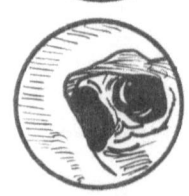

Zustand postop.

Blutgase 10.4.75 unter 0,5 1 O_2

pO_2	92 mmHg
pCO_2	38 mmHg
pH	7,38
BE	+ 3

Nach Resektion der Stenose und End-zu-End-Anastomose gesund. Bald darauf erneuter, zum Tode führender Suicid.

Die operativen Korrekturmethoden der Trachealstenosen sind heute weitgehend standardisiert. Dennoch existieren - wie Sie alle wissen - genügend ernste Probleme. Erstens, die Gefahr der Verlegung des Lumens zumeist durch Granulationen, Borken, zähes Sekret oder Fadenmaterial. Exzessiver Anstieg des Widerstandes, Verminderung des Luftdurchsatzes auf ca. 10 % der Luftmenge bei freiem Lumen, steiler

Anstieg des Verbrauches an kinetischer Energie (z.B. bei 7 % freier Fläche der 100-fache Energieaufwand gegenüber der Norm), sie sind die Ursachen der klinisch sofort augenfälligen, vitalen Bedrohung dieser Patienten.

Das 2. Problem, die Gefahr der Restenose, wird nur dann frühzeitig genug erkennbar, wenn der Patient zu regelmäßigen funktionellen und, wenn nötig, endoskopischen Kontrollen motiviert werden kann. So erkannte beginnende Restenosen können mit weitaus besserer Effizienz angegangen werden als in einer evtl. dramatischen Notsituation.

Drittens ist die Funktionsfähigkeit des tracheo-broncho-pulmonalen Systems und hier speziell die Atemmechanik der Thoraxorgane von entscheidender Bedeutung für Erfolg oder Mißerfolg. Zwerchfellparesen, Pleuraschwarten u.ä. bewirken Störungen im atemmechanischen Wechselspiel und führen daraus folgend zu z.T. erheblichen Belastungen der Trachealnaht. Hierbei kommt dem extra- oder intrathorakalen Sitz der Stenose große Bedeutung zu.

Autoren wie Konietzko, Sommerwerck u.a. zeigen, daß extrathorakale, das obere Drittel der Trachea betreffende Stenosen durch eine vor allem inspiratorische Störung der Funktion betroffen werden. Der "equal pressure point", sofern man für diesen speziellen Fall den Begriff von Mead aufrechterhalten will, liegt hierbei außerhalb des Thorax. Das heißt, daß auch bei forcierter Exspiration alle Trachealabschnitte vor Kompression geschützt sind.

Bei Stenosen der endothorakalen Trachea steht der Bereich des sog. "downstream-Segmentes" unter einem erhöhten extratrachealen Außendruck, der den Innendruck des Trachealrohres übersteigt. Hier wird neben der exspiratorischen Kompression der pars membranosa auch die Anastomose erhöhten Drücken ausgesetzt. Im postoperativen Verlauf sind daraus nachteilige Folgen möglich.

Abschließend sei bemerkt, daß Pathophysiologie und Chirurgie der Trachealstenosen in ihrer engen Verknüpfung zur Atemmechanik unsere volle Aufmerksamkeit mehr noch als bisher verdienen. Dies umso mehr, als bei der steten Zunahme erfolgreich respiratorbehandelter Intensivpatienten in Zukunft eine weitaus größere Zahl an Patienten mit aus der Vorbehandlung resultierenden Trachealstenosen unserer Behandlung bedarf.

Literatur bei den Verfassern.

VIII.6.

TRACHESCOPY FINDINGS AFTER PROLONGED INTUBATION WITH THE NL-TRACHEO-
STOMY TUBE

S. Borgeskov, B. Kirkby, N. Lomholt

From the literature it is a well known fact that high-pressure, low-vol-
ume cuffs usually produce ulceration of the tracheal mucosa during prolonged
intubation. It was a great step forward in preventing serious tracheal complications that low-pressure, high-volume cuffs were introduced some 10 years
ago.

In the NL tube (Lomholt, 1971), the cuff is inflated to a constant pressure of 30 mbar by a cuff-inflator. The cuff-inflator contains a precision
reduction valve and is supplied with compressed air or oxygen. It corrects
a too high or too low cuff pressure within a fraction of a second. This is
important in order to prevent aspiration and to allow perfusion of mucosa.

The tube has a flexible tip so that the cuff is able to center the tube
in the trachea, and thereby prevent the tip from damaging the mucosa.

During ventilation with high pressures, the cuff-inflator tube is closed
by a small valve inside the connector. A tight seal of the trachea is obtained
because the airway pressure is transmitted to the cuff through the cuff membrane (Figure 1).

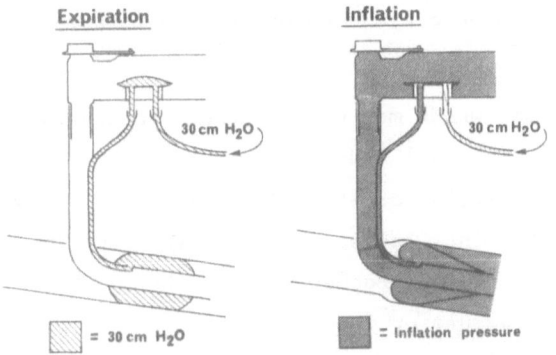

Figure 1. Functioning principle of the NL-tube.

J.A. Nakhosteen and W. Maassen (eds.), Bronchology: Research, Diagnostic and
Therapeutic Aspects. All rights reserved.
Copyright 1981. Martinus Nijhoff Publishers bv, The Hague / Boston / London

OWN SERIES

A consecutive series of 85 patients, submitted for head and neck surgery during a 4-year period, were all tracheostomized during the surgical procedure. The material consisted of 58 men and 27 women. The mean age was 56 years (14-79 years). At operation all patients were intubated with the NL-tracheostomy tube. The tubes were often left in place for several weeks (mean 2 weeks). At extubation the trachea was examined every time, using an Olympus BF 5B2 fiber-optic bronchoscope.

RESULTS (Table 1)

38% of the patients were without mucosal changes of any kind. Even in patients intubated for more than 3 weeks, about 50 per cent showed no damage and in the rest very slight changes dominated: scattered fibrin spots and slight hyperemia throughout the trachea, not particularly accentuated at the cuff area.

Hyperemia and fibrin formation was often more pronounced above the cuff than at the cuff area. This picture changed after a line for suction above the cuff was included in the tube design.

In 8 patients small superficial ulcerations (1-2 mm) were noted. Two of these patients were intubated for less than one week, three were intubated 1-2 weeks, and three for more than 3 weeks. Four were located in the rear or side wall of the trachea about the level of the tip of the tube. None of the ulcerations was seen at the cuff area. Three of the patients with possible tip lesions had skin flaps from shoulder to face to cover surgical defects. Four were located at the carina and probably were produced by suction catheter.

CONCLUSION

The background for serious lesions which may be caused by tracheostomy tubes is damage to the tracheal wall. Tracheal stenosis is produced by scar contraction, following deep mucosal necrosis resulting from excessive and pro-longed pressure. Fistulas penetrating either the esophagus or the innominate artery also begin as pressure necrosis of the trachea. So, in short, when a major necrotic ulcer caused by cuff pressure or the tip of the tube is pre-vented, as in this study, serious complications are prevented as well.

Table I. Endoscopic findings in 85 patients with tracheostomy and NL-TUBE

Days of Intub.	Total no. of Pts.	Pts. with mucosal changes	Fibrin	Hyper-emia	Ulcer	Normal Mucosa
3-7	20	11	9	6	2	9
8-14	35	25	19	16	3	10
15-21	12	6	6	4	-	6
22-28	10	5	3	2	3	5
28	8	5	1	5	-	3
Total	85	52	38	33	8	33

VIII.7.

USE OF FLEXIBLE FIBEROPTIC BRONCHOSCOPE IN PALLIATIVE TREATMENT OF TRACHEAL STRICTURES AFTER ASSISTED RESPIRATION.

A.GALLINARO, A.LAPINI-SACCHETTI (Florence, Italy)

The resection of the obstructed segment of the trachea with an end to end anastomosis represents the best treatment in the tracheal obstruction following assisted ventilation with or without tracheostomy.

But also another procedure, apparently only palliative, such as that proposed by Fantoni (1974), may produce complete recovery with a minimal risk for the patients.

The method consists in the introduction of a prothesis (a Silastic tube with an interior diameter of 9,5 mm) in the obstructed space of the tracheal lumen, which has been previously dilated. Connected to the major tube is a small Silastic tube (diameter 3,2 mm., length 10 cm.) which serves to anchor the major tube to the front surface of the neck.

The anchorage tube passes through the anterior wall of the trachea and is taped on the surface of the neck.

This tube is firmly glued to the interior surface of the major one with the Silastic adhesive type A and its chemical composition allows a good tolerance and avoids the production of infected breaches on the tracheal walls and of fistolous cutaneous sinuses.

In order to guarantee a correct position of the prothesis in the tracheal lumen, it is necessary to determine previously some reference points which correspond respectively to the tracheal carina, to the maximum level of the obstruction, to the point where the small anchorage tube must be extracted, and finally to the vocal cords.

These findings depend on the introduction of a flexible fiberoptic broncho-scope as far as the tracheal carina which is afterwards slowly extracted marking the various reference points on the instrument's sheath at the level of the superior incisors.

J.A. Nakhosteen and W. Maassen (eds.), Bronchology: Research, Diagnostic and Therapeutic Aspects. All rights reserved.
Copyright 1981. Martinus Nijhoff Publishers bv, The Hague / Boston / London

The prothesis is well tolerated and the patients don't feel at all the presence of the tube in the trachea, and in one or two days time they can speak perfectly.

An inspiratory resistence is felt only under physical effort, but usually the patients are able to live quite normally, the only inconvenience being the small bandage on the neck.

The main complications that could occur would be the obstruction of the lumen of the prothesis provoked by the inspissated endotracheal secretions and the dislocation of the prothesis with the risk of suffocation.

The first complication is avoided with daily vaporizations to correct the lack of umidity; and the second will not occur if the anchorage tube is firmly attached after each medication.

It is by all means very important to control periodically the perviety of the lumen of the prothesis and its correct position using a flexible fiberoptic bronchoscope.

After periods which vary from a minimum of sixty days to a maximum of fourteen months, the prothesis can be extracted and the obstruction appears controlled, even in cases in which the conditions of the tracheal cartilages could lead to some doubt on this subject.

In the last eight years, 17 cases of tracheal obstruction have been treated personally :

14 were males and 3 females, and the age ranged from 17 to 74 years.

7 patients had previously had a tracheotomy. The extension varied from 3 cartilaginous rings to four-fifths of the trachea.

5 patients were operated with the resection of the obstructed segment and the end to end anastomosis.

1 patient died postoperatively, but was a very ill subject who had a very serious chest trauma.

The other four patients had a complete recovery.

12 patients were treated with the endotracheal Silastic prothesis and 8 obtained a total restoration of the continuity of the lumen of the trachea.

1 patient had a relapse of the obstruction and bore the prothesis for an additional three months, and another had to be treated with a tracheal resection. Both are now quite well.

There are 2 other patients still bearing the prothesis : a man age 26 with a long obstructed segment (7 cm.) who has always refused the resection and who has been living normally for more than 3 years, and another young patient age 17 with the damage of the entire length of the tracheal walls who was treated with the prothesis only three months ago.

In conclusion, the method of the endotracheal Silastic prothesis can by itself restore the continuity of an obstructed tracheal lumen, and by all means its previous adoption can facilitate the further resection.

REFERENCES

1. A.Fantoni, G.Frova, T.Gaietta,
   A.Guarino, G.Oriani e A.Ottaviani ; Il trattamento conservativo delle ostruzioni laringo tracheali. Ediz. Anestesia e Rianimazione/Milano 1974

Chapter VIII

Section 2
OPERATIVE PROCEDURES

VIII.8.

TRAUMATIC LARYNGOTRACHEAL DISRUPTION ASSOCIATED WITH CRICOID FRACTURE AND
RECURRENT NERVE INJURY

L. COURAUD, C. MARTIGNE, P.J. DUMAS

1. INTRODUCTION

The number of thoracic tracheal injuries has markedly decreased with increased use of seat-belts. However laryngo-tracheal avulsions with fracture of the cricoid arch and paralysis of the recurrent laryngeal nerves have become more frequent. Some of them are in fact caused by seat-belts. We have treated 8 cases in the last 7 years.

2. ANATOMICAL LESIONS

These cases present the following tableau :

2.1. Laryngo-tracheal avulsion of the lower edge of the cricoid cartilage with considerable retraction of the distal tracheal segment into cervico-mediastinal tissues : of our 8 cases, 6 involved complete avulsion and 2 hemispheric only.

2.2. Elongation or disruption of the recurrent laryngeal nerves which causes paralysis in adducted position of the vocal cords : of our 8 cases, 4 were found to have permanent bilateral disruption and 4 unilateral.

2.3. Comminuted fracture of the cricoid arch, which can cause collapse of the laryngeal structures.

2.4. Retraction of laryngeal mucosa which leaves the cricoid ring denuded.

3. MECHANISM

These lesions are always caused by the same mechanism : a frontal blow to the neck (2 cases), strangulation by the seat-belt (4 cases). It should be noted that because of bad positioning of anchorage points in relation to the size and shape of the wearer, the diagonal strap of a seat-belt can inflict serious cervical injury.

4. CLINICAL ASPECTS

Acute dyspnea is caused by retraction of the trachea and tracheal bleeding. Immobilisation in adducted position of the vocal cords fortunately occurs with a delay of several hours after disruption, the only immediate sign being marked speech difficulties. Cervical subcutaneous emphysema occurs in the peri-tracheal tissues and indicate the airway laceration. Contusions on the neck point to the site of the

J.A. Nakhosteen and W. Maassen (eds.), Bronchology: Research, Diagnostic and
Therapeutic Aspects. All rights reserved.
Copyright 1981. Martinus Nijhoff Publishers bv, The Hague / Boston / London

258

lesion. At this level diagnosis is not difficult, but determination of the exact
location and type of the lesion requires endoscopy, which is at the same time the
first step in treatment of respiratory distress. If respiratory distress is cured
without the real nature of the lesion being determined, decanulation becomes
impossible and treatment of these sclerotic and possibly infected lesions becomes
much more difficult.

5. TREATMENT OF RESPIRATORY DISTRESS

Emergency management of respiratory distress involves freeing the larynx and
trachea, and preventing the airway from being flooded with blood.

Tracheotomy is traditionally indicated and is of undeniable effectiveness [1,5].
We used it in our first observation. The cervical trachea being retracted at the
base of the neck, its distal extremity must be catheterised.

Orotracheal intubation is also rapid and effective and quite easy to perform
despite the avulsion of the main airway. The catheter passes through the cellular
space of the neck before entering the extremity of the trachea. In cases of acute
respiratory obstruction, this is the first step in emergency resuscitation. If the
respiratory condition permits, intubation should be preceded by endoscopy : either
bronchoscopy, which allows diagnosis, aspiration, tracheal catheterism and per-
endoscopic ventilation, or fibroscopy. In 3 cases the ventilation tube was guided
into place using the optic of the instrument.

6. SURGICAL MANAGEMENT
6.1. Laryngo-tracheal repair

The retracted trachea is easily mobilised into its normal position and
anastomosed to the larynx. This is so even with chronic lesions. We refer elsewhere
to the need for very meticulous suturing with resorbable thread in order to achieve
good mucosa-to-mucosa apposition [3,4].

6.2. Reestablishment of a perfect covering of mucosa.

The cricoid cartilage has been denuded by retraction of the mucosa. This
denudation increases with delay in treatment with the mucosa becoming oedematised,
hyperhemic and friable. Perfect mucosal covering is absolutely fundemental and its
absence doubtless explains the high percentage of failures in published observations.
In our 5 recent cases, the mucosa necessary for this procedure was obtained by
sub-perichondral horizontal resection of part of the cricoid ring. In delayed cases,
an oblique section of the entire anterior arch was necessary in 2 cases and sub-
perichondral resection of the whole cricoid in 1 case. We attribute our excellent
results (first time healing of all patients operated on and restoration of 90 %
to 100 % of the diameter of the airway) to close attention to this technical
point, whose importance cannot be overestimated.

6.3. Reduction of fractures of the cricoid arch

Early reconstitution, if necessary on an endolaryngeal stent, has largely replaced emergency tracheotomy. The fracture is easily reduced by perichondral suture. The support provided by the stent also assists in the reduction.

We have already noted the almost invariable presence of a median vertical fracture of the posterior plate of the cricoid. In cases of bilateral recurrent laryngeal nerve paralysis this fracture can be of great use. Far from being reduced it should be enlarged. If no fracture exists cricotomy should be performed. The greater separation thus created between the two arytenoid cartilages is maintained by the stent and filled by cartilaginous growth with the result that diastasis of the vocal cords paralysed in adducted position is obtained even when the stent is removed. The large number of supplementary procedures (cordopexy, cordectomy, arytenoidectomy) mentioned in published observations underlines the importance of the technique here advocated which renders term unnecessary. Having neglected it on one occasion we were ourselves obliged to perform later cordectomy on a patient referred for dyspnea at effort.

6.4. Restoration of a patent glottis

Bilateral disruption of the laryngeal recurrent paralysis the vocal cords in adducted position causing functional stenosis which must be corrected in order to avoid permanent intubation or tracheotomy. Insertion of a transglottic tube solves the immediate problem. For the longer them we have already seen how the interposition of a fibrous growth in a vertical fracture of the posterior cricoid plate keeps the cords separated (in the manner of Rethi's operation) and the larynx patent after an intubation of variable duration, (2 weeks to 3 months) depending on the extent of the lesions or chiefly of total resection of the cartilage. Intubation is unnecessary when one cord remains functional. The prosthesis might be a T tube with exit established by subjacent tracheotomy. We however have a clear preference for a naso-tracheal tube in Silastic. This has the multiple advantages of serving as a laryngeal tutor, avoiding unnecessary and possibly dangerous tracheotomy below the anastomosis and enabling artificial ventilation if necessary (cranial traumatism).

7. CONCLUSION

We were able to restore normal main airway and respiratory function in all 8 of our cases. Speech function was also restored in all cases but sometimes with sequelae of varying degrees. For the achievement of good laryngo-tracheal viability and complete healing in a single operation the main imperatives are : establishment of a perfect mucosa covering by means of partial resection of the cricoid cartilage, consolidation of a glottal enlargement in bilateral paralysis of the recurrent laryngeal nerves.

VIII.9.

BRONCHOPLASTIC PROCEDURES FOR LUNG CANCER

T. NARUKE

PATIENT: During a 17 year period up to December, 1979, 1011 patients with carcinoma of the lung underwent resection in the National Cancer Center, Tokyo, Japan. Bronchoplastic procedures were performed on 40 patients, 4.3 per cent received bronchoplastic procedures from 1965 to 1979 and 7.1 per cent received the same procedures from 1973 to 1979.

There were 39 men and 1 woman, varying in age from 33 to 73 years. 19 were in their sixties and 5 in their seventies. The clinical stages of disease were as follows: 12 cases of Stage I disease, 8 cases of Stage II disease, and 20 cases of Stage III carcinoma.

Table I

BRONCHOPLASTIC PROCEDURES FOR LUNG CANCER
1965 - 1979

Site	Type of procedure	No. of patients
RIGHT UPPER LOBE	Sleeve, right main bronchus	16
RIGHT UPPER LOBE	Sleeve, right main bronchus with partial resection of S.V.C.	1
RIGHT UPPER LOBE	Wedge, right main bronchus	5
RIGHT UPPER LOBE	Wedge, lower trachea, right main bronchus	1
RIGHT UPPER LOBE	Resection of right lung, lower trachea, carina. Reconstruction by transverse suture.	1
RIGHT UPPER LOBE	Resection of lower part of trachea, carina and right main bronchus.	1
RIGHT LOWER LOBE	Wedge, right main bronchus	1
RIGHT MAIN BRONCHUS	Resection of right lung, lower trachea, carina. Reconstruction by transverse suture.	2
LEFT UPPER LOBE	Sleeve, left main bronchus	1
LEFT UPPER LOBE	Sleeve, left main bronchus with S6 segmental resection.	1
LEFT UPPER LOBE	Sleeve, left main bronchus with sleeve pulmonary artery.	2
LEFT UPPER LOBE	Sleeve, left main bronchus with partial resection of pulmonary artery.	2
LEFT UPPER LOBE	Wedge, left main bronchus	3
LEFT LOWER LOBE	Wedge, left main bronchus	2
LEFT LOWER LOBE	Sleeve, left main and left upper lobe bronchus.	1
TOTAL		40

Various bronchoplastic procedures have been done, including 25 for right upper lobe lesions and 9 for those involving the bronchus of the left upper lobe. A sleeve resection and anastomosis were performed on both the left main bronchus and pulmonary artery combined with the left upper lobectomy in 2 cases. A sleeve resection of the left main bronchus and a partial resection of the pulmonary artery combined with the left upper lobectomy were also performed in 2 cases (Table I).

Table II

Histologic Type of Lesion in 40 Patients performed Bronchoplastic Procedures for Lung Cancer.
(1965~1979)

Histology	Number of patients	Nodes involved		
		pN 0	pN 1	pN 2
Squamous	32	11	13	8
Adenoca.	5		1	4
Large cell ca.	1			1
Adenoid cystic	2		1	1
Total	40	11	15	14

Histological types and lymph node metastases in 40 cases in which bronchoplasty was performed are shown in Table II. 32 of the 40 tumors (80 per cent) were squamous cell carcinoma, 5 adenocarcinoma, and 2 adenoid cystic carcinoma. Of the 32 patients with squamous cell carcinoma, 8 had mediastinal lymph node metastasis. Of the 5 with adenocarcinoma, 4 had mediastinal lymph node metastasis (Table II).

DIAGNOSIS: Tomograms and bronchograms are helpful in locating the lesion. However, cancers of the bronchial mucosa can be localized exactly with an endoscope, and metastasis in the bronchial wall and lymph nodes can be located with bronchial arteriograms.

ANESTHESIA: Intratracheal anesthesia was used for all patients. Double-cuffed armored endotracheo-bronchial tube (Naruke tube) is used during the procedure. Another small tube for children is prepared to ventilate the reconstructing lung after sleeve resection of the bronchus. However, this small tube is not necessary to use routinely because only 15 to 20 minutes are spent on resection and anastomosis.

TECHNIQUE: The patient is placed in the lateral position and posterolateral skin is incised. The chest wall is opened through the fifth rib bed. Pulmonary vein ligation and dissection, complete mediastinal lymph node dissection, and pulmonary artery ligation and dissection are carried out in that order. The pulmonary ligament is cut to move the lung upward. The bronchial reconstruction was performed by single interrupted sutures by means of 3 to 4-0   Ticron, used from 1965 to 1975 and 4-0   Dexon sutures, used from 1976 to the present. The atraumatic needles are inserted through submucosa except for the membranous portion which is inserted through the full thickness. The membranous portion of the bronchus is sewn up later to join together with the calibers. It is important to keep the mucosal surface smooth when bronchial suture is performed to avoid needless suture and to keep the thread out the bronchial lumen. Pathological examination of the bronchial stump by frozen section is always necessary.

POSTOPERATIVE CARE AND COMPLICATION: Careful attention must be given to the removal of bronchial secretions with the fiberoptic bronchoscope during the early postoperative period. Regular bronchoscopic suction is necessary in the postoperative period, particularly within 4 to 5 post operative days, because the patient cannot expectorate through the site of anastomosis. The surgeon who performs the procedures must be expert in handing the fiberoptic bronchoscope. Threads protruding into the bronchial lumen from the anastomosis must be removed bronchoscopically. No deaths occured within 30 post operative days. Post operative stenosis occured in 5 cases because of granulation at the site of anastomosis. One patient required pneumonectomy. 2 cases required removal of sutures and granulation tissue. Stenosis at the site of anastomosis is usually caused by operative, especially suture, technique. frequent suctioning with the fiberoptic bronchoscope during early postoperative days and removal of sutures if they are projecting into the bronchial lumen are necessary to prevent stenosis from suture granulation (Table III).

Table III

Complications of Bronchoplastic Procedures in 40 Patients

(1965~1979)

Operative mortality ★	0
Suture granulation	5
Pneumonectomy completion due to granulation tissue obstruction	1
Stenosis	3
Stenosis & empyema without fistula	1

★ Death within 30 days of the operative procedure

RESULTS: Relative survival rates for all 40 cases indicates 37.8 per cent survival after 5 years. 20 patients died: 12 patients died of cancer from 7 months to 4 years and 3 months after operation, and 8 patients died of other causes. The remaining 20 patients are alive and well from 1 month to 14 years and 3 months after operation. Adjuvant therapy was performed on 30 cases, including preoperative infusion of MitomycinC into the bronchial arteries or postoperative irradiation or both. B.C.G. was also used in 5 cases. preoperative infusion of Mitomycin C into the bronchial arteries of patients with Stage III carcinoma showed 37.9 per cent survival at 5 years compared to 24.9 per cent of the non bronchial arterial infusion group (Table IV).

264

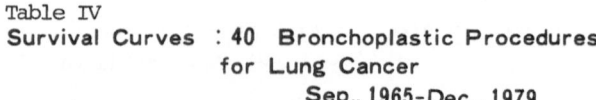

Table IV
Survival Curves : 40 Bronchoplastic Procedures
for Lung Cancer
Sep., 1965–Dec., 1979

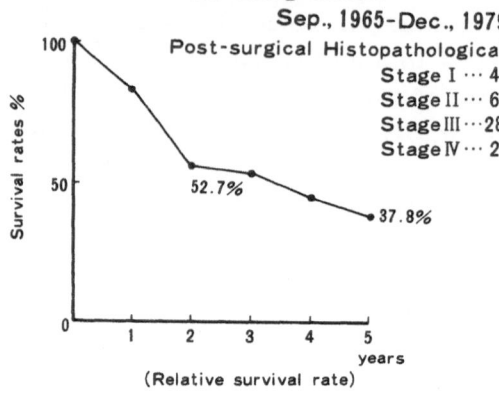

Post-surgical Histopathological
Stage I ··· 4
Stage II ··· 6
Stage III ···28
Stage IV ··· 2

Survival rates %

100

50

52.7%

37.8%

0

1   2   3   4   5
years
(Relative survival rate)

CONCLUSION: The bronchoplastic procedures are free from the risks and dangers accompanying the operation, reducing the postoperative mortality to nil. For the prevention of postoperative complications, careful attention and effort are given in suture technique, and postoperative bronchoscopic suctioning of intrabronchial secretions is absolutely necessary.

Preoperative bronchial artery infusion of Mitomycin C to Stage III patients to be beneficial prevent recurrence as well as increase in survival.

The bronchoplastic procedures assure good post-operational life and advancement in survival rate because of their pulmonary function preservation, enhancement of curability and applicability to many kinds of patients. The operation is, therefore, highly valuable.

VIII.10.

THERAPEUTIC APPROACH TO LARYNGO-TRACHEAL INJURY IN POST-TRAUMATIC AND POST-INTUBATION MAIN AIRWAY STENOSIS

L. COURAUD, C. MARTIGNE, B. PANCONI

1. INTRODUCTION

Since naso-tracheal intubation has replaced tracheotomy in respiratory resuscitation, laryngo-tracheal stenosis is encountered more frequently. Treatment of these stenoses often presents great difficulties, unlike that of isolated tracheal stenosis which is simple and gives excellent results (Table 1).

TABLE 1. Comparative treatment and results in 121 stenosis with or without involvement of the larynx.

Permanent tracheotomy (Respiratory or neurological causes)		5
Cure by endoscopic treatment		23
Isolated tracheal resection anastomosis		51
Successes	50 (98 %)	
Failures	1	
Surgery of laryngo-tracheal stenoses (Length of hospitalisation x 4)		42
Successes	38 (90 %)	
Failures (including deaths : 2)	4	

2. PRINCIPLES

The two main problems of laryngo-tracheal stenosis are :

2.1. avoidance of injury to the recurrent laryngeal nerves which enter the larynx at the lower border of the cricoid cartilage.

2.2. The need to ensure rigid skeletal support for the larynx in order to maintain patency. For this one must conserve the cricoid ring and the posterior cricoid plate on which rest the arytenoid cartilages and the muscles controlling glottal function. Experience has shown that resection of the anterior arch of the cricoid (Gerwat – Bryce [4], Pearson [5]) can be performed without immediate undesirable effects on respiratory or vocal function. However traumatisms or procedures which cause recurrent laryngeal nerve paralysis or ablation or dislocation of the posterior plate of the cricoid require stenting of the larynx until it is consolidated [3]

J.A. Nakhosteen and W. Maassen (eds.), Bronchology: Research, Diagnostic and Therapeutic Aspects. All rights reserved.
Copyright 1981. Martinus Nijhoff Publishers bv, The Hague / Boston / London

3. TREATMENT AND RESULTS

In 42 cases of stenosis affecting the larynx to a greater or lesser degree we have used various procedures according to the type, origin (traumatic or iatrogenic) and age of the lesion, the existence or otherwise of associated tracheal lesions and the experience progressively acquired.

3.1. Maximal resection-anastomoses

3.1.1. partial, horizontal sub-perichondral cricoid resection (5 cases, 5 successes)

3.1.2. oblique resection of the anterior arch of the cricoid (6 cases, 6 successes)

These procedures are mainly reserved for fibrous iatrogenic or post-traumatic stenoses. The results are excellent. The usual requirement of good tracheal surgery must of course be observed : previous reduction of infected lesions, good mucosa-to-mucosa apposition and use of resorbable sutures in order to avoid granulomatous, hypertrophic scar tissue on the suture line. These techniques cannot however be used if the stenosis continues beyond the upper border of the cricoid ring.

3.2. Laryngeal plasties

The best known of these is Rethi's operation. We prefer a more complex procedure including : resection of fibrous tissue, anterior cricotomy and posterior cricotomy with interposition of perichondral graft covered by a mucous flap.

This plasty is held in place by a T tube or naso-tracheal tube left for 3 months[2] (14 cases, 14 successes after 2 tempory failures requiring reoperation).

Indication for these plasties is not limited by the height of the stenosis but the procedure is very long (a minimun of 4 months) and there are sometimes considerable phonation sequellae. After having at one time performed plasties fairly frequently, we neglected them in favour of resections. However our present thinking is that the procedure is worth retaining.

3.3. Combined resection and plasty

3.3.1. Partial horizontal resection of the cricoid followed by laryngo-tracheal reanastomosis and stenting on a T tube or nasotracheal tube for from 20 to 45 days was applied 8 times with 8 successes to a well-defined type of traumatic lesion combining : complete laryngo-tracheal avulsion, comminuted fracture of the larynx and paralysis of vocal cords caused by disruption of the recurrent laryngeal nerves.

3.3.2. Laryngo-tracheal resection anastomosis, with total sub-perichondral exeresis of the cricoid cartilage combined with a laryngeal stent on naso-tracheal or T tube for 3 months, was performed 3 times with 2 successes and 1 death during the 5th week post-operative. Chondritis with lysis of the cricoid cartilage during the evolution of an iatrogenic or post-traumatic stenosis is a mandatory indication.

3.4. Complex resection-plasties

In 6 cases with complex and extensive mucosal and cartilaginous lesions and laryngeal obstruction, usually the result of one or two failed operations, were treated in improvised operations which combined resection of the cartilaginous, plasty with skin rotation flaps and laryngo-tracheal stenting. In 3 cases a patent main airway was achieved but phonation sequellae were marked ; there were 3 failures including 1 delayed death.

4. CONCLUSION

Involvement of the larynx in stenoses of the main airway is a cause of grave complications. Management is sometimes very long (3 to 4 months) and uncomfortable (prolonged stenting) and failure, even including death, is not uncommon (Table 2.).

TABLE 2. Treatment of main airway stenosis involving the larynx.

Partial horizontal cricoid resection	5 Successes	5 Failures 0
Resection of the anterior arch of the cricoid	6 Successes	6 Failures 0
Laryngo-tracheal plasties on stents	14 Successes	14 (2-2) 0
Partial resection with plasty	8 Successes	8 Failures 0
Total cricoid resection with plasty	3 Successes	2 Failures 1
Complex resection-plasties	6 Successes	3 Failures 3

Results are better when very typical lesions can be treated in planned procedures (19 cases, 19 successes). However with extensive, infected and already-operated lesions the indications are very difficult and should be the object of consultation and discussion (8 cases : 4 successes, 4 failures including 2 deaths). With complex lesions, laryngeal plasties without resection seem to us worth retaining despite their unasesthetic anatomical and functional results and the length of time that they demand (14 cases : 14 successes).

Difficulties in managing laryngeal stenoses are often the result of over-long intubation or of tracheotomies performed too late after intubation. This suggests rehabilitation of early low tracheotomy whenever lengthy respiratory resuscitation can be foreseen.

VIII.11.

INDICATION OF TRACHEOBRONCHIAL PLASTY FOR LUNG CANCER.

M. MAEDA, Y. KOTAKE, Y. SAWAMURA, A. MASAOKA, AND Y. KAWASHIMA

1. INTRODUCTION

This paper aims to establish how to apply the tracheobronchial plasty for lung cancer.

2. MATERIALS AND METHODS

2.1. The peribronchial region of cancer cells

In 47 patients operated the direct extension and metastatic lesions in the bronchial wall were examined histologically.

The distance of the peribronchial infiltration from primary lesion was examined in 7 lungs resected. The range was measured by using the transverse blocks of bronchi calculating the number of serial sections in 6 micron thick.

The metastasis along the bronchial wall was observed in 533 bronchi and 121 peribronchial lymph nodes of 40 lungs resected. Histologically the peribronchial metastases were divided into 3 types located at the intramucosal and paraserosal lymph vessels, and the peribronchial lymph nodes.

The positive rate was indicated as the ratio of bronchi with some type of metastasis to all examined.

2.2. The actual survival rate of cases

The follow-up studies were done using materials consisting of 3 groups, of which 41 were the plastic surgical group(B-Gr.), 422 the operated lung cancer including the B-Gr., and 37 the potential plastic surgical cases(BX-Gr.). The last group consisted of cases experienced before the bronchoplasty began to apply for lung cancer, and had been treated as lobectomy in 11, pneumonectomy in 14, and conservative treatments in 12. The later 2 groups were applied as controls for comparing with

J.A. Nakhosteen and W. Maassen (eds.), Bronchology: Research, Diagnostic and Therapeutic Aspects. All rights reserved.
Copyright 1981. Martinus Nijhoff Publishers bv, The Hague / Boston / London

the B-Gr.

3. RESULTS

3.1. The peribronchial region of cancer cells

The longest peribronchial infiltration measuring from serial sections was detected at the site of 20mm directly extending from the primary lesion in the bronchial wall.

The metastatic lesions in the bronchi were found in 32 of 40 cases(80.0%) and
in 129 of 533 bronchi examined(24.2%), the rate of which increased to 64.5% in
selecting the bronchi toward central direction. In addition the bronchial metastasis
was detected in 41.7% at the site 2 generations away from the primary lesion and
even at the bronchi toward a retrograde direction.

In 40 lungs examined, there was a case which had two cancerous lesions separately located at the left upper bronchus and the left B_6 bronchus.

The above-mentioned results indicate that lung cancer may have a certain region
along bronchi, and that the plastic operation must be carefully applied. Thus the
application of this operation was decided as follows.

    (I) Absolute indication(AI-Gr.)

        (1) Pneumonectomy patients for removal of tumor, who can not be done
            because of the limitation of pulmonary function.

        (2) Patients who have infiltration of cancer to the trachea.

    (II) Relative indication(RI-Gr.)

        (1) Patients who are able to be done pneumonectomy functionally.

In the case of the RI-Gr., the bronchoplasty instead of pneumonectomy was applied to the patient whose cancer was histologically diagnosed as the squamous cell
carcinoma, and whose lesion infiltrated as far as the segmental bronchi. Another case
of RI was early cancer located at a hilar bronchus.

3.2. The actual survival rate of cases

At present we have experienced 14 mehtods of 41 plastic operations,

In 422 operated lung cancers, plastic operations were done in 41 cases(9.0%). The AI encountered in 14 while the RI in remainder 27. In B-Gr., the ratio of squamous cell carcinoma was significantly higher than LC-Gr., and many more cases could be done curative operation compared with LC-Gr. However, the surgical stage was almost the same between the two.

The survival rates of the B-Gr. were higher than those of the LC-Gr. and the BX-Gr. The same analysis was done restricted to the squamous cell type. Twenty nine cases of the B-Gr. revealed better survival than that of 207 cases of LC-Gr., the result of which was the same in comparison with 52 cases, whose location of the lesion was similar to the B-Gr. endoscopically.

The above-mentioned results indicate that the high survival rates of the B-Gr. do not always relate to the high percentage of squamous cell carcinoma in the B-Gr.

The AI-Gr. would be the inoperable cases if the bronchoplasty could not be applied. The survival rate of this group was clearly higher than that of the inoperable cases and also that of the pneumonectomy cases in the BX-Gr. In addition, the survival of the RI-Gr. was compared with both the pneumonectomy and lobectomy groups by selecting the cases of squamous cell carcinoma who showed endoscopically similar localyzation to the RI-Gr. The RI-Gr. revealed the higher survival than that of the two groups.

4. CONCLUSION

(1) In the histological observation in 47 cases of lung cancer, cancer cells may have an extensive region along the bronchi in the way of direct infiltration, metastases, and multicentric growth. (2) The two standpoints of indication were established as the AI and RI. (3) As far as the bronchoplasty was applied to lung cancer on these criteria, the actual survival rate showed the higher levels than that of groups treated by other operations as lobectomy or pneumonectomy.

REFERENCE

1. Weisel, RD, Cooper, JD, Delarue, NC, Theman, TE, Todd, RJ, Pearson, FG:Sleeve lobectomy for carcinoma of the lung. J.Thorac. Cardiovasc. Surg. 78:839, 1979.

VIII..12.

TRACHEAL RECONSTRUCTION WITH PERICHONDRIAL GRAFTS

U. NORDIN & L. OHLSEN

Since 1972, a series of experiments performed at the Departments of Plastic Surgery and Otorhinolaryngology, University Hospital, Uppsala, Sweden, has elucidated the neochondrogenesis of perichondrium, both as a flap bridging a defect and as a free graft (ref. 1). The pathogenesis of iatrogenic tracheal injuries leading to tracheal stenosis and methods to prevent these injuries have been studied at the Department of Otorhinolaryngology, University Hospital, Uppsala (ref. 2). Anyhow, tracheal stenosis still appears and thus, there is a need for methods to reconstruct the trachea. A successful reconstruction of the tracheal wall implies normalization of the tracheal function within the reconstructed section. The lining of the reconstructed part should consist of ciliated cells to prevent accumulation of mucus below this area. Since the trachea must remain permanently open, a stable frame-work is necessary.

In rabbits a tracheal section containing two cartilages and the covering mucous membrane was removed and replaced with a free perichondrial graft taken from the ear. The animals were sacrificed after five weeks. New cartilage had formed in all animals giving support and full compensation for the removed cartilages. A tendency to stenosis was observed, but at light microscopy, the mucosa of the reconstructed area had after five weeks regenerated and was seen covered by cuboidal cells differing only slightly from the normal traceal mucosa. As observed by scanning electrone microscopy, the reconstructed part of the trachea was partly covered with ciliated cells of normal appearance but in the central parts patches of low epithelium with microvilli were still seen. It seems that the mucous membrane of the reconstructed trachea first became covered by low epithelial cells which then transformed into ciliated columnar epithelium.

J.A. Nakhosteen and W. Maassen (eds.), Bronchology: Research, Diagnostic and Therapeutic Aspects. All rights reserved.
Copyright 1981. Martinus Nijhoff Publishers bv, The Hague / Boston / London

The study was continued in two series of dogs.

In four dogs a tracheal section of two cartilages with the covering mucosa was completely removed. The circumferential defect was then reconstructed by free perichondrial grafts from rib cartilage. They were placed on two fascial flaps which had been raised from the adjacent muscles, rotated into the defect and sutured for complete coverage. The strap muscles of the neck were sutured in the midline giving complete coverage to the grafts. Regeneration of cartilage occurred in all four dogs producing a biologic frame-work already within two weeks. Section through the newly formed cartilages showed after two weeks still immature, but after six weeks more matured (Fig. 1).

The lining of the reconstructed tracheal section was restored by epithelialization, as it seemed, from the surrounding mucosa. Low epithelial cells were successively replaced by columnar ciliated cells typical of the respiratory tract. Scanning electron microscopy of the reconstructed tracheal portion demonstrates a mucous membrane with ciliated cells, similar to the normal epithelium of the respiratory tract, and low epithelial cells with microvilli. In the central parts of the reconstructed portion different types of cells can be seen, some flat and covered by short microvilli, while others are more cuboidal and covered by cilia in different degrees of protrusion. Some cilia have acquired normal appearance and length (Fig. 2).

In all these four dogs a stenosis occurred. Because of the stenosis another experiment was carried out in four dogs subjected to the same operative procedure though up to five cartilages were removed. Postoperatively, a Montgomery T-tube was inserted to maintain expansion of the reconstructed portion. By this, stenosis could be prevented and when the tube was removed after about four months, the dogs were kept alive without respiratory distress up to another four months.

The trachea was very stable within the reconstructed portion with solid cartilaginous tissue where the perichondrial grafts had been positioned. The supporting structure had all the characteristics of matured cartilage. Scanning electron microscopy of the reconstructed portion showed regeneration of the mucous membrane with a covering epithelium which did not differ from the columnar cells of normal trachea. A bronchoscopic appearance of the reconstructed part of the trachea showed the dimensions corresponding to the outer diameter of the Montgomery T-tube extracted about four months before the examination. There was an active transport of mucus stained with cardiogreen across the reconstructed section which was recorded by filming.

In summary, the tracheal wall can be reconstructed by means of free perichondrial grafts in order to produce a biologic support comparable to that offered by the normal tracheal cartilages. Reconstruction does not necessarily require

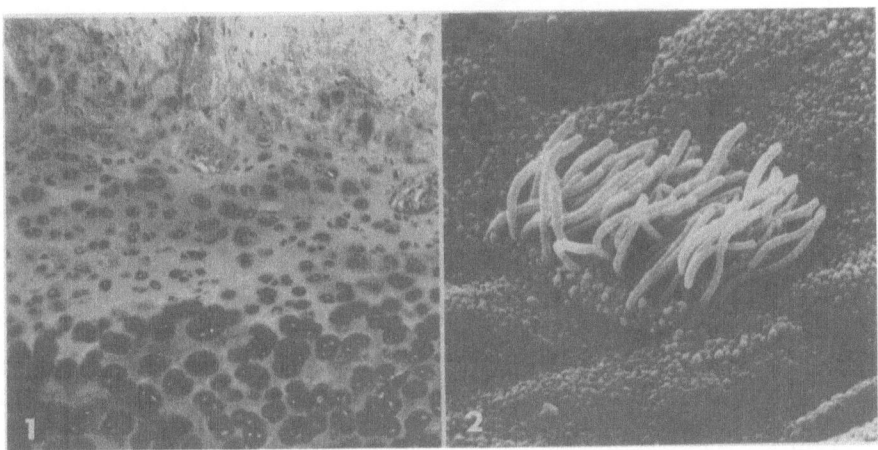

Fig. 1   Fig. 2

transplantation of mucosa. In all the presented series, regeneration of mucosal
lining occurred by ingrowth from the bordering epithelium which gradually covered
the entire defect. This epithelium, initially presented as low cuboidal cells,
transformed to columnar cells with cilia. This regenerated lining possessed
normal function allowing fairly normal mucus transport across the reconstructed
area preventing an accumulation of mucus below the reconstructed section. The
complication of stenosis was prevented by keeping the reconstructed section
distended with a silicon tube inserted in the trachea until healing was completed.
However, if the presented technique also includes transplantation of mucosa it
might shorten the healing process and maybe also diminish the tendency of scar
tissue formation causing stenosis within the reconstructed section.

VIII.13.

SURGICAL TREATMENT AND BRONCHOSCOPIC FINDINGS IN PATIENTS WITH
TRACHEAL INVASION BY THYROID CARCINOMA

T. ISHIHARA, S. YAMAZAKI, K. KOBAYASHI, S. FUKAI, A. TAKESHI

When thyroid carcinoma grows and protrudes intratracheally
tracheal stenosis occurs and the trachea is finally obstructed,
although the tracheal invasion by thyroid carcinoma is not often
encountered. Therefore thyroid carcinoma with tracheal invasion
should be appropriately treated before it causes severe dyspnea
due to tracheal stenosis.

Up to January 1980, we surgically treated 20 patients with
thyroid carcinoma invading the trachea. Five were male and 15 were
female. Their ages ranged from 31 to 77 with a mean age of 53 years.
In 14 of 20 cases, thyroid carcinoma invaded the trachea in the
course of several recurrences. In the remaining 6 cases, thyroid
carcinoma had already invaded the trachea when they were seen for
the first time.

Main symptoms of the tracheal invasion by thyroid carcinoma are
hemoptysis and dyspnea. Hemoptysis was noticed in 18 of 20 cases
and dyspnea in 9 cases.
In 20 cases surgically treated by us, 10 cases were diagnosed
by x-ray films and 10 cases were diagnosed bronchoscopically to
have tracheal invasion by thyroid carcinoma. To diagnose tracheal
invasion by thyroid carcinoma, lateral x-ray films, xeroradiograms
of the neck and bronchoscopy were useful.

Fig. 1 shows a xeroradiogram of the neck. This patient underwent
right hemithyroidectomy in September, 1975. In 1979 the patient
noticed hemosputum. Xeroradiograms revealed the tracheal invasion
by thyroid carcinoma. This xeroradiogram shows the tumor protruding
from the inner surface of the cricoid cartilage and upper trachea
into the limen.
Fig. 2 shows the resected specimen of this patient.

J.A. Nakhosteen and W. Maassen (eds.), Bronchology: Research, Diagnostic and
Therapeutic Aspects. All rights reserved.
Copyright 1981. Martinus Nijhoff Publishers bv, The Hague / Boston / London

Fig. 1

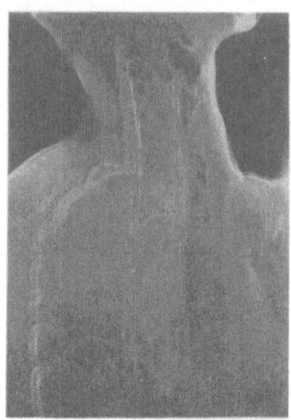

Fig. 2

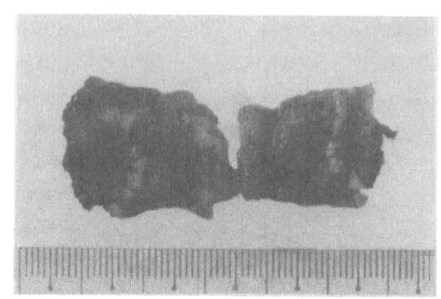

Fig. 3

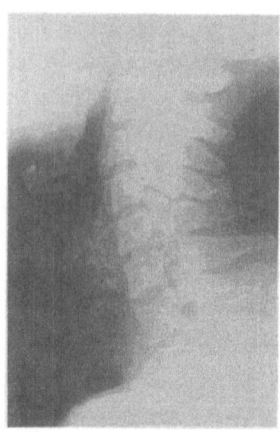

Fig. 4

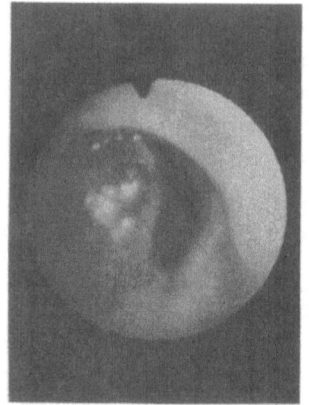

Fig. 3 is a lateral x-ray film of the neck of another patient. A round tumor shadow which overlaps the carcified tracheal cartilage is seen. This patient underwent thyroidectomy for thyroid carcinoma fourteen years ago and resection of recurrent thyroid carcinoma 7 years ago. Last year hemosputum was noticed and lateral x-ray films of the neck showed the tracheal invasion by thyroid carcinoma.

Fig. 4 is a bronchoscopic view of this patient. A tumor is protruding intratracheally from the left side wall of the trachea. The round shadow seen on the lateral x-ray film of the neck was bronchoscopically revealed to be the tracheal invasion by thyroid carcinoma.

We circumferentially resected the tracheal lesion along with thyroid carcinoma around the trachea and anastomosed in end to end fashion in 20 patients with thyroid carcinoma infiltrating the trachea.

The results of surgical treatment in 20 patients are as follows ;

There were two operative deaths. Five patients died of progression of thyroid carcinoma to the brain, vertebrae and lungs.

Complications occurred in nine cases. In one patient recurrence of thyroid carcinoma occurred in the trachea and this patient underwent reoperation. Thereafter, there has been no sign of recurrence 3 years and 6 months postoperatively.

Stenosis at the anastomosed site occurred in two cases. In one case reoperation was done but in the other case no special therapy was performed to the stenosis because there was no dyspnea.

Laryngeal stenosis occurred in 6 cases. In all these cases operative procedure extended the subglottic area. In 5 out of these 6 cases tracheal fenestration was performed and in the remaining one case tracheostomy was done.

Thirteen patients are alive three months to 7 years postoperatively.

By demonstrating several cases, I presented 20 cases of thyroid carcinoma invading the trachea and the results of surgical procedure were also reported.

Although it is generally said that thyroid carcinoma is a slow growing tumor, thyroid carcinoma which invaded the trachea did not always grow slowly.

Therefore, when a patient who underwent operation for thyroid carcinoma has hemosputum it is necessary to examine the trachea in detail by taking lateral x-ray films of the neck and performing bronchoscopy.

Reference
1. T. Ishihara, K. Kikuchi, T. Ikeda, H. Inoue, S. Fukai, K. Ito, and T. Mimura: Resection of thyroid carcinoma infiltrating the trachea. Thorax 33:378, 1978.

VIII.14.

Surgical Management of Collar Tracheal Stenoses

K. Sesterhenn, K.-G.Rose

Most of the cricotracheal or tracheal Stenoses which come
up for treatment are results of prolonged intubation whereas
in the pre-antibiotic era inflammatory and traumatic causes
played the main role.

In the Ent-Clinic in Cologne 142 stenoses have been treated
since 1950. Stenoses caused by prolonged intubation have
increased in number since 1963 at the same time as development
of intensive care in Germany began. 89 cases, that is 63%, have
been caused by intubation alone; 41 cases, that is 29%, result
from faults in tracheotomy or tracheotomy into a trachea already damaged by intubation; finally 12 cases, that is 8%, have
other causes.

The special anatomical structure of the upper respiratory tract
leads to a contact of the tube with certain mucosal aereas,
particularly the posterior wall of the pharynx, the laryngeal
surface of the epiglottis. The arytenoid region, the arch of
the cridoic cartilage and the tracheal wall at the level of the
cuff. This can be demonstrated by a post-mortem specimen of a
trachea as a typical example, the permanent contact with the
tube produces a local ischemia of mucosa, infected and accumulated mucus favours inflammatory ulcerations sometimes with
mycoses, lateron the regenerating granulation tissue will be
transformed into narrowing scars. In this context it is
necessary to point out that almost all of our patients with
tracheal-stenoses showed a tendency to produce keloid in the
skin.

Conservative procedures in therapy of tracheal-stenoses like
bouginage were abandonned at the beginning of the century and
replaced by surgical treatment. The surgical procedure is
determined by the form, the localisation and the extent of
the stenosis. Laryngo-tracheal stenoses are best treated by
plastic reconstruction of an open mould which is held open
with a suitable stent until it is completly stabilised. The

J.A. Nakhosteen and W. Maassen (eds.), Bronchology: Research, Diagnostic and
Therapeutic Aspects. All rights reserved.
Copyright 1981. Martinus Nijhoff Publishers bv, The Hague / Boston / London

anterior wall is reconstructed with skin pedicle grafts after some weeks or months.

Narrowing of the trachea by tracheomalacia is cured by laterofixation of the side walls of the organ.

For cicatricial strictures of the trachea the following therapeutical strategy has proved to be successful:
stenoses of less than 2 cm in extent on the condition that the wall is still stable are removed by submucosal resection, while the mucosa is replaced in its original position and fixed with fibrin seal.

Stenoses between 2 and 5 cm long are treated by circular resection and subsequent end-to-end anastomosis. With increasing extension of the excised stenotic tracheal segment the tension of the tracheal stumps has to be reduced by several mobilisation procedures. According to Dedo and Fishman the tension of the upper stump can be reduced by transsection of the infrahyal muscles or according to Grillo the tension of the lower trachea can be reduced by intrathoracal mobilisations. The success of the resection mainly depends on a lack of traction in the anastomosis.

Therapy of strictures which are longer than 5 cm has always been very problematic. Up to now the only possibility has been an open-mould treament which is technically difficult and time consuming. Replacement of the trachea by implantation of synthetic prostheses have been just as unsuccessful as denaturalised tracheal grafts. In 1978 we transplantated for the first time a fresh allogeneic trachea in man, the theoretical background we obtained by experiments on animals published elsewhere. After HLA-Typing of the recipient who had a tracheal stenosis extending over 8 segments Eurotransplant in Leiden provided a suitable donor. The tracheal graft, which was 2 hours old, was first prepared on the following manner: the upper and lower openings were closed by flaps prepared from the neighbouring pars membranacea. To guarantee optimal revascularisation, not disturbed by mechanical or inflammatory alterations, the graft was implanted into the

right sterno-cleido-mastoid muscle. And was left there for
6 weeks. Finally the transplant was isolated from the muscle
with the exeption of a muscle-bridge which carried the new
blood vessels. The 8-ring-tracheal graft was integrated iso-
peristaltically into the tracheal gap which remained after
the excision of the strictured part of the organ. The graft
healed well and still is vital. Occasionally we had to remove
granulations from the upper anastomosis.

In conclusion we suggest the following procedure for surgical
treatment of tracheostenosis:
Laryngotracheal stenoses should be reconstructed with plastic
surgery in the manner of an open mould.
In the case of tracheomalacia the laterofixation of the side
walls may be sufficient to guarantee an open airway.
Strictures up to an extent of 2 cm should be treated by submucosal resection.
Stenoses from 2-5 cm in length can best be removed by resection
followed by end-to-end-anastomosis.
In the case of stenoses longer than 5 cm the hetero-orthotopic
allotransplantation can be attempted without risk.
An alternative is the difficult plastic repair of a new trachea.

References may be requested at the authors
Priv.Doz. Dr. med. K. Sesterhenn, Prof. Dr. med. K.-G.Rose
Univ.Hals-Nasen-Ohrenklinik Köln
Josef-Stelzmann-Straße 9
5000 Köln 41

VIII.15.

RECONSTRUCTION OF THE STENOTIC AIRWAY - A NEW APPROACH

C.E. Lindholm

INTRODUCTION

Stenosis of the upper trachea and the larynx may be caused by external trauma to the neck, internal trauma caused by tracheal tubes, neoplastic disease, infection, auto-immune conditions, etc.

Resection of a stationary, stenotic part of the airway and primary end-to-end anastomosis is usually the method of choice (Grillo, 1979). Partial resection of the cricoid cartilage and part of the upper trachea and end-to-end anastomosis has also successfully been performed in selected cases (Pearson et al., 1975). If the stenosis comprises both the upper trachea and the larynx or the larynx alone, it is, however, often impossible to use this technique.

In reconstructioning the upper trachea and the larynx, a graft may be required to replace defects of the airway wall. The graft should be well vascularized and be composed of firm supporting tissue, covered on one side with mucous membrane.

PROCEDURE

A three-stage procedure was used to reconstruct stenosis of the larynx and upper trachea. Buccal mucosa was first transplanted to a position immediately outside the cartilaginous skeleton of the airway, with the epithelial lining turned inwards (Fig. 1 a). In some cases, a thin, silicon film was interposed between the epithelial side of the mucosa and the underlying tissue, in order to prevent adhesions.

The second stage of the procedure took place after 1.5 to 2 months. Now a cyst lined with mucous membrane had formed. The cyst was dissected free from the surrounding, superficial tissue with great care, so as not to rupture its thin wall. A free, arched, periostium-bone graft from the iliac crest (Fig. 1 b) or a slice of bone taken from the clavicle left attached to the clavicular head of the sternocleid-mastoid muscle was grafted immediately outside the described cyst (Fig. 1 c). The grafted bone was carefully trimmed and provided with multiple holes, through which ingrowth of nutritive vessels into the bone and the

J.A. Nakhosteen and W. Maassen (eds.), Bronchology: Research, Diagnostic and Therapeutic Aspects. All rights reserved.
Copyright 1981. Martinus Nijhoff Publishers bv, The Hague / Boston / London

mucosa was expected (Wilflingseder, 1972). Finally, the strap muscles·
were placed superficially on the bone graft and the subcutaneous tissue
and skin were closed.

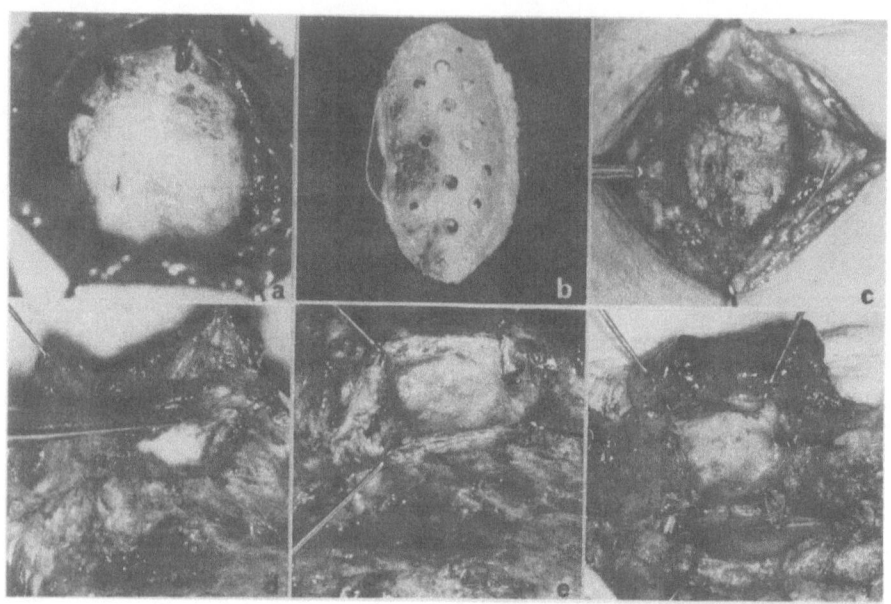

FIGURE 1 (a-f) See text.

At a third session 2 months later, the bone graft had been lined
on the inside with part of the well-vascularized mucosa of the cyst.
The cyst was opened up with a midline incision in the wall closest to
the airway. The cyst was emptied of its milky, sterile content (Fig.
1 d) and a nice, pink, mucosal membrane was found (Fig. 1 e) firmly
attached to the bone disk. The stenotic part of the airway was incised
along the anterior midline (Fig. 1 e). Fibrous scar tissue was removed
from the interior of the airway and the surface was covered with a free
transplant of trimmed, buccal mucosa. Finally, the composite graft was
interposed between the two edges of the incised larynx and/or trachea
to widen the circumference of the stenotic airway (Fig. 1 f).

RESULTS

Six patients, 3 of whom had combined laryngotracheal stenosis, have
had their airways reconstructed by the described technique.

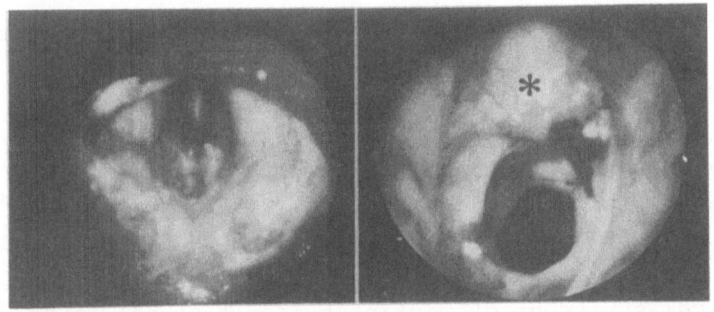

FIGURE 2. a) Stenosis of the larynx in a 26-year-old man. b) Result after surgery. * Transplanted area.

A 26-year-old man had for the last 7 years before surgery been suffering from a rare, auto-immune disease, causing multiple airway stenoses, including the larynx and the trachea. His disease had been fairly well controlled for a year when he was admitted for surgery. By that time, he had had a tracheostomy tube for 7 years, and two attempts to widen his larynx surgically had been made without success. His subglottic, laryngeal stenosis had a diameter of about 2 mm (Fig. 2 a). After the three-stage, surgical procedure, his airway had a diameter of 8-9 mm (Fig. 2 b) at the site of transplantation. At follow-up 1 year after surgery, his airway diameter was unchanged. The radiogram of the larynx and upper trachea showed an irregular contour, but he was able to go biking and cross-country skiing and, in spite of the irregular airway contour, the operation had had a functionally satisfactory result.

In addition to the patient presented above, 4 other patients had improved airways, both radiographically, endoscopically and functionally, at follow-up 1 year after the procedure. The operation was a failure in 1 patient (a woman). She suffered from a laryngotracheal stenosis, which had been slowly developing for a few years. After reconstructive, three-stage surgery, the result was satisfactory at first, but after some months re-stenosis occurred and she is now having a Montgomery T-tube inserted permanently.

DISCUSSION

The advantage of this method is that a vascularized tissue consisting of the desired components is obtained, in contrast to transposition of the hyoid bone (Wong et al., 1978), muscle-periostium-bone flaps (Lindholm, 1977) or free grafts of cartilage (Wilflingseder, 1972)

A disadvantage is that the procedure has to be carried out in stages and therefore takes a long time.

In its present form, it is thus not possible to use this method to replace defects, for instance, of the laryngeal wall produced at partial laryngectomy, but reconstruction of chronic stenosis of the upper trachea and larynx has been successful.

REFERENCES

1. Grillo CH: Surgical treatment of postíntubation tracheal injuries. J Thorac. Cardiovasc. Surg. 78:860-875, 1979.

2. Pearson FG, Cooper JD, Nelems JM, Vannostrand AWP: Primary tracheal anastomosis after resection of cricoid cartilage with preservation of recurrent laryngeal nerves. J Thorac. Cardiovasc. Surg. 70:806-816, 1975.

3. Wilflingseder R: Rekonstruktion der Trachea durch ein Segment-transplantat von Nasenseptum. Wien. Kling. Wschr. 84:226, 1972.

4. Wong ML, Kashima HK, Finnegan DA, Jafek BW: Vascularized Hyoid Inter position for Subglottic and Upper Tracheal Stenosis. Ann.Otol.87:491-197

5. Lindholm CE: Tracheal Reconstruction with Muscle-Periosteum-Bone Flap. Chir Plastica (Berl.) 4,35-40 (1977).

VIII.16.
Eine experimentelle Studie über Anastomose im Tracheo-bronchialbereich in Hinsicht auf die Ultrastruktur

M. Ohata,M.D.,M. Iida,M.D.,H.Endo,M.D.,A.Niino,M.D.,N.Hashimoto und
K.Omori.

1. Einführung

 In letzter Zeit sind viele Berichte von erfolgreichen Resultaten
bei Anwendung der End-zu-End-Anastomose im Tracheo-bronchialbereich
erschienen. Als Nahtmaterial für die Anastomose haben wir früher
nichtabsorbierbares Material wie Seide, Nylon oder Tevdeck benutzt.
Jedoch ergeben sich dabei einige Probleme wie z.B. Granulationsbildung
und die daraus ergebende Stenose der Luftwege. Um diese Probleme zu
lösen, haben wir eine experimentelle Studie über die tracheo-bronchiale
Anastomose mit einem absorbierbaren Material "Dexon" durchgeführt,
und dabei haben wir die Regenerationsvorgänge des Flimmerepithels im
Bereich der Anastomosenstelle mit dem Scanning-Elektronenmikroskop
beobachtet.

2. Methodik

 Bei 10 Hunden(1. Gruppe) wurde die Halstrachea freigelegt,und nach
Resektion von 3 bis 4 Trachealringen wurde End-zu-End anastomosiert,
und die Anastomose in der ganzen Schicht mit Knopfnähten mit 4-0
Dexon versorgt. Bei 8 Hunden (2. Gruppe) wurde eine Manschettenresektion
des rechten Oberlappens durchgeführt. Die Anastomose wurde wieder
ganzschichtig mit Knopfnähten mit 4-0 Dexon versorgt. Nach 1.,2.,
3.,9. Woche und dem 4. Monat nach Anlegung der Anastomose wurde der
Anastomosenbereich lichtmikroskopisch und elektronenmikroskopisch
untersucht.

3. Ergebnisse

 Die Oberfläche im Bereich der Anastomosenstelle eine Woche nach der
Operation im Lichtmikroskop: Die Kontinuität des Epithels ist verhält-
nissmäßig gut erhalten. Im SEM haben wir zwei verschiedene Zellgruppen,
die eine mit Mikrovilli und die andere ohne Mikrovilli, im Bereich
der Anastomose beobachtet (Fig.1). In der zweiten Woche fanden wir
eine geringfügige Mikrovillibildung (Fig.2) bei den Zellen, die Anfang
keine Mikrovilli aufwiesen. In der dritten Woche fanden wir im SEM
ein lockeres Gefüge der Epithelialen Zellen mit langen Zilien und
dazwischen eine geringfügige Anzahl von Becherzellen mit feinen Mikro-

villi (Fig.3). In der neunten Woche fanden wir in der Ultrastruktur, kein Nahtmaterial mehr. In Fig.4 sehen wir eine vom Anastomosengebiet abgespaltene Fläche;wir haben fast normales Flimmerepithel mit kuglige Kernen beobachtet. Im der neunten Woche fanden wir in der Umgebung von 100 μ um die Anastomosenlinie nur flache Zellen mit wenig Mikrovilli ohne Zilien. Bis zu einer Entfernung von 750 μ von der Anastomosenlinie fanden wir locker gelegene Epithelzellen mit Zilien. Jenseits dieser Stelle fanden wir zahlreiche normale Zellen.

4. Diskussion

Im Jahre 1884 haben Gluck und Zeller zum erstenmal eine erfolgreiche End-zu-End-Anastomose im Bereich der Trachea durchgeführt. in der letzten Zeit hat die Lungenresektion bei Bronchialkarzinom unter Verwendung der Bronchialplastik mehr und mehr zugenommen. Trotzdem gibt es nur wenig Grundforschung über die Anastomosentechniken und Nahtmaterialien. Die Anastomose versorgen wir bisher mit bis in die muscularis mucosae reichenden Nähten. Jedoch ist es praktisch unmöglich mit dieser Technik in der pars membranacea zu nähen. Um diese Probleme zu lösen, haben wir eine experimentelle Studie über die tracheo-bronch- ale Anastomose mit einem absorbierbaren Nahtmaterial "Dexon" durch- geführt, und dabei haben wir die Regenerationsvorgänge des Epithels im Bereich der Anastomosenstelle im SEM beobachtet. Über die Regenerat- ionsvorgänge des Epithels im Bereich der Anastomosenstelle nach der End-zu-End-Anastomose hat D.L. Wilhelm umfangreiche experimentelle Studien durchgeführt. D.J. Ferguson gat auch berichtet,daß beim Tier- versuch mit Hunden, 5 Tage nach der Anastomosierung der Trachea, keine Epithelbildung lichtmikroskopisch nachgewiesen werden konnte. 14 Tage nach der Operation zeigt sich erstmals eine Neubildung des Epithels in der Umgebung von 1 cm von der Anastomosenstelle. Wir haben bei der Beobachtung des Epithels mit SEM eine Woche nach der Anastomos- ierung, zwei verschiedene Zellgruppen, die eine mit und die andere ohne Mikrovilli, beobachtet. Aufgrund dieses Befundes haben wir vermutet, daß es sich bei den Mikrovilli um kleinste Zellfortsätze handelt, die keine echten Mikrovilli sind, sondern eine Regeneration des Flimmer- epithels in der Bildungsphase zu sein scheinen. Wir beobachten drei Wochen nach der Anastomose zwischen dem Flimmerepithel einige Goblet Zellen mit feinen Mikrovilli. In dem vierten Monat finden wir fast normales Flimmerepithel nicht nur in der Umgebung der Anastomose, sondern auch direkt auf der Anastomosenlinie. Dieser Befund stimmt mit einer Beobachtung von Wilhelm und Ferguson überein.

Bei "Dexon", als Nahtmaterial benutzt wird, beginnt am Anfang der

dritten Woche nach der Anastomose die Resorbierung des Fadens.
Ausserdem fanden wir, das Dexon, das innen in der Trachea oder Bronchus
bloßlegen hatte, bereits drei Wochen nach der Operation aufgelöst war.
In dem nach vier Monaten untersuchten Probestück haben wir kein Dexon
mehr gefunden. Wir möchten empfehlen, daß bei der Anastomose im Bereich
der Luftwege ganzschichtig mit absorbierbarem Nahtmaterial genäht wird.

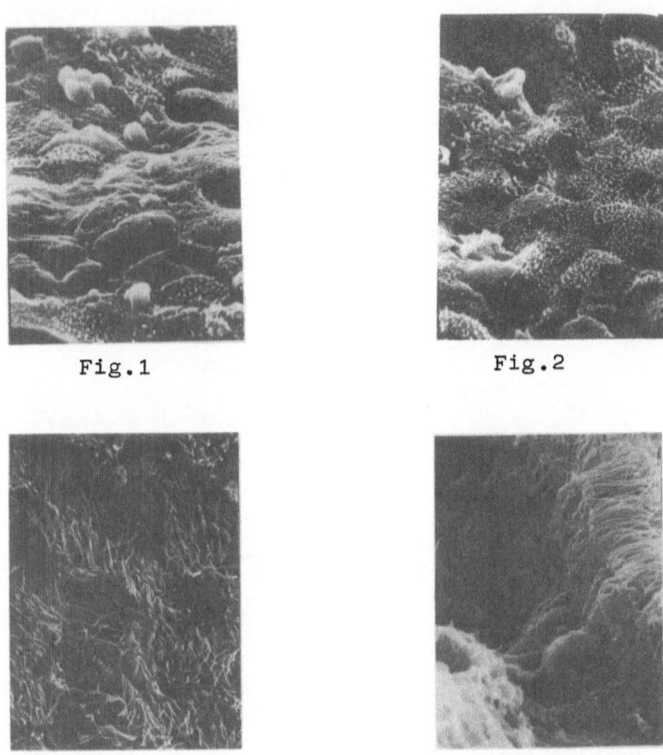

Fig.1   Fig.2

Fig.3   Fig.4

Schrifttum

1. Ferguson,D.J., Wild,J.S.,and Wangensteen,O.H.: Experimental
    resection of the trachea. Surg.,28:597,1950
2. Wilhelm,D.L.: Regeneration of Tracheal Epithelium.
                                J. Path.Bact.,IXV:543,1963
3. Hioki,K.: Zytologische Untersuchungen über das Flimmerepithel
    der menschlichen Trachea mit besondere Berücksichtigung der Beziehung
    zwischen Flimmer- und Becherzellen.   Cytologia,12:326,1942

Chapter VIII

Section 3
POST-OPERATIVE ENDOSCOPIC MANAGEMENT

VIII.17.

STUDIES ON THE EFFECT UPON PULMONARY FUNCTION OF DENERVATION AFTER TRACHEO-BRONCHOPLASTY

R. Abe, K. Tamura, H. Ikushima, T. Teramatsu, H. Higashi, M. Ito

INTRODUCTION

There are many factors concerning the effect of severing the autonomic nerve branch in the bronchial wall during bronchial reconstructive surgery. The effect has yet to be explained completely. To clarify some of these factors, we investigated the dynamic respiratory functions of patients who had undergone bronchial reconstructive surgery.

MATERIALS AND METHOD

Bronchial and tracheal reconstructions were done on 12 cases. The trachea was reconstructed in 7 patients, the left main bronchus in 3, and the right main bronchus in 2. Diagnoses included 9 neoplasms, 2 pulmonary tuberculosis, and one other. Two cases are presented here, one right and one left main bronchus.

Changes in internal diameter of airways were measured and recorded during cough, using bronchography.

Ventilation and pulmonary blood flow were examined using inert gases (^{133}Xe, ^{99}Tc, and ^{81m}Kr).

RESULTS

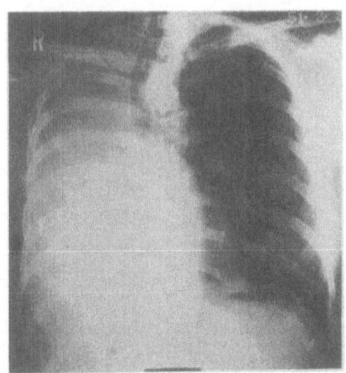 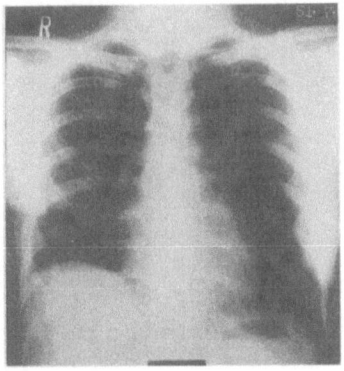

Figure 1   Figure 2

J.A. Nakhosteen and W. Maassen (eds.), Bronchology: Research, Diagnostic and
Therapeutic Aspects. All rights reserved.
Copyright 1981. Martinus Nijhoff Publishers bv, The Hague / Boston / London

292

Figure 1 shows atelectasis of the right lung due to a fibrotic tubercle occluding the right bronchus.

Figure 2. In this case, reconstruction was performed on the right bronchus where an occlusion was removed and an end-to-end anastomosis was performed. This is the post-operative chest film.

Table 1 shows the changes in the inside diameter of the airway. Of the reconstructed left bronchus, virtually no contraction is evident, whereas the right bronchus, which was not operated, the diameter has contracted to almost 50% of its original size.

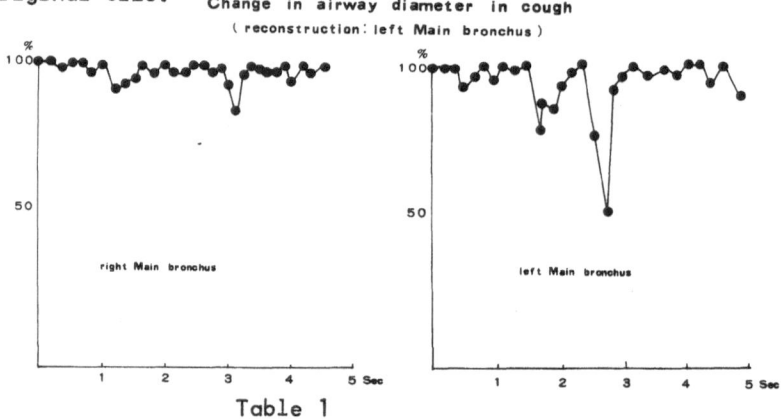

Table 1

Table 2. The reconstruction of the right bronchus has caused the comparative change to be the reverse of the first case.

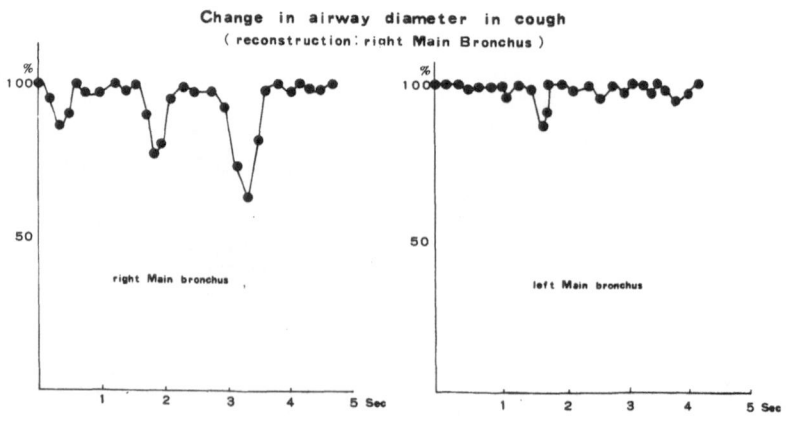

Table 2

Tables 3 and 4. Pulmonary blood flow count ($\overset{\circ}{Q}$) using $81m_{KR}$, and distribution and wash-out ().

	Left main bronchial reconstruction			Right main bronchial reconstruction	
	Right lung	Left lung		Right lung	Left lung
$\overset{\circ}{Q}$	11947 count	6672 count	$\overset{\circ}{Q}$	6548 count	12541 count
λ	0.430	0.556	λ	0.301	0.665

Tables 3 and 4

DISCUSSION

This paper reports results of studies on ventilation and pulmonary blood flow using radioactive inert gases (133_{Xe} and 99_{Kr}), and changes in the inside diameter of airways following tracheo-bronchial reconstructive surgery.

Tables 1 and 2 show that there is almost no contractile force in the reconstructed bronchus. These data suggest that this is due to the effect of denervation.

Tables 3 and 4 show that in the reconstruction of the right bronchus, pulmonary blood flow count (Q) was 6,548 for the right lung and 12,541 for the left. Distribution and wash-out of inert gases () was 0.301 for the right and 0.665 for the left lung. This indicated that there is reduced blood flow on the operated side.

The same holds true for the reconstruction of the left bronchus. $\overset{\circ}{Q}$-count was 6,672 for the reconstructed left lung and 11,947 for the unoperated right lung. The count for the left lung was approximately one-half that of the right.

The distribution and wash-out of inert gases in the left lung was far slower than in the right lung.

CONCLUSION

1. Respiratory movements on the operated lung were slower than those of the unoperated lung.

2. Broncho-motor tone was altered by the operation, and the cough effect was weakened at the bronchus peripheral to anastomosis.

3. Ventilation and pulmonary blood flow distribution of the operated lung were reduced, compared to the unoperated lung.

VIII.18.

POSTOPERATIVE USE OF FIBEROPTIC BRONCHOSCOPE FOR BRONCHOPLASTIC
SURGERY ON LUNG CANCER

KENJI NAKAMURA, KENJI SAWAMURA, KIYOYUKI FURUSE, SOGO IIOKA,
SOICHI HASHIMOTO, TAKASHI MORI, YUTAKA NAGAOKA, MASAAKI KAWAHARA,
MASAZUMI MAEDA*

1. INTRODUCTION

Recently in many instances, bronchoscope has come to be the
method of choice in order to obtain as much curability and reserve
as much pulmonary function as possible in the treatment of lung cancer.
After the procedure therapeutic use of bronchoscope is indicated
often in the postoperative period. Here we discuss about the
experience of our postoperative use of bronchoscope.

2. PROCEDURE
2.1. MATERIALS

Twenty six out of 183 patients were treated by bronchoplastic
procedure during the period of Jan. 1, 1976 through Dec. 31, 1979.
(Table 1)

Their age ranged 35 to 73 averaging 57, and recently more
the number of elderly who receive surgical intervention are increasing
so the elderly are increasing in this series. Histologically 21 cases
were with squamous cell carcinoma, 4 with adenocarcinoma, and one with
small cell carcinoma.

TABLE 1. RESECTED CASES OF LUNG CANCER (1976 - 1979)

Year	Cases	Broncho-plasty	Rate (%)
1976	37	5	13.5
1977	51	6	11.7
1978	45	6	13.3
1979	50	9	18.0
Total	183	26	14.2

*J.A. Nakhosteen and W. Maassen (eds.), Bronchology: Research, Diagnostic and
Therapeutic Aspects. All rights reserved.
Copyright 1981. Martinus Nijhoff Publishers bv, The Hague / Boston / London*

2.2. METHODS

In order to reduce postoperative pulmonary complications, bronchoscope was made use of soon after operation, and in the early postoperative period. That is to remove pooled blood in the bronchi soon after operation and to remove increased bronchial secretion with difficulty of expectoration in the early postoperative period.

In another instance after bronchoplasty bronchoscope was also used for the long term follow up evaluation of anastomosis.

3. RESULTS

When bronchoplastic procedure was applied, accumulated blood in the region is likely to flow into the bronchi during the process of anastomosis. So soon after the bronchoplasty, pooled blood in the bronchi had to be removed in 7 cases, in order to prevent atelectasis or pneumonia.

Increased bronchial secretion that was difficult to expectorate was noted in 8 cases, and among them atelectasis was noted in their chest X-ray in 4 cases.

After removal of bronchial secretion atelectasis was cured and no pneumonia was found thereafter.

For the follow up evaluation after bronchoplasty, stenosis at the level of anastomosis is the greatest matter of problem. So, fiberoptic bronchoscope was used in order to remove ơranuloma, and hitological examination was made to the materials obtained through bronchoscopical aid.

Granuloma at the level of anastomosis was found in 4 cases and removed successfully through bronchoscope.(Fig. 1a, b)

FIG. 1.a.   FIG. 1.b.

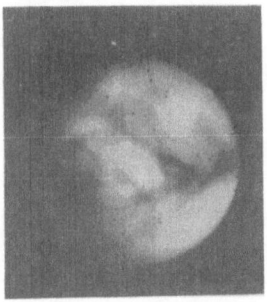
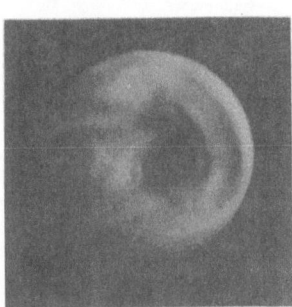

Another case of annular constriction was treated in the same way but in vain. (Fig. 2a, b)

FIG. 2a

FIG. 2b

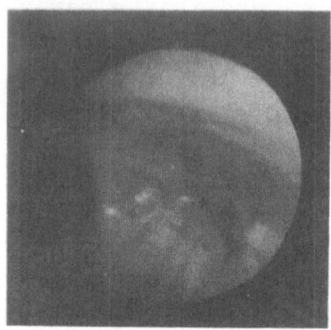

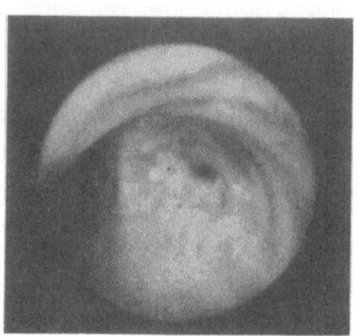

Regional recurrence was found through bronchoscope and confirmed histologically in one case.

4. SUMMARY

According to our experience mentioned abouve, we consider that fiberoptic bronchoscope is essential in the management of postoperative patients soon after operation and in the early postoperative period, and furthermore for the long term follow up evaluation.

REFERENCES

1. Tsuchiya, R., Ogata, T., et al: Prophylactic fiberoptic bronchoscope suction to prevent postoperative lung complications in lung cancer surgery. Bronchoscopy. 97-99, 1978. World Association for bronchology, Tokyo.

2. Nakamura, K., Iioka, S., Sawamura, K., et al.: Postoperative use of fiberoptic bronchoscope after Tracho- and Broncho-plasty. Jap. J. Thor. Dis. 18,2,130, 1980. (Japanese)

Chapter IX

PERBRONCHIAL FINE NEEDLE ASPIRATION

IX.1.

THIRTY YEARS EXPERIENCE WITH PERBRONCHIAL FINE NEEDLE ASPIRATION

R. LODDENKEMPER, H. GROSSER, H. -J. BRANDT

(Chest Hospital Heckeshorn, Berlin - W , Germany)

1. INTRODUCTION

Perbronchial or pertracheal needle biopsy via the rigid bronchoscope was performed ten years earlier than mediastinoscopy. SCHIEPPATI (4) described the method in 1949 as first but it started simultaneously in different pneumologic centres. Early results from our hospital were published by BRANDT (2). The technique was at first used only in patients where lymph node enlargement was suspected macroscopically or roentgenologically. Because of the easiness, the low risk and the relative good diagnostic yield (1), since 15 years the perbronchial needle puncture is performed routinely near the carina of the main bifurcation in all patients suspicious of neoplasm. Up to now the procedure has been applied in 9.000 patients, during the last years comprising constantly about 60% of all diagnostic bronchoscopies.

2. TECHNIQUE

The aspiration needle used has a diameter of 0.9 mm at the free end of 9 mm. Above is a thicker coating preventing a too deep penetration and providing stability and easy guidance of the needle 55 cm in lenght. The perbronchial puncture is performed under visual control in local or general anaesthesia. After traversing the bronchial wall the mandrin is removed and suction is applied with a 20-cc syringe. The obtained material is investigated cytologically (3).

As complications only minor bleedings are seen at the point of puncture. In some cases pericardial effusion can be aspirated at the main bifurcation. A pneumothorax or mediastinal emphysema is an extremely rare event. Tumor cell implantation is theoretically possible but we have no own observations. The risk is certainly smaller than in mediastinoscopy.

3. RESULTS

As representative we evaluated 785 needle aspiration biopsies performed 1978 routinely in 655 patients. The table shows the results in the diseases with possible lymph node involvement. 25% of the aspirations were diagnostically positive and 25% revealed lymphatic tissue. 50% gave only inadequate tissue. The best yield

J.A. Nakhosteen and W. Maassen (eds.), Bronchology: Research, Diagnostic and Therapeutic Aspects. All rights reserved.
Copyright 1981. Martinus Nijhoff Publishers bv, The Hague / Boston / London

was found in sarcoidosis, in mediastinal lymph node tuberculosis and in malignant lymphomas. In 238 patients with diseases without possible lymph node involvement inadequate tissue was seen in 64%. This demonstrates the higher probability of getting adequate lymphatic material by aspiration in diseases with lymph node enlargement.

3.1 Bronchogenic carcinoma

The 318 cases comprised 41% epidermoid, 25% adenoid, 19% small cell, 11% aplastic solid and 4% other carcinomas. The needle biopsy gave positive results in 23% of the cases allowing lymph node staging, and was diagnostic as sole method in 12%. The highest yield was obtained in small cell carcinoma (52 resp. 21%), followed by adenocarcinoma (18 resp. 14%), aplastic solid (32 resp. 9%) and epidermoid carcinoma (12 resp. 7%). These numbers reflect the regional spread of the different cell types. Positive results were found 16 times in paratracheal, 57 times in carinal and 11 times in hilar nodes.

Of the 13 patients with superior vena cava syndrome the diagnosis was established exclusively by needle biopsy in 31%. 5 of the 7 cases diagnosed by aspiration had a small cell carcinoma.

Needle aspiration was positive in 31% of the central and 19% of the peripheral bronchogenic carcinomas.

Cases with roentgenographic and/or bronchoscopic suspicion of lymph node involvement were confirmed by needle aspiration in 55%, whereas the biopsy gave positive results in 12% of inconspicuous cases.

In cases where needle biopsy was negative, an involvement of lymph nodes was found later in 6 of 18 mediastinoscopies and 29 of 93 thoracotomies suggesting false negative results in about 30%. No case with a false positive result was registered.

3.2 Metastatic neoplasms

The results in the 43 patients with metastases of extrathoracic primary neoplasms were almost identical. Here, the yield of needle biopsy was especially high in breast carcinoma (50%), which metastasizes very often into the lymph nodes.

3.2 Sarcoidosis

The group of 45 patients was enlarged by 75 patients from a controlled therapy-trial of the years before. All 120 patients underwent bronchoscopy with a positive diagnostic yield in 66%. 20% were diagnosed exclusively by perbronchial needle aspiration. The total yield was 37.5%, being highest in stage I with 63% and declining in stage II (35%) and stage III (10%). The diagnosis of the 19 patients in stage I was confirmed exclusively by needle biopsy in nearly the half (47%) performing routinely the perbronchial aspiration of the carinal and both hilar areas.

Results of perbronchial fine needle aspirations

Disease groups	No. of pts.	No. of aspirations	diagnostic results (%)	lymphatic tissue (%)
Bronchogenic Carcinoma	318	369	24	24
Metastatic Neoplasm	43	52	23	25
Sarcoidosis	45	77	31	30
Malignant Lymphoma	6	13	23	31
Tuberculosis	5	8	37. 5	25
Total in diseases with possible lymph node involvement	417	519	25	25

4. SUMMARY

  – The overall diagnostic yield of perbronchial fine needle aspiration performed as a routine method was **25%** in diseases with possible mediastinal lymph node involvement.

  – In **23%** of the patients with bronchogenic carcinoma a positive diagnosis was made allowing lymph node staging.

  – In **12%** the needle biopsy was diagnostic as the sole method.

  – The highest yield was obtained in small cell carcinoma (52%).

  – The results in metastatic neoplasms were quite similar, here the highest yield was found in breast carcinoma (50%).

  – Of 120 patients with sarcoidosis positive results were obtained in 37. 5% (stage I 63%, stage II 35%, stage III 10%).

  – Other valuable indications are seen in malignant lymphoma and mediastinal tuberculosis with diagnostically helpful results in 23 % resp. 37,5 %.

5. CONCLUSIONS

  Perbronchial fine needle aspiration is indicated routinely during rigid bronchoscopy

– at the main bifurcation in suspected pulmonary or metastatic neoplasms,

– at the main and both hilar bifurcations in suspected sarcoidosis,

– in all cases with roentgenographic or bronchoscopic suspicion of paratracheal or parabronchial masses.

IX.2.

POSSIBILITIES AND LIMITATIONS IN THE CYTOLOGICAL INTERPRETATION OF PERBRONCHIAL FINE NEEDLE BIOPSIES

H. PREUSSLER   (Chest Hospital Heckeshorn, Berlin – W , Germany)

1. INTRODUCTION

The purpose of aspiration biopsy is to obtain cell material for the cytological examination which does not reach the outer or inner surface of the body by desquamation. This method became especially important with the thin biopsy needle introduced by FRANZÉN (5). The puncture through the walls of the airways covers with the paratracheal and parabronchial region an area which is to a very high degree either directly or indirectly through the lymph nodes involved in the diseases of the chest.

Neccessary bases for the cytopathological interpretations are :

1) Exact knowledge of the anatomy and pathology of the biopsy region.

2) Exact description of the biopsy location.

3) Information about previous clinico-roentgenographic findings for expert discussion.

2. TECHNICAL WORK - UP

The value of the examination depends essentially on the biopsy technique and the direct preparations of the material. The aspirate should be squirted, if possible, on 4 – 6 glasses and immediately be spread in a thin layer with the aid of a thick coverslip. We recommend air-drying of the smears because different stainings, cytochemical and enzyme-cytochemical reactions can be performed subsequently. As standard we use the May-Gruenwald-Giemsa stain which in thin smears is superior to the Papanicolaou stain because the orthic cell material originates from lymph nodes allowing a better cell differentiation (1). For electron microscopic or scanning electron microscopic examinations a cytocentrifugate can be obtained after dispersion in physiological saline and after fixation in glutaric aldehyde.

J.A. Nakhosteen and W. Maassen (eds.), Bronchology: Research, Diagnostic and Therapeutic Aspects. All rights reserved.
Copyright 1981. Martinus Nijhoff Publishers bv, The Hague / Boston / London

3. MICROSCOPIC INTERPRETATION

The method of perbronchial biopsy is suitable for search but not for exclusion. Therefore any aspirated material is representative if it is well prepared. In this case it can be interpreted microscopically without objections.

A cytopathological interpretation consists of :

1) A comprehensive description with information about technical faults and about all elements on the glass.

2) A subsequent expert assessment including the clinical informations. Sometimes a final opinion can be given only after common consultation with the clinicians.

The cytological evidence has to be integrated critically as one mosaic piece into the clinical and roentgenological findings.

Examples for the difficulties of interpretation of aspirated cell material are:

1) A small reticular lipoid cell complex or single lipoid crystals may be either part of a lipoma or particles of the normal mediastinal fat tissue.

2) Complexes of ciliated epithelium may originate from the traversed trachea, but occasionally from a paratracheal cystic teratoma.

With these precautions for the cytopathological interpretation the dignity of the perbronchial fine needle biopsy is very high (4).

4. RESULTS

According to the frequency our own aspiration material can be divided roughly into three groups of diagnosis (6) :

1) Tumours, mostly metastasized tumours.

2) Epitheloid cell granulomatoses.

3) Primary lymphomas.

The differential diagnosis between these groups poses no problems if one proceeds in this way of diagnostic separation.

ad 1): Benign tumours, as already mentioned, can often be assessed not primarily by cytology but only epicritically. One has to consider dystopic organs too, for example a possible thyroid gland in the mediastinum. Malignant tumours occur mostly in metastasized form in the biopsy region. In the recognizable tumours we determine the type cytologically. We use the WHO-classification mostly without further subgrouping. In given cases we try to make a differential diagnosis pointing to the possible organ of the primary tumour which may be achieved by additional stainings and chemical reactions, for example by reactions of the acid or alkaline phosphatase in the differentiation of the prostatic carcinoma and the seminoma. Other possibilities are differentiation of cellular pigments by bleaching with hydrogen superoxide, by hemosiderin test or by Sudan test. Mucopolysaccharides can be demonstrated in cell vacuoles by the Alcian-PAS-reaction.

Often typical morphic changes can be seen like the formation of atypical epithelia in follicles with a central colloidal plug in thyroid carcinoma.

ad 2): In our own biopsy material (6) we find amongst the epitheloid cell granulomatoses the sarcoidosis and the tuberculosis which cannot be distinguished cytologically with certainty. It is not possible to determine the numerous morphic variants of the epitheloid cell reactions and to give a definite diagnosis by cytology, nor can it be the purpose of practical cytology to find the agens of the granulomas. All attempts to discover disease-specific characteristics failed until now with all known possibilities of examination. The cytodiagnostic differentiation between sarcoidosis and tuberculosis by sappy or lean forms of epitheloid cells (2) appears to us as a too uncertain feature, too.

The cytopathological interpretation can only state : Complexes of epitheloid cells or parts of an epitheloid cell granulation tissue.

ad 3): Primary lymphomas are easy to recognize but a distinction between Hodgkin's lymphoma and non-Hodgkin's lymphoma cannot be made. The exstirpation of a lymph node is neccessary for further histological evaluation. The cytological method cannot give a subgrouping of Hodgkin's lymphoma because no exact statement is possible about the degree of sclerosis or about the portion of lymphocytes, both being important for the treatment of the disease. In non-Hodgkin's lymphomas cytoenzymatic reactions in air-dried smears are a valuable addition to the histological examination.

5. ERROR POSSIBILITIES AND QUALITY CONTROL

If one pays attention to these shown groups of diagnosis this is often already sufficient and decisive for the treatment. False positive findings occur rarely, at most in the 0/00 - range. False negative cytological results are practically negligible because the obtained small amount of material can be surveyed easily so that only technical faults may be responsible.

Tentative diagnoses in tumours are the results of metaplastic epidermoid changes which can be seen at the carina of the bronchial bifurcations. Here, difficulties can exist in the distinction between well differentiated carcinomas. In addition, predominantly necrotic cell changes often allow only the suspicion of a tumour.

Sometimes the classification of tumours may be quite difficult, especially the distinction between adenocarcinoma and large cell aplastic carcinoma, and between the spindle cell (squamous) and the large cell aplastic carcinoma (3).

Quality control of the cytopathology of perbronchial biopsies is already given by the fact that the method is combined as a rule with other procedures including histopathologic examinations. In order to obtain an appropriate quality, retrospective controls should be performed routinely.

6. SUMMARY

The perbronchial fine needle biopsy offers favourable material for the cytopathological interpretation contributing often to the diagnosis by comprehensive work-up and critical utilization. Because of the relative easiness of the aspiration, the fast and easy technical preparation and the good interpretation of the material there is at present no alternative to this procedure.

TRANSBRONCHIAL NEEDLE ASPIRATION BIOPSY VIA THE FIBEROPTIC BRONCHOSCOPE
IX.3.

H. Kato, K. Nishimiya, J. Lay, J. Ono, K. Yoneyama, N. Kawate, I. Iimura, T. Hayashi, H. Iwahashi, I. Kawamura, Y. Hayata

INTRODUCTION

The definitive diagnostic rate of lung cancer has improved remarkably due to recent methods such as fiberoptic bronchoscopic brushing and biopsy as well as percutaneous needle biopsy. In our department, about 1,400 primary lung cancer cases have been treated over the past 30 years. From 1972-79 the preoperative diagnostic rates of central type and peripheral type lung cancer were 97.5 and 95.5% respectively. However, in a small number of cases diagnosis is still not possible. Many of such cases are tumors originating beyond the normal bronchial wall, covered by normal epithelium and cases in which it is anatomically difficult to insert forceps or bruches to the tumor. We developed a new needle for aspiration biopsy via the fiberoptic bronchoscope, TBAB.

PROCEDURE

The needle consists of a flexible catheter 111 cm in length and covered with a stainless steel spiral coil, and with a retractable needle at its extremity. There are two varieties of tips, 8mm and 10mm in length and 0.6mm and 0.8mm in internal diameter. Once the target site has been brought under observation with the fiberoptic bronchoscope, the catheter, with the needle retracted to prevent damage, is inserted via the instrumentation channel. After the tip of the catheter is visible endoscopically the needle is projected and inserted through the lesion into the bronchial wall. Aspiration resembles other aspiration biopsy methods, and the aspirated material is expelled on a glass slide immediately and fixed with isopropyl alcohol, after which it is sent to the cytology laboratory.

RESULTS

This method was employed in 17 cases in which lung cancer was suspected and in 8 cases of possible lymph node involvement. In the former group a definitive diagnosis was obtained in 14 cases (82.4%), 10 of which were primary lung cancers (5 adenoca., 2 small cell ca., 1 large cell ca., 1 mucoepidermoid ca. and 1 carcinoid). In the latter group a diagnosis of lymph node involvement was established in 3 cases. All cases suspected of lung cancer showed normal mucosa except 1 case of mucoepidermoid tumor. In 6 out of the 10 cases of lung cancer diagnosed, the diagnosis could not be obtained by any other method and the other 4 cases were also diagnosed by punch biopsy but not by brushing cytology. In 2 benign tumors (hamartoma), fibrotic cells alone were aspirated under TV control, and these cases were diagnosed as benign tumors. After tumor resection, a histologic diagnosis of hamartoma was obtained in both cases. In the 2 inflammatory disease cases, caseous material was aspirated in a tuberculosis case, and pus was aspirated in a case of lung abscess. In 1 out of 3 cases in which TBAB did not yield a diagnosis, a diagnosis of tuberculosis was made, but the other 2 cases are still being followed up without a definitive diagnosis. According to the lymphnode examinations, 3 were positive.

DISCUSSION

This method was highly effective for tumors beyond the bronchial wall and covered by normal epithelium. We have experienced no complications whatsoever up to now. Bleeding due to puncture of the pulmonary artery, especially in cases with arteriosclerosis, arteritis or a tendency to bleed, must be considered and bleeding time should be measured before the procedure. Pichlmaier et al[1] and Törzsök[2] reported on transbronchial biopsy with the rigid bronchoscope and got good results but there were problems due to discomfort caused by the rigid instrument. Our new needle is flexible and can be used with the fiberoptic bronchoscope. No patient complained of discomfort. When performed with care this method results in: 1. Good diagnostic results in tumors beyond the bronchial wall, 2. Effective examination for bronchial tumors covered with normal bronchial epithelium, 3. Estimation of lymph node involvement.

REFERENCES
1. Pichlmaier H, Erpenbeck R, Finsterer H: Der Lungen Diagnostik durch transtracheal transbronchiale Lungenpunktion und gezielte segmentale Absaugang. Thoraxchirurgie, 18: 410, 1970.
2. Törzsök L: Die transbronchiale Punktion. Praxia Pneumo., 29: 162, 1975.

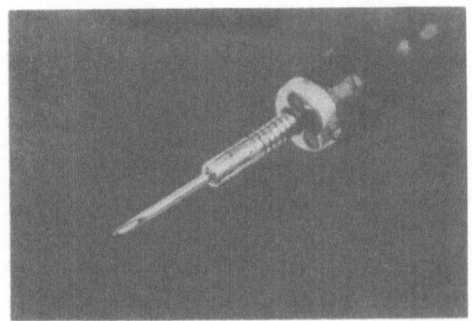

Fig. 1   Tip of needle inserted
through Olympus B3

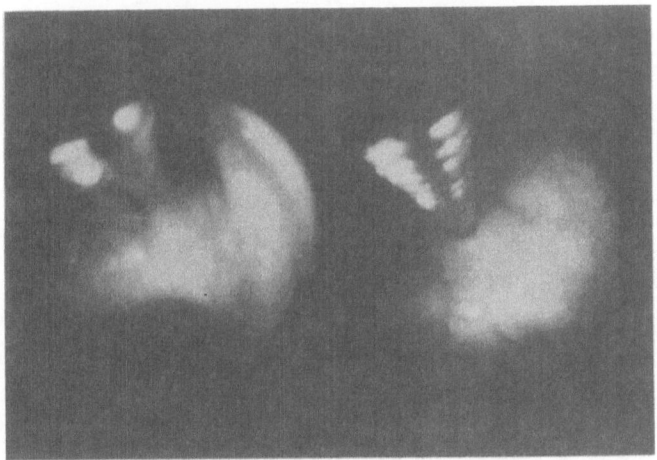

Fig. 2   Transbronchial aspiration biopsy: fiberoptic bronchoscopic findings

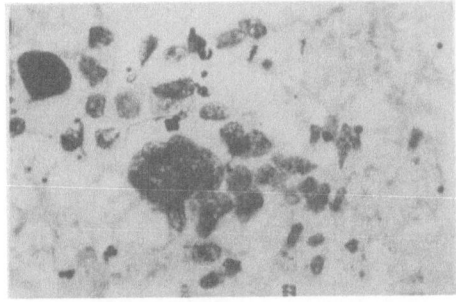

Fig. 3   Large cell carcinoma cells
obtained by TBAB

CONTRIBUTION   OF DIAGNOSTIC NEEDLE ASPIRATION IN BRONCHOSCOPIC
INVESTIGATION

C. Šimeček

IX.4.

1. INTRODUCTION

Diagnostic puncturē aspirations used in the course of bronchoscopic investigations are very important complementary procedures. The material obtained serves for passive tranfer of tub-
erkuline hypersensitivity and for bacteriogical proof in the
diagnosis of tuberculosis, but above all for cytological investigation in differential diagnosis of lymph nodes enlargement
and in the staging of lung carcinomas.

Previous anatomical studies on the right topography and the
average diameter of considered normal intrathoracic lymph nodes
are an important presumption for the results obtained in our
study.

2. METHOD

The puncture aspiration is done in the course of bronchoscopy, mostly for examinations of the lymph nodes in the hilus and
in the tracheal bifurcation. Right tracheobronchial lymph nodes
and thouse under the middle lobe bronchus are investigated only
if they are enlarged by radiological examination.

The material obtained is examined cytologicaly by different
methods, in urgent cases also in the course of bronchoscopy by
phase contrast microscopy with the possibility to repeat immediately, in the case of failure, the needle aspiration. In tuberculosis, sarcoidosis and lymphogranulomatosis mostly multiple
lymph nodes are investigated.

3. RESULTS

In this study we are analyzing the results of 4075 intrathoracic lymph nodes puncture aspirations. In 1366 observations
the reason for this procedure was the staging of the lung carcinoma, where metastasing was discovered in 58,7%. Needle aspirations from hilar lymph nodes in small cell carcinoma of the
left lower lobe were the most profitable by detecting 83% metastases. The least profitable, 15% proved metastases, were lymph
node punctures of the tracheal bifurcation in the epidermoid

*J.A. Nakhosteen and W. Maassen (eds.), Bronchology: Research, Diagnostic and
Therapeutic Aspects. All rights reserved.*
Copyright 1981. Martinus Nijhoff Publishers bv, The Hague / Boston / London

carcinomas of the left upper lobe.

Our results in lymph node sarcomas were published in the past years (Ref.2).

The recent results in sarcoidosis are almost the same as published before (Ref.1).

In 27,2% of intrathoracic lymph nodes puncture aspirations we did not succeed. In 2 patients a small pneumothorax was discovered on subsequent x-ray examination with spontaneous resorption. In cases of venectasis and hyperaemia of the mucosa small bleeding may be present, but this was only in 14 patients the reason for stopping the investigation without need of any other treatment.

4. DISCUSSION

In comparison with mediastinoscopy cytological lymph node examinations by puncture aspiration in sarcoidosis are, with 92% positive results, nearly identical. In the staging of the lung carcinoma our results with proved metastases in 58,7 exceed those of mediastinoscopy. The reason for these differences is the fact that the most profitable in this study are punctures of the hilar lymph nodes, which are not attainable by mediastinoscopy.

In cases of silicosis mediastinoscopy is more profitable, but this fact is not so important because of other methods mostly used in the diagnosis of silicosis.

All these facts support our opinion that cytological examinations of intrathoracic lymph nodes by means of puncture aspiration are a very important procedure, above all, in the differentiall diagnosis of lymph nodes enlargement and in the staging of lung carcinomas.

REFERENCES
1. Šimeček,C.: L`importance des méthodes bronchologiques dans le diagnostic des maladies du médiastin, Les Bronches 1967, 17, 257.
2. Šimeček,C.: Nemoci mediastina a nitrohrudních uzlin, Avicenum Praha 1981.

IX.5.

TRANSTRACHEALE UND TRANSBRONCHALE ASPIRATIONSPUNKTION IN DER
DIAGNOSTIK DER INTRATHORAKALEN ERKRANKUNGEN

M. Mrakovčić, M. Roglić, D. Grozdek, I. Pongrac

Durch die Einführung der transtrachealen (TTP) bzw. transbronchalen Aspirationspunktion (TBP) in der Bronchoskopie, wurden
Lymphkonten neben dem Trachealbaum der zytologischen Analyse zu-
gänglich. Auf diese Weise wurden grosse Möglichkeiten für die Diagnostik der Mediastinal – und Lungenerkrankungen geboten, egal ob
es sich dabei um eine Systemerkrankung, Metastasen der malignen
Tumoren, Tuberkulose, Sarcoidose oder anderen Krankheiten handelt.

Besonders wichtig ist die Transtrachealpunktion in der Bestimmung der Operationsmöglichkeit beim Bronchuskarzinom.

Methode und Material

Eine Transtrachealpunktion der Karina machen wir bei jedem
Verdacht auf Malignom und Veränderungen der mediastinalen Lymphknoten.

Eine transbronchale Punktion und transtracheale Punktion der
Trachealwand führen wir dort durch, wo die radiologischen Befunde
auf eine Vergrösserung der anliegenden Lymphknoten hinweisen, oder
wo der bronchoskopische Befund (extramurale Kompression) eine solche
Punktion erfordert.

Um geeignetes Material für die zytologische Untersuchung zu bekommen, punktieren wir mehrmals auf derselben Stelle. Mehrere Punktionen auf einer Stelle während der Bronchoskopie stellen wir in
den Tabellen als eine Punktion dar.

Wir bronchoskopieren mit rigidem Bronchoskop um die transmurale
Aspirationspunktion ausführen zu können.

Die transmuralen Punktionen machen wir mit sehr dünnen Kanüllen
(Kanülle Nr.18, Diameter o,45, Länge 26 mm).

Unsere erste Transtrachealpunktion führten wir im Jahre 1959.
durch, und bis zum Ende des Jahres 1979. hatten wir über 6ooo
Punktionen.

In diesem Vortrag bringen wir unser Material aus der Klinik für Lungenkrankheiten "Jordanovac" Zagreb – Yugoslawien vom Jahre 1976. bis 1979.

Auf der Tabelle 1. sehen wir:

Patienten	2928	
Bronchoskopien	4o38	
Transmuralpunktionen	343o	
für die zytologische Analyse		
geeignetes Material	22o4	66,26%
Malignomdiagnosen aus den transmuralen		
Punktionen	593	27%

Tabelle 2. zeigt 343o transmurale Punktionen mach Lokalisation:

Karina der Trachea	2928
Trachealwand	88
Bronchialwand	414

Auf der Tabelle 3. sehen wir die Resultate von 22o4, für die zytologische Analyse geeigneter Materiale

Malignome	593
Granulomatöse Reaktion	254
Hyperplasie des Lymphknotens	452
Elemente des Lymphknotens	81o
Elemente des Pleuraergusses	3o
Verschiedenes:	

Mesotelzellen
Extramedulläre
Haematopoesis   65
Struma

Tabelle 4. zeigt 593 Malignomdiagnosen aus transmuralem Punktionsmaterial

	nur in TTP und/oder TBP	in transmuralen Punktionen und anderen bronchoskopischen Materialen
Carcinoma	98	181
Carcinoma epidermoides	14	59
Carcinoma anaplasticum	53	126

Adenocarcinoma	lo	31
Neoplasma malignum	3	4
Hypernephroma metastaticum	3	-
Lymphoma malignum	4	-
M.Hodgkin	2	5
	187	406

Damit haben wir bestätigt, dass 187 Befunde aus dem transmuralen Punktat der einzige Beweis für die Diagnose waren.

Diskussion

Wenn es sich um einen Bronchialkarzinom handelt beweist der Befund bösartiger Zellen im Aspirat der transbronchalen Punktion die Propagation in die hilären Lymphknoten, der Befund aus dem Aspirat der transtrachealen Punktion aber die Ergreifung der anderen Seite, und schliesst damit die Möglichkeit eines radikalen chirurgischen Engriffes aus.

Der besondere Wert der transbronchialen Punktion liegt in der Diagnostik isolierter hilären Adenopathien. Dadurch sind alle Systemerkrankungen welche sich intrathorakal befinden eine ideale Indikation für die Transbronchialpunktion weil damit ein überflüssiger chirurgischer Eingriff vermieden wird.

Der Befund einer granulomatösen Reaktion im transmuralen Punktat ist ein wichtiter Beitrag zur Diagnose der Sarcoidose und tracheobronchialen Lymphknotentuberkulose.

Zusammenfassung

Die Bronchoskopie ist heute eine Methode die uns ermöglicht wertvolles Material für die zyto-hystologische Diagnose zu bekommen, und deshalb soll man sie soviel wie möglich ausnützen. In unserer Routine-Arbeit machen wir häufig transtracheale und transbronchale Punktionen weil uns diese Methode bischer sehr gute Resultate in der Diagnostik und Bewertung des Verlaufes intrathorakaler Erkrankungen ermöglicht hat.

IX.6.

"Morphologie der Atemwegsobstruktion: Die Bedeutung der perbronchialen Biopsie"

H.Blaha, H.Thieme, U.Cronemeyer, D.Müller-Wening

Auf vielfachen Wegen versuchen wir, dem Problem "Morphologie
der Obstruktion", das im Augenblick so brennend ist, nachzugehen.
Einmal, indem wir 26 Sektionen mit entsprechenden Diagnosen aus
der Klinik verfolgen; dann haben wir 40 Resektionen, bei denen
eine Obstruktion nachweisbar war, nachuntersucht. Schließlich
haben wir die Qualität der perbronchialen Biopsie grundsätzlich
verfolgt und,anhand dieser Kenntnisse, die perbronchialen Biopsien
bei bestehender Obstruktion analysiert (Abb. 1). Insgesamt handelt
es sich um ein heuristisches System, fortschreitend vom großen
Material zu sehr kleinen bioptischen Proben.

Aus 1026 Sektionen wurden 26 Fälle ausgewählt mit den Haupt-
oder Nebendiagnosen asthmoide Bronchitis, Asthma und ähnliches
(Abb. 2). Diese Sektionen wurden aufgeteilt in zwei Gruppen. In
der ersten Gruppe fanden sich bei der Sektion Veränderungen, die
auf eine schwere obstruktive Lungenkrankheit zu beziehen waren:
9 Fälle; in der zweiten Gruppe fanden sich andere pathologisch-
anatomische Befunde im Vordergrund: 17 Fälle. Die klinischen
Diagnosen lauteten auch hier wie oben (Abb. 3). In Abb. 4 sind
die neun Sektionen bei den "Asthmafällen", Gruppe 1, aufgeführt.
Ein einziges Merkmal ist konstant: die Eosinophilie. 1 Kranker
ist an dem gestorben, was die ältere Literatur "Schleimschlag"
nennt, nämlich die sehr plötzliche Verstopfung des gesamten Bronchialsystems mit Todesfolge. Aus dieser Gruppe ist auch erwähnens-
wert, daß Begleitleiden und zusätzliche Befunde für den Tod mit
verantwortlich waren (Abb. 5). Bei den 16 Sektionen der Gruppe 2,
klinisch obstruktive Bronchitis bei pathologisch-anatomisch überwiegend anderen Veränderungen, fanden sich zahlreiche Zustände,
angefangen von der Tuberkulose bis zur Thrombose und Embolie. Die
Verwechslung mit der Embolie, auch die Ähnlichkeit des klinischen
Bildes, ist eindrucksvoll. Eindrucksvoll sind auch die über lange
Jahre einem Asthma bronchiale gleichenden Symptome einer Lungen-
fibrose (Abb. 6). - In Summa ist das klinische Bild "asthmaähnliche

*J.A. Nakhosteen and W. Maassen (eds.), Bronchology: Research, Diagnostic and
Therapeutic Aspects. All rights reserved.
Copyright 1981. Martinus Nijhoff Publishers bv, The Hague / Boston / London*

Zustände" mit vielen krankhaften Zuständen bei der Sektion korreliert (Abb. 7).

Wir kommen zum zweiten Teil, den "Resektionen bei nachgewie-
sener Obstruktion". Es wurden einige Hundert Sektionsfälle durch-
gesehen und diejenigen Kranken ausgewählt, bei denen die Resistance über 0,3 kPa/l/sec. lag. Insgesamt handelte es sich um
40 Thorakotomien. Zur Beurteilung wurden Areale herangezogen, die
vom Hauptbefund ferngelegen waren und die vermutungsweise mit
dem Hauptbefund nicht in Zusammenhang standen. Wie bei den Sektionen handelt es sich auch bei Thorakotomien nicht um sichere
Aussagen, sondern um einen heuristischen Ansatz (Abb. 8). Die
Operationen sind in Abb. 9 aufgelistet. Die histologischen Haupt-
befunde zeigt Abb. 10. Interessant ist nun, daß an den Bronchien
nur in der Hälfte der Fälle "obstruktionskorrelierte Befunde" ver-
zeichnet sind (Abb. 11). Diese obstruktionskorrelierten Befunde
sind mit Veränderungen der Bronchialwand, Ektasien, Becherzellvermehrung, Muskelhypertrophie und Fibrosen umschrieben. Es handelt sich um häufige, schwer quantifizierbare Befunde. Dabei waren diese Befunde überhaupt nur in der Hälfte der Fälle zu er-
heben (Abb. 12). Ein wenig besser sind die Verhältnisse in bezug
auf das Lungengewebe selbst: hier waren nur in einem Viertel der
Fälle "normale" Verhältnisse anzutreffen (Abb. 13). In Abb. 14
finden wir die histologischen Ergebnisse, hauptbefundfern bzw.
hauptbefundunabhängig, wiedergegeben. Fibrosen, interstitielle
Entzündung, zellige Infiltrationen und Emphysem stehen im Vordergrund. - Es zeigt sich auch hier, daß bei bestehender Obstruktion
die Veränderungen an den Bronchien vielfältig, schwer zu deuten
und nicht mit Regelmäßigkeit vorhanden sind; ähnliches läßt sich
über das Lungengewebe aussagen. Die dem Schulwissen, dem allgemeinen Konsens entsprechenden Veränderungen kommen zwar vor, sie
müssen aber eher als selten gelten.

Im dritten Teil kommen wir zu der Frage, ob die perbronchiale
Biopsie in der Lage ist, Auskunft über etwa relevante Verändeerun-
gen zu geben. Herr CRONEMEYER hat dazu sehr genau 50 hinterein-
ander folgende Biopsien herausgegriffen. Lungengewebe fand sich
in 80%, Bronchialelemente mit Lungengewebe in 52%, Gefäße in
16%, isolierte Bronchialelemente in 18% (Abb. 15). Es läßt sich
also über wesentliche Strukturen durchaus etwas sagen. Wir haben
weiterhin die Biopsien ausplanimetriert. Der Pathologe unserer
Anstalt, Herr SCHNELLER, geht dabei so vor, daß die einzelnen

Exzisate zusammen verarbeitet werden, die Fläche der Proben addiert
sich somit. Es handelt sich überwiegend um sehr kleine "Flächen".
Ein Vergleich mit den Normalstrukturen der Lunge zeigt jedoch,
daß Aussagen durchaus möglich sind (Abb. 16).

Dem entspricht auch das, was in der letzten Abbildung ver-
deutlicht wird. Wir haben 98 perbronchiale Lungenbiopsien, bei
denen eine Resistance präoperativ von $>$ 0,35 kPa/l/sec. gemessen
wurde, verfolgt und dabei zahlreiche Veränderungen gefunden, darunter 27 Fibrosen, 20 "Sarkoidosen", 23 alveoläre Prozesse und
zahlreiche zellige Infiltrationen und Pigmentablagerungen (Abb.17).
Es ergibt sich aus diesem Ansatz, daß die Vermutung erlaubt ist,
daß es ein mehr oder minder singuläres Substrat der Obstruktion
nicht gibt. Der Weg zur Morphologie der Obstruktion heißt, daß
wir vermutungsweise auf weite Strecken von vorne anfangen müssen
und wohl auch Lunge, kleine Luftwege und große Luftwege in gleicher Weise in unsere Studie mit einbeziehen müssen.

Zusammenfassung: 26 Sektionen mit Obstruktion; 40 Resektionen mit Obstruktion und 98 perbronchiale Biopsien mit Obstruktion
werden vorgelegt. Es zeigt sich, daß der Begriff "Obstruktion"
mit vielfachen pathologisch-anatomischen Zuständen korreliert.
Es gibt kein einheitliches Substrat. Die herrschende Lehrmeinung
ist zu überprüfen.

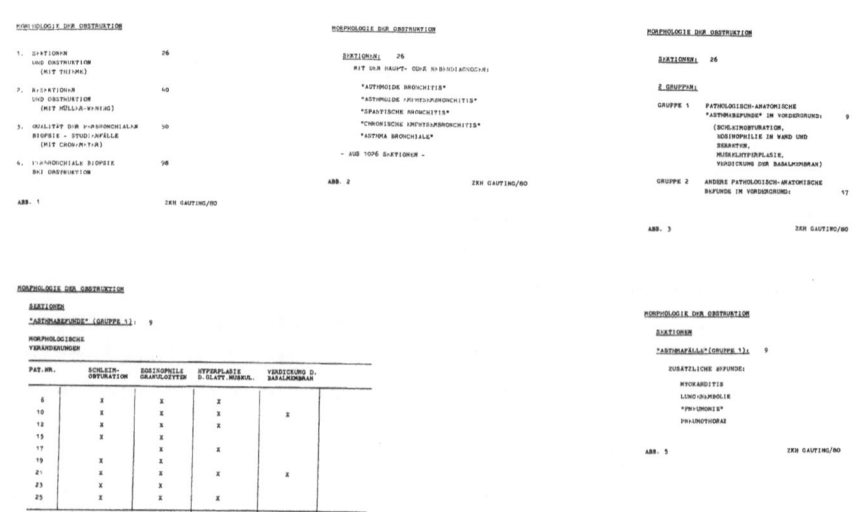

MORPHOLOGIE DER OBSTRUKTION

SEKTIONEN: %

DAVON 16 SEKTIONEN ("GRUPPE 2"):

KLINISCHE DIAGNOSE (ASTHMOIDE BRONCHITIS),
PATHOLOGISCH-ANATOMISCH ...

TUBERKULOSE   10
"FIBROSE"   3
(KLINISCHE DIAGNOSE:
CHRON. ASTHMOIDE BRONCHITIS
STATUS ASTHMATICUS
ASTHMA BRONCHIALE)
...ASTHMA...   8
KARZINOM   2
TUBERKULOMAEHNLICH   7

ABB. 6   ZKH GAUTING/80

MORPHOLOGIE DER OBSTRUKTION

SEKTIONEN

SUMME:

DAS KLINISCHE BILD "ASTHMAAEHNLICHE ZUSTAENDE"
HAT VIELE, OFT MEHRFACHE SUBSTRATE,
(Z.B.: EMBOLIE, FIBROSE, REDUKTION DER ATEM-
FLAECHE UND DES GEFAESSBETTES).

ABB. 7   ZKH GAUTING/80

MORPHOLOGIE DER OBSTRUKTION

OBSTRUKTION UND RESEKTION

40 THORAKOTOMIEN

RESISTANCE ≥ 0,3 kPa/l/sec.

HAUPTBEFUNDFAMILIE GEWÄHLT
("HEURISTISCHER ANSATZ")

ABB. 8   ZKH GAUTING/80

MORPHOLOGIE DER OBSTRUKTION

OBSTRUKTION UND RESEKTION

ART DER DURCHGEFÜHRTEN OPERATIONEN:

LOBEKTOMIE   24
PNEUMEKTOMIE   6
OFFENE LUNGENBIOPSIE   3
SEGMENTRESEKTION   2
ATYPISCHE RESEKTIONEN   2
BULGEKTOMIE   1
...EXSTIRPATION   1
...   1

N = 40

ABB. 9   ZKH GAUTING/80

MORPHOLOGIE DER OBSTRUKTION

OBSTRUKTION UND RESEKTION

HISTOLOGISCHER HAUPTBEFUND:

PLATTENEPITHELKARZINOM   11
ADENOKARZINOM   7
TUBERKULOSE   4
PNEUMOKONIOSE   3
KLEINZELLIGES KARZINOM   2
GROSSZELLULÄRES KARZINOM   2
INTERSTITIELLE FIBROSE   2
CHONDROM   2
SARKOIDOSE   1
BRONCHIEKTASEN   1
STENOSIERENDE BRONCHITIS   1
SCHIMMELPILZMYZETOM   1
POLYPÖSES BRONCHIALSCHLEIMHAUTPOLYP   1
EMPHYSEMBLASEN   1
HAMARTOM   1
SIEGELRINGMETASTASEN   1
METASTASEN EINES FOLLIKULÄREN SCHILDDRÜSEN-KARZINOMS   1
BRONCHIALADENOM   1

(Z.T. MEHRFACHZÄHLUNG)

ABB. 10   ZKH GAUTING/80

MORPHOLOGIE DER OBSTRUKTION

OBSTRUKTION UND RESEKTION

HISTOLOGISCHES ERGEBNIS: BRONCHIEN
40 PATIENTEN

NORMALER HISTOLOGISCHER BEFUND   9 PATIENTEN
PATHOLOGISCHER HISTOLOGISCHER BEFUND   20 PATIENTEN

ABB. 11   ZKH GAUTING/80

MORPHOLOGIE DER OBSTRUKTION

OBSTRUKTION UND RESEKTION

HISTOLOGISCHES ERGEBNIS: BRONCHIEN

20 PATIENTEN MIT PATHOLOGISCHEM HISTOLOGISCHEM BEFUND:

ZYSTISCHE BRONCHIEKTASEN,
EKTATISCHE BRONCHIEN,
DEFORMIERENDE BRONCHITIS,
SCHLEIMRETENTION   10
RUNDZELLSEWIKTRATE (STRATUM PROPRIUM, ADVENTITIA)   6
KRÄFTIGE BZW. HYPERPLASTISCHE BRONCHIAL-MUSKULATUR   5
BECHERZELLVERMEHRUNG   3
EOSINOPHILE GRANULOZYTEN (LAMINA PROPRIA, SCHLEIM)   2
WANDSCHICHTEN DER BRONCHIEN VERBREITERT   2
BASALMEMBRAN VERDICKT   2
PERIBRONCHIALE NARBENFELDER, FIBROSE DER BRONCHIENWAND   2
DRÜSENAUSFÜHRUNGSGÄNGE VERBREITERT   1

ABB. 12   ZKH GAUTING/80

MORPHOLOGIE DER OBSTRUKTION

OBSTRUKTION UND RESEKTION

HISTOLOGISCHES ERGEBNIS: LUNGE
40 PATIENTEN

NORMALER HISTOLOGISCHER BEFUND   9 PATIENTEN
PATHOLOGISCHER HISTOLOGISCHER BEFUND   31 PATIENTEN
(OBSTRUKTIONSBEZOGEN)

ABB. 13   ZKH GAUTING/80

MORPHOLOGIE DER OBSTRUKTION

OBSTRUKTION UND RESEKTION

HISTOLOGISCHES ERGEBNIS: LUNGE
(HAUPTBEFUND-FERNE BZW. HAUPTBEFUND-UNABHÄNGIGE BEFUNDE - OBSTRUKTIONSBEZOGEN -)

31 PATIENTEN MIT PATHOLOGISCHEM BEFUND:

KLEINBLASIGES, VESIKULÄRES, ZENTRI-LOBÄRES EMPHYSEM   17
RUNDZELLINFILTRATE   7
FIBRÖS VERBREITETE GERÜSTSTRUKTUREN   7
VERBREITERTE ALVEOLARSEPTEN   7
FIBROSE DER STÜTZGEWEBE   1
CHRONISCH INTERSTITIELLE ENTZÜNDUNG   1
MUSKULÄRE ZIRRHOSE   1

ABB. 14   ZKH GAUTING/80

MORPHOLOGIE DER OBSTRUKTION

BIOPSIEQUALITÄT

QUALITATIVE BEWERTUNG PERBRONCHIALER LUNGENBIOPSIEN:

N = 50

LUNGENGEWEBE (ALVEOLARHALTIG)   80%
BRONCHIALELEMENTE
A) OHNE LUNGENGEWEBE   16%
B) MIT LUNGENGEWEBE   52%
GEFÄSSE   16%

ABB. 15   ZKH GAUTING/80

MORPHOLOGIE DER OBSTRUKTION

BIOPSIEQUALITÄT

QUANTITATIVE AUSWERTUNG PERBRONCHIALER LUNGENBIOPSIEN:

N = 50

DURCHSCHNITTLICHE GEWEBEFLÄCHE   4,70 mm²
KLEINSTES PRÄPARAT   0,18 mm²
GRÖSSTES PRÄPARAT   15,40 mm²

VERGLEICHSGRÖSSEN (NACH HAYEK):
DURCHSCHNITTLICHER ALVEOLAR-DURCHMESSER   200 - 250 µ
ALVEOLARKAPILLARE   10 - 12 µ
DURCHSCHNITTLICHE WEITE EINES BRONCHIOLUS RESPIRATORIUS   0,4 mm

ABB. 16   ZKH GAUTING/80

MORPHOLOGIE DER OBSTRUKTION

ERGEBNISSE PERBRONCHIALER BIOPSIEN

AUSWAHL JAHR 1978

1700 BRONCHIOSKOPIEN, DAVON AUSGEWÄHLT:

98 GESICHERTE OBSTRUKTIVE ATEMWEGSERKRANKUNGEN
(RESISTANCE 0,35 kPa/l/sec.)

FIBROSE   27
"SARKOIDOSE"   20
ALVEOLÄRE PROZESSE   23
GRANULOME   4
"EITRIGE INFILTRATIONEN"   16
RUNDZELLINFILTRATIONEN   12
DESQUAMIERTE ALVEOLARMAKROPHAGOZYTEN   14
EISENPIGMENT   5
ANTHRAKOSE   18
"OHNE PATHOLOGISCHEN BEFUND"   24

(Z.T. MEHRFACHZÄHLUNGEN)

ABB. 17   ZKH GAUTING/80

IX.7.

"Bronchiale und perbronchiale Biopsien bei obstruktiven Lungen-
bzw. Bronchialerkrankungen"

R.Eckert, O.Karg, K.Lorrmann, H.Pabst, H.Blaha

Seit längerem widmet sich ein Arbeitskreis am Zentralkrankenhaus Gauting der Landesversicherungsanstalt Oberbayern der Frage
"Morphologie der Obstruktion". Auf diesem Kongreß haben wir anhand
von Sektionsmaterial, von Resektionen bei Obstruktion und auch
anhand von perbronchialen Biopsien darüber berichtet. Weitere
Arbeiten sind im Gange: EDV-Verbindung zwischen endoskopischem
Befund und Lungenfunktionsbefund; Studien zur Reversibilität der
Obstruktion und klinisch-pathologisch-anatomische Korrelations-
studien insgesamt.

Zwei Arbeiten werden hier vorgestellt: Einmal Untersuchungen
aus einem Jahrgang von Bronchoskopien mit den Auswahlkriterien
Bronchialexzision, perbronchiale Biopsie und Obstruktion. Es
handelt sich um 98 Fälle, bei denen die Voraussetzungen erfüllt
waren. - Im zweiten Teil wurden 136 Fälle ausgewählt, bei denen
die bronchiale und die perbronchiale Biopsie vorgenommen wurde
und bei denen "obstruktionsassoziierte pathologisch-anatomische
Befunde" erfaßt wurden.

Im ersten Teil fanden sich an Diagnosen überwiegend granulo-
matöse und fibrotische Lungenerkrankungen, daneben Asthma bronchiale und Bronchitis. In allen Fällen bestand eine, zum Teil
nur grenzwertige Obstruktion (Resistance > 0,35 kPa/l/sec.)
(Abb. 1). In Abb. 2 werden die pathologisch-anatomischen Haupt-
bezeichnungen aufgeführt. Wie bereits auf diesem Kongreß von
BLAHA erwähnt, ist das Substrat der "Obstruktion" vielfältig.
Abb. 3 zeigt die Obstruktionsgrade aufgeschlüsselt: Leichtere
Obstruktionen bis 0,45 k:a/l/sec.; schwerere Obstruktionen, die
darüber liegen. Die Verteilung entspricht etwa der Erwartung.
Die "Obstruktion" ist ein Symptom vielfacher krankhafter Zustände.
Sie kann unabhängig hinzutreten.

Im zweiten Teil ist die Frage ganz anders gestellt: Wie oft
finden sich im Exzisionsmaterial Befunde, die auf eine Bronchitis
bzw. auf obstruktive Bronchopneumopathien zu beziehen sind? Die

Verteilung der Gruppe mit 136 untersuchten Fällen ergibt Abb. 4. In Abb. 5 sind die Merkmale mit ihrer Häufigkeit aufgelistet, die in Zusammenhang mit der "Bronchitis" genannt werden, wobei natürlich die Epitheloidzellgranulome ihre besondere Bedeutung haben. In Abb. 6 werden aus demselben Krankengut die pathologischen Lungenbefunde aufgelistet.

Auch aus dieser Studie, die nicht der Analyse der Wirklichkeit dient, sondern der Konkretisierung der Fragestellungen: wo soll man bei Obstruktionen was suchen, was ist generell häufig, was ist unspezifisch, zeigt sich, daß wir mit unserer Arbeit "Morphologie der Obstruktion" an einem Neubeginn stehen, der dadurch erleichtert wird, daß uns Lungengewebe nunmehr ausreichend zur Verfügung steht. Über die Repräsentanz des dabei gewonnenen Materials wäre zu sprechen: Es ist selbstverständlich, daß punktuelle Methoden an globalen Methoden geprüft werden.

BIOPSIE UND OBSTRUKTION

98 PERBRONCHIALE BIOPSIEN MIT OBSTRUKTION
(RESISTANCE > 0,35 kPa/l/sec)

ÜBERSICHT "DIAGNOSEN":

SARKOIDOSE	27
FIBROSE	15
ASTHMA	21
BRONCHITIS	10
PNEUMONIE	5
NEOPLASMA	11
LUNGENTUBERKULOSE	2
SILIKOSE	2
PLEURITIS	1
PNEUMOKONIOSE	1
LUNGENEMBOLIE	1
LUNGENEMPHYSEM	1
	98

ABB. 1   ZKH GAUTING/80

BIOPSIE UND OBSTRUKTION

ERGEBNISSE PERBRONCHIALER BIOPSIEN
AUSWAHL JAHR 1978

1/00 BRONCHOSKOPIEN, DAVON AUSGEWÄHLT:

98 GESICHERTE OBSTRUKTIVE ATEMWEGS-ERKRANKUNGEN
(RESISTANCE 0,35 kPa/l/sec)

FIBROSE	27
"SARKOIDOSE"	20
ALVEOLARE PROZESSE	23
GRANULOME	4
"ZELLIGE INFILTRATIONEN"	16
RUNDZELLINFILTRATIONEN	12
DESQUAMIERTE ALVEOLARPHAGOZYTEN	14
EISENPIGMENT	5
ANTHRAKOSE	18
"OHNE PATHOLOGISCHEN BEFUND"	24

(Z.T. MEHRFACHZÄHLUNGEN)

ABB. 2   ZKH GAUTING/80

BIOPSIE UND OBSTRUKTION

SCHWEREGRAD DER OBSTRUKTION NACH "DIAGNOSEN"

	0,35 - 0,45 kPa/l/sec		> 0,45 kPa/l/sec	
SARKOIDOSE	22 =	81,4%	5 =	18,6%
FIBROSE	13 =	86,6%	2 =	13,4%
ASTHMA	9 =	42,8%	12 =	57,2%
BRONCHITIS	6 =	60,0%	4 =	40,0%
PNEUMONIE	4 =	80,0%	1	
NEOPLASMEN	7 =	63,6%	4 =	36,4%
LUNGENTUBERKULOSE	1		1	
SILIKOSE	1		1	
PLEURITIS	1		-	
PNEUMOKONIOSE	1		-	
LUNGENEMBOLIE	1		-	
LUNGENEMPHYSEM	1		-	
O.B.	2		-	

ABB. 3   ZKH GAUTING/80

BIOPSIE UND OBSTRUKTION

OBSTRUKTIONSASSOZIIERTE BEFUNDE

N = 136

ÜBERSICHT "KLINISCHE DIAGNOSEN"
(UNTERSUCHUNG OSWALD)

SARKOIDOSE	50 PAT.	=	36,0%
LUNGENFIBROSE	22 PAT.	=	16,2%
CHRONISCHE BRONCHITIS	18 PAT.	=	13,2%
PNEUMONIE	11 PAT.	=	8,1%
KARZINOM	10 PAT.	=	7,4%
ALVEOLITIS	8 PAT.	=	5,9%
LUNGENTUBERKULOSE	7 PAT.	=	5,1%
SILIKOSE	2 PAT.	=	1,5%
ANDERE	8 PAT.	=	5,9%

ABB. 4   ZKH GAUTING/80

BIOPSIE UND OBSTRUKTION

HISTOLOGISCHE BEFUNDE BEI 136 BIOPSIEN
(Z.T. MEHRFACHZÄHLUNGEN)
OBSTRUKTIONSASSOZIIERTE BEFUNDE

BRONCHUS
(NACH OSWALD)

BACHBARZELLVERMEHRUNG	55,9%
BASALMEMBRANVERDICKUNG	74,3%
EPITHELMETAPLASIE	11,8%
MUKÖSE TRANSFORMATION DER SCHLEIMDRÜSEN	48,5%
BETEILIGUNG VON EOSINOPHILEN GRANULOZYTEN	33,1%
VERMEHRUNG VON PLASMAZELLEN	29,4%
VERMEHRTE EINLAGERUNG VON LYMPHOZYTEN	26,5%
VERMEHRTE EINLAGERUNG VON SEGMENTKERNIGEN	0,7%
VASKULITIS	13,2%
EPITHELOIDZELLGRANULOME	20,5%

ABB. 5   ZKH GAUTING/80

BIOPSIE UND OBSTRUKTION

HISTOLOGISCHE BEFUNDE BEI 136 PERBRONCHIALEN BIOPSIEN
(Z.T. MEHRFACHZÄHLUNGEN)
OBSTRUKTIONSASSOZIIERTE BEFUNDE

LUNGE
(NACH OSWALD)

INTERSTITIELLE LUNGENFIBROSE	16,9%
INTERSTITIELLE PNEUMONIE	11,0%
ANTHRAKOTISCHES LUNGENGEWEBE	9,6%
LYMPHANGIOSIS CARCINOMATOSA	5,7%
PERIBRONCHITIS	1,5%
STAUUNGSLUNGE	1,5%
EPITHELOIDZELLGRANULOME	25,0%
PROLIFERATION DER ALVEOLAREPITHELIEN	3,7%
VERMEHRTE ALVEOLARSEPTEN	7,4%
ALVEOLARFELDERDESQUAMATION	16,9%
ÖDEMATÖSES STROMA	1,5%
NARBEN	1,5%
INFILTRATION VON LYMPHOZYTEN	18,4%
INFILTRATION VON PLASMAZELLEN	9,6%
INFILTRATION VON GRANULOZYTEN	7,4%

ABB. 6   ZKH GAUTING/80

322

IX.8.
Diagnostische Fragen Der Perbronchialen Lymphknotenpunktion

I. Kertes, I. Gyenei, G. Nagy, S. Moldvai /Budapest/

Die Perbronchiale Punktion /PBP/ - in der Heute ausgeübten
Form - wurde von BROUET in 1953 in die Reihe der bronchobioptischen
Verfahren eingeführt. Viele Bronchologen berichteten seither über
ihre Ergebnisse, wie SCHIESSLE, OTTE, SWIERENGA, HELBICH, SIMECEK,
KIRSCH, WETZER, KERTES usw.

Die PBP ist an die hinter der ausgebreiteten Carinae liegende
und vergrößerte Lymphknoten gezielt. Indikationen der PBP sind:
1./ Hiläre Lymphknoten Erkrankungen wie Sarkoidose, Lymphogranu-
lomatose oder Lymphosarkom;
2./ Hiläre Lymphknoten Metastasen, häufigsten bei Mammakarcinom;
3./ Bei dem Bronchialkarcinom zur a./ Diagnosestellung und/oder
b./ Klärung der Operabilität.
Es ist wohlbekannt, daß die zwei häufigsten Krankheiten wo die
PBP zur Anwendung kommt, der Bronchialkrebs und die Sarkoidose
sind.

Bei Lungenkarcinom liegen die Ergebnisse zwischen 23% /HELBICH
u. TOMANEK/, und 70% /OTTE/, in eigenem Material bei 39%. Dagegen
bei der Sarkoidose zwischen 45% /KIRSCH/, und 93% /SIMECEK/, in
eigenem Material in den Jahren 1977-78 bei 57%. Im Durchschnitt
von sechs Autoren bei 689 PBP-en bei 69,6%.

Wie ersichtlich zeigen die Ergebnisse der einzelnen Untersuchern
wesentliche Unterschiede, wir aber sollen bei dieser Feststellung
nicht stehen bleiben, sondern die Gründe aufklären.
Unsere Erfahrungen nach wird das Ergebnis von den folgenden Um-
ständen beeinflußt:
1./ Setzt sich das Patientegut aus Kranken mit Beschwerden zusammen, oder aus Patienten die beschwerdenfrei aus Röntgen Reihen-
untersuchungen kommen;

J.A. Nakhosteen and W. Maassen (eds.), Bronchology: Research, Diagnostic and
Therapeutic Aspects. All rights reserved.
Copyright 1981. Martinus Nijhoff Publishers bv, The Hague / Boston / London

2./ Stellt man die Indikation der PBP nach den am Tomogrammen
sichtbaren Lymphknoten, nach bronchoskopisch ausgebreitete Carinae,
oder auch bei normale Carinae auf;

3./ Technik der PBP abhängig vom Durchmesser der Nadel , Stärke
des Sauges oder Übung-des Untersuchers;

4./ Die cytologische Methodik der Fixation und der Färbung;

5./ Die Pathologie der Erkrankung bei dem Bronchialkarcinom;

a./ Bei Tumorstadium T 1-2 PBP Positivität 23%, bei T 3-4 49%;

b./ Bei Bronchoskopisch sichtbarer Tumorausdehnung in der Trachea
und Bifurkation PBP Positivität 46%, im Haupt-, oder Lappenbrochus
41%, im Segmentbronchus 33% und Perifär, mit Optiken unsichtbar
34%;

c./ Der endoskopisch sichtbare Charakter der Wucherung. Beim
intraluminalen Wachstum PBP Positivität 33%, beim infiltrativen
39% und bei gemischten Formen 48%;

d./ Die Ausbreitung der Lymphknotenerkrankung:

Lymphknoten	Verfizierte Sarkoidose N 60				Karzinom			
	N	%	PBP pos.	%	N	%	PBP pos.	%
Keine	-	-	-	-	53	35,6	22	41,5
Einseitige	10	16,6	6	60	81	54,4	36	44,4
Zweiseitige	50	83,4	29	58	15	10,0	6	40,0
Zusammen	60	100,0	35	-	149	100,0	64	-

Bei der Sarkoidose versuchten wir Zusammenhang zwischen bronchoskopisch sichtbaren Veränderungen und PBP Positivität zu finden.
Bei 109 Kranken sahen wir insgesamt 201 Symptome: breite Carinae
94, Kapillar Ausbreitung 49, Deformitäten der Bronchien 27, Dissemination 15 und Entzündung 16 - mal.

Die höchste PBP Positivität sahen wir bei Dissemination, dann
folgen Deformitäten, ausgebreitete Carinae und Kapillarisation.
Mit der Häufung der einzelnen endobronchialen Symptome erhöht
sich die PBP Positivität von 49% bei einem Symptom bis 100% bei
4-5 Symptomen.

Zusammenfassend ist die PBP - einstimmend mit der Literatur - und nach eigenen Erfahrungen - eine geeignete Methode zur schnellen Diagnosestellung bei mediastinalen Lymphknotenerkrankungen, Lymphknotenmetastasen und bei dem Bronchialkrebs. Mit Hilfe dieser bronchobioptischen Methode können wir häufig die Mediastinoskopie ersparen, oder die Inoperabilität bestätigen.

IX.9.

Technique for transmural lymphnode aspiration biopsy during fiberbronchoscopy in local anesthesia in sarcoidosis

E. Boehm, W. Hartmann

Many methods have been described for diagnostic procedures in sarcoidosis with different rates of success. Complications depend upon the
skill and experience of the examiner. Since in sarcoidosis usually
there are no great consequences therapeutically, those diagnostic procedures are prefered with minimal discomfort and risc for the patients.
One of these methods is the transmural lymphnode aspiration biopsy of
the carina. This is possible with a long needle which is pushed forward
by the guidance of the rigid bronchoscope into the lymphnode of the
carina (Fig. 1). By forced aspiration material for cytologic examination
can be obtained. This material is ejected and smeared on a preparation
slide. The macroscopic appearance of the aspirate already showes its
effectivity. In case of aspiration of blood or aspiration of aquous material the biopsy has to be repeated. A sample of opaque and pink material demonstrates that lymphatic material is obtained.

Technique for lymphnode aspiration biopsy during rigid broncoscopy

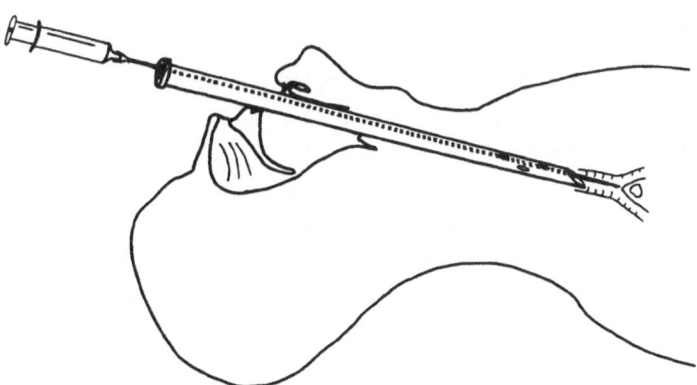

Since this method is only possible using the rigid-bronchoscope all disadvantages of rigid-bronchoscopy have to be taken into account. Therefore we tried to biopsy central lymphnodes during fiberbroncho- scopy in local anesthesia. Through the instrumentation channel of a fiberbronchoscope armed needles may be passed. However, these needles often are too thin and too short to obtain lymphatic material from the lymphnodes. Therefore, we tried to proceed in a different way as fol- lows:

The bronchoscope was inserted into a flexible tube, larynx and trachea were carefully anesthetized during intubation with the flexible bronchoscope. When the bronchoscope reached the trachea the tube was led by the bronchoscope forward into the trachea (Fig. 2).

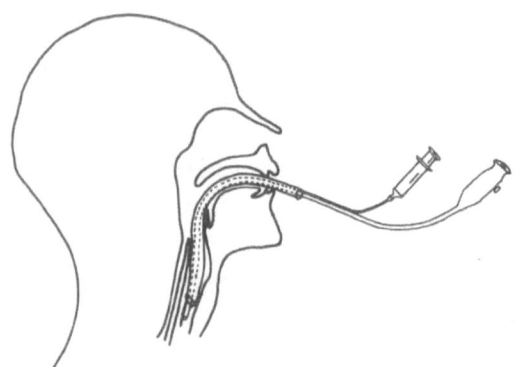

Technique for lymphnode aspiration biopsy during fiberglassbroncoscopy
in lokal anaesthesia

A needle of 1.5 cm in length and 1.1 mm in diameter was fixed to the end of the fiberopticbronchoscope so that the end of the needle exceeded the end of the bronchoscope by 1.5 cm. The needle was coupled to a tef- lon tubing for aspiration purposes. In this way it is possible to guide the needle under the control of the bronchoscope and to puncture the lymphnodes of the carina.

The results of 91 patients with suspected sarcoidosis were evaluated The x-ray in 12 out of these patients showed a diffuse infiltration of the lung. In 79 patients diagnostic was carried out because of enlarged hilar lymphnodes partly with additional infiltrates of the lung. 20 pa- tients were investigated by fiberbronchoscopy while in 71 patients the rigid-bronchoscope was used.

The group of patients consisted of 50 males and 41 females in the age between 21 und 69 years averaging 37.3 years.

Out of the total of 91 patients sarcoidosis was proven by lymphnode aspiration biopsy in 37 patients. Only in 4 patients diagnosis was verified by the histological examination of a bronchus biopsy.

Out of 71 patients investigated by rigid-bronchoscopy sarcoidosis was diagnosed in 28 patients. Three further patients had tumor metastasis in the lymphnodes. Two additional patients showed tuberculosis. Only in 15 patients we were not successful in aspiration of lymphnode tissue. In 21 patients we got lymphatic material without specific alterations.

In those 20 patients we biopsied lymphnodes by fiberbronchoscopy the diagnosis of sarcoidosis could be certified in 9 patients. In this group no other disease was found.

In about half of all cases we were able to aspirate representative material from lymphnodes. Only in a few cases the biopsy of mucous membranes was diagnostic for sarcoidosis.

In rigid as well as in fiberbronchoscopy the lymphnode aspiration biopsy is easy to perform. In the technique described the needle is long enough and bears a sufficient diameter, so cells from the lymphnode can be aspirated. Though the number of investigations in fiberbronchoscopy is still not high the method seems to be as successful as in rigid-bronchoscopy. We saw no complications and the technique enlarges the diagnostic repertoire in sarcoidosis. Besides this, the lymphnode biopsy is a valuable technique for the detection of lymphnode metastasis and systemic lymphnode diseases as well.

TABLE 1: Number of lymphnode aspiration biopsies in patients submitted to the clinic because of suspected sarcoidosis

	positive for sarcoidosis	positive for tumor or tbc	negative	total
A	28	5	38	71
B	9	0	11	20

References

Atay, Z., H.-J. Brandt: Die Bedeutung der Zytodiagnostik der perbronchialen Feinnadelpunktion von mediastinalen oder hilären Tumoren. Dtsch.med. Wschr. 102 (1977), 345 - 348.

IX.10.

THE ROLE OF COMPUTED TOMOGRAPHY IN THE SELECTION OF PATIENTS WITH BRONCHOGENIC
CARCINOMA FOR FLEXIBLE BRONCHOSCOPY AND REGID BRONCHOSCOPY.

T.D. TAN, W.J. KÜHLER, P.P.M.F. BUYINK, J.P.M. WAGENAAR, HOLLAND

INTRODUCTION

   The ability of taking biopsy of tracheobronchial lymph-nodes via a rigid
bronchoscope is a distinct advantage over the flexible bronchoscope, especially
in the assessment of mediastinal metastases. Recent reports stress the importance
of computed tomography (C.T.) in the diagnosis of mediastinal metastases in patients
with bronchogenic carcinoma (1.2.3.4.). This report discusses the role of C.T. of
the mediastinum in the selection of patients with suspected bronchogenic carcinoma
for flexible fiberoptic bronchoscopy and rigid bronchoscopy.

MATERIALS AND METHODS

   Between december 1977 and december 1979 we studied 45 patients with potentially
resectable bronchogenic carcinoma. Initial evaluation of each patient includes
chest X-ray, local tumour mass tomograms and rigid bronchoscopy examination, at all
bronchoscopy procedures routinelly a transbronchial needle aspiration subcarinal
lymph node biopsy was taken. One week before any patient underwent an invasive
staging procedure C.T. scan of the mediastinum were performed. All scans were made
in an EMI 5005 total body scanner. The mediastinum was considered to be abnormal
(scored positive) if a tracheobronchial lymph node larger than 1 cm in diameter
was demonstrated on the scan. The findings were graphically documented in a
written standard report.

RESULTS

   Table I shows the results of C.T. scanning in comparison with the histological
findings. 'C.T. POSITIVE ' signifies mediastinal nodes larger than 1 cm in diameter.
C.T. detected II abnormal tracheobronchial lymph-nodes, which at surgery all proved
to be enlarged and of these 4 by transtracheal biopsy and the other 4 cases by
mediastinoscopy proved to be malignant. In the other 34 cases, the C.T. scans were
interpreted as showing a normal mediastinum; all proved to be benignant. So there
were 34 (76%) nonproductive transbronchial subcarinal node biopsy. In our patients
C.T. had a sensitivity for tracheobronchial lymph node metastases 100%.

J.A. Nakhosteen and W. Maassen (eds.), Bronchology: Research, Diagnostic and
Therapeutic Aspects. All rights reserved.
Copyright 1981. Martinus Nijhoff Publishers bv, The Hague / Boston / London

Our findings suggest that:

1. C.T. scan is a highly sensitive method in detecting abnormal tracheobronchial lymph nodes.
2. C.T. scan is useful in the selection of patients with suspected bronchogenic carcinoma for flexible bronchoscopy and rigid bronchoscopy.

The results of this study lead us to recommend the following approach to evaluate patients with suspected bronchogenic carcinoma.

1. If the C.T. scan suggests mediastinal spread, the patient should have trans-bronchial or and transtracheal biopsy or mediastinoscopy to obtain tissue confirmation of such spread.
2. If the C.T. suggests normal mediastinum, the patients don't need to have lymph node biopsy or rigid bronchoscopy examination.

TABLE I   TRACHEOBRONCHIAL LYMPH-NODES.

ASSOCIATION BEWEEN COMPUTED TOMOGRAPHY (n = 45) AND PATHOLOGICAL FINDINGS BY MEDIASTINOSCOPY OF BRONCHOSCOPY

C.T. \ P.A.	Histologically metastatic nodes	Histologically normal nodes
Positive n (%)	8 (18%)	3 (7%)
Negative n (%)	0 (0%)	34 (75%)

REFERENCES

1. Crowe J.K., Brown L.R. and Muhm, J.R.   computed tomography of the mediastinum. Radiology 128; 75-87 (1978)
2. Heitzman E.R., Radiologic analysis of the mediastinum utilising computed tomography. Radiol.Clin.North.Am. 15; 309-329 (1977)
3. Mintzer R.A., Malawe S.R., Neiman H.L., Michaellis L.L., Vanecko R.M. and Sanders J.H.   computed V.S. Concentional Tomography in evaluation of primary and secondary pulmonary neoplasms. Radiology 132; 653-659 (1979)
4. Tan T.D., Kühler W.J., Taconis W.K., Frensdorf E.L., Zienkowicz B. and Wagenaar J.P.M.   computed tomography scanning of the mediastinum in the staging of bronchogenic carcinoma, ACTA Tuberculosea et Pneumologica Belgica, in press.

Chapter X
TRANSBRONCHIAL BIOPSY

7.7.

TRANSBRONCHIAL LUNG BIOPSY (TBB) IN 433 PATIENTS

D.M. MITCHELL, C.J. EMERSON, J.V. COLLINS, D.E. STABLEFORTH

We report our experience with transbronchial biopsy using the
Olympus BF-B$_3$ fibrescope in 433 patients, who had 456 procedures
performed at Brompton Hospital between April 1976 and July 1979.
Two thirds of the patients were male; the mean age was 52 years.
The transnasal route was used in the majority. In each case an
appropriate subsegmental bronchus was selected and the biopsy
forceps were pushed to the lung periphery or into the abnormal
mass. A single plane x-ray image intensifier and Rotacor
rotating table were used to enable accurate placement. Six to
ten biopsies were taken in each case. Oxygen was administered
by nasal cannula during the procedure. Blood was crossmatched
routinely before each procedure and platelets and prothrombin
time were checked.

In 183 patients there was a diffuse bilateral chest
radiograph abnormality and a histological diagnosis was
established by TBB in 121(66%). In 225 there was a discrete
peripheral lesion and diagnosis was established by TBB in
135(60%). The remainder (25) had multiples opacities and in
13(52%) TBB provided diagnostic histology. Overall, 269(62%)
patients of 433 had positive histology provided by TBB.

Of 183 patients with diffuse radiographic changes, 74 were
finally found to have sarcoidosis and in 58(78%), positive
histology was provided by TBB, whereas in 45 patients with
fibrosing alveolitis, only 18(40%) had positive histology on TBB.
Those with negative histology required trephine or open lung
biopsy to establish the diagnosis. In 22 patients who had
diffuse radiographic changes and who were finally found to have
carcinoma (primary or secondary), 14(64%) had diagnostic
histology on TBB. In 19 patients no diagnosis was made by TBB
or any other means. In the remaining 22 patients a wide range

*J.A. Nakhosteen and W. Maassen (eds.), Bronchology: Research, Diagnostic and
Therapeutic Aspects. All rights reserved.
Copyright 1981. Martinus Nijhoff Publishers bv, The Hague / Boston / London*

of less common diagnoses were made by TBB in 15(68%), including
idiopathic pulmonary haemosiderosis, pneumocystis carinii pneumonia
and pulmonary tuberculosis.

In 130 patients a final diagnosis of bronchial carcinoma was
reached; the majority having peripheral discrete radiographic
abnormality. In 82(63%) diagnostic histology was obtained by TBB.

In this series of 433 patients, a definite diagnosis was
established on the basis of histology obtained by TBB in two thirds
of the patients. In ten per cent, other investigations were
required including open lung biopsy, percutaneous needle biopsy
or thoracotomy. In the remainder no tissue diagnosis was
established, either because the diagnosis was felt to be
relatively secure on clinical grounds and further invasive
procedures were unwarranted, or the patient was too ill for, or
refused further investigations.

In seven patients, haemorrhage of 50 to 100ml occurred
following the procedure. None of the patients suffered
respiratory embarrassment nor needed blood transfusion.
Bleeding stopped in all 7 cases spontaneously without additional
manoevres apart from suction. Three patients developed a
pneumothorax and one required intercostal drainage. One patient
had a period of apnoea following intravenous diazepam. This
patient required hand ventilation for a few minutes and then
recovered.

In conclusion, we found that TBB yielded diagnostic or
supportive histology in 66% of patients with diffuse bilateral
chest radiograph abnormality. The diagnostic yield was
particularly good in sarcoidosis (80%), whereas in fibrosing
alveolitis it was only 40%. This lower figure reflects the
patchy nature of this disease. In peripheral carcinoma a
diagnostic yield of 63% was obtained. There were few
complications and none were serious. TBB using the fibrescope
is a simple and safe way of obtaining pulmonary tissue for
diagnosis. The chances of success for interstitial lung
diseases and peripheral carcinomas are high, and may spare the
patient more invasive diagnostic procedures.

X.2.

DIAGNOSTIC ACCURACY IN PERIPHERAL LUNG CANCER USING FLEXIBLE FIBEROPTIC BRONCHOSCOPE

K. MATSUI, M. FUKUOKA, S. TAMAI, M. TAKADA, N. OKUNAKA AND N. SAKAI

For definitive diagnosis of peripheral lung cancer, we use cytologic examination by small curet throgh the biopsy channel of flexible fiberoptic bronchoscope. The present study shows definitive diagnosis of peripheral lung cancer resected 107 cases and assess the accuracy of transbronchoscopic curettage (curettage).

Under the fluoloscopic guidance, curettage was carried out (Fig.1) and the specimen obtained upon curettage had been stained by the method of Papanicolaou (Fig.2).

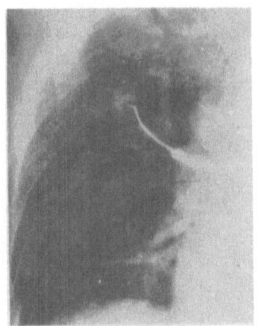

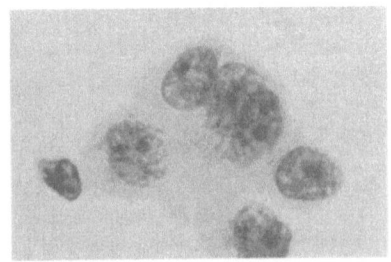

Fig.1   Fig.2

Out of 107 cases curettage performed during this study, there were 30 cases of squamous cell carcinoma, 68 cases of adenocarcinoma, 4 cases of small cell carcinoma and 5 cases of large cell carcinoma.

71 cases had tumors of 3 cm or larger, and 36 cases had those smaller than 3 cm in diameter.

The positive rate of curettage was 88.7% with tumors of 3 cm or larger, and 80.5% with those smaller than 3 cm in diameter.

Histologically, the positive rate was 93.3% with squamous cell carcinoma, 83.8% with adenocarcinoma, 75% with small cell carcinoma, 80% with large cell carcinoma and 86.0% for over all (Table 1).

The relationship between number of drainage bronchi read by bronchography and positive rate of curettage was studied.

J.A. Nakhosteen and W. Maassen (eds.), Bronchology: Research, Diagnostic and Therapeutic Aspects. All rights reserved.
Copyright 1981. Martinus Nijhoff Publishers bv, The Hague / Boston / London

336

The positive rate was 68.8% with cases of one drainage bronchus, 75.9% with two drainage bronchi, 96.3% with three, and 94.3% with more than four drainage bronchi. The positive rate became higher as number of drainage bronchi increase (Table 2).

In the correlation with the performances of curettage and positive rate, the positive rate upon one curettage was 80.4% which turned to 93.7% with two performances and 99.0% with three times (Table 3).

The coincident rate of cytology by curettage and post-surgical histology was 90.2%. There were 9 cases of non-coincidence, including 7 cases of adenocarcinoma, one case of squamous cell carcinoma and one case of large cell carcinoma.

The relation of the order of drainage bronchi and positive rate was studied. The positive rate was 74.1% with the third order of bronchi (subsegmental bronchi), 85.7% with fourth, 96.5% with the fifth, and 87.5% with the sixth order of bronchi or over.

There were 15 negative cases of curettage. Two cases were diagnosed firmly by sputum cytology, 7 cases by percutaneous needle aspiration and 6 cases by surgery.

Table 1. Positive Rate of Cytological Examination by Curettage.

Histology	: Sq. Ca.	28/30 (93.3)
	Ad. Ca.	57/68 (83.8)
	Sm. Ca.	3/4 (75.0)
	La. Ca.	4/5 (80.0)
Tumor size	: 3 cm <	63/71 (88.7)
	3 cm ≧	29/36 (80.5)
Over all	:	92/107 (86.0)

( ) : %

Table 2.
Relationship Between Number of Drainage Bronchi and Positive Rate of Curettage

No. of Drainage Bronchi	1	2	3	4~
No. of Cases	16	29	27	35
Positive Cases (%)	11 (68.8)	22 (75.9)	26 (96.3)	33 (94.3)

Table 3.
Relationship between Number of Examination and Positive Rate

No. of Exam.	1	2	3
No. of Cases	107	95	93
Positive Cases (%)	86 (80.4)	89 (93.7)	92 (99.0)

Summary
1) Reffering to the peripheral lung cancer, the positive rate of curettage was 86.0%.
2) The positive rate was as high as 99.0% when curettage was performed three times.
3) the positive rate became higher as number of drainage bronchi

increase.

4) The coincident rate of the cytology by curettage with the post-surgical histology was 90.2%.

REFERENCES

1) Ikeda, S.: Atlas of Flexible Bronchofiberscopy, Igaku Shoin, Tokyo, 1974.
2) Stringfield, J.T., et al : The Effect of Tumor Size and Localization on Diagnosis by Fiberoptic Bronchoscopy. Chest 72: 474-476, 1977
3) Radke, J.R., et al: Diagnostic Accuracy in Peripheral Lung Lesions. Chest 76: 176-179, 1979
4) Cortese, D.A., et al: Biopsy and Brushing of Peripheral Lung Cancer with Fluoroscopic Guidance. Chest 75: 141-145, 1979

X.3.

OUR EXPERIENCE WITH TRANSBRONCHIAL SEGMENTAL BIOPSIES
DR. A.H. SAEED — PAKISTAN

Ever since the application of radiology as a diagnostic technique, — lung is one vital organ which has presented maximum information. This is not confined to the pulmonary disease only, but the lung also acts as a mirror reflecting other systemic manifestations. However this spectrum is so broad that radiology alone has presented its limitations.

A study of 1600 cases suffering from pulmonary diseases revealed that 40% of our patients present a fairly clear cut radiological picture. Like fibro-cavernous tuberculosis involving apical segments. (Fig 1)

Another 25% are diagnosed accurately with the additional help of laboratory and clinical investigations. For example hydated cysts, and typical malignant metastasis. (Fig 2, Fig 3).

The remaining 35% cases are diagnostically problematic. The clinician's dilemma. These are usually reported by the radiologists as "Fibrotic Disease", "Miliary Mottling", "Alveolitis", "Migratory Pneumonias" or one of the various syndromes.

A fairly accurate diagnosis of this group of cases can be established with the help of "lung Biopsy". One of its recent methods is "Trans-Bronchial Segmental Biopsy" with the help of a flexible biopsy forceps, introduced under direct visual control through a Bronchoscope.

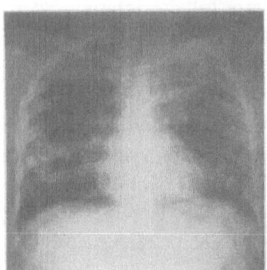

Fig 1:- Fibro-Cavernous Tbc. Involving Lt Bs 1 + 2.

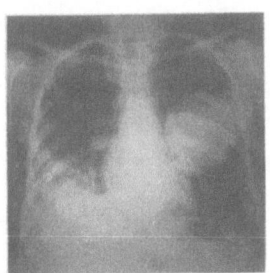

Fig 2:- Hydated Cyst, Cassonis positive. Removed surgically.

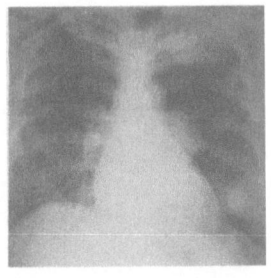

Fig 3:- Malignant Metastasis.

J.A. Nakhosteen and W. Maassen (eds.), Bronchology: Research, Diagnostic and Therapeutic Aspects. All rights reserved.
Copyright 1981. Martinus Nijhoff Publishers bv, The Hague / Boston / London

We use a rigid Bronchoscope with fiberoptic light, straight, oblique and lateral telescopes, a deflecting device to guide the flexible biopsy forceps, an optical Bronchus Biopsy. Forceps and other related equipment. The procedure is carried out under, both local and General Anaesthesia.

In the beginning we used direct visual and flouroscopic control to introduce the forceps accurately, but we found it equally easy with out flouroscopy.

After indentifying the correct segmental Bronchus, the forceps is introduced, when the pleural resistance is felt it is with drawn a couple of centimeters before the bite. (Fig 4) As a routine we take multiple Segmental Biopsies from different segments, take a couple of Bronchus Biopsies, and collect Bronchial aspirate.

We studied 146 cases who were never reported A.F.B. positive but having anti-tuberculous treatment, ranging from 2 weeks to one year, radiologically diagnosed as "Tuberculous".

Our results based on histo-pathologic examination revealed —

46% = Inflammatory Lung Disease.
38% = Neo-Plastic Disease.
16% = Pneumoconiosis and Miscellaneous.

as per details (Fig — 5).

Chronic Bronchitis	=	57
Bronchiectasis	=	6
Tuberculosis	=	2
Fungal Infection	=	1
Viral Pneumonia	=	1
Acute Bronchitis	=	1
Epidermoid Carcinoma	=	20
Anaplastic Carcinoma	=	16
Carcinoma in Situ	=	7
Large cell carcinoma	=	4
Adenocarcinoma	=	3
Unclassified	=	2
Anthracosis	=	6
Non Specific Lesion	=	5
Eosinophil Granuloma	=	1
Hemochromotosis	=	1
Fibrosing Lung Disease	=	1
Failed Biopsies	=	9
Total :		146

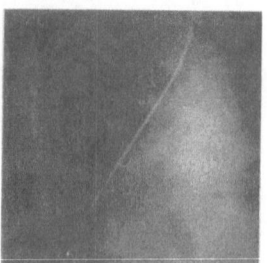

Fig 4

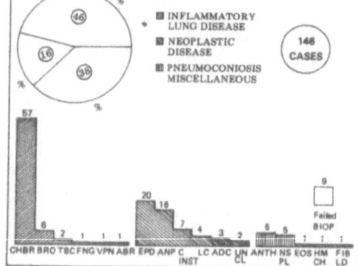

Fig 5

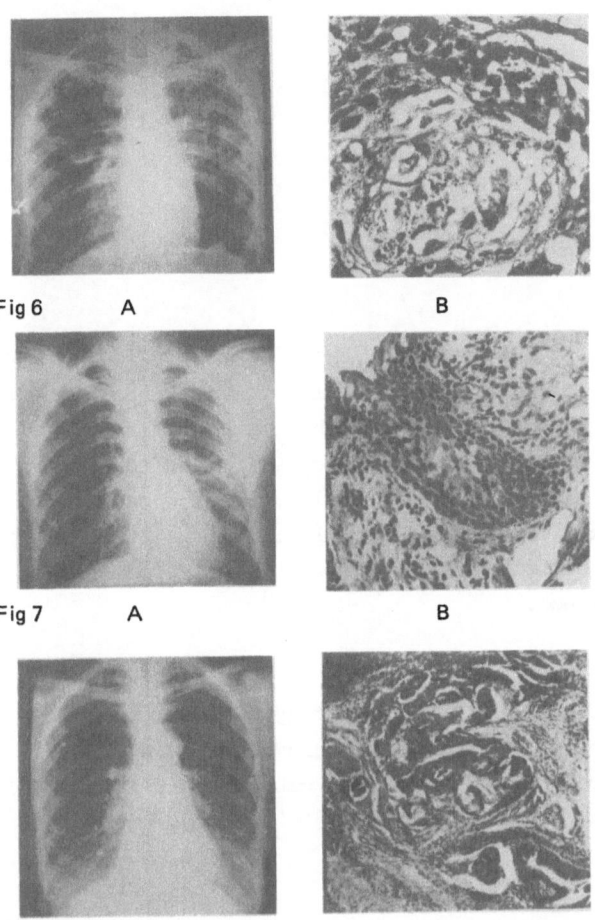

M.A. Fever, haemoptysis
cough expectoration, Anti-Tbc
therapy 4 months.
Anaplastic-Carcinoma
(Segmental Biopsy)

Fig 6   A   B

A.M. Cough, Expectoration,
Fever. Anti-Tbc therapy
6 — months. Carcinoma in Situ
(Segmental-Biopsy)

Fig 7   A   B

Mrs. G.M. Cough, expectoration, haemoptysis, anti-Tbc
treatment one year. Chronic
Bronchitis + Anthracosis.
(Segmental Biopsy)

Fig 8   A   B

Presented above are three typical examples

In conclusion this study of 146 cases shows that —

1)   35% of problematic pulmonary cases which could not be accurately disgnosed by radiology, or
       radiology and laboratory can be diagnosed with the help of lung biopsies using "Trans Bronchial
       Multiple Segmental Biopsy" method and,

2)   In countries like ours where pulmonary tuberculosis is still prevalent, majority of the cases are
       diagnosed and treated as tuberculous unless proved otherwise. This method should help in correct
       diagnosis.

Acknowledgements

Thanks to:

        Professor Werner Massen for his invitation.

        Dr. A.G. Jatoi for providing facilities at the Mideast Medical Centre, Karachi.

        Herr Karl Storz Tüttlingen, West Germany for equipment.

X.4.

A MORPHOLOGICAL ANALYSIS OF TRANSBRONCHIAL SEGMENTAL BIOPSIES

A.H.NAGI, A.S.CHUGHTAI, PAKISTAN

INTRODUCTION

The technique of transbronchial segmental biopsies using a rigid Fiberoptic Bronchoscope is not a new procedure (ref.1), however it has been used for the first time in Pakistan where lung diseases were diagnosed using superficial procedures such as biopsies of the cervical and scalene lymph nodes, sputum examination etc. The present report gives a morphological analysis of biopsies from 146 clinically nontuberculous patients who had clinical and radiological evidence of chronic respiratory disease.

MATERIALS AND METHODS

A total of 146 patients were biopsied and 2-3 tissue fragments were received from each patient. They were hand processed using ethyl alcohol, xylene and paraffin wax. The sections 3-4 micron thick were stained using haematoxylene-eosin, Ziehl-Neelsen and if required periodic-acid-Schiff's reaction, before they were examined using a Leitz Ortholux II microscope.

RESULTS

All the biopsies received after a histological examination were divided into five major groups i.e. (1) Inflammatory diseases (68 cases=46.58 per cent) (2) Neoplastic diseases (55 cases=37.67 per cent) (3) Pneumoconiosis (9 cases= 6.16 per cent) (4) Miscellaneous including atelectasis, infarction and non-specific lesions (5 cases=3.43 per cent) and (5) Failed biopsies (9 cases=6.16 per cent). The commonest amongst the inflammatory lesion was chronic bronchitis (57 cases) followed by bronchiectasis (6 cases), whereas only two cases of pulmonary tuberculosis and one each of candidiasis, viral pneumonia and acute bronchitis were seen. Amongst the neoplastic lesions squamous carcinoma (fig.1) was the commonest (19 cases= 42.22 per cent) followed by small cell anaplastic group (17 cases=37.78 per cent) (fig.2). Only four cases of large cell carcinoma, 3 of adenocarcinoma (fig.3) and two malignancies of unclassified nature were seen. In addition 7 cases of carcinoma in situ and 3 of suspicious malignancy were observed. The group of pneumoconiosis included 6 cases of anthra-

J.A. Nakhosteen and W. Maassen (eds.), Bronchology: Research, Diagnostic and Therapeutic Aspects. All rights reserved.

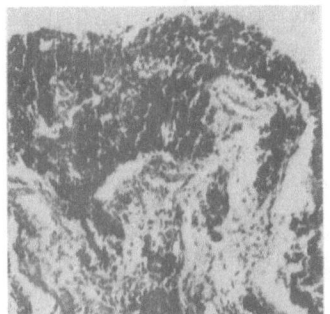

Fig.I Squamous carcinoma

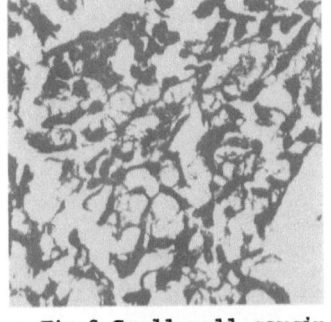

Fig.2 Small cell carcinoama

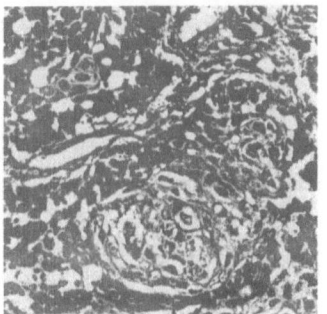

Fig.3 Adenocarcinoma

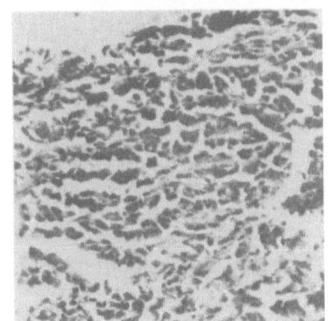

Fig.4 Anthracosis

cosis (fig.4) and one of haemosiderosis. In addition one case each of fibrosing lung disease and plumonary eosinophilia were included in this group.

The peak age incidence in the confirmed neoplastic group was between 41 and 50 years with a sex ratio of 3.5 males to 1 female.

CONCLUSIONS

a) The diagnostic yield using this technique is very high(93,84%).

b) Although inflammatory diseases form the largest number, the malignancies of lung are more common(37.67%) than what is generally considered in Pakistan.

REFERENCE

1. Andersen, H.A., Fontana, R.S. and Harrison, E.G. Jr: Transbronchoscopic lung biopsy in diffuse pulmonary disease, Dis.Chest, 48:187, 1965.

DIAGNOSTIC VALUE OF TRANSBRONCHIAL LUNG BIOPSY(TBLB) FOR DISEASES
SHOWING BILATERAL DIFFUSE SHADOWS ON CHEST ROENTGENOGRAM
X.5.
  T. SUZUKI, T.ARAI, A.NAKANO, Y.TAJIMA

1. INTRODUCTION

The open lung biopsy has proved so useful in diffuse lung diseases
presenting diagnostic problems.(1) In addition to it,transbronchial
lung biopsy(TBLB) has been introduced for the same purpose in recent
years.(2) This article describes the utility and limitation of TBLB
applied to various lung diseases with bilateral diffuse shadows on
chest roentgenogram.

2. TECHNIQUE

The lung biopsy was carried out under an x-ray TV with a flexible
fiberoptic bronchoscope aiming at the subpleural region corresponding
to abnormal shadows. The biopsied tissue was distended in physiological
saline for preparing pathological specimens.

3. PATIENTS

Our cumulative experience with this technique amounted to 165 patients
with bilateral diffuse shadows on chest roentgenogram during the period
from 1975 to 1979. The distribution of these patients was variable
with respect to sex,age,and diseases,as shown in TABLE 1..

Distribution of Sex and Age of Patients with Bilateral Diffuse Shadows

Disease	Number of case	Male	Female	Mean Age(yr to yr)
Pneumonitis	49	39	10	56.2(22 to 78)
Lung Cancer	25	9	16	59.4(30 to 81)
Chronic Bronchitis	22	6	16	58.0(26 to 78)
Sarcoidosis	11	8	3	34.3(23 to 69)
Hypersensitivity Pneumonitis	11	8	3	37.8(22 to 55)
Bronchiolitis	10	7	3	43.9(23to 68)
Allergic Pneumonia	10	6	4	41.7(16 to 57)
Pneumonia	9	4	5	51.1(32 to 71)
Pulmonary Tuberculosis	8	4	4	57.5(29 to 71)
Pneumoconiosis	5	4	1	50.2(49 to 58)
Emphysema	4	3	1	64.3(56 to 70)
Hamartoangiomyomatosis	1	0	1	51

TABLE   1

4. RESULT

Pneumonitis amounted to 49 patients,consisting of rheumatoid arthritis,progressive systemic sclerosis,systemic lupus erythematosus,
radiation pneumonitis,each,and for the remaining part,clinically
unclassified pneumonitis. The specimens showed thickening of alveolar
walls,hyaline membranes and interstitial fibrosis,but bronchoscopic
findings were within the normal limit along the area from the trachea
to segmental or subsegmental bronchi. The TBLB findings could not
disclose the etiology of pneumonitis,but TBLB was useful for detecting
histological changes and regions of them. It seemed advisable to make
the diagnosis of pneumonitis not only with the TBLB findings but also
with other clinical data.

Lung cancer amounted to 25 patients,consisting of 18 cases of
primary lung cancer and 7 cases of metastatic lung cancer. The cancer
cell could be obtained in 14 out of 18 patients of primary lung cancer
but in only one out of 7 patients of metastatic type. The biopsied
cancer cells lead directly to diagnosis of lung cancer.

Chronic bronchitis amounted to 22 patients. The bronchoscope showed
inflammatory changes of the airway from the trachea to subsegmental
bronchi and the specimens of TBLB sometimes exhibited the presence
of pneumonia. The TBLB was of complemental value for diagnosis of
this particular disease,but abnormal findings of bronchoscope were
very useful.

Sarcoidosis amounted to 11 patients who had BHL and both BHL and
diffuse shadows.The specimens showed sarcoid-granuloma in 4 patients
and interstitial fibrosis in 3 patients. Sarcoid-granuloma was the
most valuable,especially after the failure of the biopsy of super -
ficial lymph nodes. The TBLB seems to be a better method than the
mediastinoscope with regard to smaller trauma on the side of patients.

Hypersensitivity pneumonitis amounted to 11 patients. The specimens
showed thickening of alveolar walls and bronchiolitis in 4 patients,
Masson body in 2 patients and microgranuloma in 5 patients.These micro
granuloma and bronchiolitis were characteristic changes of this disease. TBLB was so useful for the diagnosis again.

Bronchiolitis amounted to 10 patients.The biopsied specimens showed
peribronchiolar round cells infiltration and lipoid pneumonia.Since
the bronchiolar biopsy was relatively difficult to perform properly,
TBLB was better tried in several different regions.

Pulmonary tuberculosis amounted to 8 patients,whose specimens
showed tuberculoma in 5 patients and interstitial fibrosis in 1 case.
TBLB was one of final methods for the diagnosis.

Pneumonia,allergic pneumonia,pneumoconiosis and hamartoangiomyoma-
tosis were in 9,10,5,and 1 patients,respectively. In each of the above
pathological conditions the specimens showed intra-alveolar neutrophil
with fibrinoid substances,pneumonia with eosinophilic infiltration,
deposition of foreign bodies surrounded by fibrosis and abnormal proliferation of the leiomyomatous element of interstitial tissue,respec-
tively. TBLB findings were as useful as other findings in these cases.

5. CONCLUSION (TABLE 2)

The TBLB was a definitive diagnostic method for lung cancer,sarcoid-
osis,hypersensitivity pneumonitis and pulmonary tuberculosis,but it
stayed as a complementary method for pneumonitis,chronic bronchitis,
pneumonia,allergic pneumonia,bronchiolitis,pneumoconiosis and hamarto-
angiomyomatosis and it was not useful for the diagnosis of emphysema
because all specimens were normal lung tissues. The TBLB was more
endurable than open lung biopsy for patients even under poor condition
in spite of adverse effects such as bleeding over 20 ml(3patients,
1.7%) and pneumothorax(12patients,7.3%).

Usefulness of TBLB in the Diagnosis of Patients with Diffuse Shadows

Disease	Average of Biopsy	Definitive	Complementary	Invalid
Pneumonittis	3.0		46/49	3/49(3bronchial)
Lung Cancer	2.4	15/25	6 /25	4/25(3normal)
Chronic Bronchitis	3.7		17/22	5/22(1bronchial)(5 normal)
Sarcoidosis	3.0	4/11	3/11	4/11(4 normal)
Hypersensitivity Pneumonitis	3.2	5/11	4/11	2/11(2 normal)
Bronchiolitis	2.5		7/10	3/10(2 normal 1bronchial)
Allergic Pneumonia	2.8		9/10	1/10(1bronchial)
Pneumonia	2.8		8/9	1/9(1 normal)
Pulmonary Tuberculosis	2.3	5/8	1/8	2/8(2 bronchial)
Pneumoconiosis	2.4		4/5	1/5(1 normal)
Hamartoangiomyomatosis	3		1/1	

TABLE   2

REFERENCES

1.J. G.Scadding: Lung biopsy in the diagnosis of diffuse lung disease.
   Brit. Med. J. 2, 557, 1970.

2. M. Shibayama, H.Miyake, E,Matsui, Y.Yamawaki, T.Kunieda, M.Goto:
   Transbronchial lung biopsy- Application to pulmonary diffuse
   diseases.- Jap. J. Chest Dis. 33(5), 340, 1974.

X.6. TRANSBRONCHOSCOPIC LUNG BIOPSY FOR DIFFUSE PULMONARY DISEASES

Hiroshi ANNO and Akira KOYAMA,

Lung biopsy combined with thoracotomy had been employed to confirm the diagnosis of pulmonary diseases having a diffuse lung shadow on chest X-ray. Establishment of the transbronchoscopic biopsy technique employing the flexible fiberoptic broncho-scope made the biopsy examination of such cases more convenient.

SUBJECTS AND METHODS

The biopsy technique was applied in 87 occasions on 78 patients having bilateral diffuse chest X-ray shadow during the past 7 years from 1973 to 1979. The trans-bronchoscopic biopsy procedure was carried out as follows: An emollient and atropine sulfate were given 30 minutes before anesthesia. Endotracheal intubation was per-formed under surface anesthesia by application of 2% or 4% xylocain solution, or under intravenous anesthesia with barbiturate and succinyl-choline. A flexible fiberoptic bronchoscope of 5 or 6 mm in diameter, is inserted through the tracheal tube for macroscopical examination of the bronchi. Insertion of a biopsy forceps of 2.0 or 2.4 mm in diameter was done through the flexible fiberoptic bronchoscope to obtain the lung tissue specimens by means of punch biopsy and using X-ray fluoro-scopy. Collected tissue specimens were put into physiological saline solution and were fixed in formaline solution to be used for histopathological examinations.

RESULTS

Bronchoscopy had been performed 225 occasions during 1973 at our hospital. Later on, bronchoscopic examination had been increased gradually year by year reaching 537 occasions in 1979 and the total number of bronchoscopic examination were 2398 occasions during the past 7 years.

The number of cases examined by transbronchoscopic lung biopsy for diffuse chest X-ray shadow was also increasing year by year and 78 cases in total had been examined during the period concerned. Among the 78 cases mentioned, two or three examinations, utilizing the biopsy technique, were performed in 7 patients making the total number of biopsies performed at 87. This figure corres-ponds to around 36% of the total performances of bronchoscopy.

J.A. Nakhosteen and W. Maassen (eds.), Bronchology: Research, Diagnostic and
Therapeutic Aspects. All rights reserved.
Copyright 1981. Martinus Nijhoff Publishers bv, The Hague / Boston /London

Of these, 54 out of 78 cases were male and 24 were female and 29 cases were younger than 50 years-old, while 49 cases were 50 years-old or more.

The diagnosis was confirmed in each of 56 cases out of 78, 71.8% in total. A definitive diagnosis rate 75.0% in the period during last two years from 1978 to 1979 was higher than the rate 69.0% in the period during 5 years from 1973 to 1977.

Final diagnosis of examined patients and definitive diagnostic rate by transbronchoscopic lung biopsy were shown in table 1.

TABLE 1. Final diagnosis and definitive diagnostic rates by transbronchoscopic lung biopsy

1. Diffuse interstitial fibrous pneumonitis	25	19	76.0%
2. Infection	5	4	80.0%
Klebsiella infection	1	0	
Fungus infection	1	1	
Tuberculosis	1	1	
Atypical mycobacteriosis	1	1	
Acute pneumonia	1	1	
3. Lung cancer	11	9	81.8%
Squamous cell carcinoma	2	1	
Adenocarcinoma	9	8	
4. Dust. physico-chemical diseases	15	10	66.7%
Silicosis	2	2	
Silico-tuberculosis	3	2	
Pneumoconiosis	7	3	
Asbestosis	2	2	
Talcosis	1	1	
5. Sarcoidosis	8	4	50.0%
6. Eosinophilic granuloma	1	0	0.0%
7. Others	13	10	76.9%
Lymphoid interstitial pneumonitis	1	1	
Bronchitis with pneumonia	7	6	
Allergic pneumonia	2	1	
Bronchiectasis	1	0	
Asthma with bronchiolitis	1	1	
Screrodermia	1	1	
Total	78	56	71.8%

In 25 cases from among the above mentioned 78, final diagnosis revealed diffuse interstitial fibrous pneumonitis, and 19 out of 25 cases 76.0% diagnosed by transbronchoscopic lung biopsy. A definitive diagnosis rate in 5 cases of infectious diseases was 80.0%. 11 cases were diagnosed finally as lung cancer. Two cases out of 11 were squamous cell carcinoma, 9 cases were adenocarcinoma. A definitive diagnostic rate in lung cancer cases was 81.8%. There were 15 cases of dust physico-chemical origin. The diagnosis of 10 cases from among 15 cases, 66.7%, were confirmed by means of the transbronchoscopic lung biopsy. In 4 cases out of 8 sarcoidosis cases, diagnosis was also confirmed by means of transbronchoscopic lung biopsy, and a definitive diagnostic rate was 50%.

In case of eosinophilic granuloma, diagnosis was not confirmed by this examination but defined after open chest biopsy. 10 cases out of 13 with other pulmonary diseases were diagnosed by transbronchoscopic lung biopsy.

Summing up the above presented results, 56 cases out of 78, 71.8% in total, could be definitively diagnosed by transbronchoscopic lung biopsy.

Chest X-ray and histological findings of a case will be presented. A 57 years-old male had an occupational history of working in an asbestos factory for many years. Diffuse linear, nodular and reticular shadows are observed in both lung fields on chest X-ray examination. Histological section demonstrated a fibrous change of the lung tissue in which the typical racket shaped asbestos body of yellowish brown colour could be observed. Based on these findings and the occupational history, this case was diagnosed as asbestosis.

The complication that accompanied the transbronchoscopic lung biopsy was a small amount of hemoptysis or bloody sputum on some occasions.

In summary, around 70% of the cases with diffuse pulmonary shadows on chest X-ray which formerly required thoracotomy for their definitive diagnosis, could be diagnostically confirmed through the use of transbronchoscopic lung biopsy and without severe complication.

REFERENCES

1. Fenessey J.J.: Transbronchial biopsy of peripheral lung lesion. Radiology, 88:878, 1967.
2. Levin D.C., Wicks A.B. and Ellis J.H.Jr.: Transbronchial lung biopsy via the fiberoptic bronchoscope. Am. Rev. Respir. Dis., 110:4, 1974.
3. Zabala D.C.: Transbronchial biopsy in diffuse lung disease. Chest, 73:727, 1978.
4. Andersen H.A.: Transbronchoscopic lung biopsy for diffuse pulmonary disease, results in 939 patients. Chest, 73:734, 1978.
5. Anno H., Koyama A., Mori J., Iwai K. and Shiozawa M.: Transbronchoscopic lung biopsy for diffuse pulmonary diseases. Bronchoscopy WCB, 37, 1978.

X.7.

RADIOLOGICAL AND PATHOLOGICAL CORRELATIONS ON THE ENDOBRONCHIAL SUBMUCOSAL LESIONS CONFIRMED BY TRANSBRONCHIAL LUNG BIOPSY

M. SHIBAYAMA, M.D., E. MATSUI, M.D., H. MIYAKE, M.D., S. YANAGAWA, M.D., H. DOI, M.D.

1. INTRODUCTION

Some kinds of broncho-pulmonary lesions which have their pathological lesions mainly in the submucosal layers with overlying normal bronchial epithelia were evaluated radio-histopathologically. By means of tomographical, bronchographical techniques and TBLB approach, we would like to report the comparative studies between radiographical and histological findings on these lesions.

2. PROCEDURE

2.1. Materials and methods

2.1.1. Studied diseases. On the study, endobronchial lymphoma 2 cases, subepithelial metastasis 1 case, lymphangitis carcinomatosa 4 cases, lung cancer 30 cases and pulmonary sarcoidosis 15 cases were included.

2.1.2. Technique of TBLB. The technique of transcatheter bronchial biopsy consists of placing a catheter as close as possible to the intrabronchial lesions under TV-fluoroscopic control in connection with the selective bronchography. Various preshaped forceps may be used according to the course of the bronchial tree in which the location of the endobronchial submucosal lesions is suspected. Prior to biopsy, the area in doubt is carefully located with the bronchographic examination or fiberoptic bronchoscopy. Thereafter, the lesion or suspected area may be biopsied directly or blindly, whether it may be visible or not.

3. RESULTS

3.1. Endobronchial lymphom. In the case of the endobronchial involvement, a partial or complete obstruction of the tracheo-bronchial lumen may be caused by the endobronchial lymphoma simulating bronchogenic carcinoma. The plain chest film showed the lobar or partial atelectasis in the lung area involved. Radiographical examinations, especially the tomogram and bronchogram were helpful to demonstrate the endobronchial involvement. The bronchogram showed the intrabronchial polypoid lesions projecting in the bronchial lumen or meniscus-like stricture in the affected bronchi. The biopsy specimen of these lesions showed a histological picture compatible with the endobronchial lymphom. This case showed the right upper lobe atelectasis and polypoid fillings defect in the right main and B-subsegment bronchi. Endobronchial giant follicular lymphoma was proved by TBLB approach.

3.2. Endobronchial subepithelial metastasis. As a rule, a number of primary malignant tumors commonly kidney, breast, and colon tumors tend to metastasize to the bronchi. It is pointed that because of the subepithelial location, smooth meniscus or incomplete obstructions are seen by the bronchogram. This case showed the right upper lobe collapse. The biopsy specimens were obtained from the strictured orifice of the right main bronchus.Histologically the subepithelial endobronchial metastases derived from renal cell carcinoma are proved.

3.3. Lymphangitis carcinomatosa. It seems to be difficult to differentiate from diffuse interstitial lung diseases. In this case, it should be emphasized that the bronchial biopsy plays an important role to differentiate this from the nonmalignant conditions. The biopsy specimen present the existence of cancer cells trapped in the capillary lymphatic vessels or blood vessels which are located in the submucosal layers of the bronchi. The bronchogram and tomogram show the smooth narrowing in the lumina of the involved bronchi in a wide length. This radiographical finding is proved to responsible for the edema and cancer cell infiltrations in the endobronchial subepithelial layers.

3.4. Lung cancer. A number of small cell cancer and adenocarcinoma(bronchiolo-alveolar type) may present the submucosal involvement of the bronchi in the affected area. The tomogram shows the diffuse narrowing of the bronchial lumina and the thickening of the peribronchial wall. The bronchogram shows the smooth narrowing of the bronchial lumina in a wide length, and so-called leafless tree picture. Consequently, we consider that it is important to assess the radiographic evidences of the involved endobronchial lesions in lung cancer. These radiographical findings are resulted from the infiltrations of cancer cells with edema and interstitial reactions in the submucosal layers of the involved bronchi. By means of TBLB, the localization and extension of the endobronchial submucosal involvement is ascertain so that it does make a difinite contribution to perform the treatment planning. This case shows diffuse mottled shadows in the right lower lobe. The bronchogram presented the narrowing of bronchial lumina in the lower bronchial trees in a wide length. The bronchial specimens presented the infiltrations of cancer cells in the submucosal layers with edema and minute interstitial reactions.

3.5. Pulmonary sarcoidosis. It is generally considered that all the bronchial layers are susceptible to sarcoidosis. The localization of the endobronchial lesions in pulmonary sarcoidosis is the most intersting. The transbronchial lung biopsy in connection with bronchography has been performed in 15 patients with pulmonary sarcoidosis. (pulmonary involvement 6 cases, BHL 9 cases)
Patients whose chest film showed hilar adenopathy without pulmonary opacities, presented submucosal granulomas of the bronchial wall in 5 of 9 cases, 55%. When

pulmonary shadows were shown with or without hilar adenopathy, pulmonary or bronchial granulomas presented the highest frequency 100%. It was found that sarcoid lesions were already found in the walls of the larger bronchi in the stage I, and also they were found in the walls of the peripheral small bronchi and in the peripheral interstitial tissues or in the alveolar spaces, especially in the sgate II.
The stage of sarcoidosis were evaluated bronchographically. It may be seen more or less unevenness of the bronchial wall and slight bronchial deformations in the stage I. In the sgate II, irregularity of the bronchial wall, bronchial deformity with slight bronchiectasis, and stenosis of peripheral bronchi may be seen.
In the sgate III, IV, there are more often bronchographically demonstrable lesions. Bronchial deformations with bronchiectasis, more or less pronounced stenosis and the finding of naked filling may be seen. It may be concluded that these findings are responsible for the grade of granuloma formations with interstitial reactions in the endobronchial submucosal layers. It should be emphasized that the bronchial mucosal biopsy may be valuable aids in the diagnosis and study of sarcoidosis.

4. CONCLUSIONS

Histopathologically, the lesions in the endobronchial submucosal layers were classified into such two groups as the localized and diffuse type. From the tomographical and bronchographical findings, polypoid filling defects, some thickening of the bronchial wall and smoothly outlined stricture of the bronchial lumen were characterized in the localized type. The diffuse type presented the diffuse thickening of the bronchial wall and smooth narrowing of the bronchial lumen in a wide length. In comparison with the pathological findings of the biopsied bronchial tissues, these radiographical findings are responsible for the amount of cell infiltrations, edema and the interstitial fibrous reactions in the submucosal layers.
As a rule, these radiographical findings are more striking in the malignant lesions. Thus they can be helpful to determine the localization and extent of the submucosal lesions in the bronchi and also to assess the treatment planning.

REFERENCES
1. Stolberg, H.O.: Hodgkins disease of the Lung. Roentgenologic-pathologic Correlation AJR, 92: 96, 1964.
2. Schoenbaum, S.: Subepithelial endobronchial Metastases, Radiology, 101: 63, 1971.
3. Shibayama, M., Matsui, E., Miyake, H., : Endobronchial malignant Lymphoma and its Roentgenologic considerations, Jap. J. of chest diseases, 37: 275, 1974.

X.8.

TRANSBRONCHIAL BIOPSY OF PERIPHERAL LUNG CANCER USING FLUOROSCOPIC GUIDANCE

DUMON Jean-François, MD[+], BALDOCCHI Gilbert, MD[+], MERIC Bernard, MD[+],
REBOUD Eugène, MD[++], and GARBE Louise, MD[+++]

Out of a total of 320 biopsies using fluoroscopic guidance, we selected 100 cases of peripheral lung cancer controlled by thoracotomy. Each case corresponds to one endoscopic examination.

Our histological classification is grouped under three headings :
- squamous cell carcinoma
- adeno-carcinoma
- small cell carcinoma and indifferenciated

In the third group we united small cell carcinoma and indifferenciated carcinoma, because there is a small number of peripheral tumors of this type.
All of these fiberscopies are realised in the same way.
The patient lies on the side that corresponds with the location of the biopsy.
The fluoroscopic surveillance is made by a mobile apparatus that shows a bidimentional view without moving the patient. This position allows for the control of an eventual bleeding.

The total results of the biopsies follow :   (table I)

ENDOSCOPICALLY INVISIBLE CANCER OF THE LUNG

	N	positive cases	%
squamous cell	48	36	75
adenocarcinoma	41	19	46.3
small cell and indifferenciated	11	6	54.3
TOTAL	100	61	61

+ Service endoscopie thoracique
  Hôpital Salvator
  BP 51-13274 MARSEILLE CEDEX 2

++ Service chirurgie thoracique
   Hôpital Salvator
   BP 51 13274 MARSEILLE CEDEX 2

+++Service anatomie pathologique
   Laboratoire Professeur PAYAN
   C.H.U TIMONE - MARSEILLE -

J.A. Nakhosteen and W. Maassen (eds.), Bronchology: Research, Diagnostic and
Therapeutic Aspects. All rights reserved.
Copyright 1981. Martinus Nijhoff Publishers bv, The Hague / Boston / London

During the same period we were able to study 257 visible tumors and had the following results : (table II)

ENDOSCOPICALLY VISIBLE TUMORS

	N	positive biopsies	%
squamous cell	171	165	96.5
adenocarcinoma	43	30	69.7
small cell and indifferenciated	43	38	88.3
TOTAL	257	233	90.6

Out of 357 cancers studied in our unit, 100 were endoscopically invisible (28 % of the cancers).

In other words, without biopsy under fluoroscopic guidance, 61 tumors out of 357 would not have been able to be diagnosed (17 %).

The results follow (Table III)

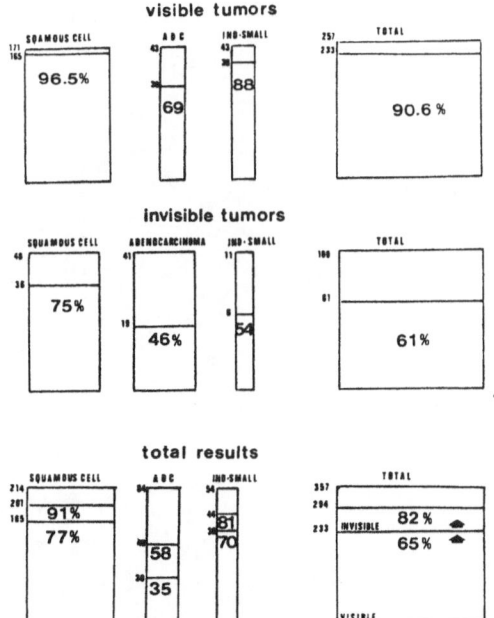

One notices ^the relative rise of adenocarcinoma in the peripheral tumors.
The quality of the results depends on three factors : the histological type, the
size of the tumor and its topography.

1. THE HISTOLOGICAL TYPE

The results are best in the squamous cells carcinoma 75 % of the squamous cells
have a positive result with only one examination.
The results are mediocre with the adenocarcinoma. This is explained by the factor of
the extrabronchial topography of the tumor (43.6 %).
The results for the small cells and undifferenciated carcinoma are slightly better,
however smaller in number (54.3 %). The 3 observations of small cells carcinoma were
all positive.

2. THE SIZE OF THE TUMOR obviously influences the results

(Fig. 1)

Table IV

Size of the tumors

			N	positive cases	%	chances of success
tumors	<	2.5 cm	33	14	42.4	1/2
tumors	>	2.5 cm	67	47	70.1	2/3

b1 rul 1/3   b1+2 lul 1/3

rul 1/2   lul 1/2

ll+rml 2/3   chances of success lll 2/3

• < 2.5 < ● < 4 < ⬤
cm

3. THE TOPOGRAPHY considerably modifies the chance of success.
The areas with the most difficult access are the apical superior right upper lobe
and the apico posterior left upper lobe (fig. 1)

incidents or accidents
The accidents noted during these examinations appear in
table V : complications of transbronchial lung biopsies

pneumothorax	bleeding ($>$ 50 ml)
2/320 (0.62 %)	12/320 (3.16 %)

SUMMARY

The study of 100 perpheral lung cancers having undergone a transbronchial biopsy
using fluoroscopic guidance give a total result of 61 % positive cases in the first
examination. The results are better in the squamous all carcinoma (75 %), in the
tumors larger than 2.5 cm (70 %) and the tumors located outside of the apical lobe.
The accidents are rare : out of 320 transbronchial biopsies, we note 2 pneumothorax
and 12 moderate bleedings.

358

X.9.

TRANSBRONCHIAL LUNG BIOPSY: PERSONAL EXPERIENCE WITH RIGID AND FIBEROPTIC
APPARATUS *

M. Freitas e Costa, J. Ruas da Silva, A. Teles de Araújo – Lisbon – Portugal.

In the Department of Lung Diseases in Lisbon Medical Faculty, we frequently use
lung biopsies, both by transthoracic or transbronchial route, in order to obtain
sufficient data on a large amount of pathologic situations.
This work summarizes our experience with transbronchial lung biopsies using
either the rigid or fiberoptic apparatus.

Material and Methods :
Our experience is based on 257 transbronchial lung biopsies performed upon 247
patients aged between 1 and 78 years old. Main incidence is in the fifties (in
about 25% of all patients).
Two hundred and twelve biopsies were performed with rigid bronchoscope and 45
with fiberoptic; two hundred and sixteen in diffuse lesions and 41 in localized
lesions.
We used rigid Storz bronchoscope with Broyle's flexible biopsy forceps of 2 mm
diameter. With it, inferior lobes, medium lobe and lyngula were easily attainable. Superior lobar biopsies were much more difficult to get because of forceps
angulation.
For fiberoptic lung biopsies (with the bronchoscope always passed through the
nasal route) we used Olympus BF-IT with the largest channel and forceps.
In patients with diffuse pulmonary lesions the zone of biopsy was choosen accor_
ding to the radiologically richest region, and preferentially where we suspected
of pleural symphisis, in order to minimize pneumothorax risk.
In majority of patients, biopsy was performed under radiological control and was
repeated when necessary or if the general macroscopic observation could lead to
suppose the non existence or scarcity of lung tissue.

Results :
Our results are summarized in the Table I. Their analysis shows that with the

---

* Centro de Investigação CnL 3 – I.N.I.C. – Lisbon – Portugal.

J.A. Nakhosteen and W. Maassen (eds.), Bronchology: Research, Diagnostic and
Therapeutic Aspects. All rights reserved.
Copyright 1981. Martinus Nijhoff Publishers bv, The Hague / Boston / London

rigid bronchoscope, technical rentability and absolute diagnostic rentability were, in all, of 79,1% and 63,6%. We want to stress that this technique revealed itself as more useful when applied in patients with diffuse pulmonary lesions in whom we obtained technical and absolute diagnostic results respectively 82,9%, 68,6%.

T A B L E   I

TRANSBRONCHIAL LUNG BIOPSIES

TYPE OF LESIONS	BRONCHOSCOPE	NUMBER OF PATIENTS	NUMBER OF BIOPSIES	R E N T A B I L I T Y	
				TECHNICAL	ABSOLUTE
Localized	Rigid	15	18	38,8 %	16,6 %
	Flexible	23	23	85,0 %	65,0 %
Diffuses	Rigid	187	194	82,9 %	68,6 %
	Flexible	22	22	65,0 %	40,0 %
TOTAL	Rigid	202	212	79,1 %	63,6 %
		247	257		
	Flexible	45	45	75,0 %	50,0 %

From our experience with the fiberbronchoscope, we can observe that the method results where, in general, worse (technical rentability 75% and absolute rentability 50%), but specially useful in localized lesions.

This situation is presumably due to our short experience with this last apparatus and to the smaller dimensions of forceps and tissue obtained with this technique. Reversely, complications were less frequent with the fiberscope (9,1%) than with rigid apparatus (19,1%) mainly concerning pneumothorax (11,2% for rigid bronchoscope and 2,4% for fiberscope).

No lethal complications were reported and the only major problems to cope with were hemorrhage and pneumthorax (Table II).

T A B L E   II

COMPLICATIONS OF TRANSBRONCHIAL LUNG BIOPSIES

BRONCHOSCOPE	PNEUMOTHORAX	BLEEDING	AIR EMBOLISM	DEATH	T O T A L
Rigid	11,2 %	8,1 %	0	0	19,3 %
Flexible	2,4 %	6,7 %	0	0	9,1 %

Discussion and Conclusions :

The problems in obtaining precise diagnosis in pneumology mainly in diffuse lung lesions, justify, in our opinion, all efforts in order to get a correct ethiolo gic definition. Histologic confirmation is, in most cases, fundamental. This is only possible through a lung biopsy.

Transbronchial lung biopsy offers an important alternative to open lung or trans thoracic biopsy. This last one, in our experience, is more productive, but in reserve, leads to more frequent severe complications.

In this connection, the preference for the transbronchial biopsy seems logic. In our's and others' experience its rentability is sufficient and the possible complications become less severe, more scarce and more easier to cope with.

Transbronchial lung biopsy through the use of the fiberscope, as in comparison to the rigid bronchoscope, has some advantages: smaller incidence of complications and easier acessibility to most lung zones, besides the known acceptabili ty for the patients. These facts are decisive in choosing the fiberscope to perform lung biopsies as it seems to be an easily appliable technique which enables us to diagnose a great number of pathologic processes specially in diffuse lung lesions without many risks.

REFERENCES :

1. Araujo, A.D.T.: Biópsia pulmonar transbrônquica - Dissertação de Licenciatu-
   ra. - Lisboa, 1967.
2. Freitas e Costa, M.: Biópsia pulmonar transbrônquica e transtorácica - Expe-
   riência de 334 biópsias. - Pneumologia 2: 163, 1971
3. Zavala, D.: Transbronchial biopsy in diffuse lung disease. - Chest 5 (Supl.)
   727-733, 1978.
4. Andersen, H.: Transbronchoscopic lung biopsy for diffuse pulmonary diseases
   (Results in 939 patients). - Chest 5 (Supl.) 734-736, 1978.
5. Poe e coles.: Sensivity and specificity of the nonspecific transbronchial
   lung biopsy. - Amer.Rev.Resp.Dis. 119-25-31, 1979.

BRONCHO-ALVEOLAR LAVAGE AND TRANSBRONCHIAL LUNG BIOPSY WITH FLEXIBLE FIBEROPTIC BRONCHOSCOPE

X.10.

S. VALENTI, C. MEREU, P. CRIMI, A. SCORDAMAGLIA

Since 1978 we started in combining broncho-alveolar washings (B.A.L.) and transbronchial lung biopsy (T.B.L.B.) in the course of the same fiberbronchoscopy. We called this technique, in which lung biopsy is performed after broncho-alveolar wash, "pulmonary luobiopsy" (from the ancient greek verb λυω which means to wash). With this method it is possible to obtain and study various lung specimens (biopsies from T.B.L.B., cells and biochemical compounds from B.A.L.). These are very useful for a more definite diagnosis in many diseases and especially in diffuse pulmonary fibrosis which are biologically characterized by an increasing of interstitial collagen and also a variable proliferation of connective cells (e.g.: macrophages, lymphocytes, fibroblasts and leuco-cytes) in interstitial septa and in alveoli.

In order to evaluate the diagnostic results from associated bronchos-copy, B.A.L. and T.B.L.B. in diffuse interstitial lung diseases we applied these investigations during the same fiberbronchoscopy in a group of 67 patients showing radiological and functional features of diffuse interstitial pulmonary fibrosis.

METHOD

We investigated 67 informed and consenting patients: 32 sarcoidosis, 8 hypersensitivity pneumonitis (H.P.), 5 idiopathic pulmonary fibrosis (I.P.F.), 4 miliary tuberculosis, 12 pneumoconiosis, 1 drug-induced fibrosis (copper-sulphate), 2 alveolar microlithiasis, 2 collagen diseases (R.A.), 1 idiopathic pulmonary hemosiderosis. Preanesthesia, local anesthesia and bronchoscopy with Olympus BF-B3 were performed as previously reported (Valenti S. et coll., 1979). B.A.L. was performed as follows: The tip of fiberoptic bronchoscope was wedged in the lateral segmental bronchus of the middle lobe; 100 ml of sterile saline solution were infused into the broncho-pulmonary segment and then aspirated by a light

J.A. Nakhosteen and W. Maassen (eds.), Bronchology: Research, Diagnostic and Therapeutic Aspects. All rights reserved.

suction after 30 sec. This procedure was repeated twice. Centrifugation at 500 g x 15' was performed. Sediment was washed twice in Hank's solution and then cells were resuspended and counted. T.B.L.B. was performed as follows: the tip of fiberoptic bronchoscope was usually wedged in the anterior segmental bronchus of right upper lobe and a 5 ml bolus of epinephrine 1:20,000 was injected into this airway. T.B.L.B. was then performed under fluoroscopic control as previously reported (Valenti e Scordamaglia, 1978).

RESULTS AND DISCUSSION

We found on the specimens from T.B.L.B.: in sarcoidosis interstitial fibrosis in 19 cases (59%), sarcoid granuloma in 18 cases (56%) and small arteries lesions in 1 case (3%); in I.P.F. interstitial fibrosis in 5 cases (100%), alveolar desquamation in 4 cases (80%) and interstitial inflammation in 3 cases (60%); in H.P. interstitial granuloma in 3 cases (38%), interstitial fibrosis in 7 cases (90%), small arteries and bronchioli fibrosis in 6 cases (75%). The total number of recovered cells from B.A.L. is increased especially in H.P. and I.P.F. when compared with healthy controls (Tabl.1). Lymphocytes in H.P. and neutrophilis in I.P.F. are prevalently responsible for this alveolar hypercytosis. In sarcoidosis the increase in mean percentage of lymphocytes is not statistically significant owing to variability of studied patients. So we divided sarcoid patients in relation to the stage and to the activity of the disease (Tab.2). The total number of cells increases in advanced and in active stages; nevertheless the increase of lymphocytes in percentage is statistically significant only in active stages.

TABLE 1. BRONCHO-ALVEOLAR CELLS

		total cells x10^6 ($\overline{X}$±DS)	macr.% ($\overline{X}$ + DS)	lymph.% ($\overline{X}$ + DS)	neutr.% ($\overline{X}$ + DS)	eosin.% ($\overline{X}$ +DS)
Controls	n. 6	6.2+ 2.2	83.5+ 6.3	13.3+ 5	2.5 + 1.4	< 1
Sarcoidosis	n.32	16.6±10.7*	71.5±21.5	26.3±21.7	< 1	< 1
H.P.	n. 8	24.2+ 5.7***	39.1±17.1***	56.3±18.3***	2.75+ 2.25	1.75±1.3
I.P.F.	n. 5	23.5+ 5.9***	57.8±13**	11.4+ 4.6	26.6 ±16.6*	2.2 ±2.9

Statistical significance (*,** ,***) of the single groups of patients versus healthy controls was evaluated by Student's test.

TABLE 2.   B.A.L. IN SARCOIDOSIS

	total cells x10^6 ($\bar{X}$+DS)	macr.% ($\bar{X} \pm$ DS)	lymph.% ($\bar{X} \pm$ DS)	neutr.% ($\bar{X} \pm$ DS)	eosin.% ($\bar{X} \pm$ DS)
I Stage n. 5	9.4+ 3.2	82.2+ 6.2	15.8+ 5.7	1 + 1	1 + 1
II Stage n.16	17.6+11.2 *	65 +24.4	32.4+25	< 1	< 1
III Stage n.11	18.3+11.6 *	74.6+20.2	22.8+18.8	< 1	< 1
Active n.16	21.9+11.3 **	60 +13.9 *	37.8+22.6 **	1.9+1.3	< 1
Inactive n.14	9.6+ 4.1	86.2+ 6.3	11.4+ 4.7	< 1	< 1

Statistical significance (*,** ,***) of the single groups of patients versus healthy controls was evaluated by Student's test.

In the patients affected by miliary tuberculosis we found a statistically significant increase of cells total number (32.8 x 10^6 cells) with lympho-cytes percentage increase (53.5% $\pm$ 23.9).

In pneumoconiosis we did not find statistically significant changes; nevertheless we found a total cells and neutrophilis percentage increase in some patients. Moreover some specific histochemical stains for B.A.L. cells or for biopsy specimens from T.B.L.B. showed to be very useful in diagnostic accuracy of particular diseases (e.g., in one case of "wine-spread lung", Okamoto-Tahamura stain showed copper-sulphate in almost all macrophages; Von Kossa and Perls stains showed to be useful respevtively in "alveolar microlithiasis" and in pulmonary hemosiderosis).

The majority of diffuse lung fibrosis follow the arrival of air poluters in alveoli. In this situation local immunological defence mechanisms are triggered so that many types of inflammatory cells can accumulate in alveolar spaces. Persisting inflammatory stimuli involve septal connective tissue with consequent fibroblast activation and production of great amounts of collagen fibres.

The structure of septa, interstitial connective tissue and vessels is well revealed in the small specimens obtained by T.B.L.B. Interstitial fibrosis was the most frequent finding observed on the specimens from T.B.L.B. in our casuastry, not only in I.P.F. but also in sarcoidosis, where sarcoid granuloma was found only in 56% of cases. This percentage of 56% differs from other authors' results. These differences of incidence of sarcoid granuloma are probably due to different stages of the diseases and also to the type of forceps employed. Nevertheless, in some patients it is impossible to study in detail alveolar cells as specimens from T.B.L.B. are too small. In these cases B.A.L., washing a lot of alveoli, allows us to recover millions of alveolar cells.

Alveolar hypercytosis is a common feature in the active stages of these diseases and testifies the arrival of inflammatory cells in alveoli as reported by Reynolds and Merryl (1979). The increase of a single alveolar cell type may correlate with the disease's etiology so that we can find an alteration of the alveolar cell ratios which, in healthy subjects, are usually as follows: 85-90% macrophages, 10-15% lymphocytes, small amounts of neutrophilis and eosinophilis.

In active stages of H.P. and sarcoidosis there are more lymphocytes such as in fibrosis following miliary tuberculosis and mycosis as reported by Niaudet et coll. (1979). In idiopathic pulmonary fibrosis neutrophiles prevail.

Moreover in sarcoidosis the amount of the increase of alveolar lymphocytes correlates to the degree in activity of the disease so that lymphocytes increase in active stage and decrease in remission stage. Reynolds and Merryl (1979) reported the same behavior regarding to neutrophiles in I.P.F..

Our results, according to those reported by other authors, prove the validity of broncho-alveolar cells study which provides useful data for diagnostic etiology and also allows to follow diseases development and therapeutic treatment.

Chapter XI

FURTHER DIAGNOSTIC PROCEDURES

XI.1.

ADVANCED BRONCHOGENIC CARCINOMA – CONTROL OF THERAPY BY BRONCHOSCOPY

N. NIEDERLE, J.A. NAKHOSTEEN, W. MAASSEN, S. SEEBER

INTRODUCTION

In small cell bronchogenic carcinoma, the results best achieved through chemotherapy are in inoperable but locally limited disease (1,4). Through aggressive induction therapy, either with or without subsequent radiotherapy, complete remission (CR) rates between 40 and 100 % are obtained. The mean life expectancy can thus be extended, from 3 months in untreated patients to 10 - 20 months. The percentage of long-time survivors or complete cures remains small, however, a major reason for this being local recurrence, re-fractive to therapy (4).

In order to reduce this rate of local relapse, a more thorough defini-tion of complete local remission is needed than that obtained through clini-cal and radiological means only. In addition to tumor marker profiles, bron-chofiberoptic serial examinations are well suited for this purpose (1, 2, 3). These examinations seem all the more important when one considers that the efficacy of localised radiotherapy and/or maintenance doses of cytostatica following remission induction has yet to be proven.

MATERIALS AND METHODS

All patients with small cell, bronchogenic carcinoma, who are not suf-fering from cardiac disease, are treated according to the "ACO II plus RT" protocol (Fig. 1) . Initially, cytostatica are administered four times, at intervals of three weeks. These consist of Adriamycin, 60 mg/m^2 i.v. on day one; Cyclophosphamide, 750 mg/m^2 as 1-hr infusion on days 1 and 2; and Vin-cristin, 1.5 mg i.v. on days 1, 8 and 15.Following the second course, pro-phylactic brain radiation with 30 Gy is given; after the second course, a consolidating radiotherapy of mediastinum, hilum and core of tumor with 30 Gy is also administered.

Pre-therapeutic staging includes endoscopic photography by bronchofiber-scopy. The bronchofiberscope (Model BF-6C, Olympus) has an extra large fiber-

J.A. Nakhosteen and W. Maassen (eds.), Bronchology: Research, Diagnostic and Therapeutic Aspects. All rights reserved.
Copyright 1981. Martinus Nijhoff Publishers bv, The Hague / Boston / London

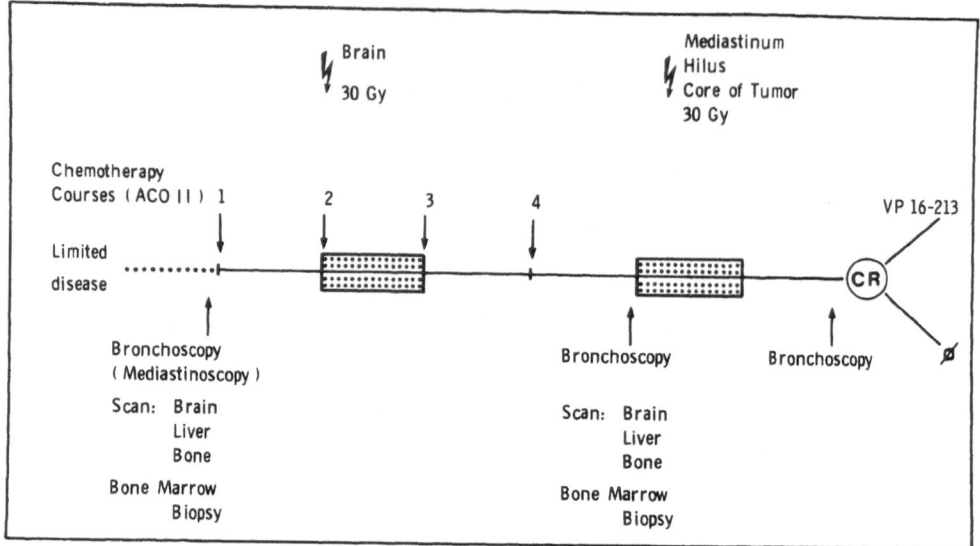

Fig. 1.   Small cell lung cancer; limited disease; treatment protocol including bronchofiberoptic
assessment of therapeutic success.

optic bundle which gives excellent endoscopic resolution (Fig. 3 and 4), but
a small internal channel of 0.8 mm diameter. The small channel allows instillation of local anesthetic and aspiration of secretions, but for biopsies a
second instrument must be used. Photographs are taken with an endoscopic
camera (Model OM-2, Olympus), fitted with a special magnifying objective-
adaptor (Model SM 4-S, Olympus). Histological verification is either through
bronchoscopy or mediastinoscopy.

After the fourth course of therapy, if complete remission is seen roentgenographically, revised staging is undertaken and bronchofiberscopy with
biopsy and photography performed. If either macroscopic or histologic residual tumor is proven, localized radiotherapy is administered. Following this,
before randomization for a maintenance dose of VP 16-213, another bronchofiberscopy is performed. All bronchoscopies were done by one examiner(J.A.N.).

RESULTS

To date, a total of 26 patients were evaluated as described (Fig. 2).
Four showed partial remission roentgenographically, residual tumor still evident in the chest film. All four were endoscopically and histologically tumor-
positive.

Radiographic complete remission was obtained in 22 (67 %) with limited
disease. Of these, 18 (82 %) showed complete remission endoscopically. Sten-

osing Tumor, initially evident, was no longer seen on control bronchoscopy, and histology was also negative (Fig. 5a and 5b).

Frequently, considerable scar tissue is evident at the tumor site following therapy, but although these lesions may be macroscopically tumor-suspect, they are usually histologically negative (Fig. 6 and 7).

In contrast, one patient, in whom macroscopically no tumor was seen, was proven histologically tumor-positive. In three further cases, residual tumor was seen macroscopically and histologically confirmed. Three of these were given radiotherapy and were shown to be in complete remission on further bronchofiberscopy.

n = 26		
	Partial Remission (n)	Complete Remission (n)
Chest x-ray (after 4xACO)	4	22
Bronchofiber-scopy (after 4xACO)	4	18
Bronchofiber-scopy (after 4xACO plus RT)	–	21

Fig. 2. Results of bronchofiberscopic assessment of of 26 patients. Following induction chemotherapy (4 x ACO), four were in partial remission and 22 in complete remission.

CONCLUSIONS

1. Exact definition of complete remission can be obtained by bronchofiberoptic assessment; the method well-tolerated, and, being virtually devoid of complications, very safe.

2. In 18 % of patients thus assessed to date, the endoscopic examination gave information on tumor status not obtained from the chest film alone. As a result further therapy, i.e., radiation, became necessary.

3. A third bronchofiberscopy following additional localized irradiation of only 30 Gy showed macroscopic remission, confirmed histologically.

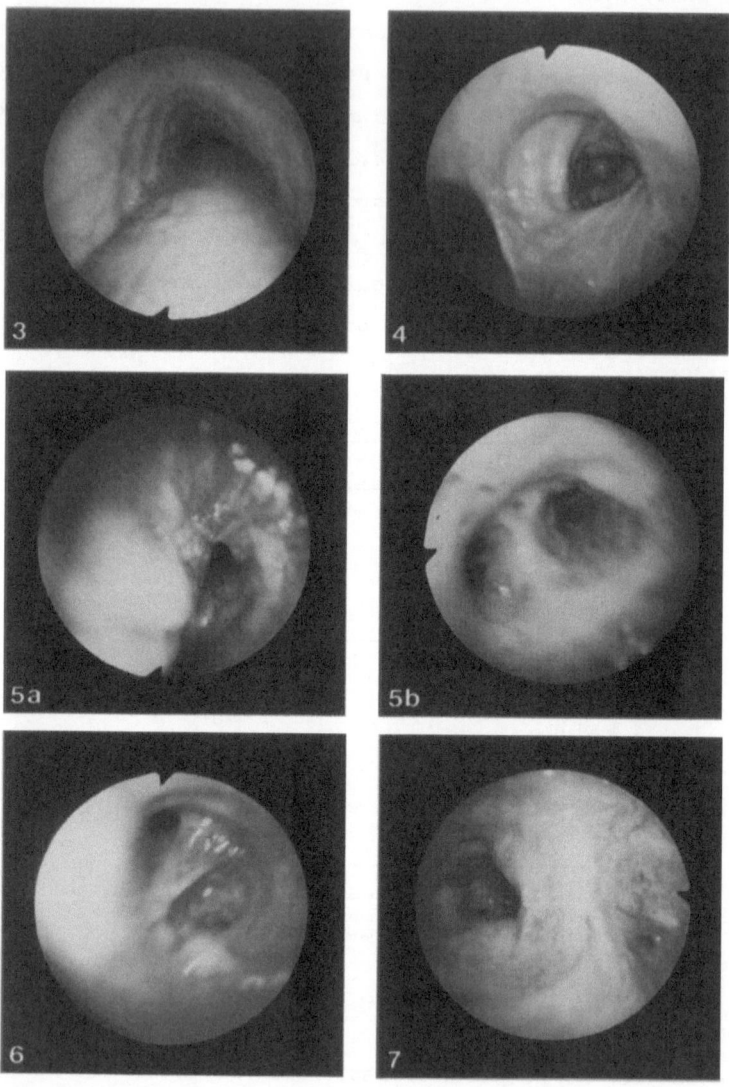

Examples of resolution of photographic system here described. Fig. 3 shows trachea of chronic bronchitic during expiration. Fig. 4 shows suspected lymph node metastatic compression of medial wall of right main stem bronchus. Small cell carcinoma of distal left main stem bronchus before (5a) and after (5b) induction therapy: complete remission.
Residual scar tissue in lingula bronchus (Fig. 6) and right upper lobe bronchus (Fig. 7) of patients in remission following induction therapy.

XI.2.

ANGIOTENSIN CONVERTING ENZYME ACTIVITY IN THE COURSE OF CYTOSTATIC TREATMENT
OF INOPERABLE BRONCHOGENIC CARCINOMA

I.Heck , N.Niederle , W.Bierbaum , G.Fricke , F.Krück ,   FRG

1. INTRODUCTION

Angiotensin Converting Enzyme (ACE) is an ectoenzyme of the endothelial layer
of all vessels and occurs in significant concentrations in lung tissue , because of the large surface of the pulmonary vascular bed.The enzyme cata-
lyses the conversion of Angiotensin I (A I) in Angiotensin II(A II) and the
degradation of Bradykinin as is expressed by the synonym Kininase II.
A further source of the enzyme are the epitheloid cells of the granulomas in
Sarcoidosis. This is of importance , if one intends to interpret the alterations in ACE-activity in serum in etiologically different lung diseases.
It is easy to imagine , that the metabolic function of the lung as concerns
A I conversion and inactivation of Bradykinin , is dependent on the quantity
or mass of functionally active lung tissue , e.g. the surface of the endothelial cells in the pulmonary capillaries. If these cells are reduced by
any reason , ACE-activity of the lung as a whole should be lowered. This
work should elucidate whether an alteration of total ACE-activity caused by
lung resections and bronchogenic carcinoma , is reflected by a simultaneous
change in ACE-activity i.s. and whether lowered ACE-activity i.s. of bronchogenic carcinoma is reversible under cytostatic treatment.

2. PROCEDURE
2.1. Material and methods

2.1.1. We compared ACE-activities i.s. before and after segment and or lobe
resections of different etiology, mainly benign tumors and injuries.
2.1.2. Furthermore we measured ACE-activities i.s. of 27 patients with inoperable small cell carcinoma of the lung under cytotoxic treatment. The
patients were staged as "limited disease" and were treated with a cytotoxic
drug combination of VINCRISTINE , ADRIAMYCINE and CYCLOPHOSPHAMIDE or CIS-
PLATINUM. To determine ACE-activity , blood samples were taken every three
weeks prior to treatment over a period of maximally 3o weeks. The clinical
course was followed up by thoracic X-ray, laboratory parameters and bronchoscopic evaluations.
2.1.3. ACE-activity was estimated by radioimmunological measurement of A II
using A I as substrate($1 U = pg A II 1o/ul^{-1} 1o min^{-1} 2.5 ng A I^{-1}$).

*J.A. Nakhosteen and W. Maassen (eds.), Bronchology: Research, Diagnostic and
Therapeutic Aspects. All rights reserved.*
Copyright 1981. Martinus Nijhoff Publishers bv, The Hague / Boston / London

3. RESULTS

The 12 patients ungergoing segmental or lobar resection showed significantly lowered ACE levels as compared to pre-operative values (Fig. 1*). The reduction was on average 31.7 %.

55 patients suffering from bronchogenic carcinoma showed initially significantly lowered ACE levels compared to normal values (Fig. 2*).

27 patients with small cell carcinoma under cytotoxic treatment showed a continuous rise in ACE activity during period of therapy in observation, i.e. 15-30 weeks (Fig. 3*). This rise was statistically significant compared to pretreatment values ($p < 0.05$ week 6, 0.05 week 9, 0.025 week 12, 0.01 week 15); the further rise up to week 24 was not significant due to the small number of patients observed.

In order to rule out the possibility that ACE activity could be influenced directly by cytotoxic drugs, we compared ACE values of patients immediately before and after cytotoxic treatment. All patients received different drug combinations and suffered from various neoplastic diseases. The results were equivocal. Most patients had a small but insignificant rise and 2 patients had slightly lowered ACE values (Fig.4*).

4. SUMMARY AND CONCLUSIONS

It may be summarized that significant changes in ACE activity in the course of cytotoxic treatment can only be found if there are definite changes in ventilation by regression of tumor mass. A normalization of ventilation by disappearance of atelectases is accompanied by a normalization of ACE activity in serum. Thus measurement of ACE activity in serum is possibly a useful parameter in the follow-up of cytotoxic treatment of bronchogenic carcinoma. It may describe the effectiveness of treatment, but further study is necessary to evaluate the sensitivity of ACE activity in serum to detect early relapse of the disease.

---

*For Figures 1-4 please see following 2 pages. Ed.

FIGURE 1. Comparison of ACE Activity before and after Lobar/segmental
Resections in 12 Patients.

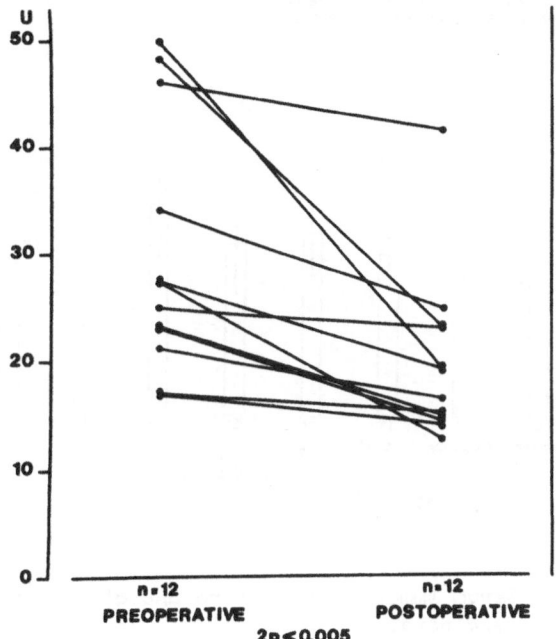

FIGURE 2. ACE Activity in Serum of 32 Normal Individuals and of 55 Patients
with Bronchogenic Carcinoma.

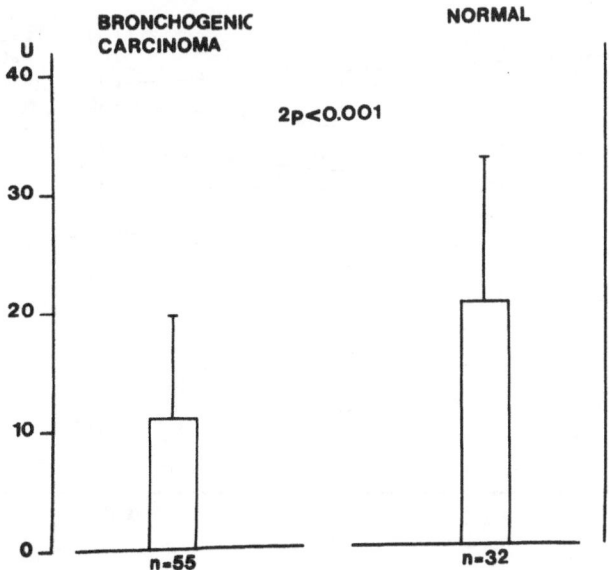

FIGURE 3. ACE Activity in Serum of 27 Patients with Inoperable Bronchogenic Carcinoma in the Course of Cytostatic Therapy.

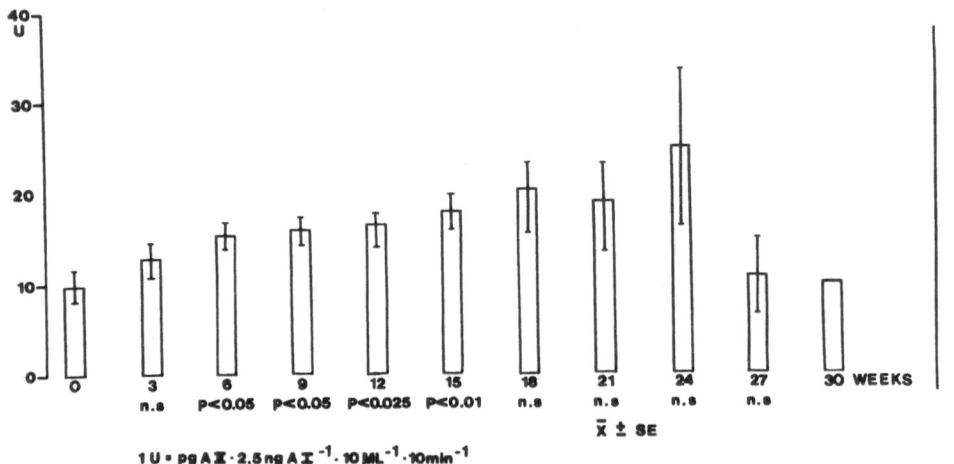

FIGURE 4. ACE Activity in Serum Immediately before and after Cytotoxic Treatment in various Neoplasms.

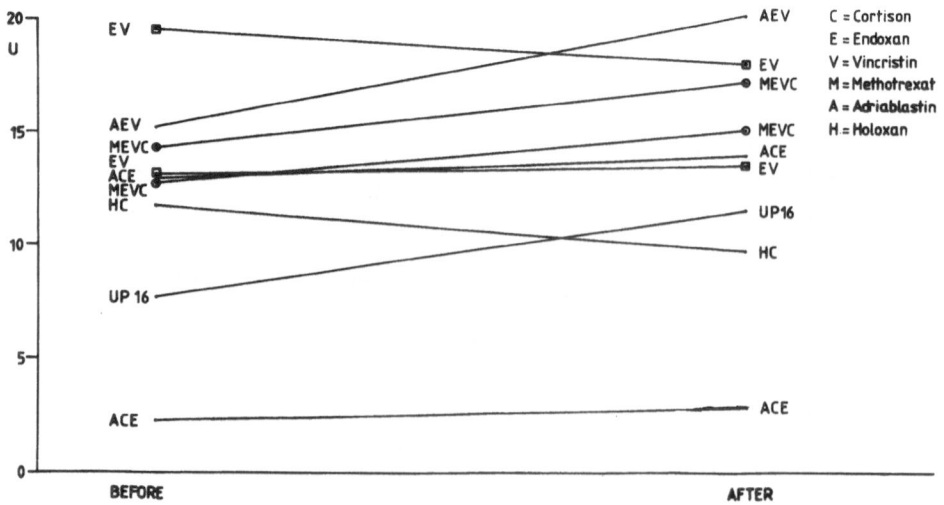

XI.3.

IMMUNOGLOBULINS IN PATIENTS WITH EVIDENCED BRONCHOGENIC CARCINOMA

VEROSLAVA MARKOVIĆ-VUKOVIĆ
I. PILIŠ
M. MOVSESIJAN

Immunological reactivity of the organism to tumorous tissue is manifested by humoral and cellular immune response. Usual approach to the study of these immunological manifestations does not give satisfactory results. However, some recent examinations with regard to the quantitation, determination and isolation of specific antibodies offers a better basis for the study of specific immunological response in an adequate way (4).

The investigations that were dedicated to the immunoglobulins in the course of some cancerous diseases gave information about quantitative changes of immunoglobulins in the circulation of patients (1, 3).

Materials and methods

The sera and broncholavates were collected from 24 patients with evidenced bronchial malignoma - 13 planocellular and 11 microcellular. Isolated sera and broncholavates were kept at -20°C, and bioptic material at +4°C. Quantitative determination of serum and broncholavate IgG, IgA and IgM was performed in RID plates. Qualitative determination of immunoglobulin was performed by the fluorescent antibody test on bioptic mucous material.

Results

On determination of immunoglobulin concentration in serum and broncholavates of patients with planocellular or microcellular bronchogenic carcinoma, it could be established that the concentration of immunoglobulin in serum approximated within the limits of normal values except for the IgA which showed a slight tendency of increase.

Total immunoglobulins in broncholavate of planocellular carcinoma amounts to 30,89 mg/100 ml, while microcellular amounts to 9,98 mg/100 ml broncholavate. On analysing the distribution of individual classes of immunoglobulin in serum and broncholavate it can be con-

cluded, on the basis of serum immunoglobulins, that there is no difference between patients with planocellular and microcellular bronchogenic carcinoma, except for the distribution of IgA in broncholavate
from patients with microcellular carcinoma which is somewhat increased (Table 1).

TABLE 1. Distribution of immunoglobulins in broncholavate and in
serum - per cent

CA	Lung	Broncholavate			Serum		
		IgG	IgA	IgM	IgG	IgA	IgM
Plano-cellular	D	57,7	39,2	3,1	73,5	22,2	4,3
	N	51,7	48,3	0,0			
Micro-cellular	D	30,6	63,5	5,9	73,7	21,7	4,6
	N	36,4	60,2	3,4			

D = diseased   N = normal

The results obtained show that the local IgA synthesis is present
in the case of both forms of carcinoma. Also by fluorescent antibody
test in bioptic material from both diseased and normal bronch, the
presence of IgA and IgG, especially IgA is proved. Using the methodological study by Johansson and Deuschel (2), on the basis of our results in lavate and serum, we can establish that IgA/IgG ratio in lavate is considerably higher than the same value in serum, which indicates the different level of the local IgA synthesis (Table 2).

TABLE 2. Concentration quotient of IgA and IgG ratio in broncholavate
and in serum

CA	Lung	IgA/IgG in lavate IgA/IgG in serum
Plano-cellular	D	2,27
	N	3,10
Micro-cellular	D	7,17
	N	5,69

Regarding the fact that IgA/IgG ratio in serum of both groups of patients is nearly identical, differences established in Table 2 show that the local IgA synthesis is higher in microcellular than in planocellular carcinoma.

Discussion

The quantity of immunoglobulin in broncholavate of microcellular carcinoma is 3 times lower if compared with findings in planocellular one, while the difference between lavate obtained from altered and non-altered bronch in this form of malignoma was not established.

Moreover, in the total quantity of immunoglobulins which are present in lavate, dominant part in the case of planocellular are IgG and in microcellular IgA.

The IgA/IgG ratio indicates to this fact showing that the local synthesis is present in all examined cases, and the results presented in Table 2 give the bounds of the level of local IgA synthesis. Data obtained for serum immunoglobulins are in agreement with the results of some other authors (1, 3), while the examinations of local synthesis gave more information about damages of bronchial micosis and its ability for local synthesis.

References

1. Hughes, N. R.: Serum concentrations of IgG, IgA and IgM immunoglobulins in patients with carcinoma, melanoma and sarcoma. Journal of the National Cancer Institute, 46, 1015-1027, 1971.

2. Johansson, S. G. O., and Deuschel, H.: Immunoglobulins in nasal secretion with special reference to IgE. I Methodological studies. Ins. Arch. Allergy, 52, 364-475, 1976.

3. Krant, M. J., Manskopf, G., Brandrup, C. S. and Madoff, M. A.: Immunological alterations in bronchogenic cancer. Cancer, 21, 623, 1968.

4. Paluch, E. and Ioachim, L. H.: Lung carcinoma reactive antibodies isolated from tumor tissues and pleural effusions of lung cancer patients. Journal of the National Cancer Institute 61, 319-325, 1978.

XI.4.

SCANNING ELECTRON MICROSCOPY AND ENERGY-DISPERSIVE X-RAY MICROANALYSIS OF
TRANSBRONCHIAL LUNG BIOPSY IN PATIENTS WITH FIBROTIC LUNG DISEASE.

H. KRONENBERGER, K. MORGENROTH, J. MEIER-SYDOW, L. SCHMIDTS and S. TUENGERTHAL

Fiberoptic transbronchial lung biopsy is known as a safe and useful method for
the investigation of diffuse interstitial lung disease. In comparison with open
lung biopsy it is preferable because of lower risk and lower costs. However the major disadvantage of this method is the difficulty of histological interpretation of
the small particles, even if multiple biopsies are obtained. In some diseases which
show a typical tissue pattern, for instance lymphangiosis carcinomatosa or sarcoidosis, this method offers a high diagnostic yield. Especially in fibrotic lung lesions however the pathologist may be unable to differentiate between a diffuse fibrosis and a focal fibrotic scar. In general, the smaller the particles and thus
the less representative the biopsy specimens are, the more clinical information is
needed for a definite diagnosis. One has to consider the whole spectrum of interstitial lung diseases, especially those caused by exogenious noxi (2).

For assessing exogenous anorganic noxi in biopsy specimens a new method has recently become available: energy-dispersive x-ray microanalysis (3). With this technique one does not only detect particles and gaines information of their type and
structure, but also can determine their chemical composition. Furthermore the topo-
graphical relation between dust deposits and local tissue reaction enables us to
assess pathogenesis of that very lesion. It should be mentioned that the method in
discussion can be performed on usual paraffin embedded material and on unstained
histological sections (3). This paper presents   three case-histories illustra-
ting the diagnostic value of energy-dispersive x-ray microanalysis performed on
transbronchial lung biopsies.

Case 1: 35 year-old male. Diagnosis: hard-metal fibrosis.

This patient was a volunteer in a study group for the early recognition of occupational pneumoconiosis in dental technicians (1). No symptoms, active in competition
sports. Six years occupied as a dental technician, formerly as a bricklayer and roo-
fer. Physical examination and pulmonary function tests are normal. Chest x-ray shows
only minimal reticulo-nodular pattern.

The histologic section of transbronchial lung biopsy reveals a few thickened alveolar walls with only sparse histiocytic infiltration. No dust deposits are visible
by light microscopy. In the scanning electron microscopy however (Fig. 1A, 1B) many
particles located between collagen fibers could be detected. Line-scan (Fig. 1B)

J.A. Nakhosteen and W. Maassen (eds.), Bronchology: Research, Diagnostic and
Therapeutic Aspects. All rights reserved.
Copyright 1981. Martinus Nijhoff Publishers bv, The Hague / Boston / London

superimposed on the dust deposit identifies silicon as a component. The energy-dispersive spectrum (Fig. 1C) reveals the chemical composition consisting of aluminum (20%), silicon (13%), chromium (20%), cobalt (29%) and traces of phosphorus, sulfur, potassium, calcium and iron.

Interpretation: It is probable, that the dust deposits in the focal fibrotic lesions are caused by occupational exposure as a dental technician. Because of the high concentrations of chromium and cobalt we believe that these hard metals are the causative agents. Since there are only small areas of fibrosis lung function and chest x-ray are essentially normal.

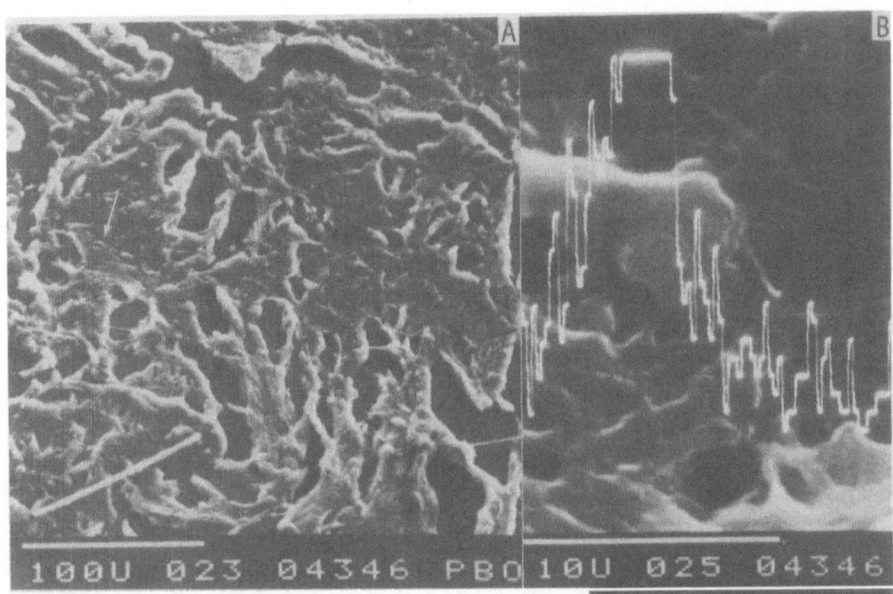

Fig.1: Scanning electron microscopy and energy-dispersive microanalysis on histologic sections.

A: Variably thickened alveolar septa with anorganic deposits (arrow).
Original magnification: x 212.

B: Higher magnification of the same dust particle. Superimposed line-scan reveals silicon concentration of anorganic material.

C: Energy-dispersive spectrum of the dust deposit showing its composition of aluminum, silicon, phosphorus, sulfur, potassium, calcium, chromium and cobalt.

Case 2: 32 year-old male. Diagnosis: early asbestosis.

This patient is also a dental technician working in his profession for 15 years. He complains of mild exertional dyspnea. Physical findings and lung function tests are totally normal. Again in this case the chest x-ray reveals only a delicate interstitial infiltration. Pleural thickenings and calcifications are not visible.

In transbronchial lung biopsy only scattered infiltration of lymphocytes and monocytes and variable amounts of anthracotic pigments are found. In scanning electron microscopy some macrophages can be recognized containing fibers highly suspicious for asbestos. The energy-dispersive spectrum demonstrates the usual composition pattern of asbestos.

Interpretation: Scanning electron microscopy and x-ray microanalysis identify asbestos fibers in lung macrophages, even though clinical findings as well as radiograph and lung function tests are almost completely normal. A detailed environmental history revealed occupational exposure to asbestos used for coating of denture moulds.

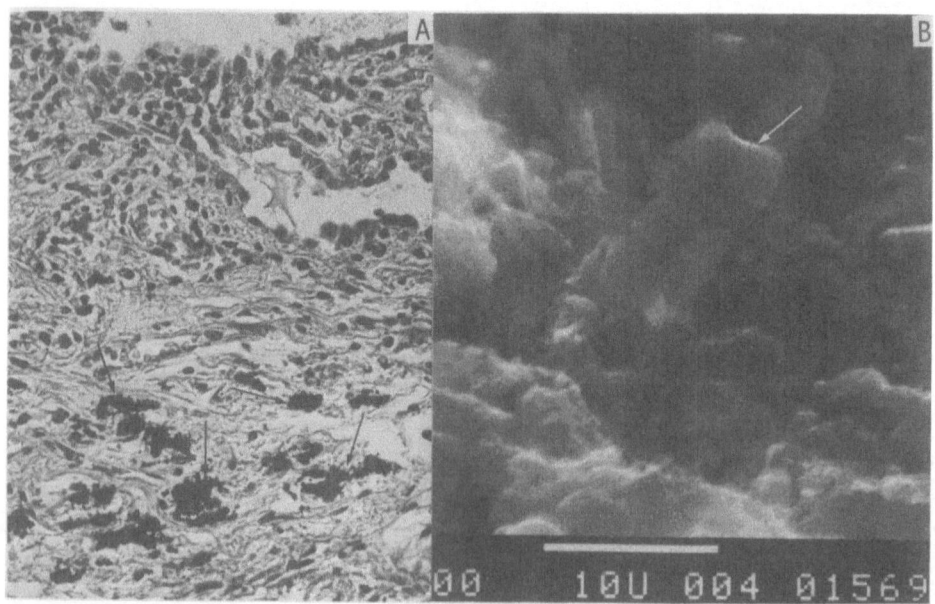

Fig.2: Histologic section of transbronchial lung biopsy specimen (Case 3).
A: Light micrograph showing fibrosis of alveolar walls with anthracotic
   pigments (arrow).
   Original magnification: x 250.
B: Scanning electron view of a fractured uncoated asbestos fiber within
   a fibrotic lesion.
   Original magnification: x 2000.

Case 3: 65 year-old male. Diagnosis: advanced pulmonary fibrosis.

For two years chronic dry cough, for two months increasing dyspnea on exertion. For 20 years occupied in a factory for plastic products. Physical findings of pulmonary fibrosis. Pulmonary function tests show considerable restriction (VC 58% of predicted normal), but no obstruction. Arterial oxygen tension at rest in the lower physiological range. The chest x-ray demonstrates a coarse reticulo-nodular pattern with honeycombing more pronounced on the right side. In addition pleural plaques and calcifications are seen on the chest wall and on the diaphragm.

Transbronchial lung biopsy (Fig. 2A) shows an advanced state of fibrotic lung disease with several dust deposits. Additionally obtained open lung biopsy provided no further information. Scanning electron microscopy (Fig. 2B) demonstrates fibers of variable size some of them fractured located within fibrotic tissue. Also in this case energy-dispersive microanalysis identified the fibers as asbestos.

Interpretation: On the base of light microscopy this case was originally regarded as idiopathic pulmonary fibrosis, although the history was suggestive for an occupational lung disease. Only with the new methods described multiple uncoated asbestos fibers could be detected, thus revealing the correct diagnosis of asbestos induced diffuse pulmonary fibrosis.

In conclusion:

1. Transbronchial lung biopsy is frequently indicated in cases with minimal radiological pathology as demonstrated in patient 1 and 2.
2. Transbronchial lung biopsy is even indicated in patients with normal radiology but with a clinical suspicion of pulmonary disease.
3. The definite diagnostic yield of transbronchial lung biopsy can be augmented by additional evaluation by scanning electron microscopy and x-ray microanalysis.
4. Using these new techniques it is possible to recognize details not detectable by conventional methods providing **increased** knowledge about etiology of diffuse interstitial lung disease.
5. Furthermore the morphological relation between the dust deposits and local tissue reactions gives a deeper insight into pathogenesis.

XI.5.

PERTRACHEAL PNEUMOMEDIASTINOGRAPHY

C. Šimeček

1. INTRODUCTION

Diagnostic pneumomediastinography is not far a method of routine examination. The reasons for this state of affairs are:

1) Unknown value of this method of investigation
2) Antagonistic reports on the results obtained by various authors
3) A number of various methods of gas insufflation as a sign of the effort of avoiding some disadvantages inherent in many of them.

In our department we started with pneumomediastinographic examinations some 27 years ago, using the method of retrosternal route of Condorelli and paravertebral method of Paolucci Giacobini (ref.1). Using these methods about each 5th examination was not successful. For this reason we developed an original method of pertracheal insufflation used in the last 25 years almost exclusively.

2. METHOD

Gas insufflation is performed after the termination of routine bronchoscopic examination with bioptic, cytologic, bacteriologic and other procedures. Only the instillation of radioopaque substances for bronchography is done after gas insufflation. A special needle is necessary because of prevention of complications, particularly in some malformations.

On the average 230ml oxygen was used for insufflation, the amount of oxygen was only exceptionally lower than 200ml and higher than 350ml. If pneumomediastinum was combined with pneumoperitoneum or with radioopaque visualisation of the oesophagus, these procedures were done after the bronchoscopic tube had been removed.

3. RESULTS

In the last 25 years we performed 2674 pneumomediastinograph-

J.A. Nakhosteen and W. Maassen (eds.), Bronohology: Research, Diagnostic and
Therapeutic Aspects. All rights reserved.
Copyright 1981. Martinus Nijhoff Publishers bv, The Hague / Boston / London

ic examinations. In 102 procedures the gas insufflation was combined with bronchography, and in 48 with radiopaque investigation
of the eosophagus. Pneumomediastinography was combined with pneumoperitoneum in 26 patients. No complications were observed. Failure due to technical reasons occurred in 0.7%, mostly in cases
of the first attempts by doctors in training.

TABLE 1. Diagnostic pneumomediastinography

Carcinoma of the lung	1171
Carcinoma of the oesophagus	58
Lymph nodes sarcoma	144
Lymph nodes sarcoidosis and tuberculosis	422
Sarcoidosis and tuberculosis of the lung	104
Mediastinal tumours benign	232
malignant	16
Cardiovascular diseases	71
Other pathological conditions	566
Total	2784

As shown in the table, pneumomediastinographic examinations
were mostly indicated for mediastinal lymph nodes visualisation.
In one of our previous studies (Ref.2) we have shown some qualitative and quantitative differences in the pictures of enlarged mediastinal lymph nodes which enable to differentiate, with
some probability, the cause of the enlargement.

Direct invasion of lung cancer into the mediastinum may be
evident, but especially in carcinoma of the oesophagus it is
already not easy to differentiate direct cancer invasion from
inflammatory reaction.

In mediastinal tumours it was possible to visualize the
state, localisation and relationship to the mediastinal structures. As shown in cases of thymomas, we were not able to distinguish benign and malignant thymomas by this examination. But
we succeeded with correct diagnosis in cases of malignant lymph-
ogranulomas arrising from the thymus, where the diagnosis was
confirmed after tumor extirpation.

They are no problems with correct appreciation of some abnormalities, as right aortic arch and megaazygos.

4. DISCUSSION

Pertracheal pneumomediastinography is a simple method of investigation without any risk of complications. It gives much important
information especially in preoperative investigation of lung carcinoma and mediastinal tumors. No less instructive is it in differential diagnosis of intrathoracic lymph nodes enlargements, where
it may be very important in localising lymph nodes before diagnostic
puncture aspiration. For these reasons the pertracheal pneumomediastinography becomes a routine method of clinical investigation in our
department.

REFERENCES
1. Šimeček,C.: Diagnostic Pneumomediastinography, Dis.Chest 1968,
   53, 24.
2. Šimeček,C.: Der Wert des diagnostischen Pneumomediastinums in
   der Differenzierung der intrathorakalen Lymphknotenschwellungen.
   Prax.Pneumol. 1974, 28, 698.

XI.6.

ABNORMAL CHEST ROENTGENOGRAM INDUCED BY BRONCHIAL INVOLVEMENT-BRONCHIAL
CAST SHADOW -

Y. OHSAKI, S. ABE, K. KIMURA, Y. TSUNETA, H. MIKAMI, AND M. MURAO.

INTRODUCTION

Bronchi are visible in the lung field radiologically in various conditions. One special condition manifesting abnormal shadow due to bronchial involvement is the replacement of the air in the bronchi by water-dense material. This type of abnormal shadow has several characteristic features, such as beeing Y or W shaped, pointing its tip toward the hilum, and fanlike distribution, because the abnormalities are based on bronchi themselves. Until recently, only two water-dense materials which produce abnormal shadow were known, namely mucus and pus. When bronchial secretion is retained and inspissated in the bronchial lumen, bronchial mucocele and mucoid impaction is the term applied for this condition. These cases are seen in bronchial atresia, allergic broncho-pulmonary aspergillosis, bronchial stenosis. Mucus retention is also caused by complete bronchial obstruction in bronchogenic carcinoma. When bronchial secretion is infected, such as in bronchiectasis and mucoviscidosis, bronchial pyocele is used for this condition, and glovedfinger or tooth-paste shadow is the roentgenological expression. Recently, we experienced cases with abnormal shadow due to impaction of cellular component in the bronchi and blood retention in the bronchial lumen.

CASE PRESENTATION

Cellular impaction of the bronchi.

Patient was a sixty year old male who complained of haemoptysis. There was a mass shadow in the right mid-lung field connected with the hilum. Bronchogram showed complete obstruction of the apical and anterior segmental bronchi of the right upper lobe, and there were rod-like shadows radiating from the mass shadow. Cut surface of the lung reveals tumor mass in the anterior segment, and also arborized tumor growth intrabronchially like gloved finger. Microscopic examination revealed that the cell type of tumor was small cell carcinoma of intermediate type. Area of intrabronchial growth of the tumor showed tumor cell impaction within the dilated bronchi which had otherwise normal architecture. We named this condition as cellular impaction of the bronchi.

*J.A. Nakhosteen and W. Maassen (eds.), Bronchology: Research, Diagnostic and
Therapeutic Aspects. All rights reserved.
Copyright 1981. Martinus Nijhoff Publishers bv, The Hague / Boston / London*

Bronchial hasmocele

Chest X-P of a fifty-three years old male who complaines of coughing spitting blood showed slight mottling in the right lung field. Bronchography revealed insufficient filling of the contrast media in the anterior bronchus. There was rod-like shadows distal to the obstructive lesion. Bronchoscopic examination revealed coagulation material obstructing the opening of the anterior bronchus of the right upper lobe. After several bouts of hemoptysis during admission, abnormal shadow cleared up completely. The second bronchography showed comlete filling of the contrast media in the bronchus occuluded previously, and no abnormalities of the bronchial structure were demonstrated. Bronchial mucus membrane was also within normal limits endoscopically.

SUMMARY (TABLE 1)

We presented four water-dense materials which could make abnormal shadow in the lung field replacing the air in the bronchi. Cellular impaction of the bronchi and bronchial haemocele are new normenclature and new entity which produce abnormal shadow.

Abnormal shadows induced by mucus or pus retention, cellular impaction and blood retention in the bronchi appear as the same pattern in the chest roentgenologically, so that differentiation of its nature is impossible. Various terms are used to describe these radiologic appearance, such as gloved-finger or tooth-paste shadow, mucus bronchography, bronchial mucocele, and mucoid impaction, although the same type of roentgenographic shadow is treated. From our experience, we propose " BRONCHIAL CAST SHADOW " as an integrated term to express radiologically these abnormal shadows induced by replacement of the air in the bronchi by any water-dense material.

Table 1.

Summary of Nomenclature for Bronchial Cast Shadow

Roentgenologic Expression	Pathogenesis		Condition of Intra-bronchial Material
Bronchial Cast Shadow Including Gloved Finger Shadow Tooth-Paste Shadow Mucus Bronchography	Retention of Following Material in the Bronchi (As general term : Bronchocele)		When inspissated or impacted
	Mucus	Bronchial Mucocele	Mucoid Impaction
	Pus	Bronchial Pyocele	
	*Blood	Bronchial Haemocele	
	*Cell	Bronchial Cytocele	Cellular Impaction

*New entity and nomenclature of bronchial pathology which makes abnormal shadow

XI.7.
A BRONCHOLOGICAL APPROACH TO THE REGIONAL FUNCTION INVESTIGATION

C. Šimeček

1. INTRODUCTION

Using an apparatus of original construction we get excellent regional spirometric curves without air pollution by isotopes. Since the mixed venous blood has in all the pulmonary capillaries the same CO_2 concentration, and the alveolar P_ACO_2 is determined by the ratio $\dot{V}_A\dot{Q}_c$, it is also possible to estimate the regional perfusion independent of radiopharmacs.

2. METHOD

In the course of a bronchoscopic or fiberbronchoscopic investigation we are recording endexpiratory CO_2 concentrations in the trachea, main and lobar bronchi by means of a rapid responding analyzer. If necessary a diagram for regional $\dot{V}_A\dot{Q}_c$ ratio determinations is used.

Present differences in endexpiratory CO_2 concentrations enable to calculate directly, from capnograms, also the regional ventilation after the following example:

$$\frac{\text{Right lung}}{\text{ventilation}} = \frac{CO_2 \text{ in the trachea} - CO_2 \text{ in the left bronchus}}{CO_2 \text{ in the right bronchus}}$$

3. RESULTS

In this study 100 capnographs are analyzed. They have been made in 92 patients in the last two years. In 6 patients the investigation was repeated, in one of them four times altogether.

Indication for regional capnographs was motly the presumption of pulmonary embolism or investigation before a surgical treatment. The third large group are such pathological conditions as lung fibrosis, diaphragmatic paralysis and congenital malformations, where disturbances of regional function have to be supposed.

In the group of 18 patients with pulmonary embolism, the correct diagnosis was confirmed in 14 patients by autopsy or, if typical clinical pictures were present, by angiography or by scintigraphy. With the exception of rider embolism CO_2 concentration was decreased by 0.5% in all these cases at least.

Differences in regional CO_2 concentrations exceeding 0.5%

J.A. Nakhosteen and W. Maassen (eds.), Bronchology: Research, Diagnostic and
Therapeutic Aspects. All rights reserved.
Copyright 1981. Martinus Nijhoff Publishers bv, The Hague / Boston / London

were not frequently found in other pathological conditions. The
greatest was seen in one of two investigated lobar emphysemas with
hypoplasia of truncus intermedius despite of expressive diminution
of regional ventilation. One of 17 lung carcinomas had decreases
regional CO_2 concentration as expression of malignant infiltration
of the pulmonary artery.

Certain diminution of CO_2 concentration was found practically
in all patients after lobectomy likewise as in lobar atelectasis,
for example in bronchial adenomas, where in the same time increased
CO_2 concentration in the upper lobe of the opposite lung is considered for a sign of pulmonary hypertension, confirmed in one of the
patients. Normalization of these conditions were observed after
tumour extirpation.

4. DISCUSSION

Clinical determination of pulmonary embolism is very difficult.
The regional capnography is not dependent on radiopharmacs, is econ-
omic and, from the point of view of air pollution, advantageous in
comparison with the xenonradiography. Regional capnography present
more accurate information on the regional $\dot{V}_A\dot{Q}_c$ ratio as that obtained by conventional xenonradiography. It represents a step in the
perfectioning of the clinical diagnostics. But it is neccessary to
keep in mind all the status where the regional CO_2 concentration
can be lowered and, in the diagnosis of pulmonary embolism, to interpret regional capnograms in connection with x-ray examinations
and anamnestic data.

XI.8.

THE VALUE OF PERFORATING THE CUSPS OF BIOPSY-FORCEPS

SVEN BORGESKOV & HENNING JENSEN

One of the problems in making diagnosis in patients with carcinoma of the lung has been the difficulty of obtaining sufficient material for the histological evaluation.

With the increasing interest and value of non-surgical treatment it has become even more necessary to get the type of the actual tumor.

By the aid of the flexible bronchoscope it is now possible to get biopsies from tumors localized in the upper lobes and even rather peripheral in the lungs.

The small diameter together with the flexibility of the instrument gave us this possibility, but it is not always easy for the pathologist to make an accurate diagnosis on the very tiny bits obtained with the biopsy forceps.

The literature mentions that a fenestration of the cusps of the biopsy forceps gives larger and better biopsies (Nozawa & Kinoshita, 1978 and Matsui et al., 1978).

It was the aim of the present investigation to see if the fenestrated biopsy forceps really was superior in the daily work of the surgeon and the pathologist.

Own series

In the present series two sizes of biopsy forceps were used, one designed for the Olympus BF-B3, the other for the 1T model. The biopsy channels measure 2.0 and 2.4 mm i.d. respectively, and the forceps have been used in a usual closed cusp fashion and in a fenestrated cusp model the fenester measuring 1 mm in the small and 1.8 mm in the large forceps (Fig. 1).

100 biopsies were taken for histological examination and evaluation. In each patient biopsies were taken with the four different forceps models.

The biopsies were evaluated according to the following criteria:

1) Absolute size

2) The presence of stroma in the preparations

3) The suitability of the preparations stated by the pathologist.

Re point 1) After cutting the whole biopsy into slices 4-5 micron thick, the largest specimen was selected. The measurement was performed in the microscope and the area calculated in sq.mm.

Re point 2) The presence of stroma in the microscopic slide was noted as

J.A. Nakhosteen and W. Maassen (eds.), Bronchology: Research, Diagnostic and Therapeutic Aspects. All rights reserved.
Copyright 1981. Martinus Nijhoff Publishers bv, The Hague / Boston / London

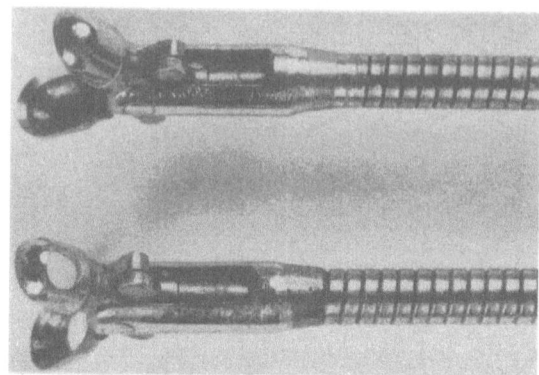

Fig. 1. Usual and perforated model af biopsy forceps.

plus og minus, thus making it possible to compare directly the value of the biopsies.

Re point 3)   For evaluation of the suitability of the biopsy the following groups were used:

Very satisfactory: Large biopsy where the epithelium measures more than 1.6 mm (which equals two arbitrary units in the microscope) in the direction parallel to the surface. There must not be any traumatized areas, and the biopsy must include sufficient amount of stroma to make it possible to exclude tumor invasion.

Satisfactory: This is a smaller biopsy than the very satisfactory one, but the size is not decisive if there is just enough epithelium to make the material representative. Furthermore it is necessary to have enough subjacent stroma to exclude invasive growth. It is acceptable that the slicing is a little oblique, but it must not be tangential to the surface. A minor traumatized area can be tolerated.

Less satisfactory: Mainly small superficial biopsies often with traumatized areas. Often the slicing is oblique or tangential making an evaluation of tumor invasive growth very difficult. The possibility for basal cells and superficial cells of being placed near each other because of tangential slicing of the biopsy can simulate dysplasia.

Not acceptable: This biopsy is very small, superficial and not representative. Very often it is traumatized and the cutting direction is so that it will be wrong to express an opinion on the slide.

Results

With the small forceps the biopsies measured in Mean 1.69 sq.mm (S.D. 0.89), and with the corresponding, fenestrated type 1.64 sq.mm (S.D. 1.28).

The large forceps gave the following results: 2.20 sq.mm (S.D. 1.58) and 2.84 sq.mm (S.D. 1.45) for the ordinary and the fenestrated type respectively.

The difference was not statistically significant.

Neither was there any significant difference in the presence of stroma in the biopsies taken with forceps with and without fenestrated cusps. For the small forceps the frequency of stroma rose from 36 to 48 per cent, when the cusps were perforated. In the large model the increase was from 60 to 68 per cent.

With different ways of calculating the results, the increase in biopsy size by fenestrating the cusps of the biopsy forceps is 15 to 30 per cent respectively for the two forceps sizes.

A statistical analysis shows, however, that it is not possible to demonstrate any significant increase. The apparent discrepancy is due to the excessive influence of a few very large biopsies on the result expressed in per cent.

THE RELATIONSHIP BETWEEN LUNG CANCER TUMORS AND THE BRONCHIAL MUCOSA
IN RELATION TO HISTOLOGIC TYPE -- BASED ON BIOPSY SPECIMENS OBTAINED
VIA THE FIBEROPTIC BRONCHOSCOPE
XI.9.

K. Oho, R. Amemiya, N. Hayashi, T. Kawauchi, K. Nagai

Different histologic types of lung cancer display different types
of development, and therefore show different characteristics on X-ray
and endoscopy. One factor related to the different clinical appearance
is the relationship between the tumor and the bronchial mucosa. In o-
ther words, the findings greatly differ according to whether the tumor
grows replacing the bronchial epithelium or whether it proliferates submucosally. When the ciliated epithelium is replaced by carcinoma the
cilial transport mechanism is disturbed, which greatly affects the clinical appearance.

We examined the relationship between the lung cancer tumor and the
surrounding bronchial wall in 199 cases of primary lung cancer and 10
cases metastatic to the lung. These cases consisted entirely of those
in which biopsy provided viable information as to the condition of the
border of malignant and normal findings.

Figure 1 shows the border of a squamous cell carcinoma lesion in
which the carcinoma has replaced the bronchial epithelium. In Fig.2
oat cell carcinoma proliferates primarily beneath the bronchial mucosa,
breaking through the epithelium on the right. Adenocarcinoma, shown in
Figs 3 and 4, is frequently observed proliferating beneath the mucosa.
Macroscopically, the edge of squamous cell carcinoma lesions is generally easily recognizable, (Fig. 5). The oatcell carcinoma in Fig. 6 was
very small, only 1.3x 0.6 cm. It grew completely covered by the bronchial mucosa. The endoscopic appearances of the different histologic
types also display various tendencies. Early stage squamous cell carcinoma exposed in right B^2b is shOwn in Fig. 7. Small cell carcinoma
proliferating beneath the bronchial mucosa typically appears as shown
in Fig. 8. Analysis of our results (Table 1) showed that squamous cell
carcinoma tends to replace the epithelium, completely exposed in the
lumen, especially in central type cases. This reflects the common
roentgen findings of inflammatory change and atelectasis.[1,2] In other
words, movement of bronchial secretions is impaired due to the loss of

J.A. Nakhosteen and W. Maassen (eds.), Bronchology: Research, Diagnostic and
Therapeutic Aspects. All rights reserved.

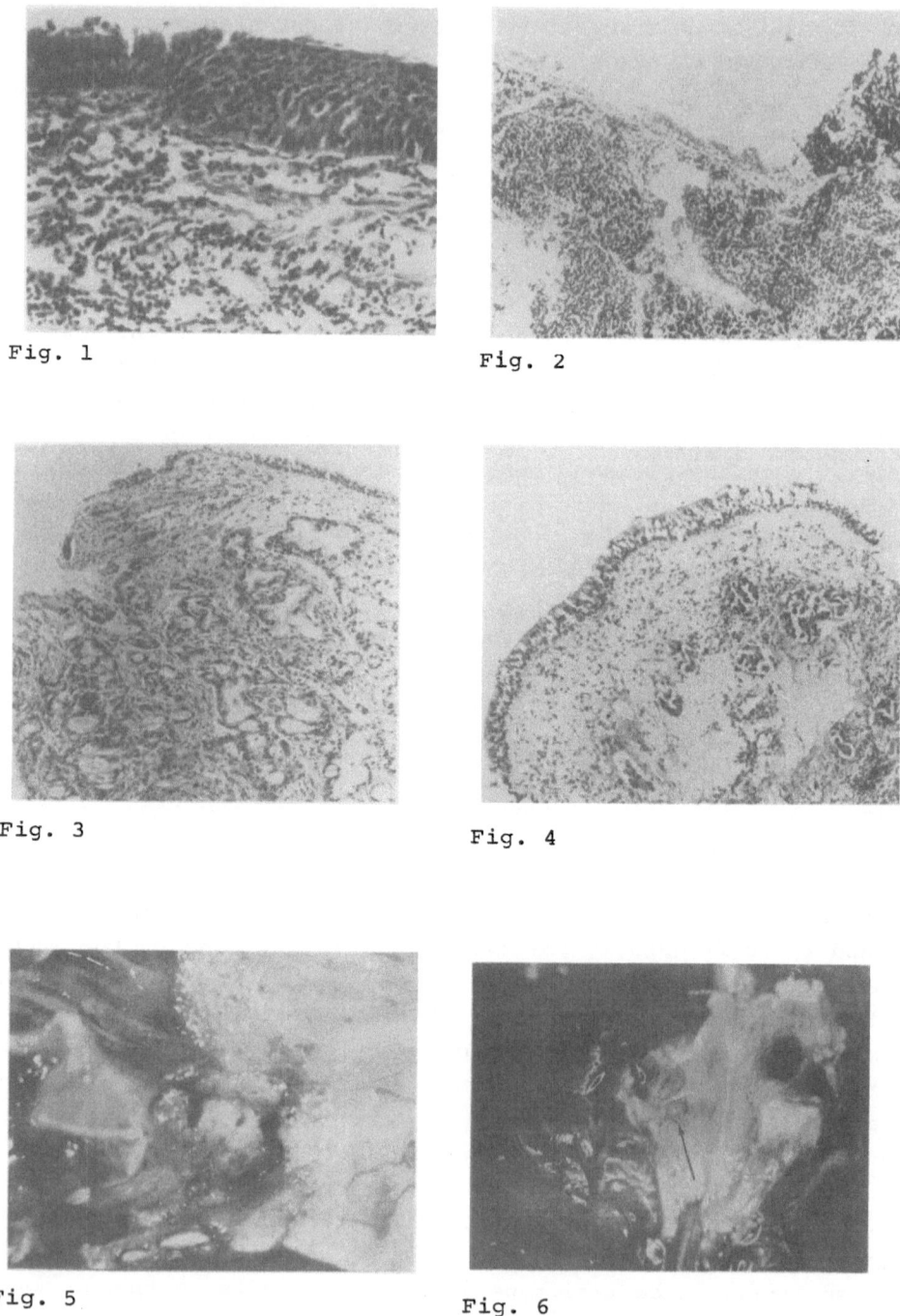

Fig. 1

Fig. 2

Fig. 3

Fig. 4

Fig. 5

Fig. 6

ciliated epithelium, while bleeding from the tumor contaminates surrounding mucosa. Mucus accumulates and secondary changes appear. The
reason it is more difficult to detect secondary changes in small cell
carcinoma, adenocarcinoma and large cell carcinoma is because they tend
to proliferate submucosally,[3] and the epithelium covering the tumor thus
retains its cilia, which allows sufficient transport of secretions.

While it may be difficult to recognize the presence or absence of
mucosa by fiberoptic bronchoscopy, examination of the blood vessels can
serve as an indicator, thus providing a suggestion as to histologic
type. Knowledge of the tendencies of the various histologic types is
essential for accurate evaluation of findings.

REFERENCES

Ikeda S, ed. Atlas of early cancer of major bronchi, Tokyo, Igaku
Shoin, 1976

Woolner LB, David E, Fontana RS, Anderson HA, Bernatz PE, In situ and
early invasive bronchogenic carcinoma, J. Thorac. Cardiovasc. Surg.,60
275-290, 1970

Oho K, Amemiya R, Practical Fiberoptic Bronchoscopy, Tokyo, Igaku
Shoin, 1980

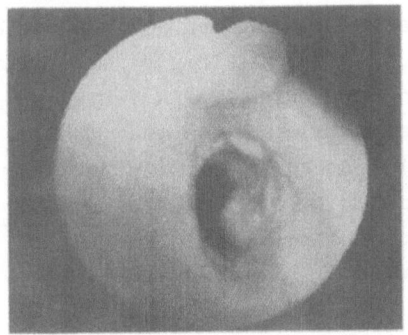

Fig. 7

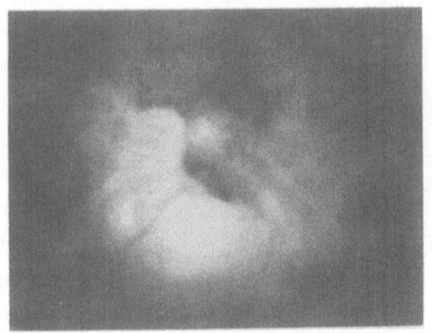

Fig.8

Table 1

**THE CONDITION OF THE TUMOR EXAMINED OF THE BASIS
OF BIOPSY SPECIMENS OBTAINED BY FIBEROPTIC BRONCHOSCOPY**

Histological type	Condition	Tumor completely exposed in bronchial mucosa	Tumor partially exposed, partially submucosal	Totally submucosal	Unclear	Total
SQUAMOUS CELL CA.	Hilar type	41	16	0	0	57
	Peripheral type	12	6	6	2	26
SMALL CELL CA.	Oat cell type	0	2	11	3	16
	Intermediate cell type	5	4	7	2	18
	Unclassified	0	0	3	1	4
ADENOCARCINOMA		6	11	48	5	70
LARGE CELL CARCINOMA		0	2	3	3	8
METASTATIC LUNG CA.		1	4	3	2	10
Total		65	45	81	18	209

Tokyo Medical Collage. (1977. 1 ~ 1979. 5)

XI.10.
STUDIES ON THE VITAL BRONCHIAL LYMPHODRAINAGE IN MAN WITH LYMPHOSCINTIGRAPHY - NEW DIAGNOSTIC TECHNIQUE

ENJO HATA, M. D. , T. Hasegawa, M. D.

Regional bronchial lymph drainage in the living individual poses still many controversies. This subject have been pursued by lympho-scintigraphy with the aid of fiberoptic bronchoscope and colloidal radionuclide. The tracer was injected into the submucosa of each segmental bronchus with specially designed fine needle under bronchoscopy. Hourly node scanning was repeated for six hours after initial injection.

As the preliminary work, the following two investigations were attempted.
1. Selection of suitable colloidal radio-nuclide.
2. Proof of accumulation of radionuclide in the regional lymphnode.

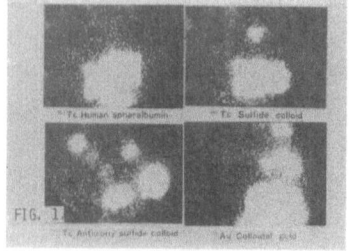

FIG. 1.

As shown in Fig. 1., examination of the adequate size of the radiocolloid particles were carried out with rabbit. Four different sized radioactive colloids were injected into the bilateral abdominal rectus muscles subcostally, six hours after injection, drainage rate of the injected agents was calculated. (Fig. 1. shows the results;) ^{99m}Tc sulfide colloid, 0.5 to 2u in particle size, 10 to 20% the injected sites and one parasternal lymph node are demonstrated, ^{99m}Tc Antimony sulfide colloid, 4 to 12mu in particle size, 30 to 50% the injected sites, parasternal and axillary lymph nodes are seen, colloidal radiogold, 3 to 5mu in particle size, 30 to 60% the injected sites and parasternal lymph nodes are seen. When ^{99m}Tc Antimony sulfide colloid or colloidal radiogold were used, lymph nodes were clearly demonstrated. Aside from clear visualization, safety of the living person is of prime importance in this procedure.

Therefore, from above mentioned results, ^{99m}Tc Antimony sulfide colloid was selected to be the most favourable agent for the purpose this study.

The segmental and sub-segmental bronchial submucosa were selected for suitable injection sites for the following reasons: (1) Lymphatic channels are well developed. (2) The injection sites can be exactly visualized via the fiberoptic bronchoscope.

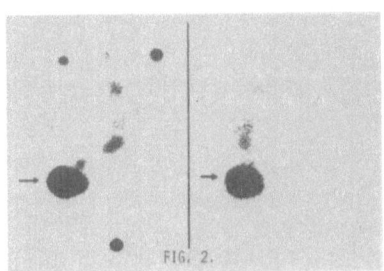 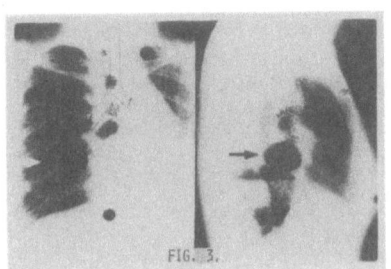

Fig. 2. The actual pictures of lymphoscintigram. In the left picture, around the edge there are two 'hot' figures. These are the marks located on the clavicles, and the lowest 'hot' figure is also the mark on the xiphoid process. The arrow indicates the injected site. The other 'hot' figures are regional lymph nodes. On the right picture the lateral image is demonstrated. Two 'hot' figures around the right edge are the marks located on the sternal angle and the xiphoid process. The arrow also indicates the injected site. The other 'hot' figures are lymph nodes.

Fig. 3. Shows lymphoscintigrams superimposed on the chest X-ray films.

To prove accumulation of radionuclide in the regional lymph nodes, after submucosal injection of colloidal nuclide of each segmental bronchus, 141 regional lymph nodes and surrounding fatty tissues were resected in 7 patients during thoracotomy and in 6 by mediastinoscopy, respectively. Radioactivities of each material collected were counted with the well counter. High degree uptake of radionuclide were confirmed in the lymph nodes along the presumed passway of lymphatic flow from the each segmental bronchus. As for the fatty tissue, though they were located very closely to the lymphatics which indicated a very high count, they indicated lower, and the result of the blood was much lower than the lowest activities of the lymphatics.

In order to determine the normal lymphoscintigram, 160 lymph node scannings were carried out with this new technique in 142 patients with neither hilar nor mediastinal lesions at Nakano National Chest Hospital from May 1976 through December 1979. In order to establish the reproducibility and reliability of the technique, 18 patients were studied with dual lymphoscintigrams. And we could confirm the complete reproducibility.

Table 1. Numbers of cases

Right	B^1	B^2	B^3	B^4	B^5	B^6	B^7	B^8	B^9	B^{10}	Total
Cases	7	6	10	9	7	5	6	7	6	10	73
Left	B^{1+2}_{a+b}	B^{1+2}_{c}	B^3	B^4	B^5	B^6	B^*	B^8	B^9	B^{10}	
Cases	4	5	5	9	9	11	2	8	8	8	69

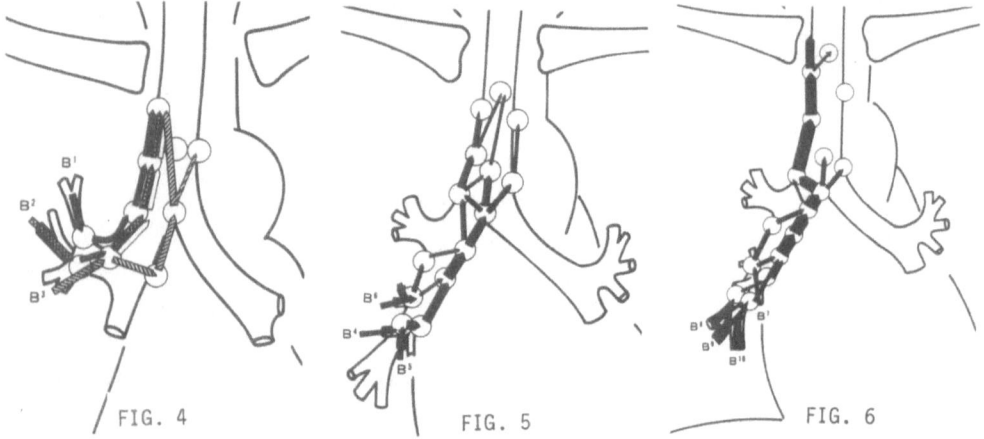

FIG. 4   FIG. 5   FIG. 6

From our analysis of these lymphoscintigrams, standard patterns of regional lymphatic drainage were obtained. Fig. 4-9 show the results. Lymph flow from right upper lobe presented very similar result to Rouviere's one. Lymph from B^1 and B^2 moved via hilar lymph nodes into the right tracheobronchial lymph nodes and then entered into the right paratracheal lymph nodes. Lymph from B^3, at first entered into the right tracheobronchial and carinal lymph nodes through hilar lymph nodes. The main flow from carinal lymph nodes into the right paratracheal lymph nodes and partialy moved into the left paratracheal lymph nodes. (Fig. 4)

Lymph from B^4, B^5 and B^6 flowed into the right tracheobronchial lymph nodes or the carinal lymph nodes via hilar lymph nodes, the latter flow was dominant in our study, the former stream proceeded into the right paratracheal lymph nodes and the latter moved into the right paratracheal, left paratracheal and pre-tracheal lymph nodes still more. Each frequency was almost the same. (Fig. 5)

Lymph from the basal segments, B^7, B^8, B^9, B^{10}, flowed via the hilar lymph nodes into the carinal lymph nodes, then still more the dominant flow moved into the right paratracheal lymph nodes and the remainder flowed into the left paratracheal lymph nodes. Current quantity of the latter was very few. (Fig. 6)

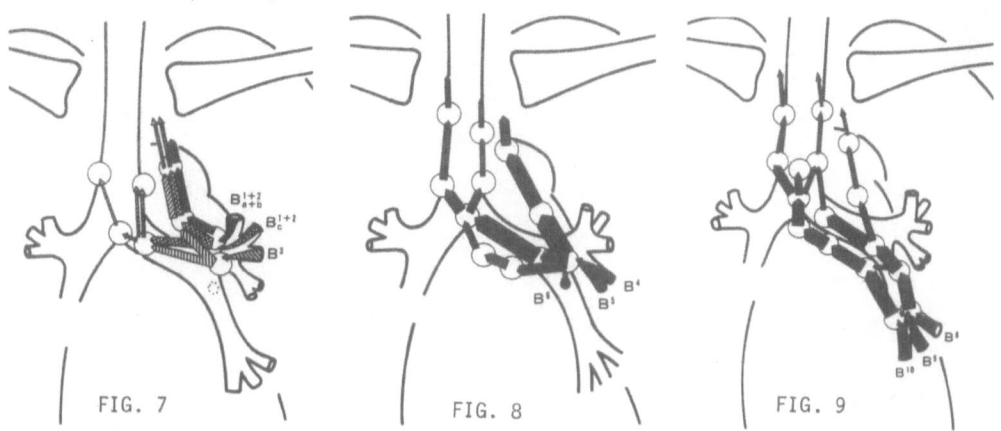

FIG. 7   FIG. 8   FIG. 9

Lymph from the left apical segment bronchus flowed via the hilar lymph nodes, further through Botallo's ligament lymph nodes, and into the aortic arch lymph nodes. Lymph from the dorsal segment bronchus in left upper lobe went into the Botallo's ligament lymph nodes and left tracheobronchial lymph nodes via the hilar lymph nodes. The frequency of these two drainages were almost the same. Lymph from the left B^3 flowed into the Botallo's ligament lymph nodes and the left tracheobronchial lymph nodes via the hilar lymph nodes, then the former stream ran into the aortic arch lymph nodes, the latter stream ran into the left paratracheal, and right paratracheal lymph nodes. (Fig. 7)

Lymph from B^4, B^5 and B^6 flowed into the Botallo's ligament, left tracheobronchial and carinal lymph nodes via the hilar lymph nodes. The former two flow were dominant in our study. From the Botallo's ligament lymph nodes, lymph moved into the aortic arch lymph nodes, and the latter two streams ran into the left and right paratracheal lymph nodes. (Fig. 8)

Lymph from the left basal segments, B^8, B^9, B^{10} flowed along the two dominant routes. One of them ran into left tracheobronchial lymph nodes via the hilar lymph nodes, and then moved into the right paratracheal lymph nodes via the carinal lymph nodes. The other route ran into the carinal lymph nodes via the hilar lymph nodes, and ran into the right and left paratracheal lymph nodes and the pretracheal lymph nodes still more. And the remaining few lymph from the basal segment brochi flowed into the Botallo's ligament lymph nodes via the hilar lymph nodes, then still more the flow moved into the aortic arch lymph nodes. (Fig. 9)

XI.11.

PLEUROSCOPY WITH THE FLEXIBLE FIBEROPTIC BRONCHOSCOPE

P.S. SHANKAR, C.L. ANDERSON, J.H. SCOTT

The etiology of pleural effusion at times presents a diagnostic problem.
closed pleural biopsy may fail to secure a diagnostic specimen due to the localised nature of a lesion. The fiberoptic bronchoscope has been used as a
pleuroscope to visualize the pleura and to perform biopsy of pleural lesions
(1-3).

The bronchoscope has been introduced through a thoracic fistula (4), a T-
shaped connector attached to a chest tube (1), a specially designed cannula
with safety stop-cocks (5) or a small thoracotomy incision with simple purse-
string sutures to the skin of the chest wall (2,3) into the pleural cavity.
We have used a trocar and cannula for the purpose.

Material and methods: Ten patients (six men and four women) with ages
ranging from 48 to 80 years (mean age 64.7 years) with pleural effusion were
studied. Four patients had an endobronchial lesion or an abnormality suggesting squamous cell carcinoma without metastasis elsewhere. The question of
pleural spread had to be answered prior to further treatment. One patient had
undergone treatment for malignancy of the colon, and another for malignancy of
the bladder. Four patients had pleural effusion of undetermined etiology.

The pleuroscopy was performed while the patient was sitting or lying in a
lateral decubitus position with the affected side up. Premedication consisted
of 50 mg meperidine intramuscularly half an hour before the procedure. The
side of fiberoptic bronchoscope insertion was in the seventh intercostal
space along the posterior axillary line.

After skin preparation, the skin, intercostal muscles and the pleura were
infiltrated with 2% xylocaine. A 1 cm incision was made in the skin. A trocar
and cannula were introduced into the pleural space. The trocar was then withdrawn and a gas sterilized fiberoptic bronchoscope was introduced through the
cannula into the pleural space. A small amount of air which entered the
pleural space helped to create a small pneumothorax and improved visualization.
Pleural fluid was aspirated through the suction channel of the bronchoscope
and the visceral and parietal pleura were systematically visualized. Biopsies

*J.A. Nakhosteen and W. Maassen (eds.), Bronchology: Research, Diagnostic and
Therapeutic Aspects. All rights reserved.
Copyright 1981. Martinus Nijhoff Publishers bv, The Hague / Boston / London*

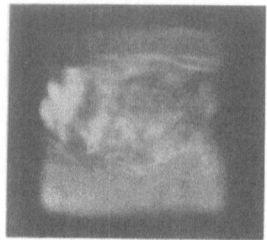

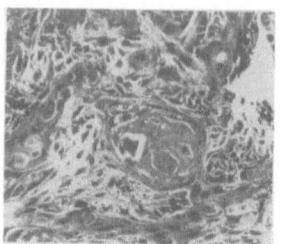

Fig. 1: Fiberscopic view of a
        growth on the pleura

Fig. 2: Squamous cell
        carcinoma

of any lesion or abnormally appearing sites were obtained for histopathologic
study (Fig. 1). Then the scope was withdrawn. The thoracotomy tube was inserted into the pleura and the cannula was removed. The tube was connected to
a vacuum bottle under low suction. A post-pleuroscopy x-ray revealed presence
of residual pneumothorax in three patients. The chest tube was removed 48
hours after the procedure. It was used to introduce tetracycline for pleurodesis in selected cases.

Results: Of four patients of histologically proven squamous cell carcinoma of the lung, two did not have any pleural metastasis, and underwent lobectomy. There was pleural metastasis in the third patient (Fig. 2). The
pleural biopsy in the fourth patient showed adenocarcinoma making it a combined
carcinoma. The patient who had undergone treatment for carcinoma of the bladder
did not show metastatic spread, and co-existent heart failure appeared to be
the cause of the pleural effusion. Another patient who had undergone treatment for carcinoma of colon revealed pleural spread of the disease.

Among four patients with pleural effusion of undetermined etiology, two
showed evidence of adenocarcinoma and subsequently underwent pleurodesis. One
patient demonstrated pleural metastasis with the primary arising in the
stomach (Fig. 3). The biopsy of the pleura and subpleural lung in another
patient with intractable cardiac failure and conduction disturbances revealed
amyloidosis (Fig. 4).

Discussion: The fiberoptic bronchoscope, used as a pleuroscope, gives an
opportunity to explore the pleura and the lung surfaces and to perform
biopsies under direct vision (5).

The cannula with an internal diameter (5.2 mm) slightly greater than the
outer diameter (5 mm) of the fiberoptic bronchoscope facilitates its entry and
maneuverability. It enables the exploration of the pleural cavity without
causing discomfort to the patient and perform pleural biopsy under direct
vision. There is no danger of development of a massive pneumothorax and the
minimal pneumothorax noted in three patients was reversed with the chest tube.

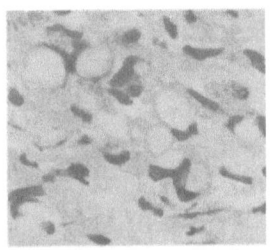

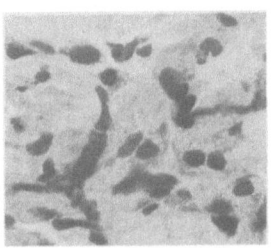

Fig. 3: Metastatic gastric adenocarcinoma showing 'signet
ring cells'

Fig. 4: Amyloid deposits in
the subpleural lung

There are no easily identifiable anatomic landmarks in the pleural cavity.
The visceral and parietal pleura can be identified easily, however inspection
is random.

Pleuroscopic study helped to identify the absence of metastatic spread
in two patients with squamous cell carcinoma so that surgical resection could
be undertaken. Earlier attempts at needle biopsy and cytological study had
failed to demonstrate the presence of pleural spread of malignancy. Presence
of a few exfoliated cells and random nature of blind pleural biopsy may fail
to prove the presence of malignant spread to the pleura. Biopsy of the pleura
established the tissue of origin of the secondary deposit in an asymptomatic
person having a primary in the stomach. Amyloidosis was noted by subpleural
biopsy in a patient with intractable cardiac failure. Pleuroscopy helped to
note the presence or absence of metastatic spread to the pleura in two patients
with carcinoma elsewhere. Adenocarcinoma was noted by its pleural spread in
two patients.

Summary: Diagnostic pleuroscopy has been done in ten selected patients
using a flexible fiberoptic bronchoscope inserted through a cannula into the
pleural cavity under local anesthesia. The procedure is performed to determine the existence of metastatic spread of bronchogenic or other carcinomas,
and to determine the etiology of undiagnosed pleural effusion by pleural or
subpleural biopsy. The procedure is safe and simple.

Chapter XII

PATHOPHYSIOLOGY IN BRONCHOLOGY

XII.1.
IMMUNOGLOBULINS IN BRONCHIAL LAVAGE FLUID *

J. Ruas da Silva, M. Agarez, M. Freitas e Costa

INTRODUCTION

Some authors reported variations in the determination of immunoglobulins in broncho-alveolar aggressions like smoking or pollutants, pulmonary extrinsic granulomatosis (sarcoidosis, pidgeon breeder lung) and lung neoplasic processes (1 - 5).

Material and Methods

16 patients were studied, 9 of them with suspected extrinsic pulmonary granulomatosis (E.P.G.) or diffuse pulmonary fibrosis (D.I.F.), 4 with localized lesions suspected of malignancy and 3 with clinical signs of COPD (chronic obstruction pulmonary disease) one of them with past exposure to copper sulphate. Olympus BF-IT was used.

In the cases when ancillary manoeuvres were performed (aspiration or biopsy) we chose a different branch for the B.A.L.

This was performed with warmed saline. Syphonage was used.

Immunoglobulins were determined by radial immunodiffusion (Mancini) in the B.A.L. fluid and in plasma.

Results - As shown in the tables.

PATIENT No. SEX AND AGE	DIAGNOSIS	SMOKERS Cig/Day	mg % Ig A	mg % Ig G	mg % Ig M	mg % C 3	mg % C 4
1	Extrinsic	–	5,5	3,0	4,0	–	18,0
M - 57	Pulm.Gran.		405,0	1325,0	157,5	69,0	80,0
2	"	20	7,0	7,5	–	–	26,0
M - 60	"		240,0	1225,0	200,0	63,0	75,0
3	"	–	–	3	3,5	–	13,5
F - 36			360,0	987,5	175,0	59,0	52,5
4							

Centro de Investigação CnL3 - I.N.I.C. Lisbon - Portugal

J.A. Nakhosteen and W. Maassen (eds.), Bronchology: Research, Diagnostic and Therapeutic Aspects. All rights reserved.
Copyright 1981. Martinus Nijhoff Publishers bv, The Hague / Boston / London

PATIENT No. SEX AND AGE	DIAGNOSIS	SMOKERS Cig/Day	mg % Ig A	mg % Ig G	mg % Ig M	mg % C 3	mg % C 4
4	Extrinsic	-	-	3,5	3,5	-	14,5
F - 49	Pulm.Gran.		290,0	2000,0	197,5	51,0	55,0
5	"	?	12,0	4,0	6,5	-	29,0
M - ?			240,0	850,0	90,0	49,0	44,5
6	"	20	-	-	-	-	7,5
M - 27			285,0	1000,0	50,0	69,0	30,0
7	"	-	-	1,1	-	-	-
M - 44			156,6	2968,0	61,0	85,5	62,0
8	"	-	5,0	2,8	-	-	30,0
F - 55			267,8	2407,0	161,1	98,5	50,9
9	"	-	-	-	-	-	-
M - 50			468,0	2407,0	116,0	67,0	28,7
10	Neoplasm	20	7,0	20,5	4	1,1	50,0
M - 49	Oat-cell		545,0	1525,0	270,0	59,0	55,0
11	Neoplasm	20	-	-	-	-	-
M - 72	Epidermoid		358,0	1401,5	258,3	128,7	32,3
12	Neoplasm	30	5,5	-	-	-	-
M - 36	Type(?)		290,6	1955,5	270,0	67,8	41,2
13	C.O.P.D.	-	-	3,0	2,5	-	20,0
F - 46			-	-	-	-	-
14	"	40	13,5	28,5	2,5	-	37,5
M - 53			345,0	1875,0	107,5	63,0	50,0
15	"	-	-	-	-	-	-
F - 43			216,8	1722,0	307,7	82,0	46,4
16	"	-	-	-	-	-	-
M - 51			514,8	1641,0	87,7	45,0	18,2

NOTE: For each patient upper values are B.A.L. values, lower are serum values.

Discussion and conclusions

The relatively scarce number of patients, the dispersion of results and, proba-bly, the non-existence of correction ratio between absolute values and potassium(K+) in the lavage fluid are factors which do not allow to confirm defined trends.

E.P.G. patients

We found in the B.A.L. fluid titrable values of Ig G and C4 in most. Ig M and Ig A were found in a smaller number of patients, without any clear correlation

with plasma values. This is probably due to a concentration of Ig the antigenic
aggression locals. The absence of C3 values could be justified by an activation
of the complement alternative pathway by inhaled pollutants and dusts, with decom-
position of C3 in fragments.

Neoplasic processes

In the oat-cell patient, we found high values of Ig G and C4, probably in
connection with defensive immune reactions or due to alterations of vascular permeability, as this patient was previously irradiated.

C.O.P.D.

In one patient with high values of Ig and C4 in B.A.L.,we cannot exclude heavy
smoking habits as an important contributing factor.
In conclusion, we think that Ig and complement factors determination in B.A.L. open
some future prospects for careful exploitation. Besides the general referred tendencies the variability of results inside the same etiology suggests different types of
immunitary evolution which could have prognostic and clinical value, in accordance
with diseases stages.

REFERENCES

1.Mandel,M.A.et al:Immunoglobulin content in the bronchial washings of patients with
   benign and malignant pulmonary disease.New Engl.J.Med.295;694-698; 1976
2.Warr,G.A.et al:Normal human bronchial immunoglobulins and proteins.Amer.Rev.Resp.
   Dis. 116: 25-30; 1977
3.Low,R.B.et al:Biochemical analyses of bronchoalveolar lavage fluids of healthy
   human volunteer smokers and nonsmokers. Ibid 118:863-875; 1978
4.Lebas,J. et al:Problemes poses par le dosage des protéines totales et des immuno-
   globulines dans le liquide de lavage broncho-alveolaire.Colloque Inserm.1979. Le
   lavage broncho-alveolaire chez l'homme - 27-35
5.Harf R. et al: Les composants proteiques du liquide de lavage broncho-alveolaire.
   Étude critique des modes d'expression des résultats. Ibid 35-48.

XII.2.

RELATION BETWEEN HISTOLOGICAL FINDINGS IN LUNG BIOPSY SPECIMENS AND THE
BRONCHO-ALVEOLAR CELL PICTURE

S. YASUOKA, T. NAKAYAMA, T. OZAKI, H. SHIMADA, K. KAWANO, H. ISHIMI AND E. TSUBURA

INTRODUCTION

To examine the diagnostic value of analysis of broncho-alveolar cells for diffuse
pulmonary interstitial diseases, we performed both broncho-alveolar lavage and
transbronchial biopsy in patients with diffuse pulmonary interstitial diseases, and
compared the broncho-alveolar cell pictures with histological findings in the biopsy
specimens.

SUBJECTS AND METHODS

Subjects

The subjects examined consisted of 20 normal volunteers aged 21 to 25 (mean
± SD, 23 ± 1) years, 50 control patients with well-localized pulmonary lesions,
the lesion-free reigions of whom were washed, aged 44 to 72 (59 ± 11) years, 35
patients with diffuse pulmonary interstitial diseases, such as idiopathic diffuse
interstitial fibrosing pneumonia (DIFP), secondary DIFP which had been associated
with collagen diseases, or induced by known causes, and hypersensitivity pneumonitis
(HP).

Method of lavage

Unless otherwise stated, segmental broncho-alveolar lavage was performed
(Method 1); namely one segment (usually B^4 or B^5) was washed 3 times with 50 ml
of saline using a flexible bronchofiberscope.

In 9 control patients, mainly the bronchial region was washed as follows.
A bronchofiberscope was inserted to the truncus bronchialis basalis without wedging
its tip, and 25 ml of saline was infused and aspirated using an aspirator (Method 2).

RESULTS AND DISCUSSION

Factors related to the broncho-alveolar cell pattern

Percentage recovery of infused saline. The percentage recovery of infused
saline was significantly higher in the young normal volunteers (67 ± 7 %) than in
the control patients, most of whom were elderly (48 ± 14 %). The percentage
recovery in patients with DIFP (40 ± 10) was significantly lower than that in the
control patients, and the values in patients with marked pulmonary fibrosis were

*J.A. Nakhosteen and W. Maassen (eds.), Bronchology: Research, Diagnostic and
Therapeutic Aspects. All rights reserved.*

very low (20-30 %). The percentage recovery of infused saline is considered to be influenced by physico-anatomical change of the lung tissue caused by disease and ageing. In nonsmokers, the broncho-alveolar cell count was in general proportional to the percentage recovery of infused saline.

Smoking. The total cell number was 1.5 to 2 times more in smokers than in nonsmokers. The difference between the total cell counts of nonsmokers and smokers was not significant in normal volunteers, but was significant in control patients and patients with DIFP. The increased total cell count in smokers was due to increase in the number of alveolar macrophages.

Method of lavage. The cell pattern of lavage fluid obtained by Method 1 was very different from that obtained by Method 2 (Fig. 1). The percentage of polymorphonuclear leukocytes (PMN) was higher in the latter than in the former. We considered that the bronchial region rather than the alveolar region was mainly washed by Method 2.

Change of the broncho-alveolar cell pattern in diffuse interstitial diseases

Figure 1 shows the broncho-alveolar cell pattern of normal volunteers (NV), control patients (CP) and patients with DIFP and HP, expressed as absolute counts per segment.

In HP, the absolute count of broncho-alveolar cells was about 10 times that of control groups, and over 90 % of the cells were lymphocytes.

The broncho-alveolar cell count seemed to increase in DIFP, considering that the percentage recovery of infused saline was decreased in this disease. As seen in Figure 1, differential counts showed that alveolar macrophages were decreased, PMN, including neutrophils and eosinophils were increased slightly and lymphocytes were not changed, in most patients. Some patients in acute stage showed percentage increase of lymphocyte. However, change in the broncho-alveolar cell pattern in DIFP was slight, compared with that in HP.

Reynolds et al. [1] reported that a percentage increase of PMN in the broncho-alveolar lavage fluid is a characteristic of DIFP. We confirmed this fact although the percentage increase of PMN in our patients with DIFP was not marked. As shown in figure 1, PMN constituted 20 to 50 % of the cells in the lavage fluid from the bronchial region, even in control patients. This indicates that the content of PMN is larger in the bronchial region than in the alveolar space, even in normal subjects. In DIFP, the percentage of cells from the alveolar region seems to decrease with increase in the percentage of cells from the bronchial region, as pulmonary fibrosis progresses because the percentage recovery of infused saline was very low in the patients with marked pulmonary fibrosis. However, infiltration of PMN in alveolar region was observed in the biopsy specimens from some patients with DIFP. Therefore both loss of normal alveolar structure associated with DIFP and increase of PMN in alveolar region are probably concerned with increase in the percentage of PMN in the broncho-alveolar lavage in patients with DIFP.

Relationship between histological findings in lung biopsy specimens and the broncho-alveolar cell pattern

Increase of lymphocytes in the broncho-alveolar lavage fluids was seen in the following 4 groups. (1) Group 1: Subjects in whom lymphocyte infiltration into the lung parenchyma was diffuse and moderate to marked. e.g. HP. In this group, histological changes in the lung are well reflected in the broncho-alveolar cell pattern. (2) Group 2: Subjects in whom lymphocyte infiltration into the lung parenchyma was diffuse but slight. e.g. idiopathic DIFP (especially acute stage), drug-induced DIFP, and sarcoidosis. (3) Group 3: Subjects in whom lymphocyte infiltration was seen in scattered regions of the lung parenchyma. e.g. sarcoidosis. (4) Group 4: Subjects in whom lymphocyte infiltration was not detectable in lung biopsy specimens. In the latter 3 groups, increase of lymphocytes in broncho-alveolar lavage fluid was slight to moderate.

On the other hand, in chronic DIFP, lymphocyte infiltration was detectable in alveolar region but lymphocyte in the lavage fluid showed no significant increase.

CONCLUSION

We conclude that analysis of broncho-alveolar cells is useful in association with histological examination of lung biopsy specimens in diagnosis of diffuse pulmonary interstitial diseases. Measurements of the percentage of broncho-alveolar cells and also of their absolute count are necessary for evaluating the nature and extent of disease accurately. It must be kept in mind that the broncho-alveolar cell pattern is influenced not only by pathological change in the alveolar reigion, but also by that in the bronchial region.

FIGURE 1. Broncho-alveolar cell pattern in normal subjects and patients. a) Absolute count of broncho-alveolar cells in the lavage fluids obtained by Method 1. b) Percentage of cells in the lavage fluids obtained by Method 1 and Method 2.

416

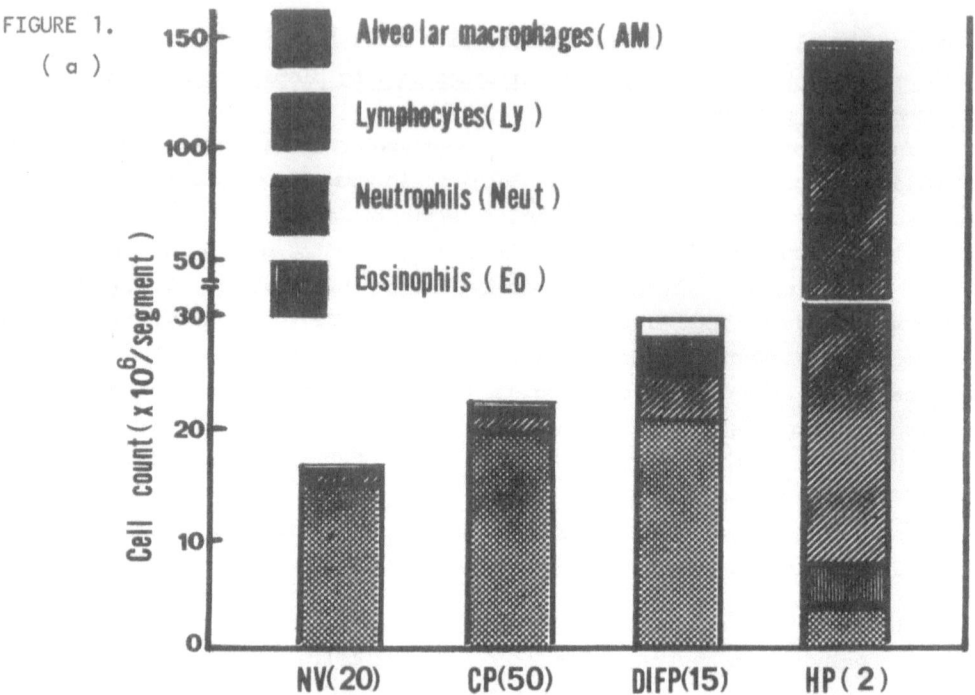

FIGURE 1.
(a)

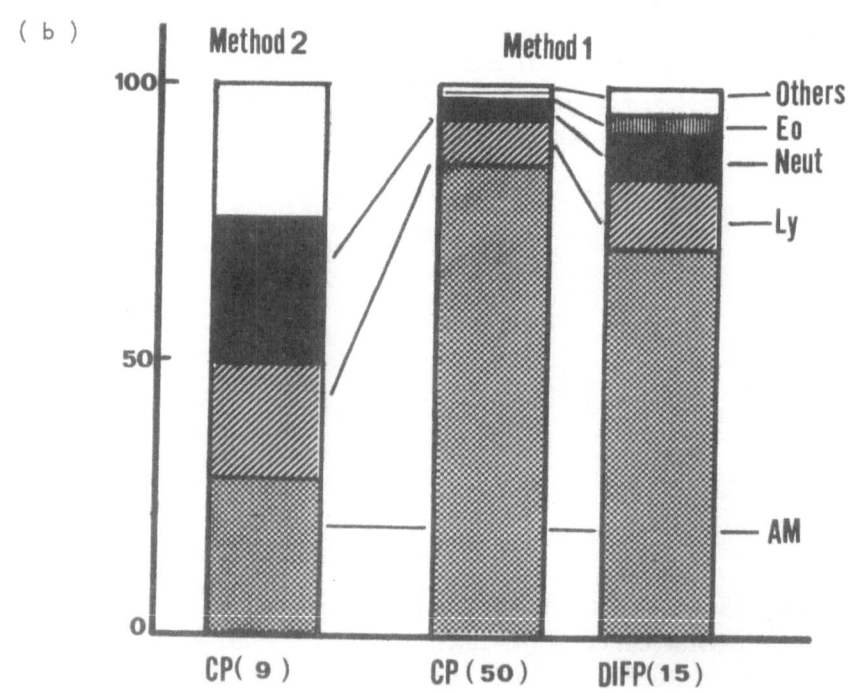

(b)

XII.3.
SELECTIVE BRONCHIAL LAVAGE.

T.TAKASHIMA,M.D. AND M.NOZAKI,M.D.,F.C.C.P.

1. INTRODUCTION

Recent studies on the function of the lungs have revealed that lungs achieved not only external respiration, but also lipid and immunoglobulin metabolism. On chest X-ray examinations the local lesion was observed in many cases of pulmonary diseases. To determine the local reactions of immunologic and lipid metabolism, the selective bronchial lavage of the normal and diseased areas were examined using flexible bronchofiberscope, and analysed the lavage fluid for cytology, bacteriology, immunology and biochemistry.

2. PROCEDURE

The selective bronchial lavage was performed on 5 patients with cancer, tuberculosis, lung abscess, emphysema and atelectasis. After premedication and local anesthesia the bronchoscopic observations were made with photographic recordings from the trachea to the peripheral bronchi taking special precautions to avoid injuring the bronchial wall. After the tip of the scope was placed at the orifice of the segmental or subsegmental bronchus, 40 ml of physiological saline was instilled through the channel using a syringe during inspiration. Lavage fluid was recovered into a mucus trap which was connected between the suction tube and a suction apparatus. To obtain enough volume of lavage fluid the procedure was repeated twice using a total amount of 80 ml of saline. The analytical procedure of the washings is shown in Fig (1).

ANALYSIS OF LUNG WASHING

Washing Fluid
Centrifugation
300G. 10min.
→ Sediment — CYTOLOGY
BACTERIOLOGY
Supernatant
Centrifugation
2,000G. 2℃. 60min.
→ Supernatant — IMMUNOLOGY
IgG, IgA, IgM
(Laser Nephrometry)
→ Sediment — BIOCHEMISTRY
● Phosphatidylcholine (PC)
● Sphingomyelin (Sph)
● others
(Phospholipid Thinchrometry)

3. RESULTS

The results of the immunoglobulin and phospholipids of the washings obtained from the normal area are shown in Table (1), and that of diseased area in Table (2) and (3). The percentage of phosphatidylcholine (PC), the main component of lung surfactant, supposed to be lower in the area of the abscess, atelectasis and severe emphysema than normal. The ratio of IgG and IgA varied from 1.69 to 4.51 and the ratio of PC and sphingomylein (Sph) varied from 6.7

Laboratory Data of Washings obtained from Pulmonary Lesions (1)

Immunoglobulin (mg/dl)	Normal Lesions		
IgG	6.63	3.01	4.51
IgA	1.47	1.36	2.67
IgG/IgA	4.51	2.21	1.69
IgM	0.57	0.55	0.43

Phospholipid (%)

PC	71.1	41.4	78.1
Sph	7.5	6.2	2.8
PC/Sph	9.5	6.7	27.9
others	21.4	52.4	19.1

Laboratory Data of Washings obtained from Pulmonary Lesions (2)

Immunoglobulin (mg/dl)	Cancer	Tbc	Abscess
IgG	1.57	2.09	4.61
IgA	0.74	1.25	0.95
IgG/IgA	2.12	1.67	4.85
IgM	0.32	0.69	0.20

Phospholipid (%)

PC	57.7	52.9	31.5
Sph	2.6	0.4	5.3
PC/Sph	22.2	132.3	5.9
others	39.7	46.7	63.2

Laboratory Data of Washings obtained from Pulmonary Lesions (3)

Immunoglobulin (mg/dl)	Emphysema		Atelectasis
IgG	0.66	2.81	1.34
IgA	2.27	3.52	3.36
IgG/IgA	0.29	0.80	0.40
IgM	0.54	1.06	0.88

Phospholipid (%)

PC	63.9	19.2	29.4
Sph	3.5	2.2	5.0
PC/Sph	18.3	8.7	5.9
others	32.6	78.6	65.6

to 27.9. As shown in Table (2) the IgG/IgA of cancer, tuberculosis and abscess varied from 1.67 to 4.85, and that of the abscess looked higher than normal. It was of interest that the PC/Sph of tuberculosis was 132.3. The IgG/IgA of emphysema and atelectasis seemed to be lower than normal and also the PC/Sph was lower.

4. SUMMARY

The selective bronchial lavage was performed on 5 patients using a flexible bronchofiberscope. According to the individual report from the laboratory, the different immunological reactions and lipid metabolism between the normal and diseased area of cancer, abscess and emphysema were observed. It was necessary to make the tip of the scope soft to avoid injuring the bronchial wall and to eliminate contamination of the blood. Our preliminary study suggested that the selective bronchial lavage would be a useful technique to obtain further information about various lung diseases in addition to cytological and bacteriological findings.

5. REFERENCES

Ramirez-R J, Schwartz B, Dowell AR, Lee SD : Biochemical composition of human pulmonary washings. Arch. Int. Med. 127:395, 1971
Ewing CW : Role of the fiber optic bronchoscope in lung lavage of patients with cystic fibrosis. Chest 73:750, 1978

XII.4.

DETERMINATIONS OF METALIC IONS IN BRONCHIAL LAVAGE FLUID *

A. Teles de Araújo, J. Ruas da Silva, I. Maulide, M.J. Halpern, M.J. Laires,
P. Rodrigues - Lisbon - Portugal.

In some of pulmonary pathology the metalic ions seem to be important and the
knowledge that bronchial lavage is an easy method and inocuous in the study of
bronchoalveolar metabolism, justified this paper (1, 2, 3, 4, 5).

Material and Methods :
We chose a group of patients suspected of extrinsic pulmonary granulomatosis or
malignancy. A few number of patients had C.O.P.D.
We use an Olympus BF-IT bronchofiberscope, and to perform the B.A.L. a syphon
was formed, with two level differences of approximately 1 meter. Ion dosage was
obtained by specific atomic absorption spectroscopy (Perkin-Elmer 360). Separation of cellular elements after lavage was not performed and we decided to get
total titles.

Results :
Total patients were 16; 11 males and 5 females, aged between 27 and 72 years old.
Eight patients had fibrosing lung processes due to extrinsic pulmonary granuloma
tosis; three had lung cancer, one of them with an oat-cell carcinoma and four
COPD, one of them with a past exposure to copper sulphate.
The results are summarized in the Table :

	DIAGNOSIS	OCCUPATIONAL EXPOS.	Mg ++ mg %	Cu ++ mg %	Cig/Day
1 M 57y.	Ext-Pulm.	Gasoil	0,30	not detect.	-
2 M 60y.	"	Silica cement dust	0,20	"	20
3 F 36y.	"	Wood dust copper sulphate	0,30	0,48	-
4 F 49y.	"	Textils synthetic fibers	0,20	0,50	-
5 M ?	"	Solderer	0,15	0,25	?
6 M 27	"	Silica cement dust	0,15	0,25	20

* Centro de Investigação CnL 3 - I.N.I.C. - Lisbon - Portugal.

*J.A. Nakhosteen and W. Maassen (eds.), Bronchology: Research, Diagnostic and
Therapeutic Aspects. All rights reserved.
Copyright 1981. Martinus Nijhoff Publishers bv, The Hague / Boston / London*

	DIAGNOSIS	OCCUPATIONAL EXPOS.	Mg ++ mg %	Cu ++ mg %	Cig/Day
7 M 44	"	Textils synthetic fibers	0,16	0,75	–
8 F 55	"	Silica copper sulphate	0,04	0,55	–
9 M 50	"	Iron, copper (founder)	0,09	0,50	–
10 M 49y.	Oat-cells	–	0,60	0,12	20
11 M 72y.	Epidermoid	–	vestiges	1,00	20
12 M 36y.	Lung Cancer (Hyst. not determ.)	–	0,57	0,85	30
13 F 46y.	C.O.P.D.	–	0,10	not detect.	–
14 M 53y.	"	–	0,15	0,24	40
15 F 43y.	"	–	vestiges	1,00	–
16 M 51y.	"	Copper sulphate	0,04	1,50	–

Discussion and Conclusions :

First we want to stress the actual non-existence of normal standards.

The manipulation of all the B.A.L. fluid is also subject to criticism due to the lack of immediate separation of cells. Nonetheless in the extrinsic pulmonary granulomatosis, there is deposition of one or more ions which are parcially eliminated through alveolar macrophages. Even with metabolic disorders, the variation in excretion of ions must reflect itself on the total amount found;

The clear cut Mg^{++} elevation in oat-cell tumour is in accordance to the concentration in tumoral mass reported in the literature. Nevertheless, we want to stress past treatment in this patient, with cobaltotherapy. This could determine epithelial lesions with cellular destruction contributting to the results. Other Mg^{++} titles are dispersed and do not allow us to get any conclusions.

Shifting to the Copper results, they are high in fluid obtained from patients with lung cancer with exclusion of the oat-cell irradiated patient. It is also increased in patients with past exposure to copper sulphate. It is hard to explain copper increases in the patients with exposition to textile and synthetic fibers. We can postulate the implication of caeruloplasmin with its enzimatic function, mobilizing copper increasing its excretion.

In the patient without Known exposures or malignancy and elevated Cu^{++} in B.A.L. fluid, we cannot discard the possibility of mistakes in collecting patient data, because she lived in a rural zone where copper sulphate is frequently used.

We would try to obtain more data, to establish the normal patterns and to determine K^{+} which is pointed as a good comparison term.

XII.5.

FUNCTIONAL EVALUATION OF HUMAN PULMONARY ALVEOLAR MACROPHAGES
OBTAINED BY BRONCHOALVEOLAR LAVAGE : EFFECT OF SMOKING

H. Shimada, S. Yasuoka, T. Nakayama, H. Ishimi, T. Ozaki, T. Kawano
and E. Tsubura

1. INTRODUCTION

To investigate the role of pulmonary alveolar macrophages (PAMs)
in the bronchoalveolar system, we examined the effect of smoking on
the biochemical and biological functions of PAMs obtained with a
bronchofiberscope by bronchoalveolar lavage (BAL) from normal
volunteers (NV) and patients (PA) with well-localized lung diseases.

2. MATERIALS AND PREPARATION OF PAMs

2.1. Subjects. Twenty-one normal volunteers (10 smokers and 11 nonsmokers) aged 21 to 25 years, and 42 patients (25 smokers and 17 nonsmokers) with lung diseases, such as lung cancer, pulmonary tuberculosis, solid benign tumors and symptomes only, aged 31 to 75 years,
were examined by BAL. The smokers had smoked more than 20 cigarettes
(1 package) per day for a minimum of 3 years. The average number of
cigarettes smoked by the NV group was about 5 pack-years, and that
of the PA group was 20-40 pack-years.

2.2. Preparation of PAMs. BAL was performed with 150 ml (50 ml x 3
times) of saline after wedging the tip of the bronchofiberscope firmly
into a segmental bronchus (usually B^4 or B^5) of a lesion-free lung.
About 50 to 65 % of the infused saline was recovered. The BAL-fluid
was centrifuged at 250 g for 10 min, and the precipitated cells were
washed twice, and then resuspended in PBS and counted. Only specimens
in which PAMs constituted over 80 % of the total cells in differential
cell counts were used.

3. RESULTS

3.1. Both the total number of cells and the number of PAMs were
more in smokers than in nonsmokers, but the difference between the
counts in smokers and nonsmokers was significant only in the PA group
(Fig. 1). The viability of PAMs, measured by trypan blue dye exclusion, was about 85 % in nonsmokers, and slightly higher in smokers,

*J.A. Nakhosteen and W. Maassen (eds.), Bronchology: Research, Diagnostic and
Therapeutic Aspects. All rights reserved.*
Copyright 1981. Martinus Nijhoff Publishers bv, The Hague / Boston / London

in both groups (Fig. 1). Oxygen consumption of PAMs, measured with
a Clark electrode, was significantly higher in smokers. The acid
phosphatase activity and protein content of PAMs were also higher
in smokers than in nonsmokers, in both groups. The acid phosphatase
activity per cell was 2-fold higher in PA-smokers than in NV-smokers
(Fig. 1). The per cent adherence as biological function of PAMs,
assayed by the nylon fiber column technique (ref. 1), was significantly
lower in smokers than in nonsmokers, in both groups (Fig. 1).

   3.2. The phagocytic activity of PAMs from the NV group was
assayed by measuring ingestion of sheep-RBC (SRBC) or ox-RBC (ORBC).
In this test, PAMs were incubated at 37°C for 60 min with 4 types of
erythrocytes : SRBC (E), ORBC coated with rabbit anti-ORBC IgG antibody (EA_G), ORBC coated with rabbit anti-ORBC IgM antibody (EA_M) and
EA_M coated with human complement (EAC). And then after lysis of free
erythrocytes in distilled water, the percentage of PAMs that had
ingested one or more erythrocytes was determined. The percentage
ingestions of EA_G were higher than those of other erythrocytes.
However, phagocytosis of EA_G by PAMs was not influenced by smoking.
The phagocytic activity of PAMs from smokers was lower than that of
PAMs from nonsmokers only when EAC was used (Fig. 2A).

   3.3. Reduction of Nitroblue Tetrazolium (NBT). PAMs were
cultured in RPMI-1640 containing 12.5 % FCS for 30 min, 4 or 20 hours
on culture chamber slides. Then the cultures were washed to remove
non-adherent cells, and NBT reduction was assayed (ref. 2). In all
cases, NBT reduction was higher after culture for 4 hours than after
culture for 30 min or 20 hours before the test. In the NV group, NBT
reduction by PAMs was similar in smokers and nonsmokers. In the PA
group, however, it was significantly higher in smokers than in nonsmokers when the PAMs were cultured for 30 min or 4 hours (Fig. 2B).
Addition of 250 g of the supernatant of BAL-fluid or human IgG to
the PAMs after culture for 30 min increased NBT reduction in all
cases (Fig. 2B). IgG was present in the supernatant.

4. SUMMARY AND CONCLUSION

   Previous investigators have reported that the number and function
of human PAMs are affected by smoking (ref. 3). We confirmed these
findings. The effect of smoking was more marked in the patients
who were older than the normal volunteers. Therefore, the effect of
smoking seems to be related to its extent. We found that biological
activities of PAMs, such as phagocytosis and adherence, were decreased
in smokers, while biochemical activities of PAMs, such as O_2 consump-

tion, NBT reduction and acid phosphatase activity were increased.

These results indicate that the functions of human PAMs were affected in different ways by smoking.

FIGURE 1.

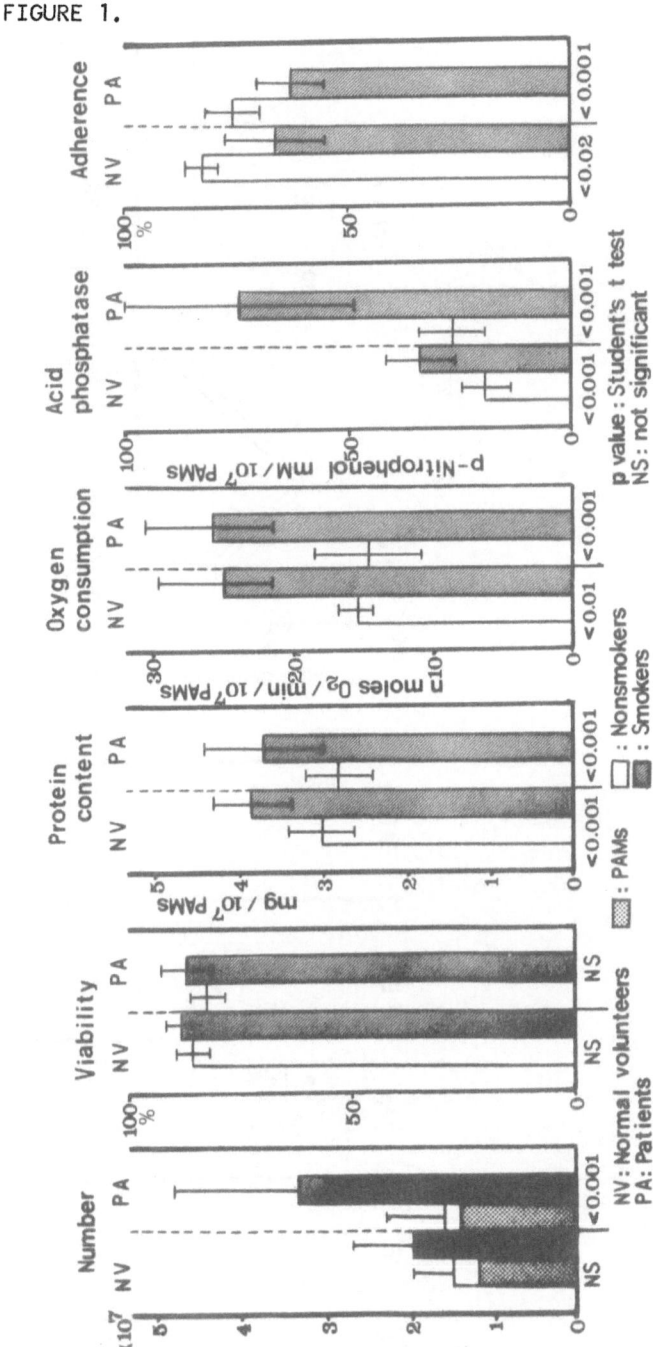

424

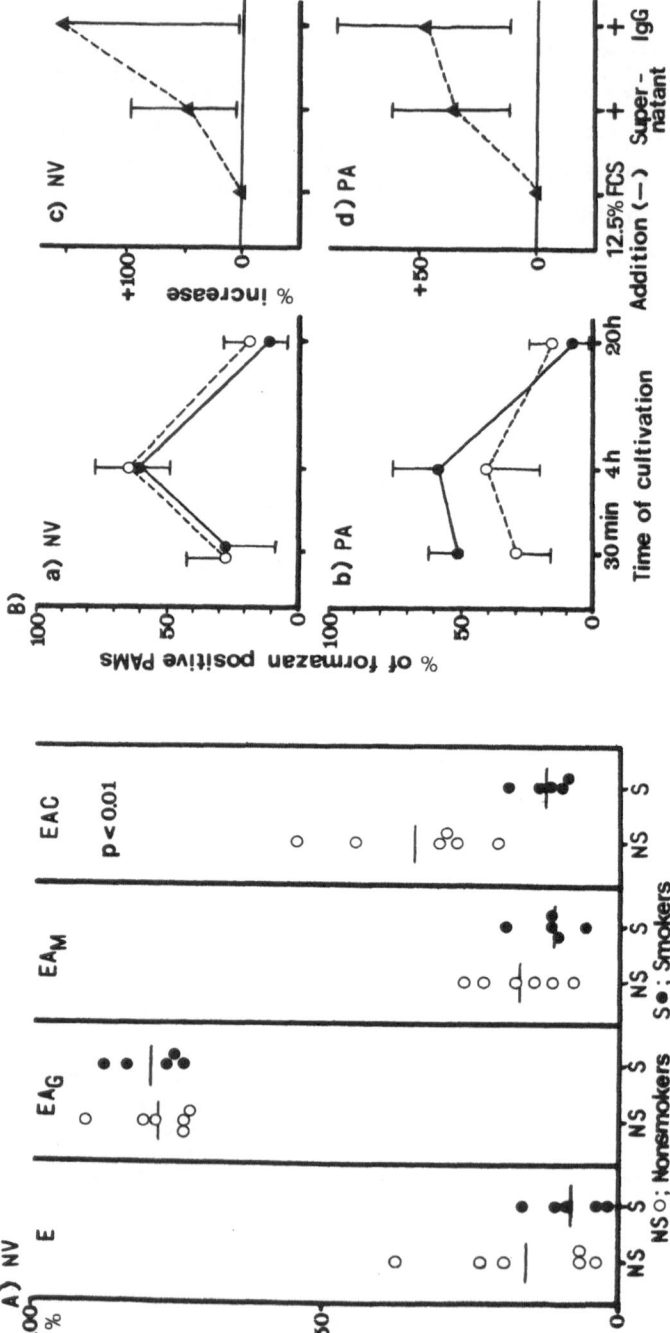

FIGURE 2. A) Erythrophagocytosis of PAMs. B) Effects of cultivation, and IgG and 250 g of supernatant of BAL-fluid, on NBT reduction by PAMs.

XII.6

ENZYMES CONTAINED IN LAVAGE FLUID FROM THE LUNG

S. YASUOKA, H. ISHIMI, T. OZAKI, T. NAKAYAMA, H. SHIMADA, K. KAWANO AND E. TSUBURA

INTRODUCTION

We examined the activities and some properties of several hydrolases in tracheal and broncho-alveolar lavage fluids from rats, and in lung lavage fluids from normal volunteers and patients with pulmonary disease, to obtain information on the biological and clinical significances of these enzymes in the broncho-alveolar system.

SUBJECTS AND METHODS

Animal experiments

Wistar strain rats weighing 150 g were used. Tracheal and lung lavages were carried out as reported previouly. [1)]

Clinical study

The subjects examined consisted of 10 normal volunteers aged 21 to 25 years, 40 control patients with well-localized pulmonary diseases, such as idiopathic diffuse interstitial fibrosing pneumonia (DIFP), hypersensitivity pneumonitis (HP) and chronic bronchitis.

One segment (usually B^4 or B^5) was washed 3 times with 50 ml of saline using a flexible bronchofiberscope. In the control patients, lesion-free segments were washed.

Enzymes analyzed

The following enzymes were measured; alkaline phosphatase (Al-P, pH 10.5), acid phosphatase (Acid P, pH 4.9), β-N-acetyl glucosaminidase (β-NAG), lysozyme (pH 6.6), lipase (pH 6.5) and phospholipase A (pH 6.5).

RESULTS AND DISCUSSION

Hydrolase activity in the trachea, lung and lavage fluids from these tissues of rats

In figure 1, enzyme activities are expressed as percentages of the activity in lung tissue and as units/mg of protein. This figure shows that the enzyme pattern of lung lavage is very different from that of tracheal lavage, and that the enzyme activities in the tracheal and lung lavage fluids are roughly proportional to those in the trachea and lung, respectively. Al-P activity was higher in the lung lavage,

J.A. Nakhosteen and W. Maassen (eds.), Bronchology: Research, Diagnostic and
Therapeutic Aspects. All rights reserved.
Copyright 1981. Martinus Nijhoff Publishers bv, The Hague / Boston / London

while the activity of lipase with a pH optimum of pH 6.5 was specifically higher
in the tracheal tissue and lavage. The activities of phospholipase A and lysophospho-
lipase were high in tracheal lavage and not detectable in lung lavage. The lipase
activity of tracheal lavage is probably that of phospholipase.

The enzymes present in the lavage from the respiratory organ at high level
in the normal state probably have some role in the broncho-alveolar system.

Hydrolase activity in human lung lavage

Enzyme activities were expressed as units per segment, and per mg protein.
The enzyme patterns of lung lavage from normal volunteers and control patients
were similar to that from rat. The Al-P activity was higher in patients with HP
and 50 % of the patients with DIFP, while the activities of acid P and β-NAG showed
no significant change in these conditions. Al-P was shown to be a high molecular
from by electrophoresis. It seems to be a parameter of the extent of disease in
diffuse pulmonary interstitial diseases, whether or not it originates from the
alveolar wall.

The lysozyme activity in lung lavage was significantly correlated with the
number of neutrophil leukocytes, but not with that of lymphocytes or of alveolar
macrophages, which were the predominant cells in lung lavage. This indicates that
lysozyme in lung lavage is mainly released from neutrophil leukocytes.

Conclusion

It is concluded that the enzyme activities in lavage fluid from the respiratory
organ serve as parameters of the function of the broncho-alveolar system, and the
extent of diffuse pulmonary diseases, such as DIFP, HP and chronic bronchitis.

REFERENCE
1. Yasuoka S, Tobiume K and Tsubura E: Lipid metabolism in rat large airway
: Tokushima J Exp. Med. 26: 19-25, 1979.

For Fig. 1 please see following page. Ed.

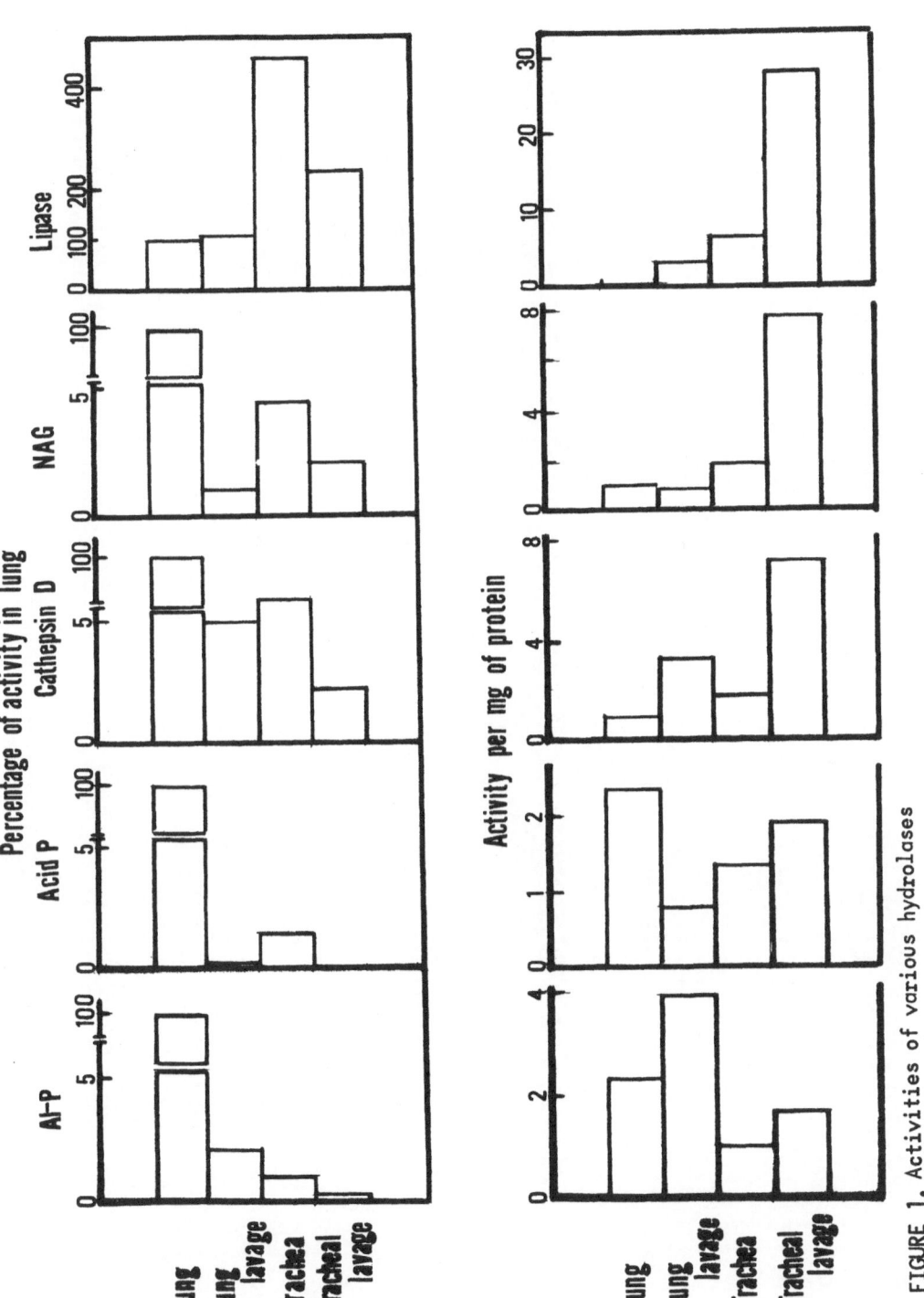

FIGURE 1. Activities of various hydrolases

XII.7.

STUDIES ON MACROPHAGES IN BRONCHIAL WASHINGS FROM THE PATIENTS
WITH BRONCHOGENIC CARCINOMA

Y. AIZAWA, T. KAWAI, T. FUJINO, R. ONO and S. IKEDA

1. INTRODUCTION

The role of macrophage in tumor immunity has recently been recognized. The Fc receptor on macrophages could be involved in the
presentation of antigen to T lymphocyte and also the antibody dependent
cytotoxicity against tumor cells. However, the role of alveolar
macrophages in immunological mechanism against bronchogenic carcinoma
is still to be elucidated. This study was performed to investigate
the immunological aspects of alveolar macrophages in bronchial lavage
from the patients with bronchogenic carcinoma.

2. MATERIALS AND METHODS

Bronchial washing studies were carried out after routine flexible
bronchofiberscopic examination in five patients with peripheral type
of bronchogenic carcinomas and in five patients with no evidence of
malignant diseases at National Cancer Center in Japan. All ten cases
were men, aged 53.2 years on an average in the carcinoma group and
49.0 years in control group. The difference of age was not significant.
All of them except one patient with cancer were smokers. Cigarette
smoking indexes of cancer patients and control were 662 and 590
respectively with no significant difference. Four patients were proved
to have adenocarcinoma while one patient had squamous cell carcinoma
localized in the periphery. One case of adenocarcinoma was under
investigation for occult lung cancer. Three of five cases with bronchogenic carcinomas were found to have advanced stage of bronchogenic
carcinoma. Five men in control group visited the hospital because
of hemosputum or cough. Two patients were found to have bronchiectasis,
while the rest of them had no obvious pulmonary diseases.

Bronchial washing of involved bronchus was performed with a
Flexible Fiberscope, equipped with two channels, model FBS-6TW,
produced by Machida Company, Japan. A total of 100 ml of sterile normal
saline was infused and aspirated by suction. The lavage fluid was

*J.A. Nakhosteen and W. Maassen (eds.), Bronchology: Research, Diagnostic and
Therapeutic Aspects. All rights reserved.*

strained through six layers of cotton gauze to remove gross mucus
and then centrifuged to separate cellular component. The cell pellet
was resuspended in Hank's balanced salt solution. The cells were
assayed for total number, viability and differential counts. Viability
of cells was measured by trypan blue dye exclusion methods. Differential counts were carried out with use of Giemsa and nonspecific
esterase staining.

Macrophages were isolated by their adhesiveness to the Labtek
chamber slides. The number of macrophages bearing receptors for Fc
portion of IgG was determined by the ability of rosette formation
with more than three ox red cells coated with rabbit IgG anti-ox red
cell antibody. Phagocytosis was assayed in the same way except incub-
ation carried out at 37°C instead of 20°C for Fc receptor assay. The
macrophages engulfing at least one red cell were regarded as positive.

3. RESULTS

The mean recovery rate of volume of lavages from the patients
with bronchogenic carcinoma was 57.5% and that from control patients
was 40.1%. The mean cell counts obtained from bronchial lavage were
3.1×10^6 in carcinoma group and 1.4×10^6 in control with no significant difference.

There was no significant difference of the percentage of macrophages, polymorphonuclear leukocytes and lymphocytes in lavage from
cancer patients and control. A patient with alveolar cell carcinoma
showed a markedly increased number of neutrophils in lavage although
no bacterial growth was proved.

The Fc receptor analysis revealed that 84.3% of macrophages
formed rosettes with sensitized ox red cells in cancer patients on
an average, while 62.0% of macrophages formed rosettes in control.
The difference of means in two groups was statistically significant
($p < 0.02$). Two patients with early stage of bronchogenic carcinoma
showed higher percentages of Fc receptor positive cells than those
with advanced stage of cancer.

The percentage of actively phagocytic macrophages from the
patients with cancer was 75.5 and that from control group was 58.5.
There was no significant difference. Two patients whose alveolar
macrophages showed high phagocytic activity had also early stages
of bronchogenic carcinoma. Therefore, mode of alveolar macrophages
may change in the course of progression of bronchogenic carcinoma.

A man with alveolar cell carcinoma, aged 40, was followed-up
for four monthes and bronchial washing studies were repeated four

times. A scattered fine nodular lesion confined initially to the right lower lung field gradually spread to bilateral lung fields. Although initial cellular analysis of lavage was almost normal, neutrophil counts in the following lavages became markedly increased. On the other hand, the number of positive Fc receptor macrophages was markedly decreased in the last lavage.

4. CONCLUSION

The number of macrophages with Fc receptor was found to be increased in the bronchial lavage of the patients with bronchogenic carcinoma. This finding became less conspicuous in the progression of carcinomatous disease. Therefore, Fc receptor on alveolar macrophage may be modified by the progression of bronchogenic carcinoma. The relation between Fc receptor assay of macrophage and antibody dependent cytotoxicity against tumor cells remained to be elucidated.

Neither macrophage counts nor phagocytosis of macrophages were found to be increased on an average in the bronchial lavage from cancer patients compared to control group. However, there was a finding suggestive of an increased phagocytic activity of alveolar macrophages as well as an increased number of Fc receptor positive macrophages in the lavages from the patients with early stage bronchogenic carcinoma.

XII.8.
Distribution and localization of immunoglobulins in bronchial
mucosa

M. Okayasu, E. Ikeguchi, M. Ekimura, Y. Nomura, Y. Hamajima,
Y. Kayama, S. Takada

We have studied the pathophysiology and immunology on the bronchi.
In the present study, distribution and localization of immunoglobulin
component in bronchial mucosa obtained from the bronchial biopsy and
from the pneumonectomized specimen were examined and these were compared with the bronchoscopic findings.

Materials and methods:
The bronchial biopsy was performed with 79 cases of lung diseases
including 25 cases of chronic bronchitis and pneumonectomy was done
with 6 cases (Table 1). By using the flexible bronchofiber scope,
biopsy specimens were obtained mainly from the truncus intermedius
of the right lung. The immunofluorescent antibody technique and the
enzyme-labelled antibody technique were employed for the immunoglobulin study. Anti-sera for human IgA, IgG, IgM, S-IgA and secretory
component used was the product of DACOPAT company. Type IV Horseradish
peroxidase was used for the enzyme labelled antibody technique.

Results:
1) The strong fluorescence of IgA was observed on the surface of
bronchial mucosa and between epithelial cells, however, small numbers
of IgA forming cell were noted in the lamina propria. On the other
hand, IgG fluorescence was found mainly in the basement membrane and
in the lamina propria. IgM was distributed in all layers of mucasal
membrane, but fluorescence was relatively weak.
2) Distribution and intensity of IgA and IgG in the bronchial mucosa
in various lung diseases were studied. Significant differences were
not seen amoung these diseases.
3) S-IgA is secreted in bronchial glands and strong fluorescence is
observed.
4) The secretory component was found in 27 cases out of 73cases
and was marked in cases of chronic bronchitis.

J.A. Nakhosteen and W. Maassen (eds.), Bronchology: Research, Diagnostic and
Therapeutic Aspects. All rights reserved.
Copyright 1981. Martinus Nijhoff Publishers bv, The Hague / Boston / London

434

Table 1. Materials

Specimen	Diseases	No.
Bronchial biopsy	Chronic bronchitis	25
	Bronchiectasis	6
	Broncho pneumonia	4
	Pulmonary tbc.	12
	Lung Ca.	26
Pneumo-nectomy	Bronchiectasis	2
	Pulmonary tbc.	2
	Lung Ca.	2
	Total	79

5)   IgA fluorescence was strongly observed on the surface of epithelium in cases of hypertrophic type of chronic bronchitis, but,
it was weak in atrophic type.   IgG was cleary seen in the lamina
propria in hypertrophic type but it was weak in atrophic type.

Discussion:
The fact that IgA was observed intensely on the surface of
bronchial mucosa, espicÅ“ally in cases of inflammation, represents
the defense mechanism for the infection at the mucosal surface.
Strong deposition of IgG in the basement membrane and in the lamina
propria indicates that IgG plays an important role when inflammation
extends into the inner part of mucosa.   Present study did not examine
the ratio of mucous amd serous glands, but, it was interested that
S-IgA and secretory component were strongly observed in cases of
massive inflammation.   Distribution and intensity of immunoglobulin
component were different between hypertrophic and atrophic type of
chronic bronchitis.   These results give us an important information
to solve pathological changes in bronchi.

XII.9.

A STUDY ON THE DIFFERENTIATION MECHANISM OF THE TRACHEAL GLANDS OF RATS AS INDICATED BY PEROXIDASE ACTIVITY

M. AOKI, M. ITOH and K. HIRAI

1. INTRODUCTION

It is well known that proliferation and hypertrophy of tracheobronchial submucosal glands are brought about in tracheobronchitis. In this study, under the state of induced tracheobronchitis, differentiation mechanism of tracheal glands was investigated using peroxidase activity as an indicator.

2. MATERIALS AND METHODS

Experimental animals were Wistar female rats. Peroxidase activities were detected cytochemically by the diaminobenzidine method.

The upper portions of the tracheas of adult rats were excised. The specimens were fixed with 2% glutaraldehyde and cut into thin sections both for light microscope and electron microscope. These sections were incubated in a solution of diaminobenzidine(0.1% of 3,3'-DAB, 0.001% H_2O_2) at 37°C for 1 hour. The specimens for electron microscope were then re-fixed with osmium tetroxide, dehydrated in the graded series of ethanol and embedded in Epon.

In order to induce tracheobronchitis experimentally, rats were exposed to 1 ppm formaldehyde gas for 10 minutes in a closed chamber. Specimens were obtained 1, 3, 14, 21 and 28 days after exposure.

3. RESULTS

Peroxidase activities were observed in the tracheal submucosal gland cells of untreated rats. These activities were demonstrated in the nuclear envelope, endoplasmic reticulum and secretory granules by electron microscope. (fig. 1) In contrast, the epithelial lining cells lacked this enzyme activity.

At 2 weeks after exposure to formaldehyde gas, moderate proliferations of basal cells had occured and peroxidase positive cells appeared in the epithelium. Basal cells lacked the enzyme activity.

At 4 weeks, groups of peroxidase positive cells were observed among a large number of proliferated basal cells and intermediate cells in the tracheal epithelium. These cell groups extended vertically to the basement membrane and seemed to be developing into submucosal glands. (fig. 2)

J.A. Nakhosteen and W. Maassen (eds.), Bronchology: Research, Diagnostic and Therapeutic Aspects. All rights reserved.
Copyright 1981. Martinus Nijhoff Publishers bv, The Hague / Boston / London

In the early stages of development, intercellular attachments were still loose and cell arrangements were irregular. Intracellular distributions of peroxidase activities were similar to those of submucosal gland cells. In these stages, peroxidase positive cells were still restricted to the tracheal epithelium. (fig. 3)

In the advanced stages of development, intercellular attachments were tight and each cell was arranged more regularly. Intracellular distributions of peroxidase activities were same as mentioned above. (fig. 4) By series sectioning, it was confirmed that these cells were continuous with the submucosal glands.

4. CONCLUSIONS

In this study, using peroxidase activity as an indicator, various stages of development of tracheal glands were observed in experimentally induced tracheobronchitis. Peroxidase activities were demonstrated even in the early stages of morphological differentiation.

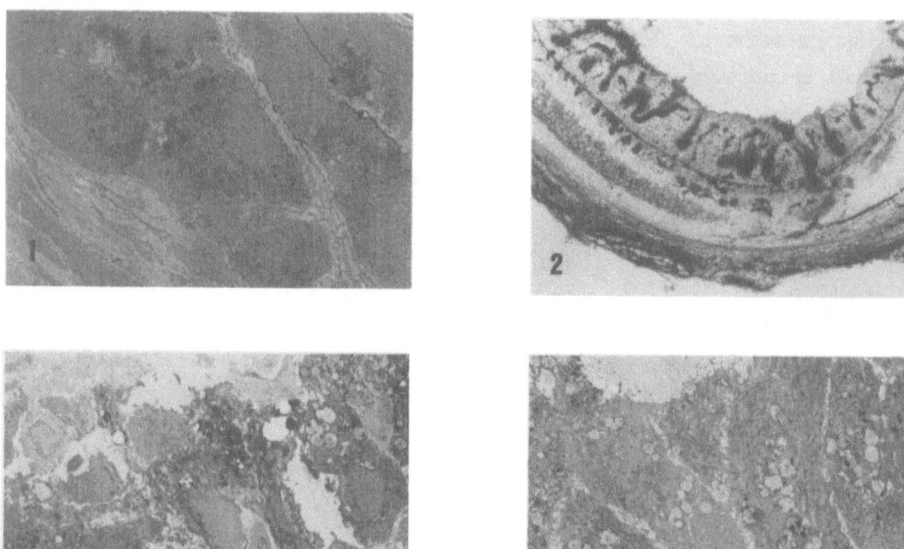

437

XII.10.

THE STUDIES OF CEA BY BRONCHO-TOILET METHOD IN LUNG DISEASE

Y. SUZUKI*, H. HIGUCHI**, E. SHIINA**, A. YAGITA**, Y. KASUGA**

Introduction

Carcino embryonic antigen (CEA) is an oncofetal proteins which has been widely ssudied as one of the clinically important substances. Since Gold and Freedman described the existence of correlation between carcinoma and CEA in 1965, a number of reports on the increase of CEA level in malignant tumor was published, and the method of radioimmunoassay has been developed.

It was generally known that 60~80% of the pulmonary carcinoma patients exhibit the increase of the blood CEA level. However the development of the cancer and the patient's clinical condition are not always in parallel with the CEA level. From these facts, Concanon concluded that the CEA level should not be applied to diagnostic nor prognostic purposes.

In the present study, we intended to investigate the presence of the CEA, and its correlation with various lung affections. For that purpose, we performed partial bronchial irrigation method on the selected patients showing the relatively limited lesion of benign or malignant affection. Then the CEA level of the fluid came our from irrigation was measured.

Materials and methods

Subjects were divided into 3 groups as follows.

Group A: Patients with malignant plumonary affections; diagnosed as malignant tumor
       with the aid of a bronchoscope, cellular examination, or surgical operation.
Group B: Chronic plumonary affections; by means of clinical records, or bronchoscope.
Group C: Acute plumonary affections; by means of clinical records. Includes also
       plumonary carcinoma patients accompany with acute inflammations, at the
       time of examination.

To collect bronchial irrigation fluid, BFS was inserted into the affected part of bronchial tree. Then injected 20 ml of physiological saline manually. The fluid was immediately recovered, and centrifuged for 10 minutes at 1,500 R.P.M. The CEA level of the liquid fraction was measured. In the case of malignant tumor group, blood CEA level was also measured simultaneously for comparative examination. Radioimmunoassay, Sandwitch method was employed for the CEA measurement. In the case of surgically operated subjects, the immunofluorescent staining of CEA-like substance

J.A. Nakhosteen and W. Maassen (eds.), Bronchology: Research, Diagnostic and
Therapeutic Aspects. All rights reserved.
Copyright 1981. Martinus Nijhoff Publishers bv, The Hague / Boston / London

in the normal lung alveoli and tumor cells was also attempted.

Results

The results of CEA measurement are as follows:
The distribution of CEA values for pulmonary disease given in Table I.

1) Chronic pulmonary affections group shows high CEA measurement in statiscally significant level. The CEA values of patients was chronic pulmonary affections. The geometric mean was 67.6 ng/ml S.D. 16.7.

2) Compare with the chronic and acute group. It is also statistically significant. (P<0.01).

3) Malignant pulmonary affection group shows the median level between the level of benign chronic and acute group. The geometric mean was 46.5 ng/ml S.D.±15.5.

4) The results shows in Fig. II. Obviously significant difference was observed between malignant and chronic group (P<0.01).

5) Some statiscally significant difference was observed between malignant and acute group (P<0.10).

6) Although most of individual shows blood CEA positive, no correlation was observed between the CEA level of blood and washing fluid in malignant group. The geometric mean was 6.7 ng/ml±S.D. 5.1.

Discussion

It is well known that blood, tissues and body fluids contain CEA or CEA-like substance[1]. Whether the CEA and CEA-like substance are the same components has not been definitely settled at present. However it has been reported that the immunological cross reaction between CEA and CEA-like substance takes place, though no such reaction was observed between CEA-like substance and NCA[2]. We consider more research on the distribution and other factors of these substances is necessary.

Present results clearly indicate that the considerable amount of the CEA or CEA-like substance is present in the fluid obtained by our bronchial irrigation method. Never the less it is extremely difficult to explain the meaning of these results, since the existence, metabolism and distribution of the CEA-like substance is not sufficiently known at present. The significant increase in some disease may indicate the pathological meaning of the substances exist even in case of the possible presence of some non-specificities in determining the level of CEA or CEA-like substance by the present method. It is now employed as an auxiliary diagnostic method to determine the degree of the extent, prognosis and relapse of malignant tumors, especially in the cases of colon, lung and breast carcinoma.

Several investigators reported the increase of blood CEA level in the cases of lung cancer and chronic lung disease. In some cases of lung cancer, 60~80 % increase was reported[3]. In our study, more than 5.0 ng/ml increase (which is believed to be pathological) was observed in 82 % of the malignant polmonary affection cases. The purpose of our study was to apply the level of CEA and CEA-like substance in the bronchial irrigation fluid to the identification and diagnosis of various pulmonary affections, based on the previously described results. The increase of CEA-like substance is most remarkable in chronic group, median in malignant group, relatively low in acute group.

Now, the range of normal CEA value in bronchial irrigation fluid is need to be determined based on above described results. Since the migration of CEA appears to be affected by many factors such as concentration in tissues, type of tissues, degree of inflammation and condition of blood circulation, the determination of normal level becomes more complicated.

Further, a fluorescent substance in normal pulmonary alveolar tissue has been shown by fluorescent antibody method; but what is this substance is not known. Some authors reported that the CEA level is not related histological type[4)5)]. In fact, we have observed in some patients, the tumor tissue which shows no fluorescent substance by the fluorescent antibody method. To explain these phenomenon is future problem. It may be suggested that the present method is further applicable to clinical purposes, because the considerably high level of CEA substance was measured in bronchial irrigation fluid obtained by radioimmuno-assay method which is clinically applicable.

Present result indicate that the level of the CEA-like substance in the irrigation fluid of malignant pulmonary affection group is significantly lower than that of chronic group, despite the blood CEA increase in malignant group. Whether these differences are due to the physiological factors or pathological affections is a problem need to be clarified, together with how the CEA is moving in blood systems and how it is metabolized.

It is generally believed that the abnormal level of blood CEA concentration is above 5.0 ng/ml, however, the normal level in irrigation fluid should be determined depends on the factors such as the part of bronchi or the age of patients. It should be pointed out from the present results that the necessity of continuous study to establish the pathological range of CEA level, as well as to improve the differential diagnosis of various tumors, with the combined application of CEA measurement and sputum examination.

Table I   Carcino embryonic Antigen Levels in pulmonary Disease

Subjects	Number	<30 ng/ml	<60 ng/ml	<100 ng/ml
Malignant Disease (A)	13	3(26.1)	7(41.1)	3(27.2)
Chronic Disease (B)	15	1(8.3)	5(28.2)	8(72.7)
Acute Disease (C)	12	8(66.6)	4(23.5)	0(0)
Total	40	12(30 %)	17(42.5%)	11(27.5%)

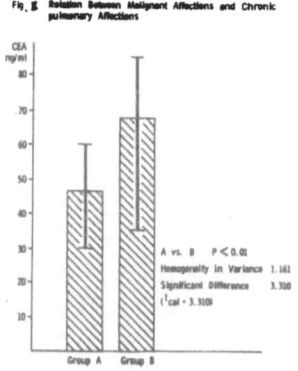

Fig. II Relation Between Malignant Affections and Chronic pulmonary Affections

A vs. B   P < 0.01
Homogenity in Variance 1.161
Significant Difference 3.310
(t cal = 3.310)

XII.11.

THE DIRECT OBSERVATION OF VOLUME-DEPENDENT DEFORMATION OF AIRWAYS BY BRONCHO-FIBERSCOPE

A. NAGAI, T. TAKIZAWA, K. KONNO, M. KAWAKAMI, T. FUJIKAWA, H. KAWADA

INTRODUCTION

This study was aimed to estimate the characteristics of the volume-dependent deformation of airways at different lung volumes, including Total Lung Capacity (TLC) and Residual Volume (RV) in different pulmonary diseases. The direct observation of a cross-sectional changes of airways were performed by a flexible bronchofiberscope.

MATERIALS and METHODS

Subjects were 45 patients with chronic pulmonary emphysema, bronchial asthma and lung cancer. After intramuscular premedication with 0.5mg of atropine sulfate and 15mg of pentazocine, flexible bronchofiberscopic examinations were performed in a supine position. A flexible bronchofiberscope was introduced through a tracheal tube using occasionally 4% xylocaine spray anesthesia and the cross-sectional changes in airways from trachea down to segmental bronchi were observed at TLC and RV respectively.

RESULT

In normal subjects slight bulging of membranous parts of main bronchi were observed symmetrically at RV (Fig. 1b) and these bulgings were also symmetrically dissolved at TLC (Fig. 1a).

In asthmatics during a period of remission, the remarkable bulging was observed at RV mostly in the membranous part of trachea (Fig. 2b), which were well patent at TLC (Fig. 2a). No significant deformations in carina (Fif. 3) and segmental bronchi (Fig.4) were noted in patients with emphysema at any lung volumes including TLC (Fig. 3a and 4a) and RV (Fig. 3b and 4b). In patients with lung cancer in the hilar region, a bulging of the membranous part of un-affected main bronchus at RV (Fig. 5b on the left) was relatively greater compared to that of the affected (Fig. 5b on the right). At TLC, no significant cross-sectional changes were observed in both main bronchi (Fig. 5a).

J.A. Nakhosteen and W. Maassen (eds.), Bronchology: Research, Diagnostic and Therapeutic Aspects. All rights reserved.
Copyright 1981. Martinus Nijhoff Publishers bv, The Hague / Boston / London

DISCUSSION

Several factors to affect cross-sectional changes have been proposed. Among these factors, bronchomotortone and pulmonary recoil pressure seem to be significantly important in pulmonary diseases. As seen in Fig. 2b, a marked bulging of trachea at RV in asthmatics can be attributable to the increase in bronchomotortone at this lung volume. On the other hand, no significant cross- sectional changes in emphysematous patients at TLC and RV are mainly due to the decrease in pulmonary elastic recoil pressure, which operates as distending force to airways. In lung cancer, relatively marked bulging of membranous part of unaffected main bronchi at RV is resulted in a mechanical restriction of deformation in the affected, which, in turn, indicates infiltration of cancer into the bronchial wall.

CONCLUSION

The differences in volume-dependent deformation of airways can be attributable to the different pathophysiological basis, therefore the direct observation of the cross-sectional changes in airways at two extreme lung volumes seems to be clinically useful.

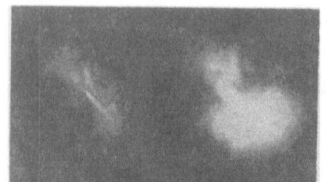 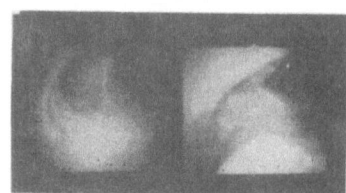 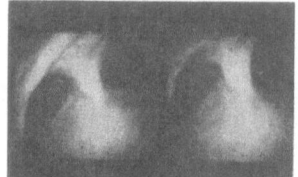

Fig. 1a Fig. 1b   Fig. 2a Fig. 2b   Fig. 3a Fig. 3b

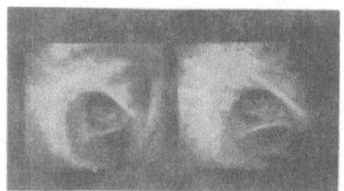 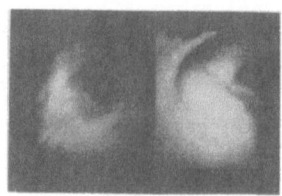

Fig. 4a Fig. 4b   Fig. 5a Fig. 5b

XII 12
BRONCHIAL RESPONSE TO ASTHMATIC ATTACK WITH REFERENCE TO HISTOLOGICAL CHANGES

Tohru Natsuizaka,M.D.,Akira Suzuki,M.D.,Kenzo Okamoto,M.D.,Miyasu Kamiya,M.D.

Bronchial asthma is a disease of significant functional changes which vary
from severe repiratory distress during acute attacks to an asymptomatic state
during remission.

This study was conducted to show the morphological changes of normal bronchial mucosa endoscopically in patients who showed various degrees of functional disturbances from severe acute attack to remission. We correlated the severity of each patient's attack with endoscopic findings in the relationship between morphology and pulmonaly function.

At the same time,biopsy was taken for histological study.

Materials

Twenty patients diagnosed bronchial asthma and treated at Sapporo Medical
College were used;11 male and 9 female,from age 18 to 59,with length of history
ranging from 5 months to 10 years.

Method

Since bronchial irritability is present in bronchial asthma,general anesthesia was employed to minimize morphologic changes which might be induced by
mechanical irritation during endoscopic manupilation. Observations and a 16 mm
cinefilm were made via endoscopy as quickly as possible. A biopsy of segmental
bronchial spur was done by forceps,Olympus made FB-3K.

Results

On the normal main bronchi,the truncus intermedium,and a part of the upper
and lower lobe bronchi,cartilageous rings are observed,and in the membranous
portion,the elastic fiber bundles are observed as longitudinal folds. These
folds usually appear finer in the more distal bronchi around the entire circumference. At the same time, the fine circular folds of the smooth muscle rings
are identifiable.

Analysis based on the morphological changes of the fine,longitudinal folds,
the fine,circular folds,the segmental and subsegmental bronchial spur thickness,
and the presence or absence of the narrowed lumen was made. The patients were
classified into five groups according to the following characteristics. Group-I
-thick,longitudinal folds in the lower lobe bronchi with unidentifiable fine
circular folds,and thickened spur with narrowing of lumen in the segmental and
subsegmental bronchi;Group II-moderately thick,longitudinal folds and a thickened spur without narrowing of lumen;Group III-near-normal,thin,longitudinal
folds and thickened spur;Group-IV-partially thickened spur;Group V-no thickened

J.A. Nakhosteen and W. Maassen (eds.), Bronchology: Research, Diagnostic and
Therapeutic Aspects. All rights reserved.
Copyright 1981. Martinus Nijhoff Publishers bv, The Hague / Boston / London

spur.

In relation to the patients' clinical condition,Group I was correlated with cases showing acute attacks until the day of examination. The severity of attacks decreased from Group I to V,with Group V showing the remission stage. Therefore,we noted that endoscopically,in bronchial asthma,segmental and subsegmental bronchi were involved in mild attacks,and larger bronchi became involved ,as the attacks increased in severity.

Analysis of the spur thickness in Group I,II and III,in which all spurs showed thickening,revealed that the thicknesses differed,and that the difference appeared locally in the segmental and subsegmental bronchi. In other words,the bronchial response to asthmatic attacks was not uniform but differed locally in intensity.

Histologically,in Group I,hypertrophy of the smooth muscle,swelling of the bronchial glands with predominant mucous glands and the infiltration of eosinophils were observed characteristically(Fig.1),but these characteristics were not observed in Group V,the remission group (Fig.2). The above characteristics were observed in Group II ,III and IV in various degrees and combinations. Thickening of the basement membrane was observed in all cases. Goblet cell hyperplasia of the bronchial epiyhelium was not associated with the severity of attack.

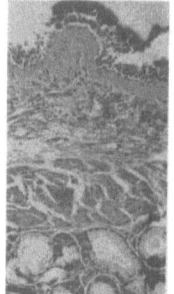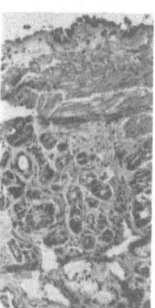

Fig.1(x70,H.E.)Fig.2(x70,H.E.)

Conclusion

This study revealed corresponding endoscopic findings according to the severity of attacks. No abnormalities were observed during the remission period; thickening of the segmental and subsegmental bronchial spur was observed during mild attacks. As the attacks increased in severity,thick,longitudinal folds appeared in the lower lobe bronchi with spur thickening accompanied by narrowing of the lumen. More specifically, a reaction is first observed endoscopically in the segmental and subsegmental bronchi,and as the attacks become more severe,larger bronchi become involved. This reaction is not uniform in the entire lung but differs locally.

The commonly accepted histological pattern of bronchial asthma was not observed during remission period;therefore,we concluded that these changes occur only during the asthmatic attack. Case 4,which was examined both during a severe attack and during remission,confirmed this finding. Also,this finding suggests that histological changes from the epithelium to inner perichondrium are reversible except for thickening of the basement membrane.

No relationship was observed between the length of history and the endoscopic or histological findings

XII.13.

HISTOLOGICAL CHANGES OF THE BRONCHIAL MUCOSA FOLLOWING PROLONGED TREATMENT WITH BECLOMETHASONE DIPROPIONATE IN PATIENTS SUFFERING FROM BRONCHIAL ASTHMA

B. Molnár, S. Ferenczy, L Mészáros

Since the first report by Hodson and Williams aerosols of steroid compounds and beclomethasone dipropionate have been widely used in the treatment of bronchial asthma.

Several reports confirmed that 400 mcg/day beclomethasone dipropionate, which equals to 6-9 mg/day Prednisolon doses decreases bronchial asthma symptoms without causing systemic side effects. The question, however, arises whether chronic administration of these small beclomethasone dipropionate doses would not lead to pathological changes of the bronchial mucosa as observed on the skin following chronic steroid treatment. Histological and longitudinal studies will help to clear the problem.

Here we report on 18 cases of bronchial asthma having been verified by allergological and respiratory functions tests. The duration of treatment is shown on the table.

Table I.

7 patients from 6 to 12 months
5 patients from 12 to 24 months
6 patients more than 24 months

The patients received beclomethasone dipropionate treatment in average for 19 months.

The patients were given daily 400 mcg beclomethasone dipropionate. Other steroids or antiasthmatic drugs /aminophylline, beta receptor stimulants/ were administered only in cases of severe dyspnea.

Before the treatment was started the following tests were performed:
1. general examination
2. respiratory function tests
3. bronchoscopy /bronchial biopsy, histological examination/
4. adrenocortical function tests

J.A. Nakhosteen and W. Maassen (eds.), Bronchology: Research, Diagnostic and Therapeutic Aspects. All rights reserved.
Copyright 1981. Martinus Nijhoff Publishers bv, The Hague / Boston / London

5. microbiological investigations

Control examinations were performed at 12 months intervals.

In the present paper we report only on the histological changes of the bronchial tissue. The biopsy material for the histological examinations was obtained before, and during the treatment at 12 months intervals. The results of histological examinations were compared with the original findings with the aim to elucidate any histological changes of the bronchial mucosa occured. Here we present a few slides on the findings.

The text of slides

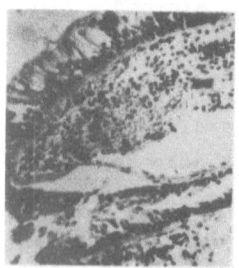
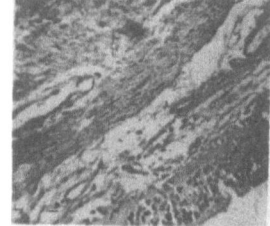

Fig. 1a   Fig. 1b

1. Patient

We can see the hypertrophy of bronchial mucosa membrane with a lot of goblet cells before the treatment. The basement membrane is widened and in the submucous layer there is an incresing inflammatory process.
After two years of treatment the edema is mild, and we can not see other alterations.

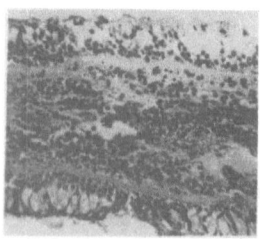
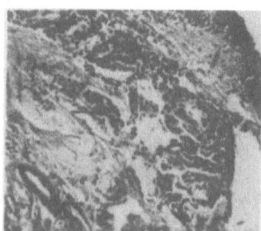
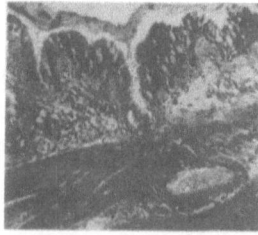

Fig. 2a   Fig. 2b   Fig. 2c

2. Patient

Before the treatment the histological examination shows the proliferation mucous membrane with a large mass of goblet cells, and with marked inflammatory infiltration.
After 2 years inflammatory tendency is decreased. After three years the mucous membrane shows hypertrophy with the proliferation of goblet cells, the submucous layer is wider than earlier, the signs of inflamma-

tion are visible in a moderate form.

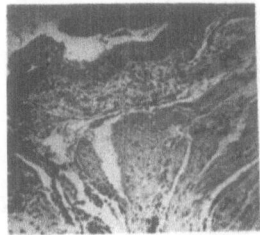

Fig. 3a

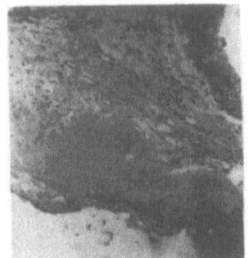

Fig. 3b

3. Patient

Before the treatment in the bronchial tissue, the proliferation of mucous membrane can be seen and the basement membrane is wider, under it there are a number of lymphocytes.

After three years besides the excess the of the goblet cells, and sparse infiltration of lymphocytes a moderate proliferation of the connective tissue can be seen.

Summary

Prolonged treatment with beclomethasone dipropionate aerosol resulted in clinical and functional improvement of 18 patients with bronchial asthma. In all patients bronchoscopy revealed the macroscopic regression of the inflammation. Histological studies verified the decrease of inflammatory reactions: that is the decrease of goblet cell hyperplasia, submucosal edema, and inflammatory infiltration. These findings are in agreement with those of Andersson and Nakhosteen. In the majority of cases, the favourable histological findings persisted 1-2 years after the treatment.

XII.14.

STUDY ON ELECTROMYOGRAM OF BRONCHIAL SMOOTH MUSCLES

Masao Ogihara, Kenichi Nagaoka, Japan

The objective of this study was to investigate through electromyography the pathophisiological aspects of bronchial smooth muscles in bronchial disturbances.

METHOD: The subjects of this study were white rabbits, healthy adult volunteers, patients with bronchial asthma and patients with chronic bronchitis. Electromyograms were taken with DISA 1500 Type Electromyograph. The electrode made of silver bipolar needles was used. The white rabbits were trachiotomized. In the case of human subjects, the bronchofiberscope (Olympus BF Type 2T) was used for electrode induction. Electromyography was performed by inserting the electrode into the posterior portion of right main bronchus and subsegmental bronchus under bronchofiberscopic control.

RESULT: In the experiment in rabbits, the electromyograms of bronchial smooth muscle and of intercostal skeletal muscle were recorded at the same time. It was found that the electromyograms of bronchial smooth muscles appeared as the grouped spikes in two parts; the later part of half of the expiratory phase and the terminal part of the inspiratory phase with respiratory rhythm. The potential of the electromyogram of intercostal skeletal muscle shows the most marked decrease in the expiratory phase (Fig. 1). The action potential of the electromyogram of bronchial smooth muscle of right main bronchus was about 30 μV (Fig. 2).

E.M.G of Rabbit's

figure 1

E.M.G of Rabbit's

figure 2

J.A. Nakhosteen and W. Maassen (eds.), Bronchology: Research, Diagnostic and Therapeutic Aspects.

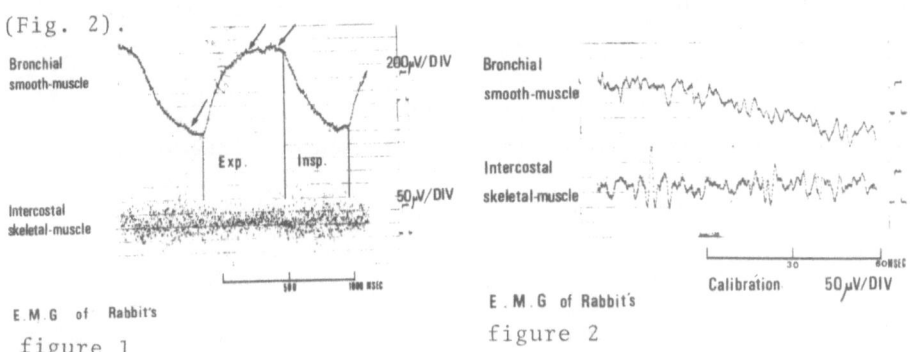

The electromyograms of bronchial smooth muscle which were recorded
in the right main bronchus and subsegmental bronchus had 30 to 60 μ V
and 3 to 8 μ V amplitudes of action potential respectively, and showed
similar patterns of diphasic or triphasic waves in healthy adult
volunteers (Fig. 3,4). The electromyograms taken on effort respiration
and coughing showed an increased in action potential. There was no
marked difference in pattern between healthy adult volunteers and
patients with bronchial asthma, but the sensitivity to acethylcholine
chloride increased in bronchial asthma. Some of patients with chronic
bronchitis showed multiphasic patterns with small amplitude

(T . S   Male   58y)

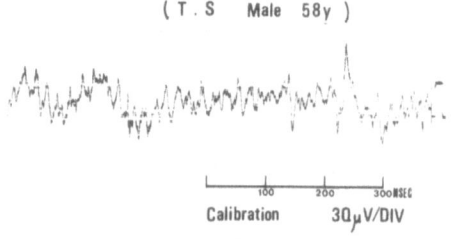

Calibration   30 μV/DIV

E. M . G of Normal- adult's Bronchial-smooth muscle

figure 3

(T . S   Male   58y)

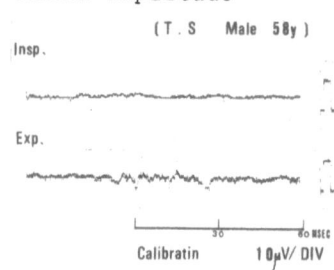

Calibratin   1 0 μV/ DIV

figure 4   E. M . G of Normal-adult's sub-Segmental bronchial
               -smooth muscle.

DISCUSSION AND CONCLUCION: The present study appears useful not only to
the pathophsiological research of bronchial smooth muscle but to the
clinical diagnosis and treatment of pulmonary diseases. A search of
the literature reveals a few studies dealing with electromyograms of
gastrointerstinal tract but no reports dealing with ones of human
bronchus. We succeeded in recording the electromyograms of bronchial
smooth muscle and those of human bronchus under bronchofiberscopic
control. This new method of ours could be used in recording easily,
accurately and safely the action potential of bronchial smooth muscles
from right main bronchus and subsegmental bronchus. This method is
expected to be particularly useful for diagnosis and treatment of
bronchial asthma, chronic bronchitis and other bronchial diseases.

REFERENCES:
1) Y. Akasaka, and I. Niki et al.: Endoscopic induction of the
electromyogram from human gastrointestinal tract. Endoscopy, 7:139-141
1975

XII.15.

SIGNIFICANCE OF THE BRONCHIAL GLAND AS A LOCAL DEFENCE MECHANISM

M. ITOH, M. AOKI, J. TAMADA and T. TERAMATSU

INTRODUCTION

The bronchial gland is an exocrine gland composed of serous cells and mucus cells, the structure of which is morphologically similar to that of the salivary gland.

Though the structure and function of the salivary gland is well known, the function of the bronchial gland is little known.

On the other hand, it is well established that in the bronchial secretion there are many defensive substances against infection such as lactoferrin, Ig-A, secretory Ig-A and lysozyme. But the origin of these defensive substances is not well known.

The purpose of this study is to clarify the origin of these defensive substances in the bronchial tree, and to investigate the relationship between the structure and function of the bronchial gland using enzyme-histochemical and immuno-histochemical technique.

During a systematic study of lactoperoxidase in the bovine exocrine gland, we incidentally found the specific fluorescence of lactoperoxidase in the serous cells of the bronchial gland.

We thought, therefore, that the bronchial gland may produce bacteriocidal substances and may play a direct role in the bronchial defence mechanism. Recently we tried to demonstrate the presence of such substances in the bronchial gland.

MATERIALS AND METHODS

Bronchus from the resected lung were used for the study of human bronchial gland. Bovine bronchus were purchased from a slaughter house.

Frozen section were cut in a cryostatt, placed on glass slides, and fixed with cold ethanol or acetone.

Direct fluorescent antibody method was used for demonstration of Ig-A and amylase, and indirect method for lysozyme.

Enzyme-antibody technique was used for demonstration of secretory component and amylase counterstained with alcian blue.

J.A. Nakhosteen and W. Maassen (eds.), Bronchology: Research, Diagnostic and Therapeutic Aspects. All rights reserved.
Copyright 1981. Martinus Nijhoff Publishers bv, The Hague / Boston / London

Enzyme-histochemical technique was used for demonstration of the activity of peroxidase, β-glucuronidase, non-specific esterase and other oxidative enzymes.

RESULTS

The specific fluorescence of lactoperoxidase in the bovine bronchial gland was concentrated near the cytoplasmic membrane of the serous cells. And these findings were also confirmed enzyme-histochemically using diaminobenzidine.

Peroxidase activity was similarily demonstrated in the serous cells of the human bronchial gland.

Specific fluorescence of lysozyme was demonstrated in the serous cells of human bronchial gland using the indirect fluorescent antibody method. A specific antibody was obtained by immunizing rabbits with human colostrum lysozyme.

As lysozyme is one of the lysosomal enzymes, the distribution of other lysosomal enzymes such as β-glucuronidase and non-specific esterase was examined enzyme-histochemically. These lysosomal enzymes were also seen in the serous cells of the bronchial gland.

The specific fluorescence of amylase was demonstrated in the human bronchial gland. The specific fluorescence seems to be limited to the serous cells.

This finding was confirmed by the enzyme-antibody method counterstained with alcian blue. The fluorescence in the foetal bronchial gland was more intense than that of the adult bronchial gland.

The antibody was obtained by immunization with amylase purified from human saliva.

The specific fluorescence of Ig-A was seen in the human bronchial gland. The fluorescence seemed to be demonstrated in the serous cells of the bronchial gland and to be concentrated in the luminal side of the cells and in the collecting duct.

The secretory component was also seen in the bronchial gland stained by the enzyme-antibody method and counterstained with alcian blue. Secretory components are thus demonstrated in the serous cells of the bronchial gland.

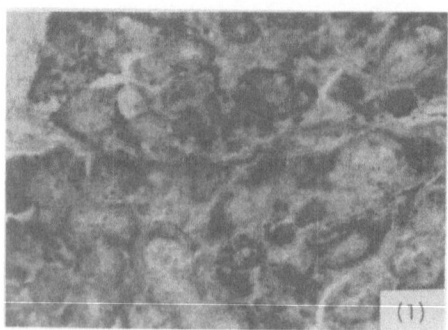 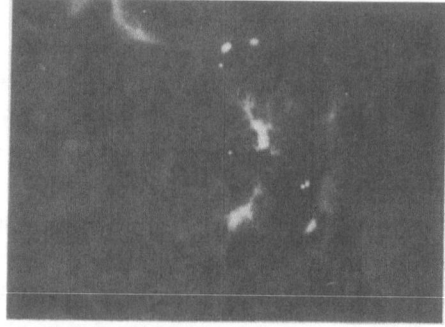

Fig 1. Peroxidase(1), Ig-A(2) in the human bronchial gland

TABLE 1. Distribution of enzymes and proteins in the bronchial gland

	Serous cell	Mucus cell
Ig-A	+	−
Secretory component	+	−
Lysosomal enzymes		
Lysozyme	+	−
β-glucuronidase	+	−
Non-specific esterase	+	−
Peroxidase	+	−
Amylase	+	−
Oxidative enzymes		
Succinic dehydrogenase	+	+
Lactic dehydrogenase	+	+

The demonstration of Ig-A and secretory component in the bronchial gland suggest that the serous cells of the bronchial gland may be closely related to the production of such defensive substances.

The results are summarized in table 1.; except for oxidative enzymes, most of the enzymes and proteins were demonstrated in the serous cells of the bronchial gland. Mucus cells seemed to produce only mucus.

CONCLUSION

From the results mentioned above, we concluded that the serous cells of the bronchial gland produce many enzymes such as lysosomal enzymes, amylase and peroxidase, and produce many local defensive substances such as secretory Ig-A and lysozyme that play a direct role in the bronchial defence mechanism.

On the other hand, mucus cells of the bronchial gland produce little or no protein, and function as a mucociliary transportation system.

So, it seems obvious that the bronchial gland functions as a bronchial defence mechanism, and that there is a differentiation of function between the mucus and serous cells of the bronchial gland.

XII.16.
THE OBSERVATION OF OZONE EXPOSED MOUSE TRACHEA BY FREEZE FRACTURE METHOD.

Hang Hsiao Hsu[*], E.I. Nakai[**], M. Kato[*] and Y. Sagawa[*].

Photochemical air pollution, first noted in Los Angeles, is now one of the big problems of the world accompanied with the industrial development. Ozone is an important factor of air pollution as a component of oxidant and it occupies over 80% of oxidant.

Ozone has been known to be a poisonous gas since its discovery (1) and it reacts with the proteins of lung tissue to produce a severe cellular irritation which alters cell wall permeability and leads to severe edema of the respiratory tract. (2)(3)

The method of freeze-fracture has some characteristics: It can remove the artifacts due to dehydration and embedding in the course of TEM or SEM, for in this method, the specimen is frozen in liquid nitrogen, freon or liquid helium after fixation. Sometimes, raw materials are freeze-fractured without any pretreatment.

In the procedure of this method, the plasma membrane of cells is cleaved in its hydrophobic discontinuous layer and membrane-intercalated protein particles are exposed on two cleaved faces of protoplasmic face (PF) and exoplasmic face (EF). (4) We used this method to observe the morphological changes of cell membrane of ozone exposed pulmonary and tracheal tissue.

Materials and methods

Six adult mice of 3D strain were divided into two groups. One group of three mice for the experiment was put in the plastic exposing chamber which was connected to ozone generator. They were exposed to 5 ppm of ozone for six hours. The concentration of ozone was determined by buffered potassium iodide method. Just after the exposure, the animals were sacrificed and total trachea was dissected. Specimen was fixed in 2.5% glutaraldehyde for over night at $4^{\circ}C$ and dipped into 40% glycerol solution for 30 minutes. Then it was carried into the ordinary procedure of freeze-fracture.

Results

Ciliary cell: In the control group, they showed numerous and regulary arranged cilia. Six to seven lines of necklace were observed in the root part of cilia. (arrows)(5) P face (PF) and E face (EF) of ciliary membrane are observed with their numerous intramembranous particles (IMP). The particles were uniformly scattered on both faces. The density of particles was $105/0.1\mu m^2$ on P face and $39/0.1\mu m^2$ on E face. (Fig. 1) In the ozone-exposed group, cilia were observed shorten and decreased in the number. The necklace was also noticed and did not show any particular changes (arrows). Ciliary membrane showed bulging, swelling and waving. Cleaved faces of ciliary membrane are observed with the decreased number of intramembranous particles. The density of particles was $67/0.1\mu m^2$ on P face and $14/0.1\mu m^2$ on E face. (Fig. 2) The particles totally disappeared on some parts and aggregated on other parts of the faces.

Clara cell: In the control group, they showed numerous microvilli along the surface. A plenty of small secretory granules (SG) were uniformly scattered in the cytoplasma. Various sized round mitochondria (M) were also observed among the secretory granules. (Fig. 3)

In the ozone-exposed group, microvilli were decreased in number. Some secretory granules (SG) enlarged, swollen and the size is various. The number of them decreased. Mitochondria (M) are well observed among the granules and did not show any particular changes. (Fig. 4)

Tight junction of ciliary cell: In the control group, each unit of the tight junction showed clear 8-shaped and many strands of the network structure. Many strands of tight junction are noticed (arrows). The strand number of the structure was usually six to nine. Intramembranous particles were clearly observed on both faces of plasma membrane. (Fig. 5)

In the ozone-exposed group, tight junctions are showing some changes in the number of strands (arrow), and the strand number decreased to four to six. The space between two strands of the network was widened and enlarged. The number of the particles of both faces decreased. Aggregation and total absence of the particles are observed on some parts of cleaved face (arrow heads). (Fig. 6)

Following results were obtained for ozone-exposed group in our experiment; decreasing and shortening of the cilia, bulging and waving of the ciliary membrane, decreasing of the intramembranous particles on both cleaved faces of ciliary membrane, decreasing of the number of microvilli, decreasing and bulging of the secretory granules of Clara cell, changes of the tight junction of ciliated cell.

Discussion: Tracheal congestion and pulmonary edema will dependent on the change of permeability of tissue and cell of the site. Decreasing of the network strand number of the tight junction may cause the change of permeability. Furthermore, decreasing of the number of intramembranous particles may also have some relations to the change of cell permeability.

Ozone is an active oxidizing agent for many organic groups, and it may have some influence to the organic groups of the membrane intercalated protein particles and the particular parts of the membrane of tight junction.
Conclusion

These changes and damages to tracheal tissue and cell were considered due to toxicity of ozone which is irritant to tissue and cell membrane.

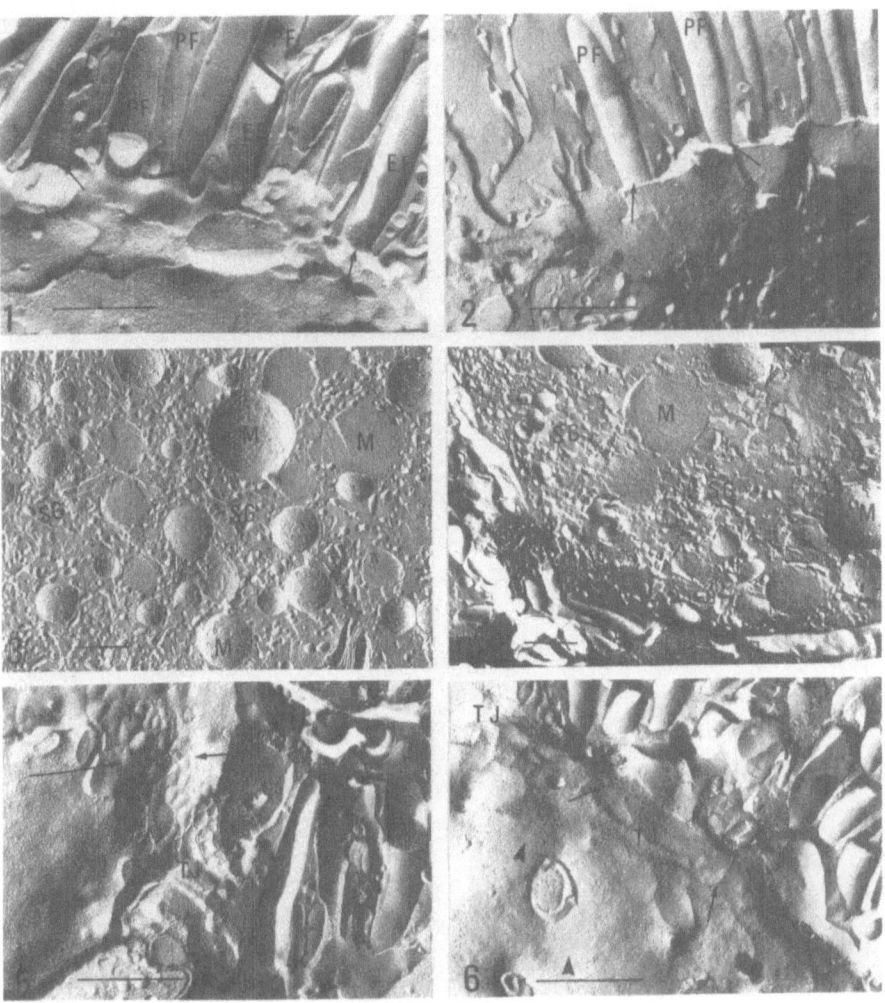

Fig. 1. Ciliary cell of normal trachea.

Fig. 2. Ciliary cell of ozone exposed trachea.

Fig. 3. Cross fractured image of a Clara cell of normal trachea.

Fig. 4. The same image of ozone exposed trachea.

Fig. 5. Cleaved plasma membrane of ciliary cells of normal trachea.

Fig. 6. Cleaved plasma membrane of a ciliary cell of ozone exposed trachea.
All the bars indicate 1μm.

BRONCHIAL BIFURCATION IN THE RIGHT UPPER LOBE AND LEFT UPPER DIVISION
BRONCHI

K. Nagai, R. Amemiya, K. Oho, N. Hayashi, T. Kawauchi, T. Saito,
I. Iimura, N. Takizawa, N. Kawate, Y. Hayata,
XII.17.

Observation and photography as far as fourth order bronchi has
been made possible by the development of the fiberoptic bronchoscope.
This has resulted in increasing encounters with cases in which it
is difficult to decide upon nomenclature. Therefore, as an aid in
analyzing pathologic findings, the authors set out to elucidate the
types of bifurcations observed in normal cases and their appearance.
Here we present the findings in 300 cases with normal left upper
division bronchi and right upper lobe bronchi.

Almost of all left upper lobe bronchi bifurcate to the upper
division bronchus and lingular bronchus, while trifurcation of B^{1+2},
B^3 and lingular bronchus was seen in only 2%. In the left upper division bronchus 3 types of branching were seen (Table 1) : 1. Bifurcation of B^{1+2} and B^3 (74%) 2. Trifurcation of $B^{1+2}a+b$, $B^{1+2}c$
and B^3 (20%) 3. Bifurcation of $B^{1+2}a+b$ + B^3 and $B^{1+2}c$ (6%)
Thus in the left upper division bronchus, bifurcation of B^{1+2} and
B^3 type was most frequent, and in this type most of the B^{1+2} bronchi
bifurcated to $B^{1+2}a+b$ and $B^{1+2}c$. Also 95% of B^3 bifurcated to B^3a
and B^3b+c. The lack of variation means that once $B^{1+2}c$ is recognized
it is relatively easy to recognize the numbers of other bronchi bi-
furcating from the left upper division bronchus.

TABLE 1. Bronchial bifurcation in the left upper division bronchi

Type of branching	Frequency	Appearance	
1. Bifurcation of B^{1+2} and B^3	74%	Blunt	43%
		Sharp	57%
2. Trifurcation of $B^{1+2}a+b$, $B^{1+2}c$ and B^3	20%	Blunt	100%
		Sharp	0%
3. Bifurcation of $B^{1+2}a+b$ + B^3 and $B^{1+2}c$	6%	Blunt	80%
		Sharp	20%

In the right upper lobe bronchus 7 types of branching were seen.
(Table 2) 1. Trifurcation of B^1, B^2 and B^3 (40%), 2. Bifurcation
of B^1 + B^2 and B^3 (22%), 3. Bifurcation of B^1 and B^2 + B^3 (17%),

4. Absolute horizontal left / right bifurcation type (B^1 + B^2 and B^3) (12%),
5. Absolute vertical upper / lower bifurcation type (B^1 and B^2 + B^3) (7%),
6. Bifurcation of B^1 + B^3 and B^2 (6%), 7. Quadrifurcation type (3%),

TABLE 2. Bronchial bifurcation in the right upper lobe bronchus

Type of branching	Frequency	Appearance	
1. Trifurcation of B^1, B^2 and B^3	40%	Blunt	71%
		Sharp	29%
2. Bifurcation of B^1 + B^2 and B^3	22%	Blunt	63%
		Sharp	37%
3. Bifurcation of B^1 and B^2 + B^3	17%	Blunt	60%
		Sharp	40%
4. Absolute horizontal left / right bifurcation(B^1 + B^2 and B^3	5%	Blunt	41%
		Sharp	59%
5. Absolute vertical upper / lower bifurcation(B^1 and B^2 + B^3)	7%	Blunt	100%
		Sharp	0%
6. Bifurcation of B^1 + B^3 and B^2	6%	Blunt	80%
		Sharp	20%
7. Quadrifurcation	3%	Blunt	33%
		Sharp	67%

There are many types of bifurcation in the right upper lobe bronchus, but types 1 + 2 + 3 accounted for 80%. Type 1 (trifurcation type) which was the most frequent type was classified into 4 sub-types, a. standard trifurcation type, b. V-type, c. inverted-V type, d. parallel trifurcation type. The standard tifurcation type was most frequent and was seen in 60% of type 1 cases. Longitudinal membranous folds from the right main-upper lobe bronchus were usually easy to detect. The longitudinal membranous folds were usually thick and run to B^2. If we use these longitudinal membranous folds as a landmark, it is easy to correctly name the right upper lobe bronchi.

In general there were two types of bifurcation, rather blunt branching in areas with cartilage, and sharper branching where the cartilage was largely replaced by elastic fiber bundles. In the left upper division bronchus Type 1 (bifurcation of B^{1+2} and B^3) blut branching and sharp branching appeared with almost equal frequency. On the other hand almost all type 2 (trifurcation type) and type 3 (bifurcation of B^{1+2}_{a+b} + B^{1+2}_{c}) were blut branching. In the right upper lobe bronchus there were many types of bifurcations. Trifurcation type varied according to the 4 subtypes. a (standard trifurcation type) and d (parallel trifurcation type) were almost all blunt branching type. On the other hand in subtype b(V-type) the sharp branching type was most frequent. In subtype c(the inverted V-type) blunt and sharp showed equal frequency. In type 2(bifurcation of B^1+ B^2 and B^3) the blunt branching type accounted for 63%, and sharp branching type for 37%. In type 3(B^1 and B^2 + B^3) the blunt branching type was seen in 59% and the sharp branching type in 41%. The bifurcations of subsegmental bronchi all showed sharp branching.

It is important to understand the findings of the normal bronchus seen the through the fiberoptic bronchoscope in order to analyze pathologic findings. We classified left upper division bronchi into 3 types, and the right upper lobe bronchus into 7 types. To look for $B^{1+2}c$ is most important for correct orientation in the left upper division bronchus whereas in the right upper lobe bronchus it is best to look for the longitudinal membranous folds. Our statistics were slightly different from those of Jackson and Huber[1] which might represent a difference in population or in examination method, as they included surgical specimens while employed fiberoptic bronchoscopic findings only.[2] A thorough knowledge of the findings in the normal bronchus, and of the type of bifurcation of each order is clinically essential for a valid evaluation of pathological findings.

REFERENCE

1. Jackson CC, Huber JF: Correlated applied anatomy of the bronchial tree and lungs with a system of nomenclature. Dis Chest, 9, 319-326, 1943.
2. Oho K, Amemiya R: Practical fiberoptic bronchoscopy, Igaku-Shoin, Tokyo, 1980.

Chapter XIII

MUCOCILIARY FUNCTION

XIII.1.
LONG-TERM EXPOSURE TO PARTICLES AND THEIR RETENTION IN THE HUMAN LUNG

R.V. LOURENÇO and T.R. GERRITY

1. INTRODUCTION

Occupational and environmental exposures of the lung to toxic particulates
are responsible for a number of lung diseases, such as pneumoconioses, and may
be important etiologic factors in others, such as pulmonary fibrosis and chronic
obstructive lung disease. The action of the inhaled substances is related to the
dose delivered to the lung tissue.

During exposure to an aerosol (a suspension of particles in air), particle
deposition and clearance occur simultaneously. These competitive processes distribute particles in the lung in such a way that different regions receive higher exposures than others. To understand how this may occur, we first consider
deposition and clearance as isolated, noninteracting phenomena and then combine
the two processes to see how they interact in the delivery of particles to lung
tissue.

2. MATHEMATICAL MODEL OF DEPOSITION AND CLEARANCE

2.1. Deposition. Particles deposit in the lung by three main mechanisms--
inertial impaction, gravitational sedimentation, and diffusion. Inertial impaction occurs when a particle slips out of the airstream and collides with the wall
of an airway. Gravitational sedimentation is the result of particles "falling"
out of the airstream under the force of gravity. Diffusion is due to particle
interactions with air molecules. In general, impaction is most effective in the
large airways, with sedimentation and diffusion being observed mostly in the
small terminal airspaces.

Detailed calculations (1) of the fraction of acutely deposited particles per
airway generation by employing these mechanisms in the Weibel A morphologic model
of the lung (2) are shown in Fig. la. If the deposited fractions are each divided
by the airway generation surface area, the relative concentration of particles
is found (Fig. 1b). The massive concentrations calculated for generations 3 and
4 may be related to the high incidence of bronchial carcinomas at these sites.

2.2. Clearance. After a single breath exposure, deposited particles are cleared
from the lung. Lung clearance has two major phases. The first phase lasts one day
during which particles deposited in ciliated airways (generations 0-15) are

J.A. Nakhosteen and W. Maassen (eds.), Bronchology: Research, Diagnostic and
Therapeutic Aspects. All rights reserved.

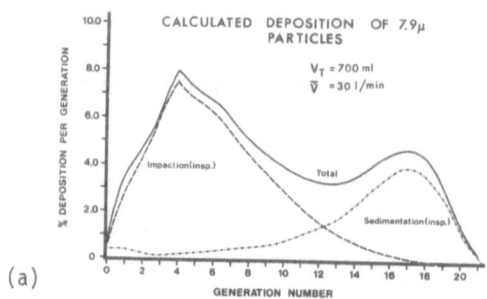

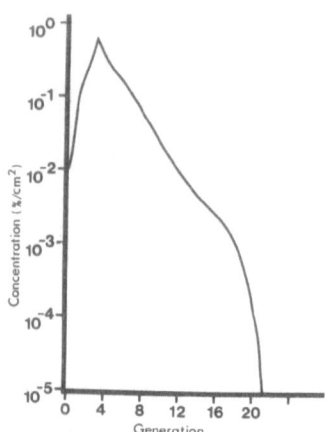

FIGURE 1. a)Calculated deposition fraction per airway generation. b)Relative surface concentration of particles per airway generation.

cleared by mucociliary transport. The second phase, alveolar clearance, lasts much longer. Iron oxide, for example, has been observed to have a clearance half-time from the alveoli of approximately 60 days (3).

Although lung clearance has been widely measured, detailed regional information on clearance is lacking. To understand more about regional mucociliary clearance, we developed a mathematical model of mucociliary clearance (4) which uses the Weibel A lung model for morphometric information. We consider the rate of change of the particle number in any generation to be the difference between the particle entry and exit rates in each generation. Particle entry and exit rates are proportional to transport rates of mucus in each generation. The formal solution to this problem depends on the initial deposition fractions per generation and mucus transport rates in each generation. The deposited fractions are calculated as previously discussed. All transport rates are related to the rate of mucus transport in the trachea by assuming that rates in distal generations are inversely proportional to the total circumference of each generation. Such a scaling of transport rates implies a uniform mucus blanket depth.

This model was tested by comparing it with mucociliary clearance data collected in our laboratory in 9 healthy, nonsmoking subjects who inhaled an 8-μm Fe_2O_3 aerosol tagged with Tc-99m. The average clearance data over 4.5 hr after inhalation and the model predictions agree well if a tracheal mucus transport rate of 5.5 mm/min is imposed. This value for the tracheal transport rate agrees well with measurements by Yeates et al (5). The model predicts transport rates as low as 4.6 μm/min in the terminal bronchioles.

2.3. Continuous exposures. Given models of deposition and mucociliary clearance, the problem of simultaneous deposition and clearance can be solved. The rate of change of particle number in a generation equals the difference between the rates of particle deposition and particle clearance.

The rate of deposition is fixed with the rate of respiration and the deposition fraction per breath; initially, it greatly exceeds the rate of clearance. During this time the particle retention increases linearly. As the number of particles in the lung increases, the clearance rate rises since it is proportional to particle number. Over long periods of time (on the order of lung clearance times), the clearance rate approaches the deposition rate, and a condition of particle number equilibrium is approached.

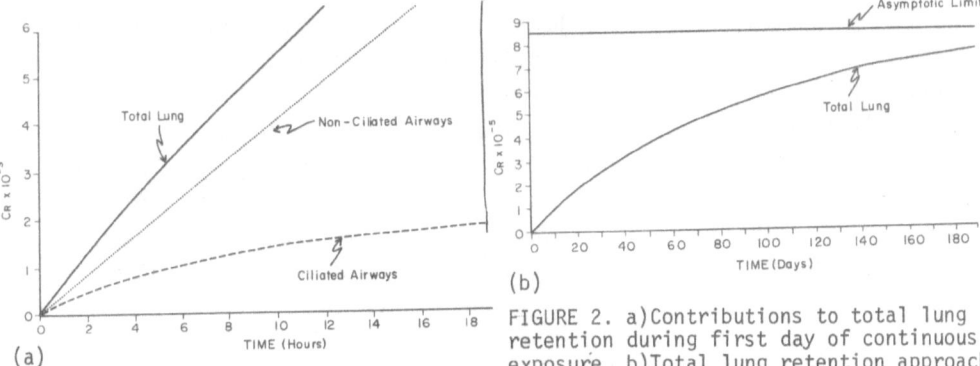

(a)

(b)

FIGURE 2. a)Contributions to total lung retention during first day of continuous exposure. b)Total lung retention approaching equilibrium (horizontal line).

Fig. 2 shows the whole lung retention of 4-μm particles as a function of time if a 60-day clearance half-time of particles is imposed on the alveoli. Fig. 2a demonstrates how the ciliated airways reach a rapid equilibrium state due to fast mucociliary clearance. Fig. 2b shows the whole lung approaching a condition of particle number equilibrium in approximately one year.

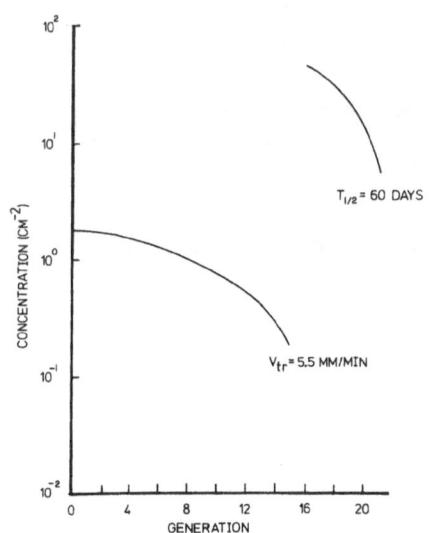

FIGURE 3. Relative surface concentration of particles per airway generation at equilibrium.

3. RESULTS

The retention represented on the vertical scale of each group of Fig. 3 is normalized to the total fraction deposited beyond the trachea in a single breath. If an aerosol with particulate concentration equal to 100 $\mu g/m^3$ enters the trachea, the amount retained at equilibrium is 60 mg. This should be compared with a total mass of 454 mg deposited in one year. Thus, the mechanisms of clearance are, in principle, very effective at keeping the lung burden of particulate low.

To compare the regional effects of a continuous exposure versus an acute exposure, the tissue surface concentration of particulate in each airway generation is graphed versus generation number in Fig. 3. The largest particle concentrations now appear in the respiratory bronchioles in contrast to the concentration distribution shown in Fig. 1b for an acute exposure.

4. SUMMARY AND CONCLUSIONS

We have demonstrated through mathematical modeling of particle deposition and clearance that continuous exposures result in equilibrium whole lung retentions that are small fractions of the total mass deposited. We have also demonstrated that when acute and continuous exposures are compared on a regional basis, acute deposition produces high concentrations in the large airways, whereas continuous exposure results in high concentrations in the respiratory bronchioles. This sharp contrast in the outcome of the two different exposure modes may relate to differences in the pathogenesis of large and small airways diseases.

REFERENCES
1. Gerrity, T.R., Lee, P.S., Hass, F.J., Marinelli, A., Werner, P., and Lourenço, R.V.: Calculated deposition of inhaled particles in the airway generations of normal subjects. J. Appl. Physiol.: Respirat. Environ. Exercise Physiol. 47(4): 867-873, 1979.
2. Weibel, E.R.: Morphometry of the Human Lung. New York, Academic Press, 1963.
3. Morrow, P.E.: Alveolar clearance of aerosols. Arch. Intern. Med. 131: 101-108, 1973.
4. Lee, P.S., Gerrity, T.R., Hass, F.J., and Lourenço, R.V.: A model for tracheobronchial clearance of inhaled particles in man and a comparison of data. IEEE Trans. Biomed. Engin. BME-26(11): 624-630, 1979.
5. Yeates, D.B., Aspin, N., Levison, H., Jones, M.T., and Bryan, A.C.: Mucociliary transport rates in man. J. Appl. Physiol. 39(3): 487-495, 1975.

XIII.2.

COMPARISON OF TECHNIQUES FOR MEASURING TRACHEAL MUCOUS VELOCITIES IN VIVO IN MAN

S.W. CLARKE and D. PAVIA

INTRODUCTION

There are three objective methods for measuring lung mucociliary clearance in living man. The first method requires the inhalation of an insoluble aerosol firmly tagged with a gamma-emitting radionuclide, followed by subsequent monitoring with external chest scintillation counters. This 'radioaerosol method' provides a measure of mucociliary clearance effectively for the whole of the tracheobronchial tree. The second method entails the measurement of time taken for a marker placed in a well defined anatomical airway to move a set distance, giving a measure of the mucous velocity (e.g., in mm min^{-1}). There are several variations of this method. The third method requires the insufflation of a radiopaque dust (e.g., tantalum powder) and the monitoring of its subsequent progress in the lungs roentgenographically.

In this paper we review the variations of the second method for measuring tracheal mucous velocities (TMV) in man, to determine the reasons for the differences previously noted.

TRACHEAL MUCOUS VELOCITY MEASUREMENTS

There are four objective techniques for measuring tracheal mucous velocities in vivo in man.

1. Cinebronchofiberscopic technique. This technique reported by Sackner et al. (1973) utilises teflon discs (0.68 mm in diameter, 0.13 mm in thickness and weighing 0.13 mg) which are blown through the inner channel of a fiberoptic bronchoscope onto the tracheal mucosa in a circumferential distribution. The cephalad motion of these discs is filmed, the discs serving as markers of the tracheal mucous transport. As the discs approach the distal lens of the fiberoptic bronchoscope, they are magnified in size. The distance (s) traversed in a given time by the discs is obtained from the difference in the apparent sizes of the discs. This is achieved using a relationship previously ascertained in vitro between apparent size of disc and distance from lens. The time (t) taken for the discs to move a distance s is obtained from the film speed and frame numbers. Dividing s by t gives a measure of TMV. However, because of considerable but unavoidable variability in individual particle transport rates attributable to anatomical and functional characteristics of the respiratory mucosa, it is recommended that analysis be made of 10-20 particles.

J.A. Nakhosteen and W. Maassen (eds.), Bronchology: Research, Diagnostic and
Therapeutic Aspects. All rights reserved.
Copyright 1981. Martinus Nijhoff Publishers bv, The Hague / Boston / London

2. Radioisotopic technique utilising a fiberoptic bronchoscope. This technique of Chopra et al. (1979) yields a measure of the average tracheal mucous velocity. The length of the trachea, i.e., the distance between the larynx and the carina, is determined by means of a graduated fiberoptic bronchoscope. These two reference points are recorded on polaroid film from the display of a gamma camera by inserting a sealed plastic catheter tagged with 50 µCi of $^{99}Tc^m$ at its tip through the inner channel of the bronchoscope. A minute suspension (40 µl) of albumin microspheres (5-7 µm in diameter) numbering approximately 50,000 and tagged with $^{99}Tc^m$ is deposited on the mucosal surface at the lower end of the trachea via a catheter placed through the inner channel of the bronchoscope. The movement of the microspheres towards the larynx serves as a marker of mucous transport up the trachea by ciliary action. By taking sequential pictures of a gamma camera display at 1 minute intervals over an observation period of 30-60 minutes (i.e., time taken for the spheres to reach the larynx), a measure of the average tracheal mucous velocity is obtained by simply dividing length of trachea by time.

3. Roentgenographic technique. This technique is a modification of the cinebronchofiberscopic technique. In this instance, the markers, teflon discs, are mixed with the radiopaque substance bismuth trioxide and insufflated through the vocal cords via the inner channel of a fiberoptic bronchoscope (Friedman et al., 1977). The cephalad motion of these particles in the trachea is recorded with a fluoroscopic unit provided with image intensifier, television monitor and videotape. Time (e.g., from a digital clock) is recorded on the videotape to enable calculation of the distance traversed in a known time during 1-2 minutes of observation. A radiopaque reference marker can be taped on the skin of the larynx and be used to correct for magnification effects inherent in the fluoroscopic unit. The mean value of tracheal mucociliary transport velocity is obtained from measurements on approximately 20 discs. Discs which are found to move transversely or caudally are counted as zero motion and are averaged in the mean.

4. Radioaerosol boli technique. This technique of Yeates et al. (1975) involves the inhalation of an aqueous aerosol containing albumin microspheres (0.5 µm count median diameter) labelled with the radionuclide $^{99}Tc^m$ (physical half-life: 6 h). By the suitable choice of an inhalation manoeuvre, i.e., inspiring the aerosol near total lung capacity at a high flow rate, the radioaerosol deposits predominantly in local concentrations (boli) in the large airways. The boli of radioactive microspheres transferred up the trachea by ciliary action and their position can be recorded by a gamma camera. The tracheal mucous velocity can then be ascertained from the measurement of distance moved by boli in a given time.

TRACHEAL MUCOUS VELOCITY VALUES

The table lists TMV values for healthy subjects obtained by the four techniques. There appears to be a direct relationship between the value of TMV and the degree of invasiveness involved with each technique. For example, there is a four-fold difference between the mean TMV value obtained by the non-invasive radioaerosol boli technique and the most invasive cinebronchofiberscopic technique.

TABLE 1. Tracheal mucous velocities (mean ± SD) for healthy subjects.

Technique	No. of subjects	TMV (mm min⁻¹)	Invasiveness score	Source
1. Cinebronchofiberscopic	16	21.5 ± 5.5	+++	Santa Cruz et al. (1974)
2. Radioisotopic utilising a bronchoscope	6	15.5 ± 0.7	++	Chopra et al. (1979)
3. Roentgenographic	7	11.4 ± 3.8	+	Friedman et al. (1977)
4. Radioaerosol boli	11	4.6 ± 2.4	o	Spektor et al. (1979)

DISCUSSION

The measurement of tracheal mucous velocities has been used to increase our knowledge of the effect on lung mucociliary clearance of (1) physiological factors such as age, (2) environmental pollutants such as tobacco smoking, sulphuric acid mist, sulphur dioxide, hair spray, (3) pharmacological agents such as mucolytic drugs and (4) disease such as asthma, bronchitis and cystic fibrosis.

There are two main reasons for the popularity of employing these four techniques: (1) a short observation period, i.e., from a few minutes up to 1 hour, thus mini-mising artefacts due to coughing and also enabling repeat measurements to be made within a short period of time after the first assessment; and (2) precise positioning of the test material results in measurements of mucous velocity in an anatomically well defined region. It must, however, be emphasised that the application of these techniques is limited to the large airways, in practice mainly the trachea, and often only a small portion of it. Further, the results obtained from the trachea may give no indication of clearance rates for smaller airways nor necessarily for the lung as a whole. Recent studies on the effects of pharmacological agents and environmental pollutants support this view.

This review highlights the discrepancies of the reported tracheal mucous velocities in healthy man and suggests that they are related to the degree of invasiveness of each technique. In this respect, it is known that even the light touching of the respiratory mucosa by a cotton swab can result in an outpouring of secretions.

The differences in the absolute values of tracheal mucous velocities do not invalidate the use of these techniques for studying the effect of specific factors on mucociliary clearance but make direct comparison of data from various centres difficult.

XIII.3.

EFFECTS OF SALBUTAMOL AS INSTILLATION SOLUTION, INHALATION POWDER AND METERED AEROSOL ON TRACHEAL MUCOUS VELOCITY

J.A. Nakhosteen*, W. Petro*, N. Konietzko*, H. Hirche**

1. INTRODUCTION

Tracheal clearance velocities are much slower in chronic bronchitics than in normals. In 1974, Van As,[1] using a rat trachea preparation, demonstrated linear increments in ciliary rate to increased concentrations of the beta-2-agonist, Salbutamol. Hence it could be expected that this substance would improve clearance function in bronchitics, and this hypothesis was tested in a two-staged trial:

First, using a randomized, cross-over, double-blind procedure, to assess the effect of intratracheal instillation of 2.5mg Salbutamol on tracheal clearance;

Second, with a randomized, double-blind, double-dummy method, to assess its effect on clearance when given as metered aerosol or in powdered form, this dosage being only 0.4 mg.

2. MATERIALS AND METHODS

2.1. The roentgenographic method described by Friedman and Sackner. Teflon tape, coated with 50% bismuth, is fed into a specially designed punch, which is attached to a source of compressed air on one side and to a fiber-optic bronchoscope (Model BF B-3R, Olympus, Hamburg) on the other. When triggered, the punch produces individual discs which are blown through the biopsy channel into the trachea. Ten minutes following application of test substance, a total of ten tracheal x-rays are taken at one-minute intervals. Four or five discs are identified, and the distance covered noted during the procedure. Subsequently, eight to ten discs are counted out and their movement measured by two investigators independently. From these measurements an average tracheal mucous velocity (TMV) in mm/min is derived.

2.2. All patients were chronic bronchitics with increased airway obstruction, determined by whole body plethysmography, and showing an improve-

J.A. Nakhosteen and W. Maassen (eds.), Bronchology: Research, Diagnostic and Therapeutic Aspects. All rights reserved.
Copyright 1981. Martinus Nijhoff Publishers bv, The Hague / Boston / London

474

ment of at least 15% following inhalation of 2 puffs of bronchodilator. Patients with bronchogenic carcinoma were excluded from the study. Average age was 58.8 years.

2.3. The endoscopic method was identical in all patients, anesthesia of nose and throat being achieved with 2 ml of 4% Lidocaine solution, and the bronchofiberscope being introduced transnasally.

In the instillation group of 10 patients, the tip of the bronchofiberscope was positioned just inside the vocal cords, either placebo or 2.5 mg Salbutamol in 5 ml physiological solution was instilled, and the discs blown into place.

In the metered aerosol, powder inhalation or placebo group of 6 patients, three runs had to be made: one each with placebo as inhaler and aerosol, inhaler with active substance, and aerosol with active substance: the "double-dummy" method. Six further patients were tested without placebo control.

2.4. Statistical Analysis. The experimental procedure consisted of a randomized complete block design, based on a latin squares pattern, in the double-dummy group. Effects of the various modes of therapy (0.4 mg Salbutamol as metered aerosol, powder inhalation or placebo) and respective administration schedules were assessed by parametric variance analysis. Thus, influence of alterations in sequence could be eliminated. Furthermore, since in such a small collective little can be said about natural distribution, differences in effect on clearance rates were determined by non-parametric, double rank variance analysis (Friedmann), and individual differences were assessed for statistical significance by the Wilcoxon, Wilcox method.

Statistical significance in the instillation group was determined by Student's t-test.

3. RESULTS

Average tracheal mucous velocity (TMV) in the group of ten patients with endotracheal application was 3.2 mm/min under placebo. Following administration of 2.5 mg Salbutamol, TMV was 4.9 mm/min ($p < 0.025$) (Nakhosteen et al.)

No significant difference was seen in the effects of inhalation powder and metered aerosol. Both forms of active substance (0.4 mg Salbutamol) caused a statistically significant improvement of TMV compared to placebo ($2\alpha < 0.05$; rank variance analysis);(Fig. 1, Tables 1 – 3).

TABLE 1. Values for Tracheal Mucous Velocity (TMV) in Patients with Chronic Bronchitis, treated with Placebo (P), Salbutamol Metered Aerosol (A) 0.4 mg, or Salbutamol Capsule-Inhalation (C) 0.4 mg.

Patient No.	TMV (mm/min)	Therapy Form	TMV (mm/min)	Therapy Form	TMV (mm/min)	Therapy Form
1	2.7	P	3.0	C	3.6	A
2	4.3	C	0.1	P	2.0	A
3	1.5	A	2.0	C	1.4	P
4	3.2	C	4.2	A	1.8	P
5	3.3	P	3.8	A	3.6	C
6	4.5	A	4.0	P	5.0	C
7	1.6	A	2.0	C		
8	2.0	C	2.0	A		
9	1.0	A	1.0	C		
10	0.5	C	1.6	A		
11	2.5	D	2.7	D		
12	4.3	C	2.9	A		

TABLE 2. Rank Variance Analysis (Friedmann and Wilcoxon-Wilcox)

No.	Capsule Value	Capsule Rank	Aerosol Value	Aerosol Rank	Placebo Value	Placebo Rank
1	3.0	2	3.6	3	2.7	1
2	4.3	3	2.0	2	0.1	1
3	2.0	3	1.5	2	1.4	1
4	3.2	2	4.2	3	1.8	1
5	3.6	2	3.8	3	3.3	1
6	5.0	3	4.5	2	4.0	1
Totals	21.1	15	19.6	15	13.3	6
Average	3.52	R_1	3.27	R_2	2.22	R_3

n = No. of Pat's

k = No. Therapy Forms

R_i = Rank Totals

$$\bar{x}^2 = \frac{12}{nk(k+1)} \cdot \sum_{i=1}^{k} R^2 - 3n(k+1)$$

The above equation gives, for $\bar{x}^2 = 9 > X^2$ (FG = 2; 2α = 0.05) = 5.99 (from the Table), i.e., the three forms of therapy differ with a 5% probability of error from each other.

TABLE 3. Individual Comparisons using Differences in Rank Totals (Wilcoxon, Wilcox)

		Rank Totals		
Rank Totals		C	A	P
C	15	0	0	9*
A	15	–	0	9*
P	6	–	–	0

If n=6 and k=3, and 2 =0.05, then a critical difference (D_{crit}) of at least 8.1 must be exceeded.

For capsule inhalation (C) and metered aerosol (A), the respective values for $\bar{D} = 9 > D_{crit}$, hence a significant difference at the 5% level from placebo exists.

4. DISCUSSION

Beta agonists may alter the physical characteristics of respiratory secretions or reduce viscosity, and thereby enhance ciliary transport. The ultrastructure of a cilium is characterized by the "nine-two" pairing of microfilaments[2], which are connected radially by spokes and circumferentially by individual links (nexins), and arms (dynein arms). These dynein arms have characteristics similar to elementary protein units, i.e., actin and myosin, which are known to be influenced by an increased intracellular concentration of cyclic adenosine mono-phosphate (cAMP). Since beta-agonists do

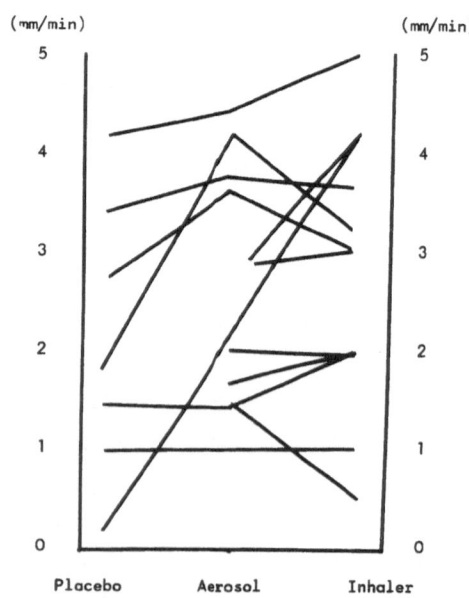

Fig. 1. Tracheal Mucous Velocity (TMV) in 12 Chronic Bronchitics: Effects of Salbutamol 0.4 mg as Metered Aerosol or from Inhaler

cause this increase, they may stimulate respiratory cilia similarly.

What are some of the more important problems encountered in the determination of TMV using the roentgenographic method? In patients where TMV was assessed three times, some developed hoarseness and showed minor traumatic lesions on the vocal cords in the third run. Since making these observations, we no longer intubate the shaft of the bronchofiberscope through the vocal cords, but position the tip just above the cords and aim through, thus lessening trauma here and reducing degree of invasiveness.

In order to reduce error in measuring disc movement, three estimations are made: one, during the procedure itself, in which 4 or 5 discs are identified and their movement noted; subsequently, two investigators measure movements in the tracheal x-rays independently. The results, when compared, find agreement to within 10% of each other, an observations also reported by Sackner.[3] The relatively high degree of inter-individual scatter is overcome here by using the patient as his own control. In an earlier study, the reproducibility of the method was found to be very good, with a correlation approaching 1 (Nakhosteen et al).[4]

The x-ray exposure of one trial run is approximately one-third that of a routine chest x-ray, because the area irradiated is confined to a portion of the trachea only.

From these studies we may conclude that in chronic bronchitics with reversible airway obstruction, administration of Salbutamol intratrachealy, and through inhalation from metered aerosol and from inhalor, improves tracheal mucous velocity, assessed by a roentgenographic method. The most effective form is intratracheal administration.

XIII.4.

MUCOCILIARY CLEARANCE IN SMOKERS AND NONSMOKERS MEASURED WITH A
BRONCHOSCOPIC VIDEO-TECHNICAL METHOD.

H. Toomes and I. Vogt-Moykopf

INTRODUCTION

The tracheobronchial mucus transport cephalad is an important cleansing system
of the bronchial tree and has been thoroughly investigated in animals. Furthermore
the influence of different drugs has been studied. The mucociliary transport shows
high sensivity to chemical stimulation. Thus it can be expected that the first disturbances of the lung function caused by cigarette smoke will appear as a decrease of
the mucociliary clearance. For human studies only indirect methods can be applied.
So far the following three in vivo methods mainly have been used: 1. bronchographic examination, 2. inhalation of radioactive marked particles and 3. bronchoscopic measurements using Teflon discs.

This study was undertaken to develop a method for clinical investigation of
the mucociliary clearance and to prove it's reproducibility. Furthermore the mucus
transport velocity should be measured in smokers and nonsmokers. Since the bronchoscopy is part of our routine examinations the endoscopic method - as described
by Sackner but modified - was selected.

Materials and methods

Standardized discs with a diameter of 1 mm and a weight of 0.2 mg were placed
upon the tracheal mucosa. Through the ciliar activity the discs are transported
cephalad with the mucus. This movement can be recorded continously. By standard-
izing the disc size and the projection factor the distance (d) of the disc to
the optic can be estimated by employing the Pythagoras theorem:

$$d = \sqrt{\left(\frac{k}{s}\right)^2 - r^2}$$

"k" is the projection enlargement, "s" the disc diameter measured on the monitor
and "r" the tracheal radius (in humans mean value 8 mm). In model tests the constant "k" was calculated and found to be 180 mm^2. By measuring two distances from
the disc to the optic and the time passed the velocity was estimated. The movement of the discs was recorded on Video-tape with a Video-camera adapted to the
bronchoscope optic. To prevent decentering of the optic in the trachea a rigid
bronchoscope - model Hopkins - was used. To simplify the calculations a tape-

J.A. Nakhosteen and W. Maassen (eds.), Bronchology: Research, Diagnostic and
Therapeutic Aspects. All rights reserved.
Copyright 1981. Martinus Nijhoff Publishers bv, The Hague / Boston / London

simultaneous Video-timer was installed.

To prove the reproducibility of this method animal experiments were performed. In 10 beagle-hounds the mucociliary clearance was measured twice at an interval of 7 days. Pentobarbital 25 mg/kg was used for the anesthesia.

In the course of routine bronchoscopies - employing the above described Video-technical method - measurements were performed in 10 smokers and 7 nonsmokers. The upper respiratory tract was anesthetized by topical application of 1% Oxybuprocain.

RESULTS

Animals measurements. Among the dogs the mucociliary clearance was to a certain extent different but could be significantly repeated in the same dog (Tab.1a).

Nonsmokers. In 7 men age 25 - 56 years (mean age 40.5 years) the mean value of the mucociliary clearance was 18.5 mm/min (SD $\pm$ 5.98)(Tab.1b).

Smokers. 10 men age 35 - 55 years (mean age 47.7 years) with an average of 15 - 40 years of smoking and with a daily consumption of 15 - 60 cigarettes were examined. The last cigarette was smoked the evening before the bronchoscopy. In this group the mean value of the mucociliary clearance was found to be 6.8 mm/min (SD $\pm$ 5.01)(Tab.1c). In 2 smokers the mucus transport had completely ceased. These findings show a significant decrease of the mucociliary clearance in smokers.

TABLE 1. Mucociliary clearance in a) 10 dogs, b) 7 nonsmokers and c) 10 smokers. Mean velocity of 10 measured particles per dog or patient.

a)

Dog No.	1.Measurement	2.Measurement
8301	7.6	7.5
8302	6.3	2.9
8305	12.0	12.3
8309	4.1	6.6
8320	7.0	8.4
8322	12.0	10.7
8325	8.3	6.0
8332	11.8	10.7
8392	14.0	14.7
8396	15.6	15.0

b)

Patient No.	mm/min
1	13.48
2	18.80
3	17.11
4	16.94
5	29.78
6	21.47
7	11.66
Mean velocity	18.46
$\pm$ SD	5.98

c)

Patient No.	mm/min
1	8.93
2	5.26
3	3.00
4	13.08
5	3.81
6	0.0
7	10.80
8	10.53
9	0.0
10	12.75
Mean velocity	6.80
$\pm$ SD	5.01

XIII.5.
A METHOD FOR MEASURING CILIARY BEAT FREQUENCY IN VITRO

H. HESSE, W. MIZERA, R. KASPAREK, J.A. NAKHOSTEEN, N. KONIETZKO

For the lung to remain healthy, inhaled toxic particles such as dust or bacteria must be removed. Ciliated epithelium of the bronchi serves this function in part. The mucociliary clearance depends on load and structure of mucus and the condition of the epithelium itself. Several methods of measuring ciliary beat frequency in animals exist, but few can measure this in man. We developed an in vitro method for measuring ciliary beat frequency of the human bronchial tree.

MATERIALS AND METHOD

Twenty healthy volunteers, aged between 20 and 40 years, were examined. All received remuneration and gave informed consent.

During bronchofiberscopy brush biopsies were obtained from trachea, left main stem bronchus and segmental (S4 left) bronchus. The brush was shaken in a nutrient solution maintained at 37°C and buffered at pH 7.4. A specimen is pipetted onto an indented slide and ciliated cells which are still viable are found under a phase contrast microscope.

The phase contrast microscope is fitted with a photo-electric cell, to which a microscope-photometer is connected. The beat of the ciliated cells interrupts the light beam to the photo-sensitive cell; and signals, thus triggered, are transmitted to an oscilloscope and registered graphically (Fig. 1).

FIGURE 1.

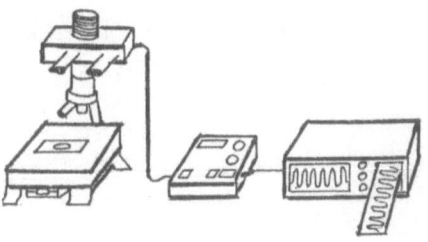

Ciliary frequency of the three anatomic regions mentioned above were measured, and the effect of temperature change assessed.

J.A. Nakhosteen and W. Maassen (eds.), Bronchology: Research, Diagnostic and Therapeutic Aspects. All rights reserved.
Copyright 1981. Martinus Nijhoff Publishers bv, The Hague / Boston / London

RESULTS

No change in beat frequency was observed over a period of 160 min, at a constant temperature of 37°C and a pH of 7.4. This was true for individual samples and for the group as a whole (Fig. 2).

FIGURE 2. Measurement of Ciliary Beat Frequency from t=0 to t=160 min.

FIGURE 3. Effect of Increase in Temp. (———:Trachea; ----Main Stem Bronchus; ••••Segmental Br.;————All Regions)

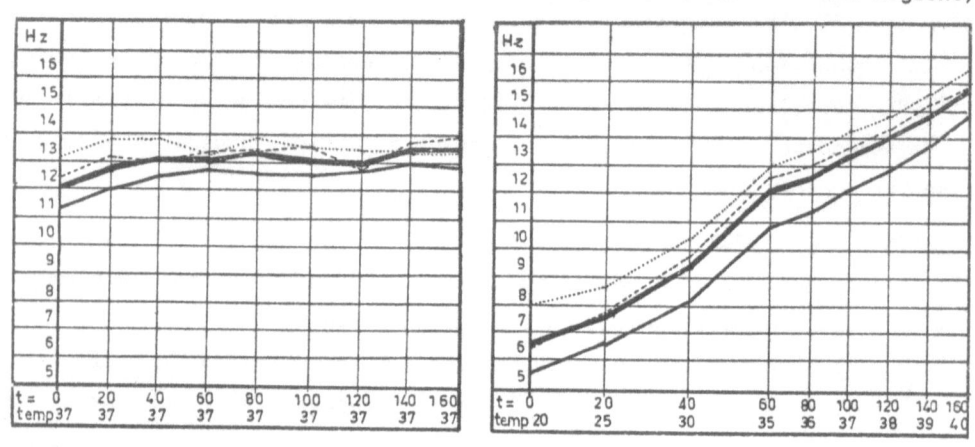

The over-all beat frequency of the trachea was 12.5 Hz (SD 2.8); the main stem bronchus 13.2 Hz (SD 2.2), and the segmental bronchus 13.6 Hz (SD 2.2). The difference is significant between trachea and segmental bronchus (Fig. 3).

Frequency was measured every 20 min while increasing temperature from 20° to 40°C (Fig. 3). Frequency at 20°C is half that at 37°C. Further temperature increments cause proportional increases.

In the 12 men and 8 women studied, the latter showed a significantly higher ciliary beat frequency. No difference was noted in smokers (Total: 10) and non-smokers (Total: 10).

DISCUSSION

This paper describes a reproducible method for measuring ciliary beat frequency in vitro.

The over-all beat frequency is approximately 13 Hz; it increases from trachea to periphery. The differences recorded between trachea and main stem bronchus or segmental bronchus are significant. These results are comparable to those reported by YAGER, who used similar methods, but are in contrast to IRIVANI, who found a halving of frequencies from trachea to periphery. Whether this difference is due to methodology or influence of local anesthetic or to some other factor is unclear.

The standard deviations of the data recorded from the group as a whole are relatively large; on the other hand, the intra-individual data was very uniform. This corresponds to the results of CAMNER, who did not find any significant difference of mucociliary clearance either intra-individually or in twins. The ciliary beat frequency increases as the temperature is raised, a fact that was observed by MERCKE in animals. At a temperature of $20^{\circ}C$ the frequency is exactly half that at $37^{\circ}C$, and it rises gradually with temperature increments from 20 to $37^{\circ}C$, finally reaching the same frequency of other control cilia maintained at $37^{\circ}C$.

No differences between smokers and non-smokers were observed; this may reflect the relatively young age of test subjects (20–40 years). A decreased mucociliary clearance in heavy smokers has been reported (SACKNER). Further investigations of ciliary beat frequence would seem indicated to examine the effect of other physical factors (medium, pH, etc.), different chemical influences (drugs, noxious substances), and the influence of bacteria and viruses, thus allowing better understanding of the processes underlying mucociliary clearance and perhaps even demonstrating connections with other lung diseases.

XIII.6.

EFFECTS OF A BETA-ADRENERGIC AGONIST (REPROTEROL) ON CILIARY BEAT FREQUENCY OF HUMAN BRONCHIAL EPITHELIUM IN VITRO

R. KASPAREK, W. MIZERA, H. HESSE

Previous investigations have demonstrated a stimulatory effect of beta-adrenergic agonists on ciliary beat frequency of animals in vitro (1). Investigations of human bronchial epithelium under the influence of these substances in vitro have not been performed. To investigate this effect brush biopsies of trachea and main bronchus of 15 patients with different lung diseases were examined.

Half of each sample was put into a nutrient medium containing Reproterol $0,9 \times 10^{-6}$ g/ml, the other part of the biopsy served as control without Reproterol. At constant temperature (25°C) and constant pH of the medium (7.4) the ciliary beat frequency was measured every 10 minutes for 1 hour. The method used is described in detail in paper 12.5.

Ciliary beat frequency was independent of biopsy site and of the time of investigation. But in both trachea and main stem bronchus a significant stimulating effect was found. Average ciliary beat frequency in the trachea increased from 7.08 ± 1.57 Hz to 8.9 ± 2.67 Hz; in the main stem bronchus, from 7.4 ± 2.55 Hz to 8.93 ± 2.9 Hz.

J.A. Nakhosteen and W. Maassen (eds.), Bronchology: Research, Diagnostic and Therapeutic Aspects. All rights reserved.
Copyright 1981. Martinus Nijhoff Publishers bv, The Hague / Boston / London

XIII.7.
RESPIRATORY MUCOSA DAMAGE AFTER BRUSH BIOPSY

R. Lundgren, P. Hörstedt, B. Winblad

INTRODUCTION

Brush biopsy through the flexible fiberoptic bronchoscope is a very valuable method in the diagnosis of bronchial carcinoma. In cases with occult bronchial carcinoma bronchial brushing from every single segment bronchus may be necessary to detect the tumour. We have studied the damage of respiratory mucosa caused by brush biopsy and the wound healing after brushing.

MATERIAL AND METHODS

30 adult rabbits were brushed in trachea through a flexible fiberoptic bronchoscope. Trachea was examined at different times after brush biopsy (table 1). Besides, another seven animals were examined without brush biopsy. Trachea was fixed in 2,5 % glutaraldehyde, critical point dried, coated with gold and examined in a scanning electron microscope (SEM). After SEM examination the gold coated biopsies were sectioned for light microscopy.

TABLE 1.
Trachea from 30 adult rabbits examined after brush biopsy

Time for autopsy	0h	1/2h	3h	6h	1d	2d	3d	5d	1w	2w	3w	4w
No. of animals	7	1	1	2	2	3	2	1	4	3	2	2

Trachea from 7 control rabbits examined without brush biopsy.

RESULTS

The normal rabbit trachea was covered by a ciliated pseudostratified columnal epithelium. Brush biopsy removed large areas of the normal respiratory mucosa (Fig. 1, 2 and 3). Sometimes the basement membrane and the small vessels in the submucosa were damaged (Fig. 4). During the first two days after brushing the deep wounded areas were covered by a fibrin and blood rich granulation tissue with inflammatory cells in the submucosa (Fig. 5). Regeneration started already within the first 24 hours from intact epithelial cells at the margin of the brushed area and from basal cells on the undamaged

J.A. Nakhosteen and W. Maassen (eds.), Bronchology: Research, Diagnostic and
Therapeutic Aspects. All rights reserved.
Copyright 1981. Martinus Nijhoff Publishers bv, The Hague / Boston / London

basement membrane (Fig. 5). Five days after brush biopsy the brushed area was covered by an epithelium but there was only a few ciliated cells in the central part of the brushed area (Fig. 6). Two weeks after brush biopsy only small areas without ciliated cells could be detected and three weeks after brush biopsy no sign of damage was observed.

DISCUSSION

Gordon and Lane (1976) studied superficial damage in the rat tracheal epithelium and noticed that basal cells became flattened and covered the wounded area within six hours. William (1953) studied deeper trauma in rat trachea and according to him regeneration of the ciliated epithelium was not complete until 6 weeks after trauma. In calf, according to Hilding (1965), a superficial respiratory mucosa damage not penetrating the basement membrane was replaced with normal pseudostratified epithelium within 7-10 days. From our studies in rabbits the following conclusions were made.

1. Brush biopsy removes large areas of the normal ciliated epithelium and the basement membrane is often penetrated.
2. During the first two days after brushing the deep wounded areas are covered by a coagulum.
3. Regeneration of the respiratory mucosa starts within six hours.
4. Normal ciliated mucosa is restored within three weeks.

REFERENCES

1. Gordon R, Lane B: Regeneration of rat tracheal epithelium after mechanical injury. Am. Rev. Respir. Dis. 113, 799-807, 1976.
2. Hilding AC: Regeneration of respiratory epithelium after minimal surface trauma. Annals of Otology, Rhinology and Laryngology 74, 903-914, 1965.
3. Wilhelm DL: Regeneration of tracheal epithelium. J. Path. Bact. 65, 543-550, 1953.

ACKNOWLEDGEMENT

This study was supported by grants from the Swedish National Association against Heart and Chest Diseases and Lions (project No. 169/80) foundation, University of Umeå, Sweden.

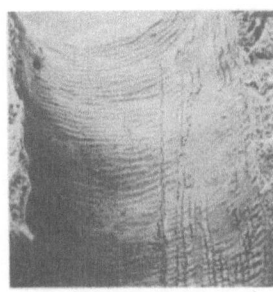 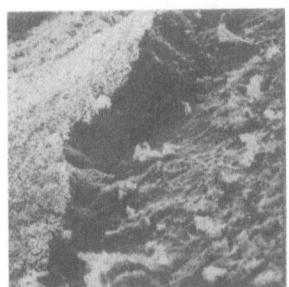

FIGURE 1. Low magnification scanning electron micrograph (SEM) of rabbit
tracheal mucosa directly after brush biopsy. The epithelium is removed in
the brushed areas (to the right) down to the basement membrane.
FIGURE 2. Higher magnification of the border between the ciliated epithelium and the brushed area.

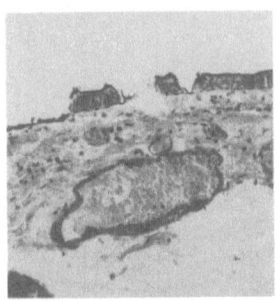 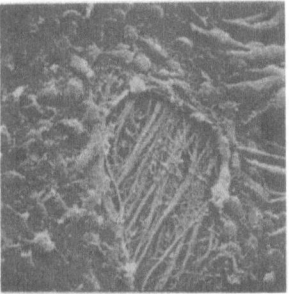

FIGURE 3. Light micrograph (LM) of the same area as in Figs. 1, 2. Notice
the remaining gold layer on top of partly damaged epithelial cells with
rifts from the brush down to the basement membrane. Htx-eosin x 120.
FIGURE 4. SEM of a somewhat deeper damage where the basement membrane is
penetrated and the underlying connective tissue is observed.

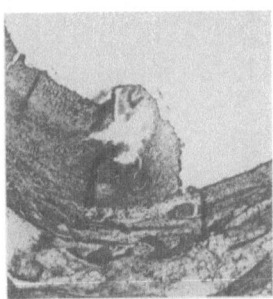 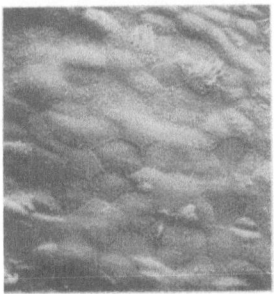

FIGURE 5. LM of trachea 24 hours after brush biopsy with a clot with
fibrin and inflammatory cells (left) and a regenerating epithelium (right).
Htx-eosin x 30.
FIGURE 6. SEM of tracheal mucosa 5 days after brush biopsy. The brushed area
is covered by an epithelium with only a few ciliated cells.

XIII.8.

ELECTRON MICROSCOPIC AND HISTOCHEMICAL STUDY OF BRONCHIAL MUCOSA OBTAINED
BY BIOPSY FROM BRONCHITIC PATIENTS

P.SZÜLE, J.APPEL and G.MISKOVITS

Bronchial mucosa obtained by bronchoscopic biopsy was studied in 52 cases.
Excisions were made from the inflammated mucosa of patients with chronic bronchitis /4o cases/ and for the purpose of controll from the normal mucosa of

patients /12 cases/. Fixation was carried out for 24
hours by glutaric aldehide, postfixation for 1 hour
by OsO_4, while contrasting by uranil acetate and plum-
bic citrate, respectively. Semi-thin sections were
stained by toluidin-blue. Photographs were taken by
a Hitachi HU-10 elektron microscope.
The following ultrastructural changes were found in
chronic bronchitis:

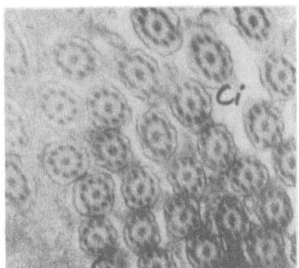

Fig.1.

1. Epithelial edema with extended extracellular space
and with increased interdigitations.
2. Increased number of mitochondria with frequent degeneration.
3. Cystic dilatation of the endoplasmatic reticulum.
4. The most conspicious changes were seen in cilia: in
the intact epithelium they were found to have regular
plasmatic covering and a normal 9+2 structure /Fig.1./,
while in the bioptic material of bronchitic patients
this plasmatic covering became dentated and racket-sha-
ped, myelin-like formations were observed /Fig.2./
The degeneration of cilia was verified by scanning
electron microscopic examinations as well: while the
cell surface of the intact epithelium was covered by
normal cilia /Fig.3./, flattening and denudated areas
were seen in cases of chronic bronchitis /Fig.4./
5. The granules of goblet cells were showing the signs
of structural changes: secretory granules of two different densities, surrounded by membranes could be well
demonstrated by glutaric aldehide and OsO_4-fixation/Fig.5./
even in the superficial excretory goblet cells of the

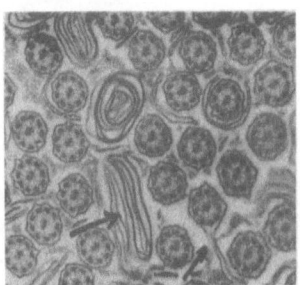

Fig.2.

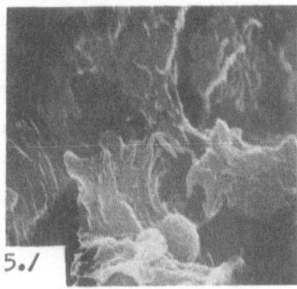

Fig.3.

J.A. Nakhosteen and W. Maassen (eds.), Bronchology: Research, Diagnostic and
Therapeutic Aspects. All rights reserved.
Copyright 1981. Martinus Nijhoff Publishers bv, The Hague / Boston / London

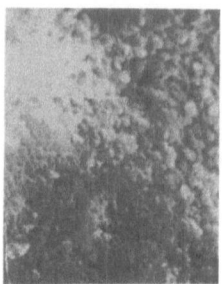

Fig.4.

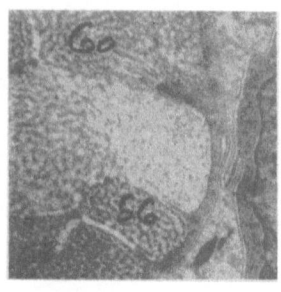

Fig.5.

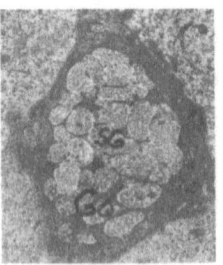

Fig.6.

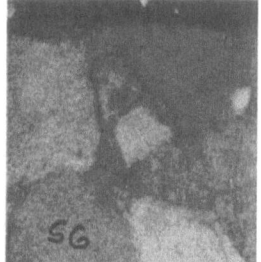

Fig.7.

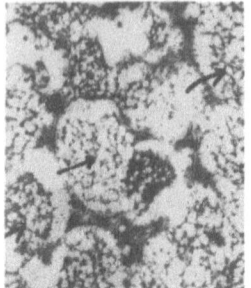

Fig.8.

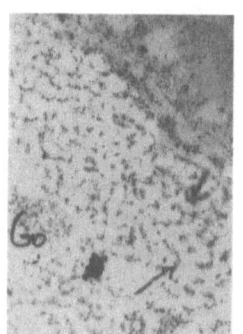

Fig.9.

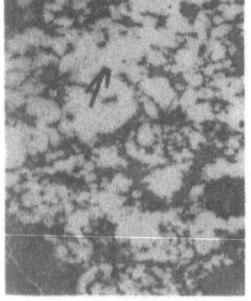

Fig.1o.

normal bronchial mucosa /Fig.6./
On the other hand, the structure of
mucous granules of bronchitic patients has shown remarkable changes, i.e. the granules were found
to merge /Fig.7./.

Different fixational and elektro-
ne-histochemical methodes were
used to demonstrate the mucopoly-
saccharides /glucose-amino-glicanes/ of the goblet cells.
Administering only glutaric aldehide fixation, the mucous granules were showing star-formation /Fig.8./.
The average diameter of the central
nucleus of these star-shaped structures proved to be 38 nanometers
and the length of the protruding
fibres l,l nanometer, respectively.

PA-silver-methenamine reaction showed a strong positivity in these materials /Fig.9./. The specificity of
the reaction was verified by controll
negativity /argentation withoud perio-
dic-acid oxidation/.

The characteristic star-shaped structure of glucose-amino-glycanes in
chronic bronchitis was loosening
/Fig.1o./, the PA-silver reaction
showed only very slight positivity,
while the alciane-blue-silver proved to be strongly positive in each
case /Fig.11./ with simultaneous controll-negativity
/argentation withoud alciane-blue staining/.

It is concluded that the carboxyl groups of mucus
are vehemently impregnated by the alciane-blue-silver reaction, suggesting the mass presence of acid
mucopolysaccharides /glucose-amino-glycanes/ in

the secretory granules of goblet cells in chronic bronchitis.

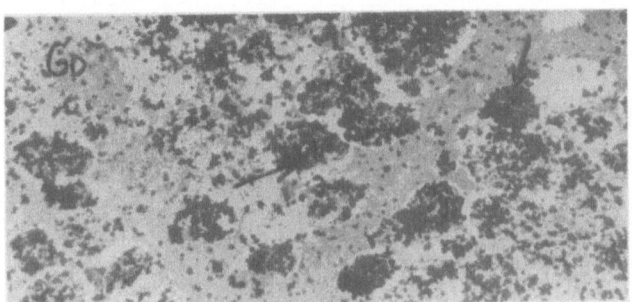

Fig.11.

Chapter XIV

BRONCHOSCOPY AS AN OFFICE PROCEDURE

XIV.1.

INDICATIONS AND CONTRAINDICATIONS FOR BRONCHOSCOPY AS AN OFFICE PROCEDURE

H. HUG

Bronchoscopy, an examination of growing importance for modern lung diagnosis can be, by itself, dangerous even fatal for the patient. It is therefore of great interest, in order to minimize the risks, to determine what patient has to undergo and what doctor is legitimated to execute this fascinating investigation. I am convinced that bronchoscopy with rigid and flexible instruments will spread over from hospital to private office, this development being catalysed by the tremendous success of fiberoptic. But we have to make a careful selection of both: patients and doctors, to avoid a decrease of accuracy and reliability in future.
Let's first see the minimal levels of experience and skill which are unabdictable for a doctor working as a responsible bronchoscopist. A large number, at least a hundred bronchoscopies must be skillfully and personally demonstrated to the student before he starts working on the patient; and I think another fifty bronchoscopies at least should be executed by himself under surveillance before he may be allowed to work alone. To some of our friends who have real industrial plants for bronchoscopy, this number might seem very small. But we attend a world congress here, and we have colleagues who are working in smaller hospital units. They will find it quite difficult to reach that number in an adequate lapse of time. As a further precaution it is needed that the results obtained by the fifty surveyed examinations give an acceptable average range of accuracy. As bronchoscopy is demanding a considerable amount of skill, a teacher should pass his instruction and his experience only to people who are actually able to handle the instruments and the patient properly. These rules for the choice of doctors are relatively transparent and easy to adopt.

J.A. Nakhosteen and W. Maassen (eds.), Bronchology: Research, Diagnostic and Therapeutic Aspects. All rights reserved.
Copyright 1981. Martinus Nijhoff Publishers bv, The Hague / Boston / London

But when we are looking at the INDICATIONS AND CONTRAINDICATIONS
FOR BRONCHOSCOPY AS AN OFFICE PROCEDURE regarding the patient, the
problem is much more complex. There are no "easy diagnosis" and
"risk-free" patients. You may meet laryngospasms, cardiac complications or local anesthesia hazards in apparently healthy people
as well as in circulatory or respiratory invalids. However the decision: office or hospital bronchoscopy can be facilitated by
performing ECG, blood-gaz analysis and general clinical check-up.
With a certain experience you get a feeling for possible complications. But being aware of imminent troubles, we should not give
way to the temptation of reducing the risks by decreasing the extent
of examination. Having a clear indication for rigid bronchoscopy
i.e. in a high risk patient, we have presumably a tendency to pass
only the fiber optic or to shorten the time of observation in order
to avoid a transfer to hospital. This is human and we all have done
so - nevertheless it is irresponsible, because it deminishes the
significance of the diagnosis. The decrease of the examinator's and
finally the method's reputation is predictable.
These considerations allow us to reckon the contraindications and
limits for office procedure. All patients who present the following
symptoms and/or diagnosis have to be examined under hospital
surveillance:

- high risk for local anesthesia
- coronary insufficiency
- arrhythmia
- respiratory insufficiency with severe change in blood-gaz levels
- severe systemic illness
- anticoagulation

For office bronchoscopy remains a large field of indications,
for diagnosis, i.e.:

- persistent caugh
- hemoptesis
- unexplained wheezing
- the necessity to obtain bacteriological and cytological samples
  by aspiration and/or brush biopsy. (The use of forceps for
  bronchial biopsy must be discussed in a further publication.
  Transbronchial biopsy is strictly reserved to the hospital.)

For therapy, i.e.:

- bronchial toilet in bronchiectasis
- removing mucus behind stenosis
- aspiration of mucus causing atelectasis
- instillation of mucolytica

Considering the fact, that office executed bronchoscopy is less frightening for the patient, much cheaper for the tax-payer and can give, in its limited field, excellent results, there is no doubt, that bronchoscopy as an office procedure will gain a world-wide increase in frequency under the condition that we resist to the "just-have-a-look-down" mentality.

XIV.2.

FIBERGLASBRONCHOSKOPIE IN DER PRAXIS

R.F. KROIDL

In dem folgenden Beitrag werde ich auf folgende Fragen eingehen:
Ist die Fiberglasbronchoskopie in der Praxis 1. Technisch möglich?
2. Medizinisch sinnvoll? 3. Forensisch vertretbar? 4. Wirtschaftlich
machbar?

Zur Frage "TECHNISCH MÖGLICH?":
Dies kann man uneingeschränkt bejahen. Die gleichen Fiberglas-
bronchoskope werden in der Klinik wie in der Praxis verwendet. Der
technische Untersuchungsablauf mit lokaler Betäubung unterscheidet
sich in der Praxis nicht von dem Vorgehen in der Klinik. Man wird davon
ausgehen, daß derjenige, der die Untersuchung ambulant durchführt, min-
destens die gleiche Qualifikation haben muß, wie der Kollege, der sie
klinisch durchführt. (Doch dies ist eine Frage der Ausbildung, die
nicht zum Thema gehört).

Die Patienten werden über Ziel und Durchführung der Untersuchung
aufgeklärt und unterscheiben eine Einverständniserklärung. Am Tage
der Bronchoskopie kommt der Patient nüchtern um 7.15 Uhr in die Praxis.
Die Assistentin gibt eine Atropin-Spritze i.m., sie appliziert Xylo-
cain-Gel in die Nase, der Patient nimmt auf einem nach hinten abklapp-
baren bequemen Sessel Platz. Zu Beginn der Bronchoskopie erhält der
Patient Valium i.v. Die Dosierung richtet sich nach dem Bedarf, sie
liegt meistens zwischen 1o und 15 mg. Zum Nachspritzen bleibt die
Nadel liegen. Routinemäßig wird nasotracheal intubiert. Nur selten
war es nötig, aufgrund besonderer nasaler Verhältnisse oral zu intu-
bieren. Bei der Bronchoskopie wird regelmäßig folgendes Material
asserviert: Spülsekret zur bakteriologischen und cytologischen Untersuchung. Bronchialbürsten-Ausstriche zur Ausstrich-Cytologie und Biopsien. Durchschnittlich dauert eine Bronchoskopie 2o - 3o Minuten. Danach verbleiben die Patienten noch zwei- bis zweieinhalb Stunden in

*J.A. Nakhosteen and W. Maassen (eds.), Bronchology: Research, Diagnostic and
Therapeutic Aspects. All rights reserved.
Copyright 1981. Martinus Nijhoff Publishers bv, The Hague / Boston / London*

der Praxis und werden dann mit dem Taxi oder einem Angehörigen nach
Hause gefahren. Bei gegebener Indikation, speziell bei peripheren Läsi-
onen wird die Bronchoskopie auf dem Durchleuchtungstisch durchgeführt.
Es kann dann unter Durchleuchtung der betroffene Herd selektiv kathete-
risiert werden. Biopsien aus der Peripherie sind dann möglich. Von
dieser Möglichkeit wird vor allem auch bei diffusen parenchymatösen
Prozessen mit perbronchialen Biopsien Gebrauch gemacht.

IST DIE FIBERGLASBRONCHOSKOPIE IN DER PRAXIS SINNVOLL?

Auch diese Frage kann uneingeschränkt mit "ja" beantwortet werden.
Zentren, die bronchoskopieren, sind bislang leider spärlich gesäht.
Die Lungenfachklinik, mit der ich häufig und gerne zusammenarbeite,
hat meistens eine lange Warteliste. Die Durchführung dieser Maßnahme
in der Praxis hat viele Vorteile: Der diagnostische Gang bleibt bis zur
definitiven Klärung in einer Hand. Ein Bronchoskopie-Termin in der
Praxis kann in wenigen Tagen, spätestens innerhalb Wochenfrist, ermöglicht werden. Viele Patienten , speziell ältere, scheuen das Krankenhaus mit neuer Umgebung, neuen Ärzten, unbekannten Schwestern. Die
diagnostische Ausbeute muß - da die Technik identisch ist - in der
Praxis die gleiche sein wie in der Klinik. Einen Überblick über 300
Bronchoskopien in der Praxis (vom Mai 1977 bis Mai 1980) gibt die folgende Tabelle:

ALTERSGRUPPEN :		INDIKATION:	
Bis 20 Jahre	4 %	Carcinom-Verdacht	74 %
40 Jahre	11 %	Tbc.	6 %
60 Jahre	24 %	Mb. Boeck	5 %
über 60 Jahre	61 %	Asthma/chron. Bronchitis	5 %
Männer 72 %, Frauen 28 %		Lymphangiosis Verdacht	2 %
Jüngster Patient: 8 Jahre		Sonstige Indikationen	8 %
Ältester Patient: 86 Jahre			

IST DIE FIBERGLASBRONCHOSKOPIE IN DER PRAXIS FORENSISCH VERTRETBAR?

Dies ist sicherlich ein Angelpunkt der anstehenden Diskussion. Man
kann ihn von verschiedenen Gesichtspunkten beleuchten: Sofern nach den
Regeln der Kunst vorgegangen wird, und die Indikation sowie die Durchführung der Untersuchung lege artis erfolgt, kann man sich juristisch
abgedeckt fühlen. Man mag einwenden, daß eine ambulante Praxis für

denkbare Zwischenfälle nicht so gut gerüstet ist wie eine Klinik. Dies
ist zweifellos der Fall. Auch vorausgesetzt, daß die ambulante Praxis
mit Notfalleinrichtung in Form technischer Ausstattung und persönlichem
know how auf Notfälle eingerichtet ist, so bleibt natürlich immer noch
die Lücke, die zur Klinik mit deren zusätzlichen Möglichkeiten nicht
zu schließen ist.

Dagegen sind die Risiken der Fiberglasbronchoskopie zu halten. An-
erkanntermaßen ist dies ein wenig riskanter Eingriff. Von den rund 300
Bronchoskopien, die ich in den letzten 3 Jahren ambulant durchführte,
hat es keinen einzigen Zwischenfall gegeben. Hierbei waren die meisten
Patienten - wie nicht anders zu erwarten - aufgrund ihrer Vorleiden
und ihrer Altersgruppe - durchaus gewisse Risikopatienten. Erwähnt sei
jedoch ein Fall, der glücklicherweise als Zwischenfall erspart blieb:
Relativ kurz nach Aufnahme der bronchoskopischen Untersuchungen in die
ambulante Praxis wurde ein Patient überwiesen, bei dem sich röntgenologisch eine knollige Verschattung im rechten Oberlappen fand. An der
Diagnose "Bronchial-Ca." wenig Zweifel; es galt, die histologische Klärung herbeizuführen. Da gerade Freitagnachmittag war, verständigte ich
mich mit dem Hausarzt telefonisch, daß die Bronchoskopie am Montagmorgen erfolgen sollte. Am Montagmorgen rief der Kollege an und sagte,
diese Maßnahme sei überflüssig, da tags zuvor der Patient spontan ver-
blutet sei. Man stelle sich vor, dieses spontane Ereignis einer Blutung
wäre zu dem Zeitpunkt eingetreten, wo mein Bronchoskop gerade den Larynx passierte! Juristische Gesichtspunkte ganz beiseite gelassen, eine
Praxis kann sich rein vom Image her eben keine Zwischenfälle "leisten".

IST DIE FIBERFLASBRONCHOSKOPIE IN DER PRAXIS WIRTSCHAFTLICH MACHBAR?
Genau so klar wie Punkt 1 und 2 eindeutig mit "ja" , Punkt 3 mit
"vielleicht" zu beantworten war, so hat dieser Punkt ganz klar die Ant-
wort "nein". Die Fiberglasbronchoskopie in der Praxis ist für den, der
sie durchführt, ein echtes und erhebliches "Zusatzgeschäft". Hierzu
die folgende Wirtschaftlichkeitsberechnung, die eindeutige Perspektiven
aufzeigt.

XIV. 3.

119. BRONCHOFIBEROPTIC EXAMINATION FOR SCREENING OF THE MALIGNANT
TUMORS

Hidehiko OKADA, M.D., Masahiko KURATA, M.D.

1. INTRODUCTION

When we perform bronchoscopy under local anesthesia, there are
still severe discomfort, but its benefit and safety are better than
its discomfort. The reason to present this paper is to report the
result of bronchoscopic examination in our hospital and to discuss
some problems through a few interesting cases.

2. CASE REPORT AND DISCUSSION

The total number of flexible fiberoptic bronchoscopy performed
at our hospital from 1974 to 1979 is 480 cases. Its detail is shown
at Table 1.

TABLE 1. Cases of flexible fiberoptic bronchoscopy from 1974 to 1979

Primary lung cancer	146
Primary lung sarcoma	5
Metastatic lung cancer	19
Benign lung tumor	8
Mediastinal tumor	8
Bronchitis, Bronchiolitis and Bronchiectasis	227
Lung tuberculosis	51
Foreign body at bronchus	1
Other	15
Total	480

When we face patients and decide to try bronchoscopic examination,
there are usually some motives like a persistent dry cough, hemoptysis
or an abnormal shadow on the chest films. All cases were classified by
hemoptysis or abnormal shadow. Table 2 shows that 186 cases were examined because of hemoptysis though 28 cases do not have abnormal shadow.

*J.A. Nakhosteen and W. Maassen (eds.), Bronchology: Research, Diagnostic and
Therapeutic Aspects. All rights reserved.
Copyright 1981. Martinus Nijhoff Publishers bv, The Hague / Boston / London*

TABLE 2. Motives of performing bronchofiberscopy

	Case
Hemoptysis	
Positive chest X-ray films	158
Negative chest X-ray films	28
	186
Non-hemoptysis	Case
Positive chest X-ray films	292
Negative chest X-ray films	2
	294

Bronchitis, Bronchiolitis and Bronchiectasis

The total of these group is 227 cases. Hemoptysis was seen often in comparison with other disease. In the case of bronchitis, bronchiolitis, it amounted to 17.5%, in the case of bronchiectasis it ran up to 76%. It repeats itself in most cases, its course is generally long term. On bronchoscopic examination, we can usually find much sputum and hyperemic, edematous bronchial mucous membrane.

Bacteriological examination is also performed together with TBLB and brushing. Bronchography is simultaneously carried out to know the degree or extent of the changes and it provides a reference to deciding future therapy. In the case with much sputum and marked inflammatory findings, bronchial toilet is also performed.

The most important thing is not to overlook the malignant changes concealed behind inflammation. It is necessary to check them over repeatedly in suspicious cases.

Lung cancer

We performed bronchoscopy in 146 cases of lung cancer. The items are shown in Table 3.

TABLE 3. Analysis of lung cancer according to its localization and histological type

	Squamous cell carcinoma	Adeno-carcinoma	Anaplastic large cell carcinoma	Anaplastic small cell carcinoma	Unknown	Total
Peripheral	33	35	4	5	9	86
Hilar	24	19	6	8	3	60
Total	57	54	10	13	12	146

One of the main reason that we perform the bronchoscopic examination is to detect lung cancer as soon as possible and to determine

the site of changes and the extent of invasion for the operation.
Two cases out of 28 cases that had only hemoptysis, were lung cancer
and one of them proved to be early lung cancer.
Case 1: 55-year-old female, Chief complaint was hemoptysis.

There is no abnormal shadow on the chest films. Bronchoscopically
whitish, edematous swelling of mucous membrane at the right B$_6$ orifice
and interruption of the longitudinal fold were observed. It was proved
to be adenocarcinoma, roentgenologically occult lung cancer, by punch
biopsy. After a right lower lobectomy early lung cancer was verified.

When the patients complain of hemoptysis without abnormal shadow
on the chest films, it is desirable to observe each bronchus carefully.
Squamous cell carcinoma that shows polypoid or nodular development is
easy to detect but when adenocarcinoma or undifferentiated small cell
carcinoma show superficial infiltrative development, it is necessary
to observe the localization more carefully.
Case 2: 63-year-old female

For one year, she has complained of a dry cough and received medication under chronic bronchitis. On September 1979 she noticed a
muscle weakness of upper extremities and clonic convulsion, so she received removal of the brain tumor under diagnosis of metastatic brain
tumor on November 1979. From the chest films we can not well observe
the left hemidiaphragm and can not follow the left basal airbroncho-
gram so we can suspect atelectasis of the left lower lobe or existence
of mass lesion on the left heart shadow. Bronchoscopy shows the invasion of the tumor at the left main bronchus. The tumor completely
obstructed the orifice of the basal bronchus. Although the left pneumonectomy was planned, the patient died of diffuse metastasis to the
bilateral lungs just before operation.

It may be said that the area near the hilum, especially the area
overlapping the heart shadow is one of the blind spots. If the
bronchoscopy had been performed ealier, the patient might be saved.

3. CONCLUSION

We have performed bronchoscopy for the purpose of screening for
lung cancer and been sometimes surprised to discover the roentgenologically occult cancer or look at unexpected changes through the
bronchoscope.

It is of course important to find out early cancer, but I think it
is also important for clinicians not to overlook the operable staged
cancer.

Chapter XV

PEDIATRIC BRONCHOLOGY

XV.1.

FIBREOPTIC BRONCHOSCOPY IN SMALL CHILDREN

J.O. WARNER, S.W. CLARKE, M.J.H. SCALLAN

INTRODUCTION

Fibreoptic bronchoscopy has revolutionised the management of adults with chest disease, but its application to paediatric practice has been very limited. Airway calibre has dictated an absolute limitation on its use, as the patient must breathe round the instrument. Furthermore, children undergoing such a procedure require a general anaesthetic which is difficult to administer and negates one of the major advantages of the procedure, namely the avoidance of general anaesthesia.

As the fibreoptic instrument has a greater visual range and produces fewer complications than the rigid, open-tube bronchoscope, we have applied a general anaesthetic technique which allows the flexible instrument to be used safely even in small children.

PROCEDURE

The children are pre-medicated with trimeprazane 2-3 mg/kg given orally two hours before the anaesthetic. One hour later they are given an intramuscular injection of papaveretum 0.3 mg/kg and atropine 0.02 mg/kg. Following pre-oxygenation, anaesthesia is induced with "Althesin" (a mixture of alphadalone and alphaxalone) and maintained with Althesin given either by continuous infusion or in small bolus doses intravenously (approximate dose 0.005 mg/kg per minute). Muscle relaxants, either short (suxamethonium) or long (pancuronium) acting are given, the choice depending on the anticipated duration of the procedure. A Portex blue line infants feeding tube size FG6-8, depending on the size of the child, is passed through the nose into the trachea. The tip of the tube lies approximately half way down the trachea, and this position is confirmed later by the endoscopist. Ventilation is achieved by an injector which includes a pressure-reducing valve. The injector is connected to a wall oxygen supply (pressure 60 P.S.I. or 4.2 kg/cm^2). The distal end of the injector is connected to the tracheal tube, and ventilation is started with the pressure-reducing valve set to minimum. The pressure is gradually increased until ventilation appears to be adequate as judged by chest expansion. Obstruction to expiration may occur, particularly in smaller children, where the difference between the internal diameter of the upper respiratory tract and the external diameter of the bronchoscope may be small. Therefore, the anaes-thetist must satisfy himself that expiration is complete before initiating the next inspiration. Respiratory frequency is maintained at approximately 20/min.

J.A. Nakhosteen and W. Maassen (eds.), Bronchology: Research, Diagnostic and Therapeutic Aspects. All rights reserved.
Copyright 1981. Martinus Nijhoff Publishers bv, The Hague / Boston / London

Adequate ventilation is achieved by the Venturi effect, which operates equally efficiently when the bronchoscope is in the airway. The pulse, blood pressure, colour and ECG should be monitored throughout the procedure. For very small children, we feel that transcutaneous oximetry should also be employed.

The bronchoscope is passed through the mouth, rather than the nose as in adults, and by direct visualisation guided into the larynx and thence the trachea. The position of the ventilating tube is checked prior to visualisation of the bronchial tree.

PATIENTS AND RESULTS

We have studied five children from 4-11 years using an adult bronchoscope (Olympus BFB3), with an external diameter of 5.3 mm. The details of the procedures on these five patients are presented and compared with the outcome on five children who had rigid, open-tube bronchoscopy over the same period of time on the paediatric unit (Table 1).

TABLE 1. Bronchoscopy in small children.

Indications	Fibreoptic				Rigid (open-tube)			
	Age	Sex	Findings	Complications	Age	Sex	Findings	Complications
? Foreign body	8	F	None seen	None	3	M	None seen	Stridor 48h
					3	F	Peanut fragments removed	Pneumonia
					4	M	None seen	Stridor 24h
? Bronchiectasis (with bronchography[1])	4	M	+ve Bilateral basal	None	5	F	+ve Left lower lobe	Pneumonia
	6	M	+ve Left lower lobe	None				
	11	M	None	None				
Persistent collapse right lower lobe	5	M	Extrinsic compression, ulcerating lesion, biopsy - tuberculosis	None				
Wheeze and stridor post-extubation			-		4	M	Tracheal stenosis - dilated	None

[1]Selective with fibreoptic bronchoscopy

An eight year old girl with a slowly resolving right upper lobe pneumonia had fibreoptic bronchoscopy to exclude an inhaled foreign body. She had a fairly prolonged procedure but had no complications and was ready for discharge within a few hours of recovering from the anaesthetic. This can be compared with two younger boys (age 3 and 4 years) who had rigid bronchoscopy for suspected foreign body and in whom distressing stridor, presumably due to subglottic oedema, persisted for 24-48 hours after the procedure, with painful cough for 7 days in one. Of four children who had suspected bronchiectasis, three had selective bronchography during the fibreoptic bronchoscopy. None suffered any complications, whilst the five year old girl who had a rigid bronchoscopy for the same reason had a post-procedure pneumonia. Very little contrast (6-8 ml) was required to provide good radiographic visualisation of the airways when selective bronchography was performed. The rigid bronchoscopies performed on a four year old boy with tracheal stenosis and a three year old girl with an inhaled peanut were probably the two situations where rigid bronchoscopy would be the preferred technique. However, with the development of appropriate instrumentation, even these problems can be dealt with via a fibreoptic bronchoscope. The five year old boy with persistent collapse of his right lower lobe had obvious hilar adenopathy on tomography, but the Mantoux test was negative. Accordingly, fibreoptic bronchoscopy was performed, and extrinsic compression of the right main bronchus was noted, with a lesion ulcerating into the airway. This was biopsied and was confirmed to be tuberculosis both on histology and bacteriology. This child suffered no complications from the procedure, and his right lower lobe completely re-expanded over the subsequent four months on anti-tuberculous therapy.

DISCUSSION

Our preliminary experience would suggest that fibreoptic bronchoscopy can be safely performed even on small children and results in far fewer complications than rigid bronchoscopy. Using the anaesthetic technique described, the adult broncho-scope can be used in children down to five years of age. With the development of smaller paediatric instruments, this procedure could be employed in infants. Post-bronchoscopy subglottic oedema did not occur using the flexible instrument, though a steroid cream was used for lubrication of the bronchoscope and manipulation of the instrument was kept to a minimum. The one complication which may be of concern is pneumothorax. This should be avoided by using the minimum inflation pressure required to achieve adequate ventilation and by not starting the next inspiration before the previous expiration is complete. The position of the tracheal tube should be carefully checked and anchored to avoid the tip slipping past the carina.

Bronchoscopy is rarely done in children but may have more extensive application if it is as safe as our preliminary experience would suggest.

XV.2.

INDIKATIONEN FÜR BRONCHOLOGISCHE UNTERSUCHUNGEN BEI KINDERN

W. THAL

Bronchologische Untersuchungen bei Kindern gehören heute zum
diagnostischen Spektrum jeder spezialisierten Kinderklinik.
Darüber hinaus werden sie selbständig oder in Kooperation mit
Pädiatern von Laryngologen, Anästhesiologen und Pulmologen
durchgeführt. In der DDR verfügen wir derzeit über 23 kinder-
bronchologische Zentren, in denen insgesamt etwa 50.000 Kinder
mit rezidivierenden und chronischen Erkrankungen der Atemwege
betreut werden. Jährlich werden etwa insgesamt 2.500 Kinder
bronchologisch untersucht. Bei 70 % wird eine kombinierte
bronchologische Untersuchung, d. h. Bronchoskopie und Bronchographie in einem Untersuchungsgang durchgeführt. Dabei werden
in 7 Zentren etwa 80 % der bronchologischen Diagnostik vorgenommen. Alle Untersuchungen werden in Allgemeinanästhesie
durchgeführt mit Barbiturat und/oder Halothan und Muskelrela-
xation. Als Kontrastmittel nutzen wir Propyliodon (Cilag),
Dionosil (Glaxo) und Visotrast B (DDR-Produktion). Als Instru-
mentarium wird das Beatmungsbronchoskop von FRIEDEL (MGB)
eingesetzt, das für das Kindesalter ideale Untersuchungsmöglich-
keiten bietet. Bei besonderer Fragestellung setzen wir in
gleicher Narkosetechnik das Bronchofiberskop ein, d. h. nicht
in Lokalanästhesie. Untersucht werden Kinder aller Alters- und
Gewichtsklassen. Kontraindikationen bestehen bei einer Kontra-
indikation zur Allgemeinnarkose und bei hämorrhagischen
Diathesen. Die häufigsten Indikationen zur bronchologischen
Diagnostik im Kindesalter sind: rezidivierende und chronische
Bronchitis und chronische Pneumonie mit 70 %, Asthma bronchiale
mit 15 %, zystische Fibrose mit 6 %, Corpus alienum mit 4 %.
Bei unseren Patienten sehen wir zu etwa 40 % chronische Fremdkörper, d. h. Fremdkörper, die länger als 2 Wochen im Bronchial-
baum waren.

Die Bronchographie ist auch heute eine Untersuchung mit
hohem Aussagewert. Schon bei sehr kleinen Kindern wollen wir
Anomalien erfassen, um dem Kind eventuell weitere komplizierte
Diagnostik und nutzlose Therapie zu ersparen. Hierzu ein Beispiel:
Neugeborenes mit Verschattung im rechten Hemithorax. Während der

folgenden Monate und Jahre immer wieder Kontrollaufnahmen,
obwohl das Kind beschwerdefrei war. Kardiologische Diagnostik
negativ. Erst im Alter von 5 Jahren wurde bronchologisch die
Diagnose gestellt: Aplasie des rechten Oberlappens. Die Bronchographie bei Kindern ist besonders wichtig zur Diagnostik der
Bronchiektasen. Ein negatives Thorax-Röntgenbild schließt
Bronchiektasen nicht aus. Nach der Operation von Bronchiektasen,
die wir in den meisten Fällen bei Kindern mit lokalisierten,
auch bilateralen Bronchiektasen vornehmen lassen, ist ebenfalls
eine bronchographische Kontrolle erforderlich, in der Regel nach
einem Jahr. Aber auch zum Nachweis einer diffusen deformierenden
Bronchitis ist die Bronchographie unerläßlich. Unsere Unter-
suchungstechnik ist so perfekt, daß wir für die Bronchographie
einer Lunge vom Beginn des Kontrastmitteleinlaufes, das wir über
ein Füllrohr durch das Bronchoskop exakt plazieren, bis zum
Absaugen des Kontrastmittels nicht mehr als 20 - 30 sec benötigen.
Die Strahlenbelastung ist also gering. Wir bevorzugen beim Kind
die unilaterale Bronchographie, schließen aber eventuell nach
Absaugen des Kontrastmittels gleich die Bronchographie der
gegenüberliegenden Seite an. Bei mehreren tausend Bronchographien der vergangenen Jahre haben wir keine Komplikationen
gesehen. Kritische Meinungen, daß in Relaxation eine Beurteilung
der Funktion des Bronchialsystems nicht möglich sei, können
wir nicht bestätigen. Die Beobachtung des Kontrastmitteleinlaufes auf dem Monitor läßt bereits erkennen, welche Segmente
das Kontrastmittel schnell aufnehmen und in welche es nur
zögernd einläuft, woraus man auf die Durchgängigkeit des Bron-
chuslumens insbesondere aber auf die Stärke des peripheren
Sogs schließen kann. Zur Beurteilung der Reinigungsfähigkeit
der Bronchialschleimhaut kann die röntgenologische Kontrolle
der Eliminationsgeschwindigkeit, d. h. des Nachweises von
Kontrastmittelresten im Bronchialbaum dienen, was wir aber nicht
generell überprüfen. Nach meiner Meinung gibt es anstelle der
Bronchographie bei Kindern noch kein anderes Verfahren, was
technisch einfacher, in der diagnostischen Aussage umfassender
und exakter und hinsichtlich der Belastung des Kindes schonender
ist. Es sei mir erlaubt, in diesem Kreis zwei Raritäten von
Bronchogrammen zu zeigen, die zwar mit dem üblichen Kontrastmittel, aber nicht in üblicher Technik gewonnen wurden. Bei dem
ersten Kind handelt es sich um ein zwei Tage altes Frühgeborenes,

bei dem eine Passagestörung des Ösophagus ausgeschlossen werden
sollte, worunter es zu einer Aspiration von Kontrastmittel kam.
Das Kontrastmittel war bei diesem Kind, was sich in Rückenlage
befand, in gleicher Weise über alle Abschnitte verteilt nachweisbar. Nach Absaugung aus Trachea und Bronchien mittels
Katheter erholte sich das Kind schnell. Bei dem zweiten,
4jährigen Kind mit Hydrocephalus internus war im Säuglingsalter
zuvor eine Ventiloperation (PUDENZ-HEYER) durchgeführt worden.
Jetzt fiel auf, daß das Kind stark hustete, wenn das Ventil
manuell betätigt wurde. Wir gaben in den distalen Schenkel des
Ventilsystems ein wässriges Kontrastmittel, wobei es zu einer
Auffüllung des rechten Bronchialbaumes kam. Der Katheter war
also in den rechten Lungenoberlappen penetriert.

REFERENCES
1. Thal W: Kinderbronchologie, Barth-Verlag Leipzig, 1972.
2. Thal W, Leupold W, Wunderlich P: Asthma bronchiale im
   Kindesalter, Thieme-Verlag Leipzig, 1977.
3. Thal W, Röse W, Christoph B: Zu einigen Aspekten inter-
   disziplinärer Zusammenarbeit bei der bronchologischen
   Untersuchung von Kindern, Z. Erkrank. Atm.-Org. (1980) im Druck
4. Wunderlich P, Thal W: Zum Stand der kinderbronchologischen
   Diagnostik in der DDR, Dtsch. Gesundh.-Wesen 34 (1979) 2335
5. Wunderlich P, Thal W: Zum Stand der bronchologischen Technik
   bei Kindern in der DDR, Z. Erkrank. Atm.-Org. (1980) im Druck

λV.3.

BACTERIAL LARYNGOTRACHEOBRONCHITIS - USE OF FIBEROPTIC BRONCHOSCOPE

W. H. PARRY, MD, LTC, USA, MC and W. A. MADDEN, MD, LTC, USA, MC

Laryngotracheobronchitis (croup) is a common cause of upper airway obstruction in children under three years of age. It is characterized by a prodrome of upper respiratory symptoms consisting of
cough and coryza, followed by signs and symptoms of upper airway
obstruction including brassy cough, inspiratory stridor, and supra-
sternal and subcostal retractions. Laryngotracheobronchitis has been
thought to be of viral etiology since Rabe's study in 1948.

Croup is, in fact, a laryngitis or laryngotracheitis rather than
a laryngotracheobronchitis inasmuch as lower airway signs or symptoms
or both are not usually present in croup. Bacterial laryngotracheobronchitis (a true laryngotracheobronchitis), on the other hand,
should be considered a distinct disease entity, and is associated
with signs and symptoms of lower airway obstruction. The clinical
history is entirely compatible with that of ordinary viral croup, beginning with a prodrome of upper respiratory symptoms followed by the
development of a brassy cough, inspiratory stridor and retractions.
There is nothing in the fever course, duration of symptoms prior to
hospitalization, total leukocyte count or differential leukocyte
count that would distinguish bacterial laryngotracheobronchitis from
ordinary viral laryngotracheobronchitis. However, there are either
signs or symptoms of lower respiratory involvement (wheezing); an
abnormal chest film revealing infiltrates or atelectasis; an abnormal lateral neck x-ray showing tracheal mucosa irregularity or a
combination of these.

Six patients with bacterial laryngotracheobronchitis have been
diagnosed at our institution in 15 months. The age range of these
patients was from 15 months to 15 years. Tracheal mucosa irregularity, indicating thick tracheal secretions, was seen on lateral neck
roentgenogram in three of six cases. The epiglottis was normal in
all. There was an abnormal chest roentgenogram in five of six. Airway obstruction was progressive and all six required intubation for

respiratory distress due to subglottic obstruction. Intubation
resulted in dramatic relief of respiratory distress. At intubation,
thick purulent secretions were obtained which revealed polymorphonuclear leukocytes and gram positive cocci on smear. Culture of the
tracheal secretions obtained at intubation grew Staphylococcus aureus
in five instances and Streptococcus pneumoniae in one. Intravenous
antibiotics were used in treatment of all cases. In one case, viral
cultures of tracheal secretions grew Influenza B; five cases revealed
no viral growth.

Serial bronchoscopic examinations were made at intubation and
during resolution of the disease process. At intubation, thick pur-
ulent-appearing secretions were found in the trachea and extended
to the lobar bronchi. The airway mucosa was fiery red. During
resolution of the inflammation, secretions became thin, watery and
less purulent in appearance. The airway mucosa became pale in a
patchy distribution, gradually returning to normal pink coloration
in approximately four days. Extubation may be accomplished at this
time. Follow-up examination has been normal in all patients and
there has been no recurrence.

XV.4.

USE OF FIBEROPTIC BRONCHOSCOPE IN THE NEWBORN INTENSIVE CARE UNIT

W. H. PARRY, MD, LTC, USA, MC and W. A. MADDEN, MD, LTC, USA, MC

Techniques of fiberoptic bronchoscopy in the newborn intensive care unit (NICU) are applicable even in the small premature infant. Limitations occur because current equipment lacks suction capacity and directional flexibility in those instruments small enough to pass through the endotracheal tubes used in the neonate. Addition of directional capability or a suction port renders the instrument too large to pass through these endotracheal tubes.

Fiberoptic bronchoscopy is useful in the NICU for the following indications: Assessing placement and patency of endotracheal tubes; positioning the endotracheal tube above the carina; assisting in selective intubation of bronchi; evaluating the lower airways; and evaluating the upper airway, particularly supraglottic structures. In the NICU, we have used the Meditech fiberscope (2.5 mm outer diameter) or the Olympus BF4C3 (outer diameter 4.5 mm). The Meditech has no suction capacity nor directional flexibility, but can pass through a 3.0 mm endotracheal tube. The Olympus bronchoscope has a small (0.5 mm) suction channel and directional capability, but cannot be inserted through the small endotracheal tube used in the neonate.

Accurate and rapid airway evaluation and management, including intubation, in the critically ill infant is paramount to avoid consequences of hypoxemia. Clinical signs available to assess a successful intubation may be inaccurate in the neonate. Inserting the fiberoptic bronchoscope through the endotracheal tube at intubation can readily confirm the correct placement of the endotracheal tube.

Moreover, in the case of a sudden deterioration in the infant's clinical condition, accidental extubation or occlusion of the endotracheal tube must be considered and ruled out. Prior to fiberoptic bronchoscopy, clinicians were often required to extubate the infant to ensure patency of the endotracheal tube, thus requiring reintubation. With the advent of the small fiberoptic bronchoscope, accidental extubation can be quickly diagnosed by passing the fiberscope through the endotracheal tube and identifying its location in the trachea or esophagus. Also, patency of the endotracheal tube can be assured without extubation. If the endotracheal tube is found to be occluded, suctioning can be attempted and its success assessed by subsequent examination with the fiberoptic bronchoscope. This capacity has relieved many infants of unnecessary manipulation, extubation and reintubation.

The location of the endotracheal tube above the carina can be ascertained and the endotracheal tube fixed in position without chest x-ray confirmation. Thus, accumulated radiation exposure to the neonate during hospitalization, is reduced. The method is simple. The fiberoptic bronchoscope is advanced to the carina and a mark made with white ink on the fiber column. The fiberscope is then withdrawn to the tip of the endotracheal tube and a second white mark made on the fiber column. The bronchoscope is withdrawn and the distance between the two marks measured, accurately determining the distance of the endotracheal tube above the carina. If the distance is inappropriate, the endotracheal tube may be advanced or withdrawn until a satisfactory distance is achieved.

One currently recommended treatment of unilateral pulmonary interstitial emphysema is selective intubation of the contralateral bronchus and ventilation of the unaffected lung. Selective intubation is accomplished by inserting the fiberoptic bronchoscope into the appropriate mainstem bronchus. The fiberoptic bronchoscope then serves as a guide over which the endotracheal tube can be advanced into proper position.

Lower airway evaluation is most easily accomplished in an intubated patient using the Meditech fiberoptic bronchoscope. However, since this bronchoscope has no directional flexibility, visualization of the upper lobes is unsuccessful. Moreover, the lack of a suction channel seriously limits its ability to expand atelectatic portions of the lung. However, it can examine major bronchi for occlusion as well as assess the success of suctioning. For lower airway evaluation, the Olympus bronchoscope's usefulness is limited to the trachea and immediate subglottic area in non-intubated neonates. Both congenital and acquired lesions can be diagnosed.

The fiberoptic bronchoscope is particularly valuable in the evaluation of supraglottic structures. The dynamics of supraglottic structures during breathing as well as identification of supraglottic lesions is greatly facilitated by the use of flexible fiberoptic laryngoscopy. Neither direct examination by laryngoscope nor indirect laryngoscopy with mirror gives the physician the detail, the magnification or the ease of study that the fiberoptic bronchoscope gives him. Some lesions identified in our NICU have been laryngomalacia, swollen arytenoids, vocal cord paralysis, tracheal webs and innominate artery compression.

In summary, fiberoptic bronchoscopy in the NICU is useful in the emergency situation, assessing placement, patency and position of the endotracheal tube, in the diagnostic examination of the upper and lower airways, and in assessment of bronchial toilet.

XV.5.

OUR EXPERIENCE WITH OLYMPUS BF TYPE 4 B2

A. PAOLINI, F. TOSATO, M. RUGGIERI, F. RICCARDELLI

We began our experience in fiberoptic endoscopy five years ago
with an Olympus BF B2 instrument, in Thoracic service of IV Surgical Clinic, Rome University.

We choose Olympus bronchoscope for many reasons but chiefly be
cause we found very easy to guide it from control section.

The 2.0 mm in diameter channel was big enough to obtain a
good suction from a simple singer compression and to take cytological and histological samples from bronchial wall.

The insertion was easy under local anesthesia both from mouth
and nose, even if sometimes we had little problems from the nose
because of the outside diameter of 5.8 mm.

The exame was without trouble for patient.

We used then since '78 the Olympus BF B3 whichlet us have a
more clear vision and consequently also better photographic results
using a round field.

The smooth and excedingly flexible distal portion considerably
diminishes the patient disconfort.

It was then possible from a new suction auto-adapter to assure
an avaiable suction for sputum removal and lens-cleaning while taking histological or cytological samples.

We had recently the opportunity to use the new Olympus fiberoptic endoscope BF4 B2.

This instrument presents an outer diameter of 4-9 mm which is
almost 1 mm less than the previous BF B3. This carachteristic is
very important if compared to the channel which is still standard,
2 mm in diameter so the patient confort is greatly enhanced during intubation both from mouth and nose.

The small diameter of the insertion tube plus the 2 mm channel
mantenance both can give us the advantage to join easely the V°
order bronchial branches without renouncing to the possibility to
have a good suction and to get mucosal cytological and/or histological samples from there - An increased angulation of 180°
up/60° down allows easier examination of the difficult - to - reach
upper lobes in more patients.

Since 1976 we performed fiberoptic bronchial endoscopy in 280
lung cancer patients histologically confirmed at the time of operation.

Positivity rate of cytological and/or histological examinations
in bronchoscoped patients is summarized in the table.

*J.A. Nakhosteen and W. Maassen (eds.), Bronchology: Research, Diagnostic and
Therapeutic Aspects. All rights reserved.*
Copyright 1981. Martinus Nijhoff Publishers bv, The Hague / Boston / London

YIELD OF POSITIVE DIAGNOSIS OF BRONCHOGENIC
CARCINOMA (280 – 1976/80) IN BRONCHOSCOPED
PATIENTS

Sputum	70%
Bronchial brushing	76%
Bronchial washing	80%
Bronchial biopsy	90%
Post bronchoscopy sputum	75%

Sputum positivity was of 70% in our experience; cytological
positivity rate increased greatly with fiberoptic deeply connected
methodics: 76% for bronchial brushing, 80% for washing and finally
75% for post-bronchoscopy sputum.

Biopsy positivity rate was of 90%. This high value is easely
explaned because biopsy is done only in case of a macroscopic endoscopical evidence of lesion. It is to be remarqued that bronchial washing has improved it's positivity rate since we begun to
connect the specimen trap from the beginning of the examination.

But both cytological and histological investigations connected
to fiberoptic endoscopy are really improving in our experience,
which is dipending formerly on the assessment of cyto-histological
technique but also, we think, on the new thinner instrument.

A final aspect we want to point out about the new Olympus
BF4 B2 instrument is the effective improvement in clarity of endoscopic field which makes possible a better definition of even minimal mucosal damages and a more faithful endoscopical picture.

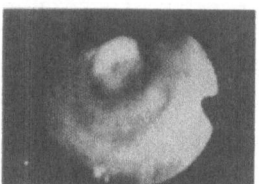

Fig. 1: clear evidence of endoluminal mass in a segmental bron-
    chial branch .

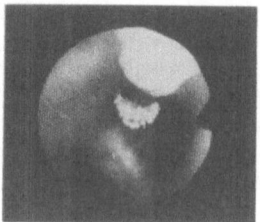

Fig. 2: instrument is brushing a suspected area.

In conclusion our four years experience with Olympus fiberoptic
bronchoscopes is really positive. Diagnostic possibilities already
high with BF B2 instrument, improved with BF B3 for better quality
of resolution power.

XV.6.

EARLY DETECTION OF ALLERGENS BY RAST IN INFANTS AND PRESCHOOL CHILDREN WITH RECURRENT BRONCHITIS

D. GLAUBITT and K. SIAFARIKAS

1. INTRODUCTION

The disclosure of allergic factors in the etiology of recurrent bronchitis may be difficult in infants (children under the age of 2 years) and preschool children (in this study children at the age of 2 to 6 years) because at this age often no acceptable results are obtained by skin tests and provocation tests (ref. 5). The RadioAllergoSorbent Test (RAST), however, as an in-vitro test determines the level of allergen-specific antibodies of the IgE class in plasma or serum and thus reveals to what extent the pathogenesis of recurrent bronchitis includes allergic reactions mediated by such antibodies.

We investigated the clinical efficacy of RAST in infants and preschool children suffering from recurrent bronchitis.

2. MATERIALS AND METHODS

Fourty-one children (27 boys and 14 girls) aged 1 month to 6 years who had recurrent bronchitis were examined. Fourteen children were infants, 6 among them being aged 2 to 12 months. RAST in plasma was performed using up to 66 allergens (foods, animal epithelia, mites, house dust, insect venoms, moulds as well as pollen of grasses, weeds, and trees, and, in addition, penicilloyl G and V). The concentration of total IgE in plasma was determined by the Paper RadioImmunoSorbent Test (PRIST). Radioimmunoassay kits for both measurements were obtained from Deutsche Pharmacia GmbH, D-7800 Freiburg. The RAST results were allocated to RAST classes; in class 0 no antibodies of the IgE class to the tested allergen were detected whereas the concentration of those antibodies was low in class 1, significant in class 2, moderate in class 3, and very high in class 4. Additional comments on the methods were given in a previous communication (ref. 3).

3. RESULTS

A positive RAST result was found in 14 children each for foods or animal epithelia, 7 for mites, 10 for house dust, 4 for honey-bee venom and 2 for yellow-jacket wasp venom (out of 34 tests), 12 for moulds as well as 20 for grass pollen, 17 for weed pollen, and 9 for tree pollen. In one child (out of 13 children examined) RAST was positive for

J.A. Nakhosteen and W. Maassen (eds.), Bronchology: Research, Diagnostic and Therapeutic Aspects. All rights reserved.
Copyright 1981. Martinus Nijhoff Publishers bv, The Hague / Boston / London

526

penicilloyl G. In 10 infants a positive RAST result was obtained for at least one of the allergens tested.

The level of total IgE in plasma was raised in 6 infants and 8 preschool children. In 3 children (one infant and 2 preschool children) RAST was normal but the concentration of total IgE in plasma was elevated. In 18 children (5 infants and 13 preschool children) RAST presented a pathologic result which was accompanied by a normal total IgE level.

Normal RAST results and a normal IgE concentration in plasma were observed in 3 infants (2 boys and 1 girl) and 6 preschool children (5 boys and 1 girl).

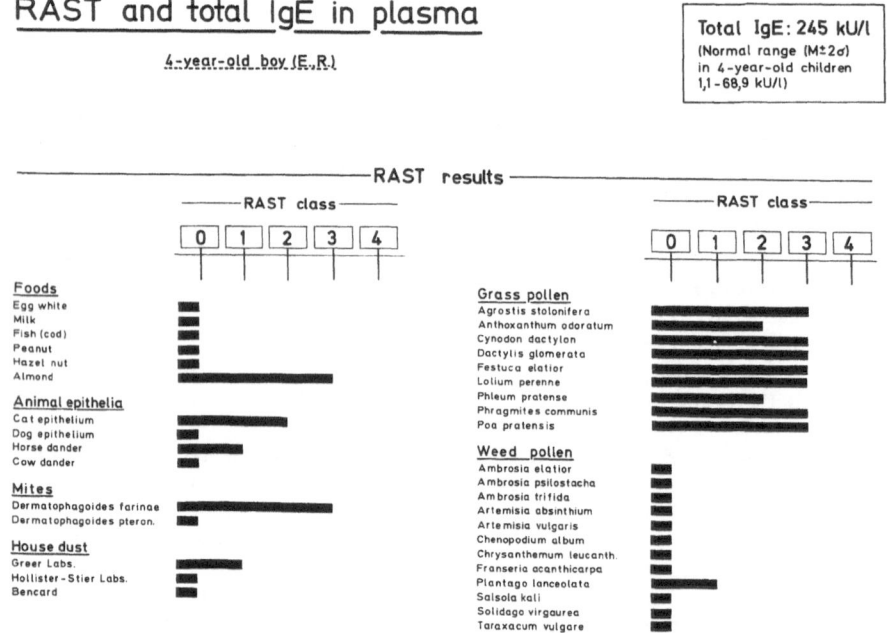

RAST and total IgE in plasma

4-year-old boy (E.R.)

Total IgE: 245 kU/l
(Normal range (M±2σ) in 4-year-old children 1,1 - 68,9 kU/l)

Fig. 1 Preschool child with pathologic RAST results and raised total IgE level in plasma.

RAST was even more valuable in infants than in preschool children because in infants skin tests and especially provocation tests can be performed only with difficulty.

An example of the high clinical efficacy of RAST was seen in a 4-year-old boy who suffered from recurrent bronchitis. Although no atopic disease was suspected clinically, this preschool child presented a positive RAST result for one kind each of foods, mites, house dust, and weed pollen, 2 kinds of animal epithelia, and all of the 9 kinds of grass pollen examined. Fig. 1 shows those groups of allergens in which one or more pathologic RAST results were found. The concentration of total IgE in plasma was elevated considerably and thus was concordant with the pathologic RAST results. These findings in the boy demonstrated that allergic factors were at least a partial cause of the recurrent bronchitis and had to be considered subsequently during therapy. An atopy was assumed tentatively and confirmed.

When the same boy was examined 19 months later, RAST was pathologic for 62 allergens. It may be supposed that with increasing age of this child more allergic reactions became manifest although in this comparison the possibility of divergent RAST results in different seasons has to be taken into account. The first RAST was carried out at the end of February, the second test in the following year at the beginning of September; the exposition to many allergens, e.g. pollen, was much higher at the end of the summer than during the winter.

4. DISCUSSION

Recurrent bronchitis requires early diagnosis and appropriate therapy. In this context it may be mentioned that in children this disease may be followed by bronchial asthma (ref. 2).

RAST assists to identify allergens which are involved in the immediate (anaphylactic) type of allergy. There is no doubt that RAST has only limited value for the assessment of the actual clinical sensitization to an allergen (ref. 3). Therefore skin tests or even provocation tests would be desirable also in infants and preschool children if these tests would provide the same meaningful information as they do in adults (ref. 5).

It appears to be a great advantage of RAST that it obviously does not render false positive results (ref. 1). RAST may be repeated without causing considerable inconvenience to the patient.

The specificity of the response of IgE to allergens is probably reduced with increasing age and rising total IgE concentration in the plasma. Specific antibodies belonging to the IgE class may be found for egg protein and milk protein already in the first years after birth whereas such antibodies to pollen antigens may be detectable not until the fourth year of life (ref. 4).

RAST showed only a loose correlation with the concentration of total IgE in plasma. This fact is intelligible because the panel of allergens used for RAST is small compared with the extremely large number of allergens conceivable to raise antibodies of the IgE class and to be reflected by the concentration of total IgE in plasma. For this reason it is recommended both to determine the level of total IgE and to perform RAST for all of the allergens suspected to be involved in the atopic disease of the patient examined.

5. SUMMARY

RAST is a useful diagnostic tool in the early identification of allergens which may play a role in the pathogenesis of recurrent bronchitis. RAST proved to have a high clinical efficacy in infants and preschool children in whom skin tests and provocation tests are less applicable.

Chapter XVI

ENDOSCOPIC LASER,
CRYO- AND ELECTROTHERAPY

XVI.1.

USE OF CARBON DIOXIDE LASER TECHNOLOGY IN LARYNGEAL AND BRONCHIAL
SURGERY

H.H. DEDO

TECHNICAL DETAILS

The patient is anesthetized with a small endotracheal tube (24
French for adults, 3 mm for children, and 2.5 mm for infants) with
aluminium foil tape protecting the tube. For lesions in the larynx
or hypopharynx my microscopic laryngoscope* is installed and then
held in place with a self-retaining arm. Distal fiberoptic
illumination is employed. The appropriate suction protector* is
installed when lesions are to be treated on the false cord or true
cord. The laser we use is a CO_2 type made by Coherent Medical
systems**.

APPLICATION WITH SPECIFIC LESIONS

Color microphotographs of laryngeal lesions will now be shown
with, where possible, follow-up photographs, along with reports
of the effect on airway and voice.

1. Papillomas of the larynx

(a) We now have eleven patients who have had their papillomas
clinically controlled (no evidence of recurrence for two to three
years) after six or fewer treatments with laser and podophyllin.
In papilloma patients, after the laser removal I paint the area
of removal with a mixture of podophyllin in 20% resin to make it
more difficult for virus particles or tumor particles to implant.
(b) There is a second group which has required six to twelve
treatments at two-month intervals to achieve clinical control.
(c) A third group with even poorer tissue resistance has required
more than twelve treatments, but we seem to be making gradual
progress.

All three groups, however, have been making much better progress
per treatment than with prior mechanical removal and, since fewer
treatments are required, there tends to be less scarring and more
normal mucosa in the larynx when clinical control has been achieved.
However, it is still important to only treat one anterior true or

* Pilling Company, Delaware Drive, Fort Washington, PA 19034
** Coherent Inc., Medical Division, 3270 W.Bayshore Blvd. Palo Alto
CA 94304

J.A. Nakhosteen and W. Maassen (eds.), Bronchology: Research, Diagnostic and
Therapeutic Aspects. All rights reserved.
Copyright 1981. Martinus Nijhoff Publishers bv, The Hague / Boston / London

false cord at a time to prevent anterior commissure scarring.

2. Singer's nodules

I have a patient in whom the singers' nodule returned in six months after cup forceps removal, but after laser removal, including shaving the underlying connective tissue away down just to Reinke's space, followed by 2 weeks of voice rest and then speech therapy, the nodule has not returned in this busy executive in over two years.

3. Polypoid cords

They can be removed with cup forceps but a prolonged period is required for vocal rehabilitation. I have the preliminary impression that with laser removal the voice ends up better and sooner than after cup forceps removal.

4. Webbing or Stenosis

(a) Anterior Commissure

Although some surgeons have reported good results with division of anterior webs with the laser beam alone, in my hands they have tended to recur. Therefore, my present preference is to incise the web with a knife or the laser beam using the special die* and place one of my teflon keels[1].

(b) Mid Glottis

Scarring between the mid portions of the cord is nicely handled with the laser beam because the epithelium at the anterior and posterior commissure prevents re-stenosis.

(c) Posterior Commissure Stenosis

Ordinarily, in my experience, this has required a mucosal advancement flap after removal of the scar tissue in order to prevent recurrence[2]. However, in two cases when the posterior stenosis was between the bodies of the arytenoids with a small mucosa lined sinus behind it, as a result of prolonged endotracheal intubation, laser division of this resulted in complete resolution in contra-distinction to stenosis of the anterior commissure.

(d) Subglottic

With posterior stenosis just below the arytenoids I have resected the submucosal scar with the laser beam and then incised the mucosa on the anterior and inferior surface of the stenosis to use it as a flap to hasten epithelialization of the treated area. In one patient it was incised in the vertical midline creating two flaps which swung to the sides.

The airway opened from a diameter of 5 mm to one of 8 mm, and the patient is quite comfortable. The technique successfully used in another patient was to make an incision where this mucosa was attached to each side wall and lay it posteriorly as a tongue of tissue reaching up into the posterior commissure. If the problem is not resolved after one or more endoscopic laser attempts, it is still possible to do the repair via a laryngofissure as in the past[2].

5. Subglottic Hemangiomas

In the past this lesion required placement of a tracheotomy tube, if there was significant airway obstruction, and waiting while hoping for the lesion to involute between 12 and 18 months of age, or else over a prolonged period for differential growth to enlarge the airway sufficiently for tracheotomy tube removal. Three sub-glottic hemangiomas have now been removed with the laser endoscopically achieving a good airway in all three. The total blood loss averaged 2 to 3 drops per patient.

6. Bilateral Vocal Cord Paralysis

In the past this lesion was treated with arytenoidectomy via an external surgical approach to the neck. I have been now done laser arytenoidectomy successfully in 7 of 9 cases. In cases where the airway has still been insufficient, it is possible to go back and repeat the procedure and remove the scar from the first operation and more tissue in order to enlarge the posterior glottic airway more.

7. Vocal Cord Thinning

In patients in whom there has been a teflon injection with either placement of too much teflon or subsequent development of a granuloma, the voice can be improved by partial removal of the teflon and scar tissue and cord substance. This can be done with cup forceps, but it is possible to do it with more precise control with the laser[3].

A highly specialized application of this thinning technique is with the occasional patient who redevelops spasticity in the voice after recurrent nerve section for spastic dysphonia. This happens between 6 and 15 months after the initial operation in approximately 5% - 8% of the patients, primarily in those who had very severe spastic dysphonia before recurrent nerve section.

8. Subglottic and Tracheal Stenosis

Circular or circumferential stenosis of the trachea, unless it is just a thin hymen-like membrane less than 3 mm in thickness, has not responded well to any endoscopic surgical technique in my experience and requires segmental resection of the trachea[4].

9. Leukoplakia of the Vocal Cord

It has been my observation that leukoplakia here, as well as elsewhere in the mouth and pharynx, tends to recur less after meticulous removal with the laser than after removal with the cold or electric knife.

10. Carcinoma of the Vocal Cord

We are approaching the laser treatment of small superficial carcinomas of the vocal cord and pharynx very carefully. However, in highly selected cases, such as people who have already received full-course x-ray therapy and medically are unable to have a long enough general anesthetic for a vertical hemilaryngectomy or total laryngectomy, treatment with the CO_2 laser has resulted in less than a 20% local recurrence rate when followed up for three years.

Another application in vocal cord cancer patients has been the removal of excess tissue from the deliberately over-filled pseudo-cord created with a mucosal advancement flap and fat implant at vertical hemilaryngectory[5]. After the initial surgery has healed the mucosal edema has cleared and the fat has atrophied over a period of four months, the pseudocord is then sculptured with the laser beam via direct laryngoscopy over one or two treatments so that it becomes a straight line from the anterior to the posterior commissure at the level of the opposite cord free edge creating a 4 to 5 mm opening at the posterior glottis during inspiration. Using this technique it has been possible to achieve a better voice and a more adequate airway without aspiration than before with conventional surgery.

11. False Cord Surgery

Cysts and amyloid deposits in the false cord and papillomas on the false cord and in the ventricle have been successfully resolved with the CO_2 laser.

12. Lesions of the Trachea and Mainstem Bronchi

The development which made laser bronchoscopy feasible is a system of mirrors and prisms in a small box which attaches to the end of the rigid bronchoscope and makes it possible to direct

both the helium aiming beam, the CO_2 laser beam, and the surgeon's
line of sight down the bronchoscope. We have found that it can
be used with bronchoscopes 9 mm x 40 cm down to 3 mm x 20 cm. The
smoke and steam are either cleared away with the tidal flow of
oxygen and anesthetic gas or a small suction line placed alongside
the fiberoptic light carrier in the wall of my laser bronchoscope
design*. In order to have sufficient light come through the prisms
and the magnifying lens a continuous fiberoptic cable was also
developed for us by Pilling Company*.

With the advent of the CO_2 laser bronchoscope we have now
confirmed that it is feasible to remove benign lesions such as
papillomas and granulomas. So far I prefer to treat circumferential
stenosis such as that caused by balloon cuffs with segmental
resection of the trachea[4]. Although it is not feasible to cure
carcinoma in the trachea with the laser, it is possible to remove
other benign lesions of the trachea which are attached to less
than 30% to 40% of the circumference of the trachea at any one
point.

REFERENCES

1. Dedo, H.H.: Endoscopic teflon keel for anterior glottic web.
   Annals of Otol. Rhinol. and Larygol., 88:467-473, 1979.

2. Dedo, H.H. and Sooy, F.A.: Surgical repair of late glottic
   stenosis. Annals of Otol. Rhinol. and Laryngol., 77:435-441, 1968.

3. Horn, K.L. and Dedo, H.H.: Surgical correction of convex vocal
   cord after teflon injection. Laryngoscope, 90:281-286, 1980.

4. Dedo, H.H. and Fishman, N.H.: Laryngeal release and sleeve
   resection for tracheal stenosis. Annals of Otol. Rhinol. and
   Laryngol., 78:172-180, 1969.

5. Dedo, H.H.: A technique for vertical hemilaryngectomy to prevent
   stenosis and aspiration. Laryngoscope, 85:978-984, 1975.

EXPERIMENTS ON TUMOR RESECTION BY LASER SURGERY VIA THE FIBEROPTIC
BRONCHOSCOPE
XVI.2.

T. Ohtani, K. Oho, R. Amemiya, O. Taira, K. Hayakawa, I. Ogawa,
Y. Hayata

The combination of endoscopy and laser technology has attracted
increasing attention of late, and our group has conducted a variety of
experiments using different lasers with the fiberoptic bronchoscope.[1,2]
Figure 1 shows the schema of one experimental layout for tumor resection in dogs. The helium-neon laser was used as a pilot beam, in
conjunction with a YAG or argon-ion laser. The lasers were transmitted
by means of a teflon-coated quartz fiber inserted through the
instrumentation channel of an Olympus 1T fiberoptic bronchoscope. Air
insufflation through the teflon sleeve is necessary to prevent tissue
fragments adhering to the tip of the fiber, which is positioned
5 - 10 mm from the target. Eye protection is required for all involved
in the procedure. Figure 2 shows the two lasers radiating from the tip
of the quartz fiber.

In Fig. 3, the tip of the quartz fiber can be seen in the upper
left hand side, pointing in the direction of a section of canine glu-
teal muscle which was impacted in the bronchus to resemble a tumor.
In conjunction with our basic research on maximizing effectiveness on
target tissue and minimizing deleterious effects on surrounding normal
tissue, we transsected the sternomastoid muscle and partially inserted
it in the trachea, in imitation of a tumor obstructing the trachea,
and injected it with black ink[2], (Fig. 4). The results after irradiation with the YAG laser are shown in Fig. 5. The argon-ion laser
operates at lower power than the YAG laser, and as shown in Fig. 6, has
less effect on surrounding tissue. Figure 6 shows the findings immediately after photoirradiation with the argon ion laser (left) and 1 week
later, (right). The method was employed to dissect a tumor which had
developed in a nude mouse after subcutaneous transplantation of a
cultured cell line of human oat cell carcinoma of the lung. No bleeding was recognized.

In our experiments, carbonized material was observed to disperse
over an area of radius 2 cm, therefore in carcinoma cases the question

J.A. Nakhosteen and W. Maassen (eds.), Bronchology: Research, Diagnostic and
Therapeutic Aspects. All rights reserved.
Copyright 1981. Martinus Nijhoff Publishers bv, The Hague / Boston / London

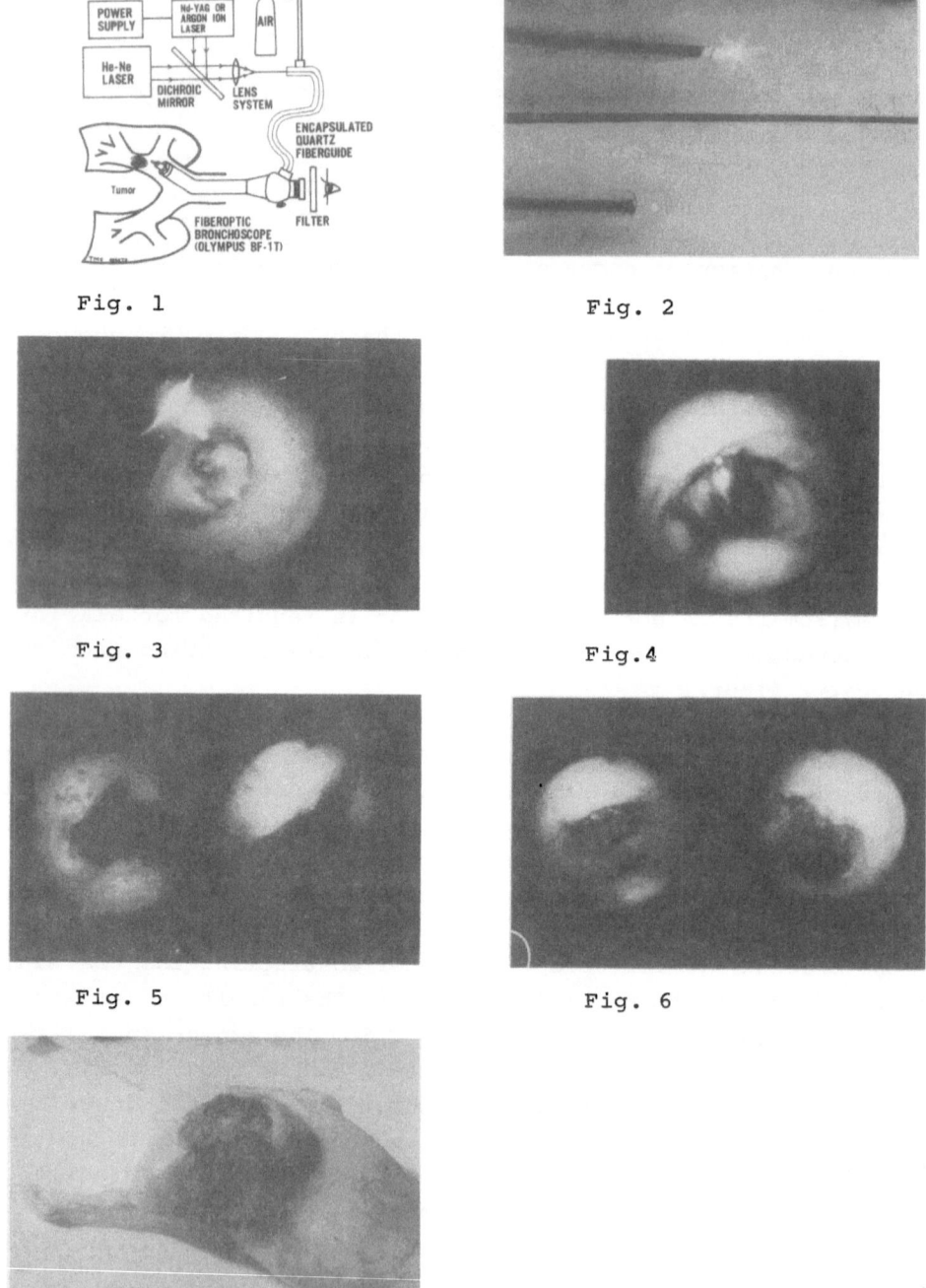

Fig. 1

Fig. 2

Fig. 3

Fig.4

Fig. 5

Fig. 6

Fig. 7

of the viability of such material is extremely important.

Although there have been reports of a CO_2 laser successfully used with the rigid bronchoscope in a case of severe stenosis of the distal trachea[3], we feel that the high power YAG laser, used through the fiberoptic bronchoscope is another therapeutic option, as it does not cause bleeding and can be performed under local anesthesia. We are beginning to employ this method clinically, and have experienced one case so far. The procedure was performed under local anesthesia and was successful in alleviating the dyspnea of the patient caused by tracheal stenosis. While more research is necessary, we feel that laser therapy through the fiberoptic endoscope holds much promise for the future, especially in the field of bronchology.

REFERENCES
1. Amemiya R, Hayakawa K, Ohtani T, Ogawa I, Oho K, Hayata Y: Laser photoirradiation via the fiberoptic bronchoscope; Effects on the tracheal and bronchial wall, J. Jap. Society for Bronchology, 1, 65-68, 1979 (in Japanese).
2. Hayakawa K, Oho H, Amemiya R, Ohtani T, Ogawa I, Taira O, Hayata Y: Photodynamic effects of laser surgery on the trachea and bronchi of mongrel dogs: 2nd World Congress for Bronchology, Dusseldorf, 1980.
3. Eugene GL, Robert LB, Charles WV: Carcinoma obstructing the trachea, treatment by laser resection, New. Eng. J. Med. 294, 17; 941, 1976.

540

LASER PHOTOIRRADIATION VIA THE FIBEROPTIC BRONCHOSCOPE: EFFECTS ON THE
BRONCHIAL WALL

R. Amemiya, K. Oho, T. Ohtani, I.Ogawa, K. Hayakawa, O. Taira, Y. Hayata

XVI.3.

The authors have been studying the effects of laser beams transmitted via
a quartz fiber inserted through the instrumentation channel of the fiberoptic
bronchoscope (Olympus 1T). The quartz fiber is in a teflon sleeve, with an
overall diameter of 2 mm. The angle of divergence from the tip is 8-14°, and
75-80% transmission efficiency is obtained for a fiber length of 4 meters[1].
In order to prevent carbonized material adhering to the tip of the fiber,
continuous air insufflation is performed through the teflon sleeve, (Fig. 1,2).

A total of 3 lasers were involved in the experiments. Because the YAG
(Yttrium, Argon, Garnet) laser is invisible, and because the indispensable
protective goggles can obscure the view of the argon ion beam (Fig. 3), a red
helium neon beam is used as a pilot guide. The power output of the argon ion
laser is 1-10 watts, while the maximum output of the YAG is 40 watts.

Although there are difficulties because of respiratory movement, we aim to
keep the tip at a distance of about 5-10 mm from the target. At a distance of
less than 5 mm there is a danger of carbonized material adhering to the tip,
or of actually touching the target itself, which would result in the fiber itself
being burned. The carina and other bifurcations were selected as targets.

We evaluated the effectiveness of this method for biopsy beyond the
bronchial wall. Fig. 4 shows the bronchial wall immediately after perforation
with the YAG laser (left), and the findings after 1 week (right). The findings
with the argon ion laser are shown in Fig. 5. The appearance on the right shows
good healing at one week. Through the perforations we were able to obtain biopsy
specimens from extramural lymph nodes, lung parenchyma and connective tissue.
The appearance via the fiberoptic bronchoscope during biopsy is shown in Fig.6,
and a biopsied lymph node can be seen in Fig. 7. The dogs were contributed by
the Tokyo Metropolitan Government, on the condition that they would be sacrificed
as they were unclaimed strays, therefore most of them were sacrificed immediately
after the experiment. In the small group (dogs) of animals which were not
sacrificed, mediastinitis was recognized, but no pleuritis was observed. As was
reported by Hayakawa[2], our group established a classification system to evaluate
the results of laser photoirradiation, and Fig. 8 shows examples of each of the
5 grades. Grade 1; grayish-white mucosal solidification, Grade 2; blackening,
Grade 3; ulcer formation (1mm), Grade 4; deep ulcer formation and Grade 5;

J.A. Nakhosteen and W. Maassen (eds.), Bronchology: Research, Diagnostic and
Therapeutic Aspects. All rights reserved.
Copyright 1981. Martinus Nijhoff Publishers bv, The Hague / Boston / London

perforation. The energy curves are shown in Figs 9 and 10, and it was seen that in the bronchus the YAG laser required 5 times as much energy, measured in joules, as the argon-ion laser to reach Grade 5. A total of 90 points in 40 dogs were irradiated, and experience 1 case of sudden death due to bleeding. In the dog that died low-power argon photoirradiation had been performed for a long time, and in such cases it has been reported that the laser loses its coagulative effect[3]. This case serves to confirm this report.

Our conclusions are summarized in Fig. 11. Our experience shows the method effective and safe, if the photoirradiation interval is short. However a thorough knowledge of bronchial anatomy and experience in fiberoptic bronchoscopy is required for the procedure in clinical cases. We feel that laser photo-irradiation, using the fiberoptic bronchoscope will soon be an important clinical procedure in certain cases.

REFERENCES

1. Frühmorgen P, Bodem F, Reidenbach HD, Kaduk B, Demling L: Endoscopic laser coagulation of bleeding gastrointestinal lesions with report of the first therapeutic application in man, Gastrointestinal Endoscopy, 23, 73-75, 1976.
2. Hayakawa K, Oho K, Amemiya R, Ohtani T, Ogawa I, Taira O, Hayata Y: Photodynamic effects of laser surgery on the trachea and bronchi of mongrel dogs, 2nd World Congress for Bronchology, Dusseldorf, 1980.
3. Amemiya R, Hayakawa K, Ohtani T, Ogawa I, Oho K, Hayata Y: Laser photo-irradiation via the fiberoptic bronchoscope; Effects on the tracheal and bronchial wall, J.Jap.Society for Bronchology, 1, 65-68, 1979 (in Japanese).

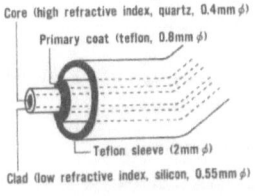

Schema of the optical fiber system

Core (high refractive index, quartz, 0.4mm φ)
Primary coat (teflon, 0.8mm φ)
Teflon sleeve (2mm φ)
Clad (low refractive index, silicon, 0.55mm φ)

Angle of divergence : 8~14°

Fig. 1

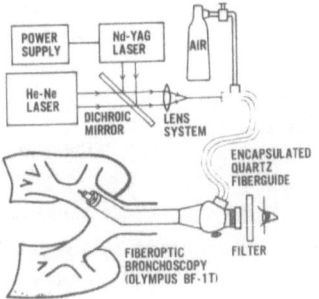

POWER SUPPLY | Nd-YAG LASER | AIR
He-Ne LASER
DICHROIC MIRROR | LENS SYSTEM
ENCAPSULATED QUARTZ FIBERGUIDE
FIBEROPTIC BRONCHOSCOPY (OLYMPUS BF-1T) | FILTER

Fig. 2

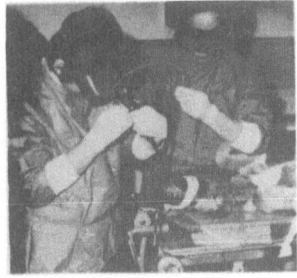

Fig. 3

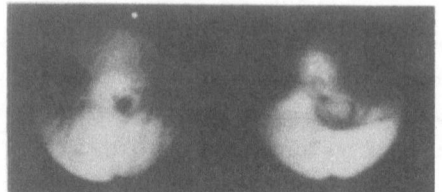

Fig. 4

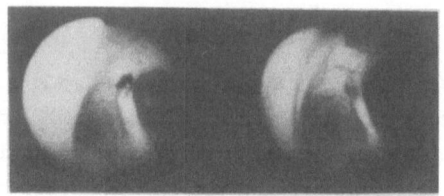

Fig. 5

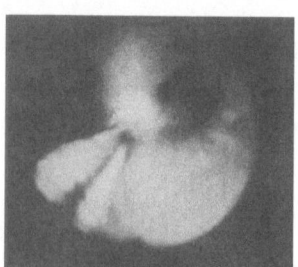

Fig. 6

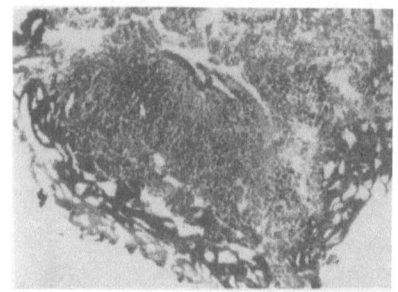

Fig. 7

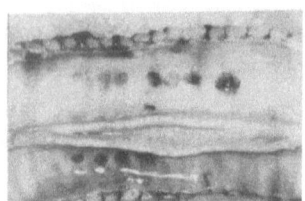

Fig. 8

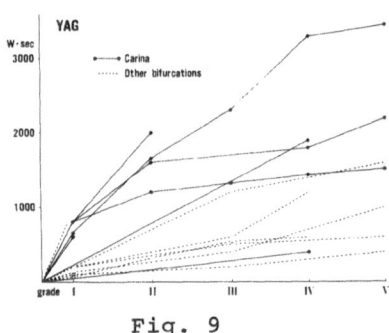

Fig. 9

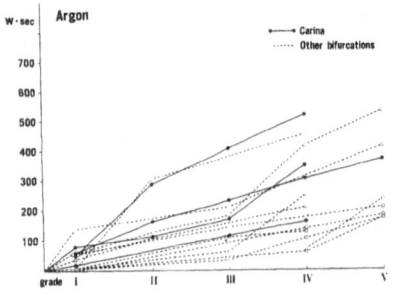

Fig. 10

CONCLUSION

1. Effective to obtain biopsies from beyond the bronchial wall, such as in cases of extrabronchial tumor or lymph nodes.

2. Safe if the photoirradiation interval is short.

3. Argon ion laser has lower effects on surrounding tissue but requires a longer period of photoirradiation.

4. Thorough knowledge of the bronchial anatomy and experience in fiberoptic bronchoscopy is necessary.

Fig. 11

PHOTODYNAMIC EFFECTS OF LASER SURGERY ON THE TRACHEA AND BRONCHI OF MONGREL DOGS

K. Hayakawa, K. Oho, R. Amemiya, T. Ohtani, I. Ogawa, O Taira, Y. Hayata

INTRODUCTION

The range of options in the treatment of pulmonary diseases continues to expand with developments in the fiberoptic bronchoscope. Photoirradiation by laser beams via the fiberoptic bronchoscope has attracted increasing attention as a future therapeutic method.

One extremely important point is how to maximize the effects of photo-irradiation in target tissue while minimizing effects in non-target tissue. Since the absorption of photoirradiation energy of a beam of given energy varies according to the color of the irradiated object and the wave length of the beam, we set up a series of basic experiments to clarify how this can be utilized to maximize effect in tumor tissue and to obtain a classification of the effects of laser photoirradiation as a means of comparing effectiveness.

MATERIALS AND METHODS

The lasers used were the YAG, argon ion and helium-neon lasers described by Amemiya[1] and Ohtani[2], and the beams were transmitted via a teflon quartz fiber which can be inserted through the instrumentation channel of the Olympus 1T. In a basic study of the color-dependency of the effects of the laser beams we used papers of 7 different colors. The colors were yellow, orange, cobalt blue, blue, green, red and black. Based on those results we then examined the effect of photoirradiation of chicken muscle injected with black ink, Congo red, and a green dye, ICG. Then tracheotomy was performed in 2 mongrel dogs, the above dyes were injected submucosally and photoirradiation was performed with the quartz fiber alone, and with it inserted through the fiberoptic bronchoscope (Olympus 1T).

RESULTS

At a power of 1 watt the argon ion laser made pinholes immediately only in red and black paper, (Table 1), while at 4 watts pinholes were opened in all papers and red paper burst into flame. With the YAG laser (Table 2), the beam made a hole in black paper only at 5 and 10 watts, but at 20 watts holes were made in red, green and blue paper, and black paper burst into flame. Even after long periods of irradiation there was no effect on orange, cobalt blue and yellow paper, and black paper burned.

J.A. Nakhosteen and W. Maassen (eds.), Bronchology: Research, Diagnostic and Therapeutic Aspects. All rights reserved.
Copyright 1981. Martinus Nijhoff Publishers bv, The Hague / Boston / London

EFFECTS OF ARGON-ION LASER IN COLORED PAPERS

Color \ Power	1 Watt	4 Watts
Black	<1˙	<1˙
Red	<1˙	<1˙
Green	1˙	<1˙
Blue	1˙	<1˙
Orange	1˙	<1˙
Yellow	1˙	<1˙
Cobalt blue	23˙	<1˙

Table 1

EFFECTS OF YAG LASER IN COLORED PAPERS

Color \ Power	5 Watts	10 Watts	20 Watts	40 Watts
Black	‖	‖	‖	‖
Red	—	—	+(1.5˙) / ‖(8˙)	+(1˙) / ‖(3˙)
Green	—	—	‖(2˙)	‖(1˙)
Blue	—	—	‖(2˙)	‖(<1˙)
Orange	—	—	—	‖(2˙)
Yellow	—	—	—	‖(2˙)
Cobalt blue	—	—	—	‖(1˙)

— : no change   + : carbonization   ‖ : perforation   ‖ : burst into flame

Table 2

EFFECTS OF ARGON-ION AND YAG LASERS IN CHICKEN MUSCLE

Color	Time required for			
	Carbonization		Deep ulcer formation	
	Argon (4W)	YAG (30W)	Argon (4W)	YAG (30W)
Natural	5˙	3˙	34˙	7˙
Red	2˙	3˙	15˙	9˙
Green	2˙	3˙	24˙	6˙
Black	2˙	<1˙	20˙	2˙

Table 3

CLASSIFICATION OF LASER PHOTOIRRADIATION EFFECTS ON TISSUE

Tokyo Med. College Hospital

Grade 1 : White discoloration due to tissue solidification

Grade 2 : Blackish changes due to carbonization

Grade 3 : Shallow ulcer formation (about 1 mm)

Grade 4 : Deep ulcer formation

Grade 5 : Perforation

Table 4

COLOR DEPENDENT EFFECTIVENESS IN DYED TRACHEAL MUCOSA

Color	Laser	Grade 1	Grade 2	Grade 3	Grade 4
Black	Argon	3	5	7	24
	YAG	1	1	3	4
Green	Argon	2	3	7	21
	YAG	4	7	21	26
Red	Argon	1	2	8	19
	YAG	1	2	4	7

Argon : 2 Watts
YAG : 10 Watts

Table 5

In chicken muscle (Table 3) it was seen that the color of the injected dye had a significant effect on the effectiveness of irradiation and the time required to reach a specific effect. The quickest results were obtained with red and black. These results showed the necessity for a categorization of the effects of photo-irradiation, and we composed the classification shown in Fig. 4 (Table 4).

We examined the effects of the laser beams on the tracheas of 2 mongrel dogs under tracheotomy. The argon ion beam had the greatest effect in red injected trachea, while the YAG had the greatest effect in trachea injected with black. The results were exactly the same with the transmission fiber inserted through the Olympus 1T fiberoptic bronchofiberscope, and there appeared to be no specific problem in using it in this manner, (Table 5).

CONCLUSION

The effects of photoirradiation were observed to be significantly affected by the color of the dye used, which means that selection of the most appropriate dye for the target site in clinical cases will significantly decrease the amount and time of irradiation required, thus minimizing possible adverse effects on surrounding non-target tissue. The method of inserting a quartz fiber through the flexible fiberoptic endoscope appears to be suitable method. The classification method we proposed appears to be suitable for classifying the effects of laser photoirradiation and making a meaningful comparison of laser beam characteristics.

REFERENCES

1. Amemiya R, Oho K, Ohtani T, Ogawa I, Hayakawa K, Taira O, Hayata Y: Laser photoirradiation via the fiberoptic bronchoscope; Effects on the bronchial wall, 2nd World Congress for Bronchology, Dusseldorf, 1980.
2. Ohtani T, Oho K, Amemiya R, Ogawa I, Taira O, Hayakawa K, Hayata Y: Experiments on tumor resection by laser surgery via the fiberoptic bronchoscope, 2nd World Congress for Bronchology, Dusseldorf, 1980.

XVI.5.

COMPARATIVE STUDIES BETWEEN CO_2 GAS LASER AND YAG LASER ON THE TRACHEAL CILLIA.

OTOHIKO TAKAYAMA

I. INTRODUCTION

Lasersurgery on the air way has progressed rapidly recently. Basis studies of laser surgery, however, have not developed completely. The author investigated effects of laser beam surgery on the bronchial cillia using the CO_2 gas laser and YAG laser beams.

Previous reports demonstrated that CO_2 laser on soft tissues using the fixed irradiation method revealed crater formation immediately after irradiation. Scanning electron microscopic observation of the crater revealed irregularity and unevenness of figures in the inside of the structures, resembling sponge forms. Numerous secondary holes on the ridge of the crater demonstrated protrusion. This report concernd only with the tracheal wall of adult dogs.

2. MATERIAL AND METHOD.

Eight adult dogs were used to examined the cillia on the tracheal wall using the CO_2 laser(2 cases) and YAG laser(6 cases) respectively.

Two kind of lasers were irradiated until perforation of the tracheal wall was confirmed. After irradiation tracheal tissues were examined by light microscope and scanning electron microscope. Examinations strictly followed three points.

1). Comparative studies between CO_2 & YAG lasers.
2). Comparative studies between 10 joules irradiation and 15 joules irradiation by CO_2 gas laser.
3). Histological alteration by defocusing irradiation of YAG laser.

3. RESULTS.

1). Histopathological studies were performed on the tissue after treated with CO_2 laser & YAG laser respectively.
   (1). The effects of CO_2 laser to the surrounding tissue when

J.A. Nakhosteen and W. Maassen (eds.), Bronchology: Research, Diagnostic and Therapeutic Aspects. All rights reserved.
Copyright 1981. Martinus Nijhoff Publishers bv, The Hague / Boston / London

examined with low power magnification(50 times) demonstrated more regularity than YAG laser when examined with low power magnification(35 times).

(2). Irradiation holes and the surrounding tissues when examined with high power magnification(150 times) revealed that the effects of CO_2 laser to the surrounding tissue were not obious. However, the effects of YAG laser when examined with (80 times) magnification, the affected areas were more obvious.

The alteration of cillia by CO_2 ⋜ YAG laser revealed that pathological changes were almost similar when compared.

(3). Cillia on surrounding area of the crater and its concentrated circle demonstrated fissure and tear. With use of the CO_2 gas laser alterations of the concentrated circle were relatively clear but the YAG laser demonstrated not only irregularity but also progressive fissure and tear.

(4). The layer of the cillia near to the crater demonstrated thick membranes and smooth protrusions of the surface area. Folds(wrinkles) were also observed in some places.

2). Comparative results between lo joules & 15 joules of CO_2 gas laser.

No significant differences between lo & 15 joules exposure of the CO_2 gas laser were demonstrated by histological comperison using low and high magnification. Morphological alteration of cillia was not demonstrated.

3). Histological alteration of defocusing irradiation of YAG laser. Defocusing irradiation revieled different alterations of the tissue, such as formation of folds or protrusions , fissure or tears of the cillia.

4.CONCLUSION.

The author investigated effects of laser beam surgery on the bronchial cillia using CO_2 gas laser & YAG laser beam. Svanning electron microscopie observed that the YAG laser beam had a stronger effect to the surrounding tissue.

We expected clinical use of CO_2 & YAG laser beam for surgical treatment. We concluded that the YAG laser beam can be expected more dehydration of the tissue, fissure and tear of the tissue.

YAG laser is more significant for the promotion of the coagulation of the tissue. Alteration of the pathological cillia, however, did not clearly demonstrated any differences between them.

REFERENCES.

1. M.Stuart Strong: Recurrent respiratory papillomatosis management with the CO_2 laser, Annals of Oto-Rhino-Laryng. 85: 508-516, 1976.
2. S.Mihashi: Histological changes after its irradiated with CO_2 laser, Japanese J. of Oto-Rhino-Laryng. 80: 1483-1487,1977.
3. S.Mihashi,M.Hirano: Laser surgery, Otologie(Fukuoka) 25: Suppl,2. March 364-377, 1979.

XVI.6.

TREATMENT OF THE TRACHEOBRONCHIAL LESIONS WITH A FIBER LASER

J.F. DUMON, E.REBOUD, R. GUIDICELLI, F.AUCONTE

THE APPARATUS : The laser used is the YAG 100 laser sold by A.L.M hospital equipment compagny. The source of YAG Neodyme lasers emets infrared radiation at a wavelength of 1.06 microns. The laser power is adjustable between 40 and 100 watts at the fiber outlet. The radiation may be continous or interrepted. It is transmetted by flexible optic fiber, 2.5 mm in diameter. The divergence of the aiming light is 10°, which focuses the impact. The fiber is cooled off by an air jet. A red aiming light obtained by HeNe laser permits a precise aim. We chose this instrument because of the transmission by flexible fiber as well as its physical properties : if the power is moderated and the time of emission relatively long, the coagulation effect is excellent ; if the power is increased, the vaporization effect is higher and the resection of the tumor is simple. The discontinued emission avoids the propagation of heat to the neigboring tissues.

TECHNIQUE : 1°) UNDER GENERAL ANESTHESIA : When the resection is high, if there must be associated dilatation, or the patient is not cooperative, we prefer to use general anesthesia. The anesthesia remains light in order to permit spontaneous ventilation. It is only ventilated in a case of depressive breathing created by the necessity of the complementary analgesy. The intubation is accomplished using a rigid open tube or an intubation tube. The laser beam is directed by a large channel fiberscope (Machida 6 TL II).

2°) UNDER LOCAL ANESTHESIA : When the resection is lower, in the case of bleeding during a fiberscopy, under local anesthesia or if general anesthesia is not indicated, we prefer to use local anesthesia, because the laser radiation is totally painless.

RESULTS : Our experience is as yet moderate as we have had this apparatus for only a short time. We have made 25 laser treatments of 18 patients. The principal indications studied were the following :

1°) TRACHEOBRONCHIAL TUMORS (table I) : They seem to be the best indication. The tumoral resection is accomplished without hemorrhaging, which is essential. Our experience is with squamous cell carcinoma, adenocarcinoma, carcinoid and cylindroma tumors.

HOPITAL SALVATOR
13274 MARSEILLE CEDEX 2
FRANCE

J.A. Nakhosteen and W. Maassen (eds.), Bronchology: Research, Diagnostic and Therapeutic Aspects. All rights reserved.
Copyright 1981. Martinus Nijhoff Publishers bv, The Hague / Boston / London

I. TRACHEOBRONCHIAL TUMORS

histology	topography	No of laser treatments	anesthesia	result
squamous cell	tr.intermedius	2	local	+ +
squamous cell	trachea	2	general	+ + +
squamous cell	right main br.	1	local	+ + +
squamous cell	b6 right L.L br	1	local	+ + +
squamous cell	trachea	1	general	+ + +
adenocarcinoma	right U.L br.	1	local	+ + +
adenocarcinoma	left lower L.br.	2	general	+
	right U.L br.	2	general	+ + +
cylindroma	left main br.	3	general	+ + +
carcinoid	left main br.	2	general	+ + +

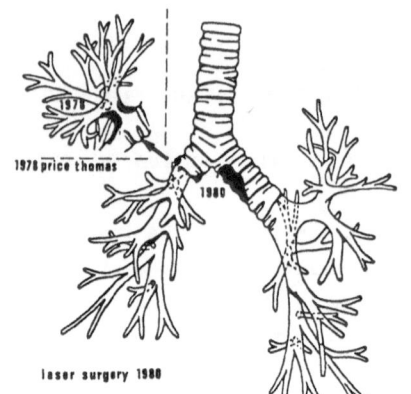

1978 price thomas

1980

laser surgery 1980

recurrent cylindroma

One observation is especially spectacular :
A 53 year old man operated for a cylindroma of the
right upper lobe in 1978, had a relapse in 1980 at the beginning of the left main
bronchus. Three laser treatments were necessary to obtain a normal calibre of the
bronchus. We are led to believe that the potential evolution of this type of tumor
will necessitate numerus resections in the future. The effet is always striking if the
tumor is strictly intrabronchial.

2°) THE TRACHEAL STENOSIS (table II) : Most of tracheal stenosis are also associated
with en external compression, which limits the efficacity of the laser. The additional tracheal dilatations are indispensable. In these conditions the results are
satifactory, but the potential evolution of the stenosis is a frequent cause of
relapse.
3°) OTHER INDICATIONS : These have not all been explored. We succesfully used the
laser in resections of granuloma, sections of sutures, and in removing implanted
foreign bodies.

CONCLUSION : The authors report their first results on the use of the YAG Neodyme
Laser in tracheobronchial endoscopy. The laser fiber is directed by a fiberscope.
The treatment is made under local or general anesthesia with spontanous ventilation.
Our experience has been 25 laser treatments for 18 patients. The effect is spectacular in tumors, squamous cell carcinoma, adenocarcinoma, carcinoid and cylindroma
tumors which were succesfully treated. The results of tracheal stenosis are only
succesful with the use of an associated dilatation. Specific indications are proposed ; resections of granuloma, sections of suture, removing implanted foreign
bodies and treatment of hemorragy.

II. TRACHEAL STENOSIS

type	associated treatments	No of laser treatments	immediat results	long term results
virole	dil.(6/8)	2	+ + +	relapse
virole	dil.(6/8)	2	+ +	relapse
ring	0	1	+ + +	+ + +
virole	0	1	+ +	+ +
virole	dil.(6/7.5)	1	+ +	relapse

XVI.7.

Bronchoscopic Cryosurgery: Mayo Clinic Experience

D R SANDERSON, R S FONTANA, H B NEEL III

Introduction

The preferred treatment for most localized endobronchial tumors
is surgical extirpation. If resection is not feasible, then radiation
therapy usually is the second choice. However there are certain
patients who, for various reasons, are not candidates for treatment by
either of these modalities, but who have localized endobronchial
lesions that threaten life. Systemic chemotherapy may not be desirable
for these patients because their disease is localized. In selected
patients with such conditions, endobronchial cryotherapy may provide
satisfactory palliation and, on rare occasions, even produce apparent
cure.

Background

It has long been recognized that freezing can injure tissue, and
this principle has been applied to a number of clinical situations.
Cryotherapy has been used by dermatologists to treat superficial
skin lesions and by surgeons as an adjunct to resection and radiotherapy for management of cancers of the head, neck and oral cavity.

In the early 1970's one of us (HBN) performed a series of
experiments that defined the prerequisites for successful application
of cryotherapy to tumors in laboratory animals. It was discovered
that the size of the tip of the cryotherapy probe correlated with
the extent of tumor destruction and with subsequent survival. The
larger the area of probe-tip to tumor contact, the better the result.
The temperature of the probe-tip was also important. Mice with tumors
frozen to -180^{0}C survived longer than mice with tumors frozen to -60^{0} C.
It was also observed that repeated freezing with intervals for spontaneous thawing produced a better therapeutic response than a single
application of the cryoprobe.

Next, a technique was developed that enabled application of a
cryoprobe to an endobronchial lesion via an open tube ventilative
bronchoscope. A Frigitronics cryosurgical unit was modified by

J.A. Nakhosteen and W. Maassen (eds.), Bronchology: Research, Diagnostic and
Therapeutic Aspects. All rights reserved.
Copyright 1981. Martinus Nijhoff Publishers bv, The Hague / Boston / London

attaching a long insulated probe equipped with interchangeable probe tips of varying shapes and sizes. The probe was inserted through the rigid bronchoscope and the probe tip applied directly to the desired area. Obviously, only lesions within the range of the rigid scope could be treated.

Materials and Methods

All cryotherapy candidates have been Mayo patients with confirmed tumors of the tracheobronchial area. Most have had prior treatment, either surgical or radiological or both, and have presented with persistent or recurrent tumor. In a few instances cryotherapy was chosen as the initial form of treatment, to palliate localized disease when there were other serious medical problems that precluded resection or radiation.

In one patient transbronchial cryotherapy was conducted under general anesthesia. In all other cases, topical anesthesia was employed. The open tube ventilating bronchoscope used was 40 cm. long and 9 mm. in diameter.

The coolant is liquid nitrogen, which boiled at -197° C. A pressurized reservoir feeds the coolant into, and recovers it from, the insulated probe, which is 55 cm. in length. Only the exposed copper probe-tip becomes cold, with surface temperatures reaching as low as -160° C. Selection of the probe-tip depends upon the configuration of the lesion to be treated, and occasionally the tip may be changed during a procedure to obtain better contact.

Results

Between 1972 and April, 1980, 24 Mayo patients were treated by means of transbronchial cryotherapy. There were 20 men and 4 women, whose ages ranged from 47 to 77 years (mean 63). Twenty of the 24 patients had squamous bronchial cancers, one had a cylindroma, one an atypical bronchial carcinoid, and one tracheopathia osteo-plastica. The remaining patient had carcinoma of the esophagus with metastasis to an anterior mediastinal lymph node which had invaded the trachea.

Three patients had not received prior treatment. One of these was the patient with cylindroma. This tumor had caused marked obstruction of the distal trachea and right main-stem bronchus. Surgical resection was not considered feasible, and a favorable response to radiation seemed unlikely. The second patient had severe emphysema with cor pulmonale and a squamous cancer obstructing the bronchus to the lower lobe of the right lung. The respiratory reserve of this patient was considered insufficient to permit either resection or radiation, so cryotherapy was applied with the hope of relieving the obstruction. The third patient was the one with tracheopathia osteoplastica. This condition had caused moderate obstruction.

In all, 55 cryotherapy treatments were performed on the 24 patients. Ten patients had only one treatment session, while the other 14 each had two or more. The maximum number of treatments in any patient was eight.

It is difficult to objectively assess results of treatment in this group of seriously ill patients. During the early cryosurgery experience at Mayo, several patients were treated who had extensive cancers that invaded the mediastinum. It was clearly evident that these tumors were not adequately controlled by endobronchial cryotherapy, and in retrospect treatment probably should not have been attempted.

Patient responses were considered favorable if treatment accomplished local control of the tumor, or reduced the amount of bleeding, or improved ventilation. To assist in evaluating therapy, color photographs were obtained of all tumors before and after each treatment session and at all subsequent bronchoscopic examinations. In 13 of the 24 patients the response to cryotherapy was considered favorable, while in the other 11 there was no evidence of significant benefit. One patient with recurrent tumor in the stump of the right main bronchus (following pneumonectomy for squamous carcinoma) remained well, with neither visual nor biopsy-verified evidence of disease more than four years after treatment. The patient with the cylindroma had a favorable initial response to cryotherapy, but later developed recurrent obstruction of the airway. A second remission was then induced by radiotherapy. Another patient had four separate cryotherapy sessions as treatment for a squamous cancer involving the tracheal bifurcation. This patient subsequently died of a myocardial infarction, and at autopsy no evidence of endobronchial cancer was observed, although serial sections of the involved area were not obtained.

Complications have been infrequent. Significant bleeding has not been observed, either during or following a treatment. Two patients became restless and complained of breathlessness as a consequence of temporary further compromise of the airway during freeze application. One other patient, who had previously undergone pneumonectomy, developed significant edema of the bronchial wall following cryotherapy to the area of the tracheal bifurcation and subsequently died. This is the only procedure-related death.

Discussion

Cryotherapy is effective in causing local tissue destruction. When applied precisely to circumscribed endobronchial tumors, control and even cure is possible. Candidates for cryotherapy should be carefully selected. Patients with extensive tumors should probably be excluded from consideration, because these lesions are too bulky to permit realistic expectation of benefit from treatment. The ideal lesion for cryotherapy would be a low-grade superficial cancer only a few millimeters in diameter that is located in the wall of the trachea or a major bronchus. Currently available probe-tip configurations and the rigidity of the probe and the bronchoscope do not allow access to upper lobe segments. Cryotherapy of endo-bronchial tumors is still in the developmental stage. Before consider-ing application other traditional forms of treatment, such as surgical resection and radiation, should be given a thorough trial.

Summary

Transbronchoscopic cryotherapy has been used at the Mayo Clinic in 24 patients, most of whom had squamous cancers. A total of 55 freezing treatments were administered. There was one procedure-related death from aggravation of airway obstruction. The treatments were well tolerated by the other patients, half of whom derived benefits in the form of local control of the tumor, or reduced bleeding, or improvement of the airway.

XVI.8.

BRONCHOSKOPISCHE KRYOTHERAPIE.

G.SCHUSTER, H.PETERS

1. EINLEITUNG

Die lokale Tumorzerstörung spielt beim Bronchial-Carcinom nur eine untergeordnete Rolle. Nur die frühzeitige Resektion kann die heute noch schlechten Spätergebnisse verbessern. Nach Diagnose-stellung sind heute immer noch ca. 40% aller Bronchial-Carcinome nicht mehr resezierbar. Diese Inoperabilität kann neben einer ge-neralisierten Tumoraussaat auch bedingt sein durch einen sehr zen-tralen Sitz des Primärtumors.

2. INDIKATION

Angeregt durch die Erfahrungen der Kryotherapie in der Aache-ner Klinik beim Rektum-Carcinom (LANGER,S. et al. 1972-79) hiel-ten wir die Vereisungsbehandlung auch beim Bronchialcarcinom in den genannten Fällen für einsetzbar. Die histologische Diagnose mußte vorliegen. Die Inoperabilität war durch verschiedene Ver-fahren wie Bronchoskopie, Mediastinoskopie sowie Lungenfunktions-untersuchungen usw. festgestellt worden. Auch wurden Operations-verweigerer in diese Behandlung aufgenommen.

3. WIRKUNGSWEISE

Sie wird einmal durch die lokale Tumorzerstörung erreicht. Der sichere Erstickungstod der Patienten durch Tumorverlegung der Trachea oder Hauptbronchien kann so möglichst lange hintangehalten werden. - Zum anderen sollte die mögliche immunologische Beein-flussung des Tumorleidens durch die Vereisungsbehandlung mitbe-rücksichtig werden. Diese zwar bisher wenig untermauerten immuno-logischen Aspekte beruhen auf einer massiven antigenen Freiset-zung aus dem tiefgefrorenen Gewebe. Die Möglichkeit einer sekun-dären, immunologisch bedingten Tumorzellzerstörung wird von meh-reren Autoren diskutiert (BLACKWOOD,G.E. et al. 1972, ABLIN,R.J. et al. 1972, LARGIADER,F. et al. 1979, LANGER,S. et al. 1978, FLAD et al. 1978.

J.A. Nakhosteen and W. Maassen (eds.), Bronchology: Research, Diagnostic and Therapeutic Aspects. All rights reserved.
Copyright 1981. Martinus Nijhoff Publishers bv, The Hague / Boston / London

4. TECHNIK

Das technische Vorgehen entspricht prinzipiell der Bronchoskopie mit starren Instrumenten in Vollnarkose. Der Gefrierkopf wird zentral auf den polypös wachsenden Tumor aufgebracht. Ein meist mehrmaliges Gefrieren mit flüssigem Stickstoff bei minus 160 - 196 Grad Celsius ist notwendig. Es muß in einer Sitzung versucht werden, so viel Tumorgewebe wie möglich zu gefrieren. - Bronchoskopische Kontrolluntersuchungen und weitere Vereisungen werden in Abständen von zunächst 2, später von 4 - 6 Wochen vorgenommen. - Auf Grund unserer Erfahrungen erscheint es wichtig, den Patienten darauf hinzuweisen, daß einige Tage nach der Vereisungstherapie verstärkt Husten mit Auswurf einsetzen kann. Dieser ist bedingt durch die dann auftretende Nekrosenabstoßung.

5. KASUISTIK

Aus dem eigenen Patientengut der inoperablen Bronchialcarcinome der letzten 2 Jahre (Gesamtzahl 74) wurden 12 Patienten mit zentral sitzendem Bronchialcarcinom der Vereisungsbehandlung unterzogen. Die Befunde von 2 Patienten sollen hier stellvertretend demonstriert werden. Bei beiden Patienten war Inoperabilität gegeben. - Der erstgenannte Patient wurde über 15 Monate in regelmässigen Abständen kryotherapiert. Es handelte sich um einen Zustand nach Unterlappenresektion 5 Jahre zuvor wegen eines Plattenepithelcarcinoms. Jetzt bestand ein inoperabler Trachealtumor. Erst nach 15 Monaten kam es zu einer generalisierten Aussaat an der der Patient ad Exitum kam. Der 2. Patient ist 75 Jahre alt und hat ein verhornendes Plattenepithelcarcinom des rechten Lungenunterlappens bei gleichzeitig ausgedehntem Tumor gleicher Histologie im Bereiche der Bifurkation. Dieser Patient wird jetzt bereits über 12 Monate therapiert.

6. DISKUSSION

Auf Grund des Gesagten ist für die kleine Gruppe der Patienten, die an einem inoperablen zentral sitzenden Bronchialcarcinom leiden, deren Erkrankung zum wahren Leiden wird durch die Zunahme der Luftnot bishin zum Ersticken, die kryochirurgische Behandlung angezeigt. Neben der genauen Dosierbarkeit der Kryotherapie ist in den letzten Jahren die Frage einer allgemein-immunologischen

Stimulation hinzugekommen. Klinische Anhaltspunkte einer Immun-
veränderung könnten darin zu sehen sein, daß über längere Zeit
das Tumorwachstum sistiert bzw. eine generalisierte Metastasie-
rung hinausgeschoben werden kann. Im eigenen Krankengut scheint
dies auch der Fall zu sein, wobei man jedoch einschränkend einmal auf die kleine Zahl hinweisen muß und zum anderen sich daran
erinnern sollte, daß selbst spontane Rückgänge von Metastasen
und auch ein sehr langsam verlaufendes Wachstum von Tumoren ohne
Kryotherapie bekannt sind. In den hier geschilderten Fällen ist
jedoch ein weitaus wesentlicherer Effekt der Kryotherapie für die
Patienten von entscheidender Bedeutung. Der letale Ausgang solcher inoperablen Carcinome kann zwar nicht verhindert werden.
Wir haben jedoch die Möglichkeit, die Lebensqualität des Patienten über längere Zeit zu erhalten. Die mögliche Lebensverlän-
gerung durch Änderung des Immunverhaltens stellt heute erst einen interessanten Nebeneffekt der Kryotherapie bei diesen Tumoren dar.

7. ZUSAMMENFASSUNG

Die Kryotherapie scheint der Elektroresektion und der reinen
instrumentellen Abtragung der Tumoren überlegen. Lokale Tumorzerstörung durch die nahezu genaue Dosierbarkeit ohne Zerstörung
umliegenden Gewebes und die mögliche immunologische Wirkung sind
so entscheidende Vorteile, daß ihr Einsatz generell zur palliati-
ven Tumorzerstörung heute nicht mehr diskutiert wird. Aus diesem
Grunde ist auch die Anwendung bei inoperablen zentralsitzenden
Bronchial-Carcinomen gerechtfertigt.

LITERATUR: Bei den Verfassern

XVI.9.

ELECTROSURGERY VIA THE FIBEROPTIC BRONCHOSCOPE

N. Takizawa, K. Oho, R. Amemiya, N. Hayashi, T. Kawauchi, Y. Hayata

INTRODUCTION

Electrosurgery via the fiberoptic endoscope was first developed in 1971.   At present its used inculde the treatment of esophageal varices and stenosis, bleeding gastric ulcer, in addition to polypectomy or extirpation of submucosal tumors in the stomach and colon, in addition to papillotomy of the papilla of Vater.   At present laparotomy is rarely chosen for polypectomy as transendscopic surgery is considered effective and less invasive, and the patient's recuperation is faster.   But in the field of bronchology, transfiberoptic bronchoscopic surgery with mechanical, laser or electrosurgical appliances is just beginning to develop.

At the Department of Surgery of Tokyo Medical College Hospital, we perform over 1,500 fiberoptic bronchoscopic procedures annually, and we have been developing both laser and electrosurgery techniques with the instrument over the past 5 years. Recently we have refined these techniques to the stage where they are now being applied clinically with encouraging results.   This describes our experience with electrosurgery.

MATERIALS AND METHOD

Figure 1 shows the Olympus UES power source which, though compact,supplies adequqte power for the procedure, and the electrode which is inserted through the instrumentation channel of the Olympus 1T is shown in Fig.2.   A close up view of the tip of the Olympus KD1-L shows it with the teflon sleeve, into which it is retracted to allow insertion through the instrumentation channel of the fiberoptic bronchoscope without damaging the latter, (Fig. 3).   The tip is only extended after the sleeve comes into the view of the bronchoschopist.

Figure 4 shows the set up for transfiberoptic bronchoscopic electrosurgery. A "patient plate", or P-plate is inserted under the patient for safety, to ensure the return of any leaking current to the power source.   The footswich control allows selection of either cutting or coagulating current, or an automatically controlled blended current.

CASE PRESENTATIONS

J.A. Nakhosteen and W. Maassen (eds.), Bronchology: Research, Diagnostic and
Therapeutic Aspects. All rights reserved.
Copyright 1981. Martinus Nijhoff Publishers bv, The Hague / Boston / London

560

Case 1. A 65 year-old male presented with dyspnea, stridor and poor expectoration of sputum. Biopsy of the tumor proliferating in the posterior trachea revealed adeniod cyctic carcinoma, which was consistent with the fiberoptic bronchoscopic appearance of the tumor. As he complained strongly of dyspnea we decided to perform electrosurgery. Figures 5 and 6 show the lateral tomography and fiberoptic bronchoscopic findings before treatment. The polypoid tumor arose from the membranous portion of the trachea, causing remarkable stenosis . After the first electrosurgery session, performed via the fiberoptic bronchoscope under the local anesthesia, his complaints were dramatically alleviated, and after the 4th procedure his general condition had improved and a curative operation was performed. The membranous portion of his trachea was replaced by a 6.6 cm graft. He is now alive and healthy 1 year postoperatively, (Fig. 7).

Case 2. Fiberoptic bronchoscopy was perfomed in a 61 year-old male who presented with bloody sputum. Figure 8 shows the glossy tumor obstructing B6b and compressing B^6c. Biopsy revealed chondroma. Electrosurgery was performed, followed by bougieing with Fogarty's catheter, and remarkable effect was obtained, (Fig. 9).

CONCLUSION

Methods for mechanical, laser, cryo- and electrosurgery via the fiberoptic bronchoscope are being developed. We perform all cases of electrosurgery through the instrument under local anesthesia. Its indications include obstruction or severe stenosis of major bronchi or the trachea, with danger of asphyxia, as the airway can be freed more safely than by emergency thoracotomy. It can also be indicated as a palliative procedure in cases of advanced lung cancer, or as an intermediary step enabling a patient to be a candidate for curative resection, as in Case 1.

Furthermore, in cases of benign tumors, such as in case 2, radical therapeutic effects can also be obtained in tumors with a low grade of malignancy if the entire tumor is extirpated. We experienced no complications whatsoever in over 100 procedures.

REFERENCES

1) Niwa H :Gastroenterlogical Endoscopy 13. (3): 297, 1971
2) Soma S et al :Endoscopicpapillotomy. Gastroenterlogical Endoscopy 16. (4):446, 1974
3) Uchida T :Endoscopic Surgery (Stomach). Stomach and Intestine 11. (11): 1431, 1976
4) Nagahama A et al : On the Transendoscopic Extirpation of Gastric Submucosal Tumor. Stomach and Intestine 11. (11). 1475, 1976
5) Nakahara A et al : The Fundamental and Clinical Studies on The Endoscopic electric current. Gastroenterological Endoscopy 18. (5) : 727, 1976.

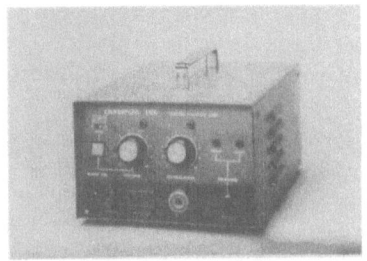

Figure 1

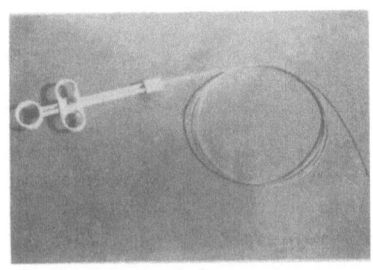

Figure 2

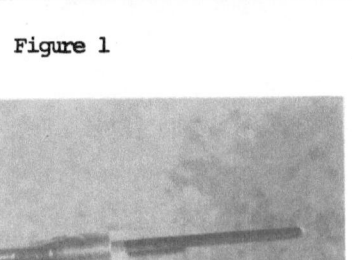

Figure 3

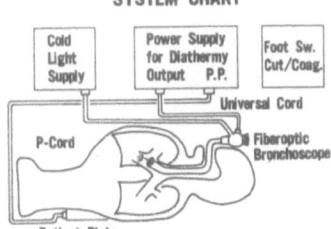

SYSTEM CHART

Figure 4

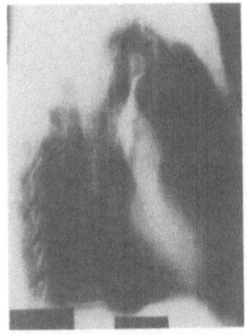

Figure 5

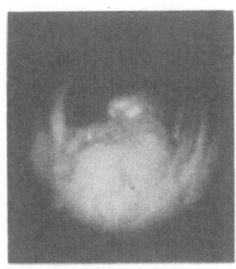

Figure 6

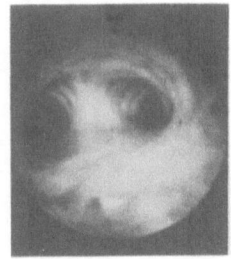

Figure 7

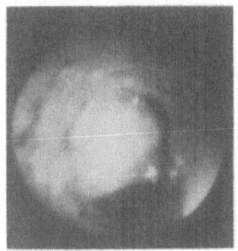

Figure 8

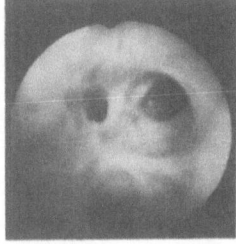

Figure 9

XVI.10.

HIGH-FREQUENCY ELECTROSURGICAL TREATMENT OF TRACHEAL OBSTRUCTION
USING THE FLEXIBLE BRONCHOFIBERSCOPE

H. TAGUCHI, T. NAGATA, H. KAWAI, K. SAITO and T. WAKABAYASHI

1. INTRODUCTION

Endoscopic electrosurgery with high-frequency diathermy has been developed since 1970, and employed widely in the field of gastroenterology, especially for polypectomy. Since 1978, we have been applying this high-frequency diathermy technique through the flexible bronchofiberscope as palliative treatment of tracheall obstruction.

2. MATERIALS AND METHODS

2.1. Materials

A total of seven procedures have been performed in four patients. One patient had metastatic thyroid cancer which was located in the tracheal wall. Another showed tracheal stenosis due to a web, which developed from granulation 3 months after tracheostomy. She had been treated for apoplexia. The other two were advanced lung cancer cases with tracheal invasion. For these two patients, this technique was performed repeatedly to prevent suffocation because the tumor regrew quickly.

2.2. Methods

In all procedures, an orotracheal tube was inserted after heavy premedication under local surface anesthesia with 4% xylocaine. The orotracheal tube more than 8.5mm in internal diameter was used to maintain ventilation. Access for intravenous infusion of sedative was established. If coughing is not controlled, danger results and the technique cannot be performed correctly.

The Olympus Co. P.S.D. and U.E.S. high-frequency electrosurgical power sources were used. These allow selection of either cutting or coagulation current or an alternating blended current. (Figure 1)

The flexible bronchofiberscope, lubricated by olive oil, is inserted into the tracheal tube and diathermy was performed by means of the high-frequency knife or snare inserted through the instrument-ation channel of the fiberscope. It is very important to perform the procedure very gradually and repeatedly. Thus the degree of bleeding can be observed and the resected fragment removed easily. This method is not curative treatment for the original disease but palliates the critical condition of suffocation. Radical treatment is a secondary choice.

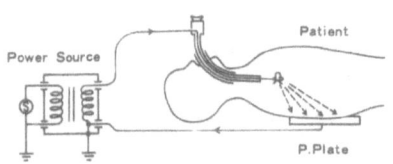

Figure 1

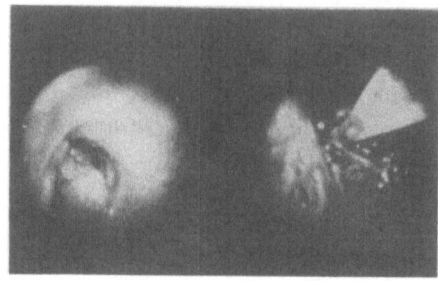

Figure 2

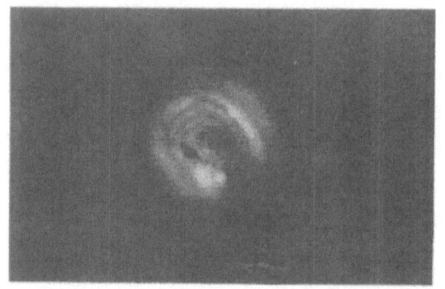

Figure 3

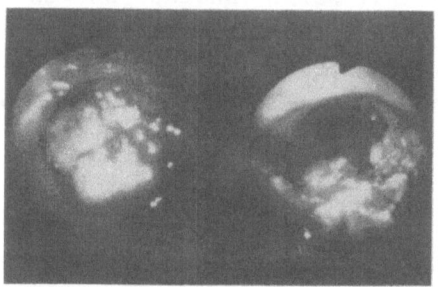

Figure 4

3. RESULTS

Figure 2 is a case of metastatic thyroid cancer. The left shows a polypoid pedunculated papillary adenocarcinoma, originating in the tracheal wall and obstructing the trachea. The right shows the stalk strangulated by the snare.

Figure 3 is the view of the trachea after resection. There is no bleeding and part of the stalk is seen in the left wall of the trachea. The dyspnea completely disappeared. Thereafter, 5,000 rad

Co^{60} radiation was administered. She is alive and well 2.5 years later.

Figure 4 is an advanced lung cancer case. He had undergone resection of the right upper lobe 4 years previously. The left shows the endoscopic finding before the procedure. The tumor with a necrotic surface occupies the trachea, with a broad base. Ventilation is possible only through a tiny crescent-shaped crevice. The right shows the postprocedure findings. Part of the broad base remains in 2/3 of the wall, but at least the bronchofiberscope can pass the stenotic portion. And the carina is observable. The dyspnea disappeared immediately. The tumor grew up to the same size again after 4 weeks. A total of 3 procedures were performed over 3 months.

TABLE ELECTROSURGICAL TREATMENT OF TRACHEAL OBSTRUCTION

Case	Age	Sex	Cause of obstruction	No. of procedures
C.W.	70 yrs	f	Intratracheal metastasis of thyroid cancer	1
R.W.	54 yrs	m	Advanced lung cancer	2
M.N.	58 yrs	f	Posttracheostomy web	1
K.U.	64 yrs	m	Advanced lung cancer	3

4. CONCLUSION

We think this method is not curative treatment for the original disease, but is significant in alleviating the critical condition due to suffocation, and radical treatment should be selected secondarily. This method must be performed carefully by operators experienced in fiberoptic bronchoscopy and one must always beware of hemorrhage due to injury of the bronchial artery, and of bronchial or tracheal formation.

The instrumentation for the procedure is not extremely conplicated. All that are required are the power supply and endoscopic surgery accessories, in addition to the usual fiberoptic bronchoscopic equipment.

We believe that this is a valuable palliative therapeutic option, and that it should occupy a definite position in the field of bronchofiberscopy.

Chapter XVII

FURTHER TOPICS AND CASE REPORTS

XVII.1.

IODINE-125 IMPLANT WITH A FLEXIBLE IMPLANT NEEDLE BY FIBEROPTIC BRONCHOSCOPE

J H HARRELL II, J R UTLEY, S L SEAGREN, K M MOSER, K ONEDA.

Symptomatic endobronchial recurrence of bronchogenic carcinoma in the previously heavily irradiated patient presents a difficult therapeutic challenge. External radiation is usually palliative when a patient is suffering from hemoptysis or airway obstruction.[1] Doses in excess of 6000 rads delivered externally to the mediastinum generally are not well tolerated. Interstitial radioactive implants allow the therapist to reduce the volume of tissue radiated and limit serious toxicity. Interstitial radiation can be safely employed after maximum external beam radiotherapy in other tumor systems.[2] It seems reasonable to employ endobronchial interstitial implantation in or near the lesion via the bronchoscope in this clinical setting.

Endobronchial implantation of radioactive seeds is not a new idea.[3] In all previous reports, sources have been introduced through a rigid bronchoscope under laryngeal block or general anesthesia. The advantage of interstitial radiation (brachytherapy, endocurietherapy) is that the fall off of radiation is rapid from the implanted source, in accordance with inverse square law. This allows delivery of a high dose of radiation to a relatively small volume of tissue. Therefore, the toxicity is generally acceptable, even though the tumor dose is high. The Volume to be implanted can be specifically defined through the bronchoscope. Only the specific region causing symptomatic obstruction will be radiated. This is not possible employing standard external beam techniques.

There are also disadvantages to implantation. In interstitial therapy one attempts to place the radioactive sources as homogeneously as possible at specific points within a tissue volume. This is difficult enough with unimpeded access to the volume to be radiated, but becomes even more difficult when these radioactive sources must be placed through a bronchoscope into the wall of the bronchus.

In permanent implant techniques we have employed iodine-125 seeds (I-125) which are inserted directly into the tissue and remain there permanently.

This radioactive source is commercially available as small cylinders 3 x 0.75 mm. It has a relatively long half life of 60 days. It allows protraction of radiotherapy which offers some biologic advantage. Its relatively low energy (30 KeV) makes radiation protection easy and limits the dose to the operating room personnel. However, disadvantages are inherent in I-125, especially in late palliative therapy of bronchogenic carcinoma. The dose rate is slow, and one may wish to deliver the radiation more rapidly than is possible with I-125 because of the urgency of symptoms, e.g., bronchial obstruction.

This paper deals with two cases in which combination implants of I-125 were done with a flexible needle via the fiberoptic bronchoscope. The right upper lobe and left upper lobe lesions were previously very difficult to implant via the rigid straight needle.

Methods and Clinical Experience: The flexible needle itself was developed in conjunction with Mr. Katsumi Oneda of Machida America and is applied through a large 2.6 mm channel Machida Fiberoptic Bronchoscope. The patient must fit the usual criteria for bronchoscopy. 1) PO_2 greater than 50. 2) PCO_2 less than 50. 3) Free of significant bronchospasm. 4) No serious arrhythmias. The patients are scoped with the radiotherapist to determine if implant is possible, determine the area of implantation and calculate the appropriate dosage.

The needle portion can be withdrawn into a flexible sheath for passage through the bronchoscope. The needle is milled to accept a radioactive I-125 pellet. This may be sealed in place with either bone wax or KY jelly. The needle is withdrawn into the flexible sheath and inserted via the fiberoptic bronchoscope. The area to be implanted is identified. The needle is advanced into the parenchyma of the neoplasm. An obturator is used to push the radioactive pellets into the tumor. The rigid needle and rigid scope can be used to implant lower lobe lesions.

CAPSULE INJECTOR

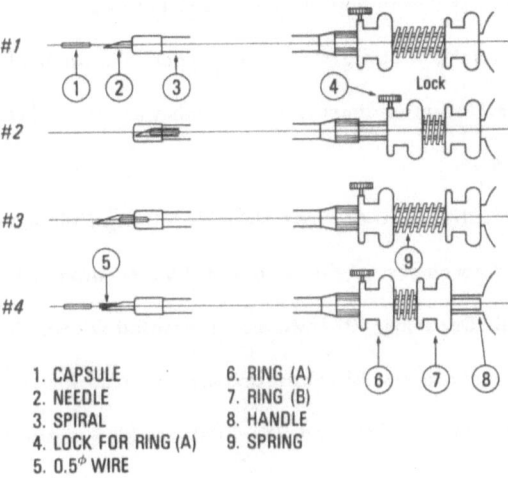

#1

① ② ③ ④ Lock

#2

#3

⑤ ⑨

#4

⑥ ⑦ ⑧

1. CAPSULE   6. RING (A)
2. NEEDLE   7. RING (B)
3. SPIRAL   8. HANDLE
4. LOCK FOR RING (A) 9. SPRING
5. 0.5$^{\phi}$ WIRE

Fig. I

572

D.G. Patient #1. The patient was a 49-year old female who in January, 1975 had a right lung wedge resection for poorly differentiated alveolar cell cancer. This was followed by radiation therapy. In March, 1975 she had a left upper lobe excision of squamous cell carcinoma followed with radiation therapy. In February, 1979 she developed pneumonia of the right upper lobe and underwent radiation to the right upper lobe again. Because of continued obstruction and maximum radiation treatment, I-125 seeds were implanted into the right upper lobe and bronchus intermedius.

L.M. Patient #2. The patient is a 66-year old male who was diagnosed in 1975 as having inoperable undifferentiated carcinoma of the lung with SVC syndrome. He was treated with 5200 rads and did well until December 1979 when he presented with aspiration pneumonia and hemoptysis. He received an additional 1200 rads and was referred for evaluation of implants. The patient was implanted with 21 I-125 seeds for a total of 14.4 microcuries administered to the right upper lobe and bronchus intermedius.

The obstructed bronchi were opened in both patients, achieving palliation.

Complications: Potential complications include bleeding, obstruction, infection, hypoxemia, as well as other known complications of Fiberoptic Bronchoscopy.

Summary: The concept of a flexible implant needle for use in a fiberoptic bronchoscope is presented. This device is used as a supplement to rigid tube bronchoscopy for implantation in difficult-to-reach upper lobe areas. This is a palliative procedure used to relieve obstruction in patients who have exhausted all other means of therapy. The patients must fit the usual criteria for bronchoscopy.

Conclusions: 1) I-125 implants with FOB appear to be a clinically useful approach. 2) This technique has application in a very specific patient population. 3) This technique is limited to those with extensive experience in FOB. 4) This is a palliative procedure.

XVII.2.

A CASE OF BRONCHIAL FOREIGN BODY (BULLET) WHICH REQUIRED LEFT UPPER LOBECTOMY

MASAMOTO NAKANO, AKIRA IKEBE, NAOFUMI SUYAMA, TAKEHIRO NAKATA

The patient, a 60 year-old man was shot in the neck on the right side, in 1944, (in World War II). He has had recurring fevers, chills and coughs several times each year since 1949. These symptoms went untreated.

In July, 1979, he was transferred to our hospital from an other hospital because of recurring pneumonia. At admission, the chest x-ray showed the finding of Atelectasis in upper lung field, where the bullet was found. Then bronchofiberscopy was performed. It showed a white coated bullet at the orifice of the left upper lobe bronchus.

Attempts to remove it by using various foreign body forceps failed. Because of this and recurring pneumonia, left upper lobectomy was performed. A schema of the bullet and the bronchus shows the location of the bullet in the bronchus which was 4 cm in length and 0.6 cm in diameter.

The bottom of the bullet was located at the orifice of the left upper lobe bronchus, and the head was found perforating the outside of the bronchus and was located in the pseudodiverticulm formed around the bronchus. The patient was discharged later, and is leading a normal life.

DISCUSSION

We think this case is quite interesting for the following reasons: First of all, this bronchial foreign body was a bullet. Second, it is relatively rare for a foreign body to be found in the left upper lobe. Third, the patient had lived 35 years without serious symptom. Fourth, it is not clear how and when the bullet had reached the orifice of the left upper lobe bronchus from the right side of the neck. Because detailed records of the gun shot incident were not available, this case appeared to be complicated.

A case of a bullet in the bronchus has not been reported in Japan. It is generally known that mineral foreign bodies are not as irritating to the bronchus as botanical foreign bodies, and it is not rare for patient with mineral obstruction to be asymptomatic. The passage route of the bullet to the left upper lobe bronchus was not determined either before or after the operation. BRENT analized pre and post operative observations on 68 cases of gun shot neck wounds, and found that

J.A. Nakhosteen and W. Maassen (eds.), Bronchology: Research, Diagnostic and
Therapeutic Aspects. All rights reserved.
Copyright 1981. Martinus Nijhoff Publishers bv, The Hague / Boston / London

17 cases had additional wounds outside the neck. 3 cases had tracheal perforations. It is possible that the patient in our report had such a tracheal perforation, that the bullet entered the bronchus through the trachea. Although we could not remove the bullet with variuos foreign forceps, we could have tried a strong magnet or powerful suction. Surgical treatment seemed to be most appropriate in this case, since **irreversible** complications had taken place in the lung.

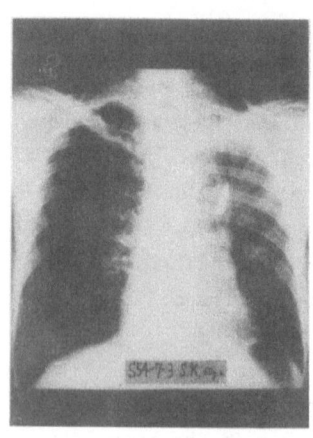

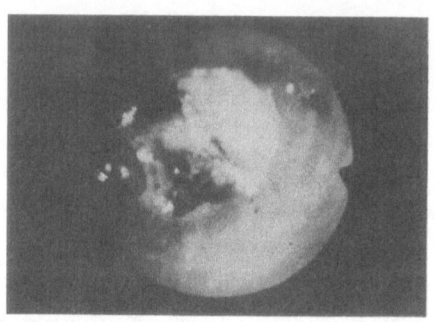

FIGURE II Bronchoscopic view

FIGURE I P-A view of chest x-p
(July 3, 1979)

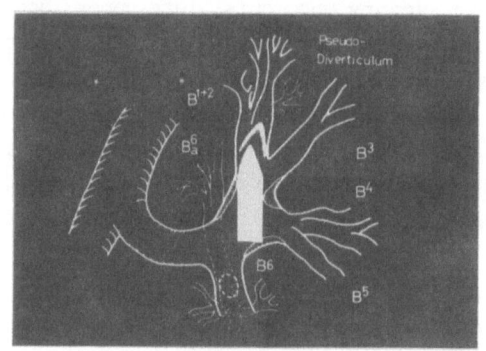

FIGURE III Schema of bullet and bronchus

REFERENCES

1. Stromberg, B.V.: Exploration of Low-velocity Gunshot Wounds of the Neck. J. Trauma, 19: 381-383, 1979.
2. Matsukura, H., et al: Surgical Removal of the Foreign Bodies from Intracardiac Cavity, Bronchial Tree and Thoracic Wall. Kyobugeka, 28: 574-579, 1975.
3. Osafune, H., et al: A case of Bronchial Foreign Body which Requred Left Upper Lobectomy. J. Jpn. Bronchoesophagol. Soc., 28: 217-221, 1977.

XVII.3.

CLINICAL, RADIOLOGIC, BRONCHOSCOPIC , AND HISTOLOGIC SIGNS IN BRONCHIAL ADENOMAS

K. NERGER, M. AMTHOR, H. KRONENBERGER, J. MEIER-SYDOW, M. RUST, H.L. SCHMIDTS, S. TUENGERTHAL

We present the clinical, radiologic, bronchoscopic, and histologic findings in 6 patients with bronchial adenomas. These tumors represent 1-6 % of all lung tumors (own results: about 2 %) and are most common in patients between 30-50 years (30-65 years). The incidence is slightly higher in females (4 out of 6). 90 % of these tumors are located in the upper parts of the bronchial tree (6 of 6), 75 % in the right lung (4 out of 6) (1,2,3,4).

About 80 % are carcinoid tumors, about 15 % are adenoid-cystic tumors, and less than 5 % are mucoepidermoid tumors (3).

Bronchial adenomas grow slowly. The time from onset of symptoms until diagnosis in the study by Roenspies (3) ranged from 2 weeks to 19 years; in our patients, 2 months to 4 years. Because these tumors tend to local invasive growth in 25 % and metastasise in 5-10%, they are classified as semi-malignant (1, 5).

We saw only carcinoid tumors. The most common clinical features are dry irritating cough (5 of 6), hemoptysis (2 of 6), and recurrent or chronic bronchitis or poststenotic pneumonias (5 of 6). Sometimes thoracic pain (2 of 6) and wheezing (1 of 6) are found. Endocrine symptoms are described in 2-7 % of all patients (3); we found none in our group, however.

Radiologic signs of chronic or recurrent local pneumonias and metastases are suspicious for an obturative tumor (Fig. 1). On tomographic sections roundish shadows, projecting into the bronchial lumen, are often found (Fig. 1, above). Sometimes air trapping is seen, especially marked during expiration, e.g. by fluoroscopy. Sometimes even a contralateral mediastinal shift can be observed (Fig. 2).

Fiberoptic bronchoscopy through an endotracheal tube with bronchial biopsy of tumor is an efficient method for the diagnosis of these tumors. We see a spherical, broad-adherent or pedunculated, flesh-colored tumor, mostly

J.A. Nakhosteen and W. Maassen (eds.), Bronchology: Research, Diagnostic and Therapeutic Aspects. All rights reserved.
Copyright 1981. Martinus Nijhoff Publishers bv, The Hague / Boston / London

obturating one bronchus (Fig. 3). Besides these findings, purulent secretions are often present. After biopsy the bronchial tree must be cleaned carefully, for bleeding can be intense. Cytologic investigations are not sufficient.

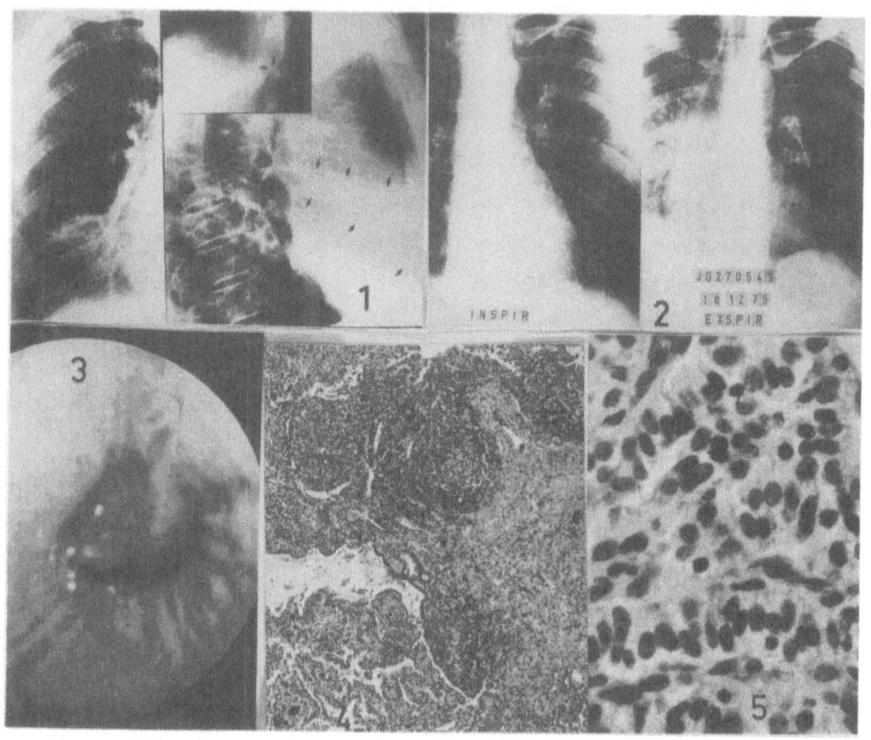

Carcinoid tumors are epithelial tumors of the bronchial mucosa. They show exophytic growth into the bronchial lumen and/or invasiveness into lung tissue (Fig. 4). If the invading part is greater than the exophytic, it is refered to as the "iceberg phenomenon". The carcinoid tumors consist of medium-sized, round or polygonal cells with regular oval nuclei and a light cytoplasm with fine granules (Fig. 5). Solid cell bands are arranged in trabecular or reticular manner. The stroma is tender.

Therapy must be surgical resection as a rule. In our opinion bronchoscopic resection and bronchoscopic laser therapy are not sufficient, because the intramural parts of the tumor cannot be assessed and eliminated with certainty. In our patients, bilobectomy of the right lower and middle lobe was necessary in 3 cases, lobectomy of the left lower lobe in 2, and lobectomy of the right upper lobe with sleeve resection of the right main bronchus in one patient. To date, no relapses have been seen. In other investigations, the 10-year survival rate is 90 % (1).

XVII.4.

CONGENITAL BRONCHOBILIARY FISTULA DIAGNOSED BY BRONCHOFIBERSCOPY

Y. OSAKABE, H. SUZUKI, K. NAKAGAMI, T. KUNIEDA, H. JONOUCHI, N. NAGAI, AND E. NOGUCHI

1. INTRODUCTION

The congenital fistula between respiratory system and gastro-intestinal system is extremely rare except the bronchoesophageal fistula.

A case of congenital bronchobiliary fistula is reported in this study in which the diagnosis was mainly taken by the bronchofiberscopy under the general anesthesia.

2. CASE REPORT

Our patient is a 1 year and 9 months old female infant. She was normally delivered with a body weight of 3.8 kg. at the department of gynecology of our hospital on August 4, 1977. She was suffering from biliary vomitting just after birth and dyspnea and cyanosis appeared a couple of days later. The strong chemotherapy was given her under the diagnosis of aspiration pneumonea and she became soon free from these complaints. Although the various clinical examinations were taken, the diagnosis could not be established. But she was discharged on December 3, 1977.

One year and 5 months later she was readmitted for the exact examination and the treatment because of the repeated biliary vomitting.

The physical findings and the laboratory findings were almost normal.

There were demonstrated the abnormal shadows in the both lower lung-fields of the chest X-ray film at the second admittion.
The nuclear scan of biliary system with 99^{m}Tc-IDA revealed the abnormal RI activity from the upper portion of the left liver to the tracheal bifurcation.

The fistula was located at the center of tracheal bifurcation having the flow of yellow juice (Fig. 1) and the green flow from this fistula after the ICG intravenous injection. The confirmation of the biliary juice was made by the chemical analysis.

J.A. Nakhosteen and W. Maassen (eds.), Bronchology: Research, Diagnostic and Therapeutic Aspects. All rights reserved.
Copyright 1981. Martinus Nijhoff Publishers bv, The Hague / Boston / London

580

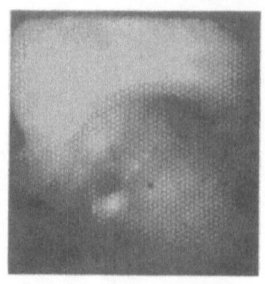

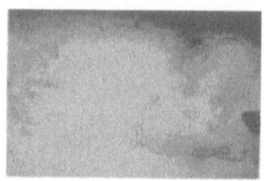

FIGURE 2. Histological findings

FIGURE 1. Bronchofiberscopic findings

The diagnosis of congenital bronchobiliary fistula was made and the operation was successfully performed according to the method by Stigol and others (Ref. 1).

The specimen of intrapleual fistula resected, was about 1 cm in diameter and about 3 cm in length. The fistula was consisted of the tissues of trachea and biliary duct (Fig. 2).

3. DISCUSSION

The first case of congenital biliary fistula was reported by Neuhauser and others in 1952 (Ref. 2) and 10 cases were reported so far.

Symptomatically, our case is extremely similar to the reported cases. The clinical symptoms occurred just after birth in our case such as others. The biliary vomitting is the most characteristic symptom.

Developmentally, there is no established theory for this anomaly.

Sane and others (Ref. 3) believe that the fistulography is most useful for the diagnosis of this anomaly. However, we believe that the bronchofiberscopy is the best method for the diagnosis of congenital bronchobiliary fistula.

After the operation she recovered well step by step. At present she is quite healthy and she complains nothing at all.

REFERENCES
1. Stigol, L. C. et al: Carinal trifurcation with congenital tracheo-biliary fistula: Pediat., 37: 89, 1966.
2. Neuhauser, E. et al: Congenital direct communication between biliary system and respiratory tract: Am. J. Dis. Chil., 83: 654, 1952.
3. Sane, S. M. et al: Congenital bronchobiliary fistula: Surgery, 69: 599, 1971.

XVII.5.

TRACHEOBRONCHOPATHIA OSTEOCHONDROPLASTICA: A clinical, bronchoscopic and spirometric study.

N. Stjernberg and R. Lundgren
Department of Lung Medicine, University Hospital, S-901 85 Umeå,
Sweden.

Tracheobronchopathia osteochondroplastica (TO) is a rare disease, distinguished by accumulation of bony and cartilaginous nodules in tracheal and bronchial mucosa. The ethiology of the disease is unknown (Magnusson and Rotemark 1974). Most cases have been diagnosed at autopsy but an increasing number have been diagnosed in vivo by bronchoscopy.

Material and methods

From 1972 untill 1979 nine cases of TO were diagnosed among 2180 bronchoscopies performed at our department. There were five men and four women with a mean age of 60 years. Seven were non-smokers and two ex-smokers. Clinical history, bronchoscopic findings and lung function were studied in these patients.

Bronchoscopic examination was performed with a rigid broncho-scope until August 1974 and after that time a flexible fiberoptic bronchoscope was used. Bronchoscopy was performed under topical anesthesia.

Lung volumes were measured with a closed circuit helium dilution method and dynamic spirometry was recorded with a Bernstein spirometer.

Results

Clinical data are summarized in Table 1. The most common respiratory symptoms were those of cough, phlegm, dyspnea, recurrent respiratory infections and haemoptysis.

582

TABLE 1. Clinical picture and spirometry patterns in nine patients
with tracheobronchopathia osteochondroplastica.

Age/ Sex	Duration of symptoms	Cough	Phlegm	Hemop- tysis	Exertion dyspnea	Recurrent respira- tory infection	Spirometry pattern
79 M	1 month	X	X				Obstructive
75 F	1 year			X		X	Obstructive
74 M	20 years	X	X	X	X	X	Obstructive
74 F	10 years	X			X	X	Not examined
63 M	45 years	X	X		X	X	Obstructive
55 M	25 years	X	X		X	X	Normal
54 M	30 years	X	X			X	Obstructive
53 F	20 years	X	X	X	X	X	Obstructive
30 F	15 years			X			Obstructive

Bronchoscopy disclosed multiple yellow-white papilla-like, hard
formations on the cartilaginous parts of trachea, main bronchi
and lobe bronchi. The extension of bronchoscopic changes is shown
in Table 2. Biopsies showed well-differentiated osteo-cartilaginous
tissue consitent with TO in all patients.

Spirometry was performed in eight of the nine patients (Table 1).
Six patients had an obstructive spirometry pattern, one had a
combination of restrictive and obstructive patterns and one had
a normal spirometry.

TABLE 2. Bronchoscopic findings in nine patients with tracheobronchopathia osteochondroplastica.

Age/ Sex	Extension of the bronchoscopic changes in the airways					Biopsy diagnostic
	Trachea	Main bronchi	Lobe bronchi	Segmental bronchi	Narrowing of the bronchi	
79 M	X	X				Yes
75 F	X	X	X	X		Yes
74 M	X	X	X			Yes
74 F	X	X				Yes
63 M		X	X			Yes
55 M	X	X				Yes
54 M	X	X	X	X	X	Yes
53 M	X	X	?	?	X	Yes
30 F	X	X				Yes

Discussion

The frequency of TO has been reported to be three per 1000 autopsies
(Ragaini and Piccoli, 1957). In the present series nine patients
with TO were found among 2180 bronchoscopies (0,4 per cent). TO is
said to have a male predominance but this can not be confirmed by
the present study. According to Martin (1974) most patients are
totally asymptomatic, but all our patients had respiratory symptoms
and most of them had an obstructive spirometry pattern.
TO is a disease with chronic respiratory symptoms and the patients
often have an obstructive spirometry pattern. Patients with TO
may be hidden among the large number of patients with chronic
obstructive lung diseases. Bronchoscopy is the only way to establish
a sure diagnosis during lifetime. The bronchoscopic findings are
typical and the diagnosis can be confirmed by biopsy through the
bronchoscope.

XVII.6.

3 CASES WITH BRONCHIAL CARCINOID

S. AWATAGUCHI

1. INTRODUCTION

Bronchial carcinoid is known as an adenomatous tumor characterized by slow growth and long primary stage without definite synptoms,but it sometimes results in malignant change with serious endocrine disturbance. During past 30 years I have encountered three cases with bronchial carcinoid.

2. CASES

Case 1. An 18-year-old male

He was complaining of persistent cough and wheezing associated with frequent episodes of acute exacerbation of pneumonitis and was treated under erroneous diagnosis of prumonary tuberculosis for 5 years. His chest radiographs showed abnormal shadow at the left hilar region, and bronchoscopy revealed a large tumor at the distal end of the left main bronchus. The tumor was red in color and had smooth and rounded surface. Histological diagnosis of the biopsy taken bronchoscopically was carcinoid. Left pneumonectomy was performed. On the resected specimen, a sessile tumor was developed from the bronchial wall at the orifice of the lingular division, growing proximally into the left main bronchus. Histochemically, argyerophile reaction of tumor cells was positive and electron microscopic view revealed granulous formation in the tumor cells. He is living a normal life over one year now.

Case 2. A 33-year-old female

She was complaining a cough, sputum and elevated temperature for 2 months. Her chest x-ray films showed an abnormal shadow in the right lower lung field, and bronchoscopy revealed a tumor growing at the orifice of the right lower lobe bronchus. Histological examination of the biopsy was not diagnostic. Right pneumonectomy was carried out under the suspicion of the bronchial cancer associ-

J.A. Nakhosteen and W. Maassen (eds.), Bronchology: Research, Diagnostic and Therapeutic Aspects. All rights reserved.
Copyright 1981. Martinus Nijhoff Publishers bv, The Hague / Boston / London

ated with suppurative pneumonitis. The resected specimen showed a thumb-tip-sized tumor growing at the bifurcation between the middle and lower lobe bronchus. Histological diagnosis was bronchial carcinoid. She has been alive over 12 years.

Case 3. A 24-year-old female

Her illness started with chills and fevers followed by a productive cough and bloody sputum. She was treated as pulmonary tuberculosis for 7 months. Her chest x-ray films showed atelectasis of the right lower lung field. Bronchoscopy revealed a large tumor occluding the orifice of the intermediate bronchus. The tumor was removed completely by forceps and repeated cauteries were done on the origin of the tumor bronchoscopically. Histological diagnosis of this tumor was carcinoid. 7 years after the bronchoscopic removal of this tumor, she noticed the gradual onset of productive cough and wheezing associated with bloody sputum and flushing of her face. Urinary excretion of 5-HIAA was 29.5mg/day. These findings were suggestive of carcinoid syndrome caused by recurrence of bronchial carcinoid. Right pneumonectomy was done, and carcinoid syndrome disappeared. However, 4 years after right pneumonectomy,Cushing's syndrome appeared and she died 12 years after diagnosis of bronchial carcinoid was first made. Necropsy revealed widespread metastases involving the regional lymph nodes, the adrenals and the pancreas. ACTH and serotonin contents of the bronchial and metastatic lesions increased markedly.

3. CONCLUSION

The bronchial carcinoid looks just like red, hard cherry on bronchoscopy and can be clearly differentiated from bronchogenic cancer by its characteristic appearances. Bronchial carcinoid is considered to originate from neurosecretory cells (Kultschitzky cells) lining the bronchial glands and characterized by slow growth and long symptomless primary stage, but it, sometimes, could potentally degenerate into malignancy and cause serious complications such as carcinoid syndrome, Cushing's syndrome, etc. Therefore, the best treatment for bronchial carcinoid seems to be lung resection.

REFERENCES
1. Bench, K.G. et al.: Studies on the bronchial counterpart of Kultschitzky (Argentaffin) cell and innervation of bronchial glands.Jour. of Ultrastructure Res. 12; 668 - 686, 1965.
2. Isawa T. et al.: Cushing's syndrome caused by recurrent malignant bronchial carcinoid. Am Rev. Resp. Dis. 108; 1200-1204, 1977.

XVII.7.

HEMOPTYSIS DUE TO IDIOPATHIC BENIGN ULCER OR EROSION OF THE
RESPIRATORY TRACT

H.Kudo*, H.Kuwabara*, K.Inatomi*, H.Homma*, H.Mochizuki**.

1. INTRODUCTION

In about 30% of outclinic patients complaining of hemoptysis, no
etiology could be found after thorough clinical investigation, and
there has been as yet no information about hemoptysis due to idiopathic
ulcers or erosions of the respiratory tract. This paper presents
bronchoscopic findings and clinical features in these cases.

2. PATIENTS AND METHODS

During the period of from 1968 to 1979, eleven patients with complaints of bloody sputum or hemoptysis were admitted and diagnosed by
bronchoscopy as having idiopathic bronchial ulcers or erosions. They
were ten males and one female and their ages ranged from twenty-one
to sixty-eight (the average age was forty-two), the majority being
men in their thirties. Bloody sputum or hemoptysis was the initial
sign. Chest pain, fever, or dyspnea were rarely noted. These patients
had episodes of bleeding lasting from several days to twenty eight
years and the amounts of blood ranged from a few milliliters to about
300 milliliters a day. They had no histories of serious illness and
occupational hazards. Forty percent smoked regularly including one
heavy smoker. Blood coagulation tests were all within normal limits.
Chest X-ray films usually revealed no changes except transient consol-
idations in only two cases wich disappeared within a week. Bronchography failed to reveal any abnormal findings except in the case of
one person who had mild bronchiectasis of the right B^9. There were no
acid-fast bacilli and malignant cells in the sputum. Rhinolaryngo-
logical disease, heart disease, and other diseases were all excluded
by a battery of clinical examinations. These patients were examined by
a Machida-6T fiberoptic bronchoscope in a supine position under endotracheal intubation after inhalation of anesthesia.

J.A. Nakhosteen and W. Maassen (eds.), Bronchology: Research, Diagnostic and
Therapeutic Aspects. All rights reserved.
Copyright 1981. Martinus Nijhoff Publishers bv, The Hague / Boston / London

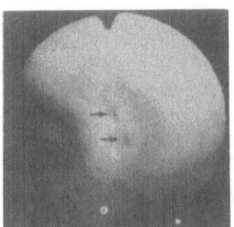

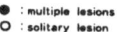

● : multiple lesions
○ : solitary lesion

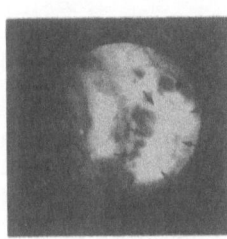

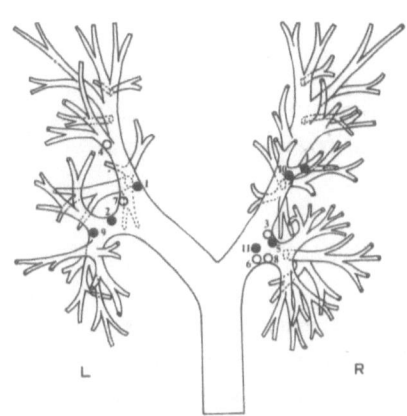

L   R

FIGURE 1. a) Case 1, b) Case 2   Figure 2. Location of bronchial
                                    ulcers or erosions.

Shown in figure 1 are the bronchoscopic findings in two cases with
typical ulcers (arrow) and location of bronchial ulcers or erosions.
a) a 47 year-old man. Two ulcers are shown without any bleeding around
the orifice of the right B^4. b) a 35 year-old woman. Bleeding and
congestion of vessels around an ulcer (arrow) at the wall of the left
main bronchus are shown. Figure 2 shows that these lesions are more
common on the right side than on the left side. All lesions are found
in areas ranging from the main bronchus to the segmental bronchi.
Half of the cases had single ulcerous or erosive lesions and the rest
had multiple lesions.

3. SUMMARY

1. Eleven cases with idiopathic benign bronchial ulcer or erosion
studied by the fiberoptic bronchoscope are reported.
2. The patients were ten males and one female of ages ranging from
21 to 68 year old, the majority being men in their thirties.
3. These lesions were located in the main bronchus and/or in the
segmental bronchi and more common in the right bronchi.
4. Half of the cases had solitary lesion and the rest several lesions.
5. These lesions of unknown etiology are considered to be of benign
nature, because all seven patients being followed up have been doing
well without recurrence or any severe consequence.

REFERENCES

1. Homma H. Jap. Med. J., 2429:3, 1970.

XVII.8.

RARE TRACHEAL DISEASES —— VIDEO TAPE RECORDING OF BRONCHOFIBERSCOPIC FINDINGS

M. KANEKO, J. HONDA, K. SOHMA, T. TAKAHASHI, N. YAMAMOTO, H. YOSHIMURA,

T. MATSUBAYASHI, and S. IKEDA,

At Kitasato University Hospital, almost all bronchofiberscopic procedures are performed with a direct connection to a TV camera, and important findings are recorded by VTR. This method is very useful for the progress of diagnostic accuracy, smooth examination and medical education. In particular, playing the VTR scene is especially valuable for the education of medical students and residents.

Here, we will present some recently-experienced cases of rare tracheal diseases.

As the tracheal lumen is wider than the bronchi, a powerful light source and special new bronchofiberscope which has more glass fibers for image and light guide than the usual type are necessary for connection to the TV camera.

Case 1. Tracheobronchomalacia

A 50-year-old male was admitted to Kitasato University Hospital because of pneumonia. In spite of the disappearance of the abnormal shadow on chest X-ray films, dry cough persisted. Bronchofiberscopy revealed that the lumina of the trachea and bronchi were enlarged in the inspiratory phase and narrowed in the expiratory phase. The convex cartilage protruded into the tracheal and bilateral main bronchial lumina.

These findings were confirmed by tracheobronchography. The tracheal cross section area was 4.6 cm^2 in the inspiratory phase and 1.3 cm^2 in the expiratory phase, as measured by C.T. scan.

Case 2. Tracheal diverticulum with cartilaginous rings

A 58-year-old female patient was admitted to Kitasato University Hospital because of chronic cough and sputum. Frontal chest X-ray film revealed marked emphysematous lungs. A tracheobronchogram showed that there was a diverticulum, at the posterior wall of the trachea, which was narrowed at the peripheral part.

Bronchofiberscopically, there was a diverticulum at the posterior wall of the mid-trachea. The distal portion of the tracheal lumen was narrowed with cartilaginous rings without the membranous portion. During coughing, the membranous portion of the proximal part of the trachea and the bilateral main bronchus were elevated, but the lumen of the narrowed tracheal section did not change.

J.A. Nakhosteen and W. Maassen (eds.), Bronchology: Research, Diagnostic and Therapeutic Aspects. All rights reserved.
Copyright 1981. Martinus Nijhoff Publishers bv, The Hague / Boston / London

Case 3. Trauma of the trachea

A 40-year-old male patient was admitted to Kitasato University Hospital because of chest trauma caused by falling from the second story of a building. There were multiple fractures of the ribs, and marked subcutaneous emphysema was noted on the chest X-ray film.

Emergency bronchofiberscopy was performed. Two granulomas were found at the distal anterior and left tracheal walls and two very tiny polypoid lesions were found at the carina.

Case 4. Adenoid cystic carcinoma of the trachea

A 63-year-old patient was admitted to Kitasato University Hospital because of difficulty in swallowing. A chest X-ray revealed a mass at the right middle mediastinum.

On C.T. scan at the lower part of the trachea, the tumor was seen as behind the trachea and compressing the tracheal lumen.

Bronchofiberscopically, the membranous portion was elevated at the distal part of the trachea, and the mucosa was partially lost, disclosing tumorous tissue. Tortuositas vasorum was seen. It was difficult to pass the bronchofiberscope through the narrowed segment. Pathological diagnosis by biopsy specimen was adenoid cystic carcinoma.

Generally, rigid endoscopy has been performed for laryngeal and tracheal lesions. Now, however, diagnosis of tracheal, laryngeal and nasopharyngeal lesions has also become possible using the new bronchofiberscope and a powerful light source for observation.

REFERENCES

1. Rayl JE, Hall CJ, Rourke D, Spindler LJ: Requirement for television-bronchoscopy. Chest, 73: 764-767, 1978.
2. Ratliff JL, Campbell GD, Reid MV: Tracheobronchiomegaly: Report of two cases with widely differing symptomatology. Ann Otol, 86: 172-175, 1977.
3. Greene DA: Congenital tracheal rings. Arch Otolaryngol, 102: 241-243, 1976.
4. Urschel HC, Razzuk MA: Management of acute traumatic injuries of tracheobronchial tree. Surgery, Gynecology & Obstetrics, 136: 113-117, 1973.
5. Baydur A, Gottlieb LS: Adenoid cystic carcinoma of the trachea masquerading as asthma. JAMA, 234: 829-831, 1975.

Derzeitige Bedeutung der Bronchialtuberkulose

R. Götz, G. Deissler, H. Blaha
XVII.9.

Folgender Beitrag gilt einer allgemeinen Orientierung. Eine Aussage zur Häufigkeit endobronchialer Veränderungen bei Tuberkulose ist an dieser Stelle nicht
möglich. Dies einerseits deswegen, weil das zur Untersuchung kommende Krankengut eine Mischmenge darstellt - Verdacht auf Tuberkulose oder ungeklärte
Bakterienausscheidung, V. a. Bronchialkarzinom, unklare Pneumonie - andererseits deswegen, weil selbstverständlich nicht bei jeder Tuberkulose eine Bronchoskopie durchgeführt wird. Die Endoskopie kommt also nur in speziellen Fällen mit gezielter Fragestellung zur Anwendung. Es handelt sich demzufolge um ein
selektioniertes Krankengut. Eine statistische Auswertung ist daher nicht möglich,
bzw. würde zu falsch hohen Frequenzen führen.
    Wir sehen die Bedeutung der Bronchialtuberkulose bzw. des Einsatzes der
Bronchoskopie bei Tuberkulose und Tuberkuloseverdacht in der Diagnostik und
Differentialdiagnostik. Relativ grob könnte man folgendermaßen unterscheiden:
Differentialdiagnose endobronchialer Befunde bei Tuberkuloseverdacht einerseits,
Entwicklung und Verlauf bei Tuberkulose andererseits.
Die wichtigste Differentialdiagnose ist zum Bronchialkarzinom zu stellen. Auch
der Nachweis von Tuberkulosebakterien kann uns nicht davon entbinden, nach
anderen Ursachen endobronchialer Veränderungen zu suchen. Auf das häufige Zu-
sammentreffen von Tuberkulose und Karzinom wurde schon früher verwiesen.
Weitere endobronchiale Veränderungen finden sich im Rahmen von Sarkoidose,
bronchopulmonaler Aspergillose, bei Fremdkörpern u. a. m.
Den zweiten wichtigen Aspekt in diesem Zusammenhang stellt die Klärung von
Entwicklung und Verlauf bei Tuberkulose dar. Als Beispiele seien ungeklärte Bakterienausscheidung und Reparationsvorgänge genannt. Wir finden das tuberkulöse
Ulkus und den Lymphknoteneinbruch oft genug nur endoskopisch. Reparationsvorgänge
können Anlaß unklarer Röntgenbefunde sein, so beispielsweise Stenosierungen,
die zu Atelektasen und Retention führen können. Weiterhin achten wir auf Resi-
duen bei Tuberkulose, es interessieren uns Zustände geringerer Rückbildungs-
fähigkeit, oft als Ausdruck von Bronchialläsionen.
Die vorliegende Zusammenstellung stützt sich auf das Krankengut aus dem Zentralkrankenhaus Gauting in den Jahren 1974 - 1976.
Bezogen auf sämtliche histologisch gesicherten Lungentuberkulosen in diesem
Zeitraum - es sind dies 370 - war eine Tuberkulose der Bronchialschleimhaut
in 42,7% der Fälle nachzuweisen, dass sind absolut 158 Fälle.
Zunächst kurz zur Morphologie. Charakteristische endoskopische Befunde bestehen eigentlich nicht. Schleimhautrötung, ödematöse Schwellung, eitriges Sekret
und Ostiendeformierung, um nur einiges zu nennen, stellen unspezifische Zeichen
dar. Granulationen mögen richtungsweisend sein, auch sie repräsentieren keinen
eindeutigen Hinweis.
Die von uns zur Erleichterung der Übersicht vorgenommene Einteilung in Gruppen stellt eine mutwillige Einengung eines Kontinuums dar.
Gruppe I   Begleitende Tuberkulosen innerhalb des Bronchialsystems bei ausge-
dehnten Veränderungen der Lungen.
Gruppe II   Fraglich isolierte Bronchialtuberkulosen bei nicht zerfallendem Parenchymbefund.
Gruppe III Schädigung des Bronchialsystems mit Geschwürsbildung und Durch-

bruch bei Lymphknotentuberkulose.

Die histologisch gesicherten Bronchialtuberkulosen gliedern sich folgendermassen in die einzelnen Gruppen auf: Den Hauptanteil hat die Gruppe I, absolut 76 Fälle, was 48% aller Fälle ausmacht. Einen eher geringen Parenchymbefund bei größerer relativer Bedeutung der Bronchialtuberkulose finden wir in Gruppe II, die bei einer absoluten Fallzahl 28 von 46 Fällen 28% ausmacht. In 23% der Fälle etwa, absolut 36 Fälle, wurde Lymphknotenkompression, Lymphknoteneinbruch oder der Verdacht auf das Vorliegen eines solchen Geschehens angenommen.

Abschließend die bakteriologischen Befunde: Bei Gruppe I 75 Mal eine positive Bakteriologie, davon 6 Mal nur aus dem Bronchialsekret. Bei Gruppe II 11 Fälle mit negativer Bakteriologie, nahezu 25% dieser Gruppe; in drei Fällen konnte ein positiver bakteriologischer Befund erst nach Bronchoskopie erhoben werden. Bei Gruppe III 6 Fälle mit negativem bakteriologischen Untersuchungsergebnis, 16,6% dieser Fälle; in 5 Fällen der Nachweis säurefester Stäbchen erst aus dem Bronchialsekret.

Insgesamt waren 140 von 158 Fällen bakteriologisch gesichert, davon 14 nur durch den Einsatz der Bronchoskopie. Dies bedeutet einer Verbesserung der bakteriologischen Ausbeute, neben der histologischen Frühdiagnose.

Zusammenfassend stellt die Endoskopie ein wertvolles Instrument in der Tuberkulosediagnostik dar. Bei der Unsicherheit der Tuberklinprobe, der Unsicherheit des röntgenologischen Befundes und der Langwierigkeit des bakteriologischen Beweises bietet die Endoskopie die Möglichkeit des raschen histologischen Nachweises.

XVII.10.
BRONCHIAL TUBERCULOSIS SIMILAR TO LUNG CARCINOMA *

J. Honda, K. Souma, T. Takahashi, H. Ohtsuka, T. Tomita, Y. Tazaki, Y. Yamamoto, H. Yoshimura, M. Kane, S. Ikeda

Although the rate of occurrence of tuberculosis is steadily falling in most parts of the world, this disease remains a significant world-wide health problem.

The purpose of this study was to clarify the bronchoscopic differences between bronchial tuberculosis and lung carcinoma, using flexible fiberoptic bronchoscopy.

Six cases, aged 33 to 51 years, with bacteriologically proven bronchial tuberculosis were reviewed and documented on video tape.

Bronchoscopic findings of these patients showed tumor-like lesions with small superficial necrosis and irregular surface, located in the large bronchus. Of six patients, four showed obstruction and/or stenosis of the segmental bronchus due to necrotic mass lesions. These findings resembled squamous cell carcinoma, hence the difficulty in differentiating these two.

Generally , in bronchial tuberculosis, the surface of the bronchial mucosa shows a tumor-like irregularity, but no actual tumor is present. Squamous cell carcinoma is apt to protude past the endobronchial surface. Furthermore, bronchial tuberculosis is characterized by smooth-surfaced, white-colored necrosis, while in the neoplasm , irregular-surfaced necrosis is seen. Small cell carcinoma of the bronchus causes bronchial stenosis, as opposed to the necrosis caused by bronchial tuberculosis. Finally, bronchial tuberculosis shows redness and swelling, and spreads more broadly, forming multifocal lesions.

---

*This is a summary of a video tape presented on this subject by these authors. Ed.

XVII.11. BACTERIOLOGICAL PROBLEMS DURING FIBEROPTIC BRONCHOSCOPY

H. MAGNUSSEN, L. KRIZEK, M. EXNER, H. LINDSTAEDT

1. Introduction

The value of bacteriological cultures of specimens collected from the lower repiratory tract during fiberoptic bronchoscopy is limited by three major factors: a. contamination with the oropharyngeal flora, b. effectiveness of the sterilization procedures and c. the effect of topical anesthetics on the micro-organisms. We have examined some aspects of these sources leading to questionable results.

2. Materials and Methods

2.1. Disinfection of the bronchofiberscope

2.1.i. in vitro studies.

The bronchofiberscope (Olympus BF – B3) was contaminated for 20 min with a suspension containing one of the following microorganisms: Hemophilus influenzae, a-hemolytic Streptococcus, Pseudomonas aeruginosa and Candida albicans. Disinfection was started by rinsing with tap water for 10 min, followed by 10 min of administration of one of the solutions: 1. succinaldehyde, 2. glutar aldehyde, and 3. povidine iodine. Before taking 6 specimens from different parts of the bronchoscope, a 10 min washing of the scope was repeated.

2.1.ii. in vivo studies.

In 10 patients transnasal fiberoptic bronchoscopy was performed in order to diagnose bronchogenic carcinoma. There was no clinical or endoscopic evidence for bacterial infection of the respiratory tract. After bronchoscopy the microorganisms growing in the cultured specimens taken from six parts of the instrument were compared before and after disinfection. Chemical disinfection was done with glutar aldehyde. In addition to the procedure described the operating channel was cleaned

J.A. Nakhosteen and W. Maassen (eds.), Bronchology: Research, Diagnostic and Therapeutic Aspects. All rights reserved.
Copyright 1981. Martinus Nijhoff Publishers bv, The Hague / Boston / London

mechanically using standard brushes.

2.2. Effect of lidocaine on bacterial growth

Suspensions of Proteus mirabilis, Klebsiella pneumoniae, Hemophilus influenzae, Staphylococcus aureus, a-hemolytic Streptococcus and Pneumococcus were each exposed to 4, 2, and 0.2 % solutions of lidocaine, respectively. The antibacterial activity of lidocaine was evaluated after 10 min and every hour for 6 hours. The data were compared to the bacterial growth in physiological saline.

3. Results

2.1.i. In vitro only the disinfection procedure using glutar aldehyde resulted in no residual contamination.

2.1.ii. In the patients within the 60 specimens cultured before disinfection, microorganisms were detected 20 times and identified in most cases as being inhabitants of the oropharyngeal flora. After disinfection only 4 of the 60 specimens showed bacterial growth.

2.2. The effect of different concentrations of lidocaine and of saline on the bacterial growth is expressed in Table 1 as the time (in hours) necessary to decrease the number of colonies to half their original value.

Table 4.

	Saline	LIDOCAINE (%)		
		0.2	2	4
Pneumococcus	2.5	1	1	1
a-hemol. Streptoc.	6	4	4	0.7
Staph. aureus	> 6	6	4	3
Proteus mirabilis	> 6	6	2	2
Klebsiella pneum.	> 6	6	2	2
Haemophilus influenzae	6	6	1	1

4. Discussion

Our data, similar to those of Bartlett et al.[1] ,indicate that the value of bacteriological cultures of specimens obtained during fiberoptic bronchoscopy is limited. 1. During passage of the upper repiratory tract, contamination of the instrument with oropharyngeal flora cannot

be avoided. As the species detected are normal and pathologic strains
(e.g. pseudomonas) found in the upper airways of several hospitalized
patients, the clinical relevance of the interpretation is unreliable.
2. During disinfection in most cases the time of exposure to the chemical
solution has to exceed 10 min, a time often proposed by the manufactu-
rers. In the clinical situation disinfection can be improved by vigorous
mechanical cleaning of the operating channel. This is based on the observation that biological materials, e.g. sputum, will offer a barrier
to the penetration of the disinfecting solutions. 3. The topical anesthetic lidocaine will influence the organismsin a time and species
dependant fashing. Though our results differ in detail from those reported by Bartlett et al.[1] the general conclusion seems to be valid in
that cultures have to be performed immediately in order to avoid errors
introduced by local anesthesia.

XVII.12.

DIAGNOSTIC VALUE OF TRANSBRONCHIAL BIOPSY IN ENDOSCOPICALLY NONVISIBLE BRONCHIAL CARCINOMA

T. ARAI, T. SUZUKI, and A. NAKANO,
Nakano National Chest Hospital, Tokyo, Japan.

The transbronchial forceps biopsy for the diagnosis of peripheral lung cancer was started in March 1976 in our hospital and it has become our major diagnostic method in the last 2 years.

Materials and methods

During the last two years, 148 patients with bronchogenic carcinoma underwent diagnostic bronchoscopy, using flexible bronchofiberscope. 70 out of those 148 patients had the tumor in the peripheral area of their lung, and endoscopically the tumor was not visible. Of those 70 cases with nonvisible carcinoma, the transbronchial biopsy was performed in 51 cases, and further, among those 51 cases, the brushing was also performed in 23 cases. In the next 10 cases, the transbronchial biopsy was tried but the forceps failed to reach the tumor; the brushing was performed in these cases instead. And, for the remaining 9 cases the brushing was chosen from the beginning. For the transbronchial biopsy and brushing, we inserted the biopsy forceps or brush through the flexible bronchofiberscope into the tumor in the peripheral lung under fluoroscopic guidance.

Results

Of the 51 cases, in which the transbronchial forceps biopsy was performed, the carcinoma tissue were obtained from 35 cases. In the remaining 16 cases, the biopsy specimen showed only the normal tissues. Therefore, the diagnostic accuracy of the transbronchial biopsy was 68.6%. The diagnostic accuracy by the size of the tumor were none out of 2 cases with less than 1.9cm in diameter, 10 out of 15 cases with 2.0cm – 2.9cm, 12 out of 17 cases with 3.0cm – 4.9cm, and 13 out of 17 cases with 5cm or more. The histological classification of the biopsied carcinomas were adenocarcinoma in 16, squamous cell carcinoma in 8, small cell carcinoma in 3, large cell carcinoma in 1, and unclassified in 7.

In the 23 cases, in which both biopsy and brushing were performed, the results of these diagnostic methods were compared. The table shows the result of those 23 cases. The result showed that the carcinoma tissue was obtained by biopsy in 14 cases, 60.9%, and by the brushing, the carcinoma cells were obtained in 17 cases, 73.9%. By either one or both methods, however, the diagnosis of carcinoma was successfully made in 21 out of 23 cases, 91.3%.

J.A. Nakhosteen and W. Maassen (eds.), Bronchology: Research, Diagnostic and Therapeutic Aspects. All rights reserved.

Table. Result of the Transbronchial Biopsy and Brushing.

Result of Histology by Transbronchial Biopsy	No. cases	(%)	Result of Cytology by Brushing	No. cases	(%)
ca. positive	14	(60.9)	positive	10	(91.3)
			negative	4	
ca. negative	9	(39.1)	positive	7	
			negative	2	(8.7)
Total	23	(100.0)		23	(100.0)

The analysis of the location of the tumor in the lung showed that all of 19 cases, with one exception, in which the forceps failed to reach the tumor or the brushing was chosen from the beginning, the tumor was located in a certain area of Segment 1, 2, 3 or 6. In these area of the lung, the insertion of the forceps into the tumor was frequently very difficult due to the lack of flexibility of the forceps. Although the brushing was performed in all of those cases instead, only 8 out of 19 cases, 42%, the diagnosis of carcinoma was successfully made by the brushing, since the brushing was also difficult in these area. The overall diagnostic accuracy for the nonvisible peripheral lung cancer by either the transbronchial biopsy or brushing using flexible bronchofiberscope was 50 out of 70 cases, 71.4%.

Discussion

The major diagnostic method for the endoscopically visible bronchogenic carcinoma has been long time the forceps biopsy. For the diagnosis of the endoscopically nonvisible carcinoma, the brushing has been the commonest method, however, the transbronchial forceps biopsy was recently begun to be used. The results of this series show that the success rate in the diagnosis of the nonvisible carcinoma by the transbronchial biopsy is as high as in brushing. Moreover, the transbronchial biopsy has a great advantage of making the histological diagnosis.

Conclusion

The transbronchial biopsy was highly evaluated as a method to make a histological diagnosis even on the endoscopically nonvisible bronchogenic carcinoma. It had some technical limitation, but it could be complemented by brushing.

REFERENCES

I.3.

1. Friedel H: Die Katheterbiopsie des peripheren Lungenherdes. Tuberkulose-bibliothek. No 99. Barth, Leipzig. 1961.

2. Friedel H: Ein Anwendungsgebiet der bronchographischen Forschung: die Katheterung der Lungenperipherie. Z Tuberk. 115:304. 1961.

3. Kirsch M, H Mucke: Die bronchoskopische Lungensondierung und ihre diagnostischen Möglichkeiten. Wien med Wschr. 116:127. 1966.

4. Wetzer K, B Preisler, D Wenzel: Konventionelle Tubusbronchoskopie oder Glasfibertechnik? Z Erkrank Atm-Org. 141:352. 1975.

5. Wetzer K, B Preisler, D Wenzel: Gefahren und Komplikationen bei der Bronchoskopie. HNO-Praxis. 4:135. 1979.

I.4.

1. Atay Z: Cytopathologische Erkennbarkeit früher Neoplasien. In A. Georgii: Frühe Tumoren in der Diagnostik und Therapie. Verh Dtsch Krebs Ges. 2. Gustav Fischer Verlag, Stuttgart, New York. 1979.

2. Atay Z, HJ Brandt: Ergebnisse cytologischer Untersuchungen des Bronchial-sekrets bei Lungentumoren im Verhältnis zum Tumorstadium (TNM-System). Dtsch Med Wschr. 100:1269. 1975.

3. Friedel H: Ein Anwendungsgebiet der bronchographischen Forschung: Die Katheterbiopsie der Lungenperipherie. 1 Tag wiss TBS-Ges d DDR. Weimar. 1959.

4. Kluge J: Die histologische Beurteilung des Katheterbiopsie-Aspirates beim Bronchialkarzinom. Zeitschr f Tuberk. 124:97. 1965.

5. Maaßen W: Katheterbiopsie - Mediastinoskopie. Beitr Klin Erforsch Tuberk. 140:238. 1969.

II.6.

1. Lawin P: Praxis der Intensivbehandlung. Thieme, Stuttgart. 1975.

2. Streicher HJ, J Rolle: Der Notfall: Atemnot. Thieme, Stuttgart. 1973.

3. Ferlinz R et al: Bronchologische Eingriffe. Thieme, Stuttgart. 1976.

III.2.

1. Zavala DC: Diagnostic fiberoptic bronchoscopy. Techniques and results of biopsy in 600 patients. Chest. 68:12. 1975.

2. Lindholm C-E, B Ollman, JV Snyder, EG Millen, A Grenvik: Cardiorespitatory effects of flexible fiberoptic bronchoscopy in critically ill patients. Chest. 74:362. 1978.

3. Pereira V Jr, D Kovnat, GL Snider: A prospective cooperative study of complications following flexible fiberoptic bronchoscopy. Chest. 73: 813. 1978.

4. Suratt PM, JF Smiddy, B Grubner: Deaths and complications associated with fiberoptic bronchoscopy. Chest. 69:747. 1976.

5. Zavala DC. Complications following fiberoptic bronchoscopy. Chest 73: 783. 1978.

III.4.

1. Gottlieb LS, R Hillberg: Endobronchial tamponade therapy for intractable hemoptysis. Chest. 67:482. 1975.

2. Sahebjani H: Iced saline lavage during bronchoscopy. Chest. 69:131. 1976.

3. Stemberger A, HM Fritsche, P Primbs, G Blümel: Fibrinogenkonzentrate und Kollagenschwämme zur Gewebeklebung. Med Welt. 29:720. 1978.

4. Zavala DC. Pulmonary hemorrhage in fiberoptic transbronchial biopsy. Chest. 70:584. 1976.

III.7.

1. Ikeda S: Atlas of flexible Bronchofiberscopy. 1974. Thieme. Stuttgart.

2. Randazzo GP, AF Wilson. Cardiopulmonary changes during flexible fiberoptic bronchoscopy. Respiration. 33:143. 1976.

III.8.

1. Albertini RE, JH Harrell II, N Kurihara, KM Moser: Arterial Hypoxemia Induced by Fiberoptic Bronchoscopy. Jama. 230:1666. 1974.

2. Harrell II JH: Transnasal Approach for Fiberoptic Bronchoscopy. Chest. 73:7045. 1978. Supp.

3. Zavala DC: Flexible Fiberoptic Bronchoscopy. Press of Pepco Litho. Iowa. 1978.

4. Kerr JH, AC Smith, C Prys-Roberts, R Meloche, P Foex: Observations During Endobronchial Anesthesia II: Oxygenation. Br J Anesth. 46:84. 1974.

5. Newman RW, GE Finer, JE Downs: Routine Use of the Carlens Double-Lumen Endobronchial Catheter. J Thoracic and Cardiovas Surg. 42 (3):327. 1961.

III.10.

1. Lutz H: Sorgfalt bei der Voruntersuchung und Vorbehandlung. Anästh- u Intensivmed. 2:31. 1979.

2. Sechzer PH, LD Egbert, HW Linde, DY Cooper, Dripp, HL Price: Effect of CO_2 inhalation on arterial pressure, ECG and plasma catecholamines and 17 OH corticosteroids in normal man. J appl Physiology. 15:454. 1960.

3. Hügin W: Die Verträglichkeit von Octapressin mit verschiedenen Narkosen. Anästhesist. 11:185. 1962.

4. Johnston RR, EJ Eger: A Comparative Interaction of Epinephrine with Enflurane and Halothan in Man Epinephrine induced PUC's and Anesthesia. Anest Analg Curr Res. 55:709. 1976.

III.12.

1. Karetzky, Garney, Brandtetter: Effect of FB on arterial oxygen tension. NY State Jour of Med. 74:62. 1974.

2. Randozzo, Wilson: Cardiopulmonary changes during FB. Respiration. 33: 143. 1976.

3. Shrader DL, S Lakshminarayan: The effect of fiberoptic bronchoscopy on cardiac rhythm. Chest. 73:821. 1978.

4. Luck JC et al: Arrhythmias from fiberoptic bronchoscopy. Chest. 74: 139. 1978.

5. Khan MA: Fiberoptic bronchoscopy revisited. Chest. 74:119. 1978.

III.13.

1. Albertini RE, JH Harrell II, N Kurihara, KM Moser: Arterial hypoxemia induced by fiberoptic bronchoscopy. JAMA. 230:1666. 1974.

2. Karetzky MS, JW Garvey, RD Brandstetter: Effect of fiberopticbronchoscopy on arterial oxygenation tension. NY State J Med. 74:62. 1974.

III.15.

1. Atocha J: Available Techniques in Foreign Body Removal. First World Cong on Bronchoscopy. Tokyo. 1978.

2. Ikeda S: Atlas of Flexible Bronchoscopy. Igaku Shoin. Tokyo. 1974.

3. Sackner MA: Bronchofiberscopy: State of the Art. Am Rev Resp Dis. 111:62. 1975.

4. Zavala DC: Flexible Fiberoptic Bronchoscopy. Press of Pepco Litho. Iowa. 1978.

V.1.

1. James DG, J Turiaf, Hosoda Y, MW Jones, HL Israel, AC Douglas, LE Siltz-bach: Description of sarcoidosis: Report of the subcommittee of classification and definition. Ann NY Acad Sci. 278:742. 1976 (b).

2. Arnoux A, C Danel, G Stanislas-Leguern, J Marsac, G Huchon, JC Saltiel, R Dufat, J Chrétien: Données cellulaires concernant 65 lavages Broncho-Alvéolaires effectués au cours de Sarcoidoses. Le Colloques de l'INSERM. Le Lavage Broncho-Alvéolaire. INSERM. 84:489. 1979.

3. Cushman DW, HS Cheung: Spectrophotometric assay and properties of the angiotensin-converting enzyme of rabbit lung. Biochem Pharmacol. 20: 1637. 1971.

4. Stanislas-Leguern G, J Marsac, A Arnoux, D Lecossier: Serum angiotensin-converting-enzyme and bronchoalveolar lavage in sarcoidosis. Lancet. 723. 1979.

5. Lieberman J: Elevation of serum Angiotensin-Converting-Enzyme (ACE) in sarcoidosis. Am J Med. 59:365. 1975.

6. Warr GA, RR Martin, CI Holleman, BS Criswell: Clissification of bronchial lymphocytes from non-smokers and smokers. Am Rev Resp Dis. 113:96. 1976.

V.2.

1. Chase MW: The preparation and standardisation of Kveim testing antigen. Am. Rev. resp. Dis. 84, 86, 1961.

2. Siltzbach LE: Significance and specificity of the Kveim reaction. Acta Med. Scand. [Suppl], 425, 74, 1964.

3. Mitchell DN, Sutherland I, Bradstreet CMP, Dighero MW: Validation and standardizaion of Kveim test suspensions prepared from two human sarcoid spleens. J. clin. Path., 29, 203, 1976.

4. Mitchell DN, Scadding JG: Sarcoidosis. Amer. Rev. resp. Dis., 110, 774, 1974.

5. Siltzbach LE: Qualities and behaviour of satisfactory Kveim suspensions. Ann. NY Acad. Sci., 278, 665, 1976.

6. Kennedy WPU: An evaluation of freeze-dried Kveim reagent. Brit. J. Dis. Chest, 61, 40, 1967.

7. Douglas AC, Wallace A, Clark J, Stepehens JH, Smith IE, Allan NC: The Edinburgh spleen: source of a validated Kveim-Siltzbach test material. Ann. NY Acad. Sci., 278, 670, 1976.

8. Bradstreet CMP, Dighero MW, Mitchell DN: The Kveim test: analysis of results using Colindale (K12) materials. Ann. NY Acad. Sci., 278, 681, 1976.

9. Bradstreet CMP, Dighero MW, Mitchell DN: The Kveim test: analysis of results of tests using K19 materials. In proceedings of the 8th International Conference on Sarcoidosis, Cardiff, 1978, in press.

10. Mikhail JR, Mitchell DN, Sutherland I, McNicol MW: Sarcoidosis presenting in a District General Hospital: In proceedings of the 8th International Conference on Sarcoidosis, Cardiff 1978, in press.

11. Mitchell DM, Mitchell DN, Collins JV, Emerson C J: Flexible-bronchoscope biopsy of bronchial wall and of lung in the diagnosis of sarcoidosis. Brit. med. J., 280, 679, 1980.

12. Mitchell DN, Siltzbach LE, Sutherland I, D'Arcy Hart P: Some further observations of the Kveim test in relation to BCG vaccination and tuberculin sensitivity. In Proceedings of the IV International Conference on Sarcoidosis, Paris 1967, p154.

13. Mitchell DN, Cannon P, Dyer NH, Hinson KFW, Willoughby JMT: The Kveim test in Crohn's disease. Lancet 2, 571, 1969.

14. Mikhail JR, Shepherd M, Mitchell DN: Mediastinal lymph node biopsy in sarcoidosis. Endoscopy, 11 (1), 5, 1979.

15. Stableforth DE, Knight RK, Collins JV, Heard BE, Clarke SW: Transbronchial lung biopsy through the fibreoptic bronchoscope. Brit. J. Dis. Chest, 72, 108, 1978.

V.3.

1. Greschuchna D, W Maaßen: Results of mediastinoscopy and other biopsies in sarcoidosis and silicosis. In: Mediastinoscopy. Jepsen O, HR Sørensen (Ed). Odense Univ Press. 1971.

2. Maaßen W, D Greschuchna: Die Biopsie bei Sarkoidose und Silikose. Kongr Ber Wiss Tag Norddtsch Ges Tbk u Lungenkrht. 13:83. 1973.

V.7.

1. Olsson T, H Björnstad-Pettersen, N Stjernberg: Bronchostenosis due to sarcoidosis. A cause of atelectasis and airway obstruction simulating pulmonary neoplasm and chronic obstructive pulmonary disease. Chest. 75:663. 1979.

2. Roethe R, F Fuller, R Byrd, D Hafermann: Transbronchiscopic lung biopsy in sarcoidosis: optimal number and sites for diagnosis. Chest. 77:400. 1980.

3. Stähle J: Bronchial involvement in pulmonary sarcoidosis. Acta Med Scand. 176:234 (Suppl 425). 1964.

606

V.10.

1. Koontz, C.H., Joyner, L.R., Nelson, R.A.: Transbronchial lung biopsy via the fiberoptic bronchoscope in sarcoidosis. Ann.Int.Med. 85, 64-66, 1976
2. Schiessle W.: La ponction transbronchique et transtrachéale des adénopathies peritrachéobronchiques. J.franç.Méd.Chir.thor. 16, 551-569, 1962
3. Leuenberger Ph., Zellweger J.-P., Solari G., Benusiglio L.N., Vodoz J.F., Domeninghetti G., Aguet F., Vejdovsky R., Favez G.: Fréquence de l'atteinte bronchique et pulmonaire aux differents stades de la sarcoïdose endothoracique. (To be published)

V.12.

1. Crowe J.K., Brown L.R. and Muhm J.R.: Computed tomograpny of the mediastinum. Radiology 128: 75-87, 1978.
2. Faves G., Willa C., Heinzer F.: Posterior oblique tomography at an angle of 55° in chest roentgenology. A.J.R. 120: 907-915, 1975.
3. Heitzman E.R.: Radiologic analysis of the mediastinum utelising computed tomography. Radiol. Clin. North Am. 15: 309-329, 1977.
4. Mintzer R.A., Malawe S.R., Neiman H.L., Michaellis L.L., Vanecko R.M. and Sanders J.H.: Computed v.s. conventional tomography in evaluation of primary and secundary neoplasms. Radiology 132: 653-659, 1979.

VI.2.

1. Commentary. JAMA. 227:5. 1974.
2. Eygelaar A, ETh Edens: Postsurgical treatment of tracheal or bronchial anastomosis. Arch Chir Neerl. 24: 329. 1972.
3. Huzly A: Bronchoskopie. Diagnostische und therapeutische Anwendung. HNO. 25:362. 1977.
4. Katz RL, G Berci: A new intubation technique for adults and children with specific reference to teaching. Anesthesiol. 51:251. 1979.
5. Oho K, R Amemiya: Practical fiberoptic bronchoscopy. 1st ed. Tokyo. Iguka-Spoin. 1979.
6. Sackner MA: Bronchofiberscopy. Am Rev Resp Dis. 111:62. 1975.
7. Zavala DC: Pers comm. 5d World Cong Broncho-esophagology. Palm Beach. 1980.

VII.6.

1. Lomholt N: A new tracheostomy tube. Acta anest scand. Suppl. 44. 1971.

VII.8.

1. Alonso WA, LL Pratt, JH Ogura: Complications of laryngotracheal diarup-tion. The Laryngoscope. 84:1276. 1974.

2. Couraud L, A Bruneteau, JR Hazera: Désinsertion laryngo-trachéale post-traumatique aven fracture du cartilage cricoide et arrachement bilaté-rale du nerf récurrent. Ann Chir Thorac Cardiovasc. 13:249. 1974.

3. Couraud L, Ph Chevalier, A Bruneteau, P Dupont: Le traitement des sténoses trachéales après trachéotomie. Indications thérapeutiques, préparation à l'intervention. Ann Chir Thorac Cardiovasc. 8:351. 1969.

4. CouraudL, C Martigne, PJ Dumas, P Houdelette: Traitement chirurgical des sténoses de la voie respiratoire après ránimation. Chirurgie. 104:74. 1978.

5. Lejeune FE: Laryngotracheal separation. The Laryngoscope. __:1956. 1978.

VII.10.

1. (Same ref. as VII.8.3).

2. Couraud L, A Bruneteau, JJ Desplantez: Le traitement des sténoses de la voie respiratoire principale après réanimation. Expérience personnelle de 81 cas. Ann Chir Thorac Cardiovasc. 15:311. 1976.

3. (Same ref. as VII.8.4).

4. Gerwat J, D Bryce: The management of subglottic laryngeal stenosis by resection and direct anastomosis. Laryngoscope. 84:940. 1974.

5. Pearson FG, JD Cooper et al: Primary tracheal anastomosis after resec-tion of the cricoid cartilage with preservation of recurrent laryngeal nerves. J Thorac Cardiocasc Surg. 70:806. 1975.

VII.12.

1. Ohlsén L: Cartilage regeneration from perichondrium. Experimental studies in rabbits and dogs. Acta Univ Upsal. 252: (page not given. Ed) 1976.

2. Nordin U: The trachea and cuff-induced tracheal injura. An experimental study on causative factors and prevention. Acta Otolaryngol (Stockh). Suppl. 345:(page not given. Ed.) 1977.

VIII.1.

1. Atay Z, HJ Brandt: The importance of cytodiagnosis of perbronchial fine needle aspiration of mediastinal or hilar tumours. Dtsch med Wschr. 102:345. 1977.

2. Brandt HJ, in Grunze H: Klinische Zytologie der Thoraxkrankheiten. Ferninand Enke. Stuttgart. 1955.

3. Preussler H: Possibilities and limitations in the cytological interpretation of perbronchial fine needle biopsies. In: Nakhosteen JA, W Maassen (Ed): Bronchology 1980. Martinus Nijhoff, The Hague, London, Boston. 1980.

4. Schieppati E: Mediastinal lymph node puncture through the tracheal carina. Surg Gynecol Obstet. 107:243. 1958.

VIII.2.

1. Atay Z, IG v Schlieben: Cytologische Diagnostik des Bronchialcarcinoms. Internist. 22:327. 1970.

2. Atay Z: Die Zytodiagnostik der intrathorakalen Sarkoidose. Verh Dtsch Ges Path. 55:572. 1971.

3. Atay Z, H Preussler: Ergebnisse der vergleichenden Zytologie und Histologie von 921 malignen Tumoren aus 2500 Biopsien im Thorax. Verh Dtsch Ges Path. 57:360. 1973.

4. Atay Z, HJ Brandt: Die Bedeutung der Zytodiagnostik der perbronchialen Feinnadelpunktion von mediastinalen oder hilären Tumoren. Dtsch med Wschr. 102:345. 1977.

5. Esposti P-L, S Franzen, J Zajicek: The Aspirations Biopsy Smear. in LK Koss: Diagnostic Cytology. Lippincott, Philadelphia. 1968. (P. 565 ff)

5. Loddenkemper R, H Grosser, HJ Brandt: Thirty years experience with perbronchial fine needle aspiration. Nakhosteen JA, W Maassen (Ed): Bronchology 1980. Martinus Nijhoff, The Hague, London, Boston. 1980.

IX.10.

1. Niaudet P, A Venet, P Even, JF Bach: Study of human alveolar lymphocytes populations obtained by broncho-alveolar lavage. Colloques de l'INSERM. 84:211. 1979.

2. Reynolds HY, WW Merril: Analysis of broncho-alveolar lavage in normal humans and patients with diffuse interstitial lung disease. Colloques de l'INSERM. 84:227. 1979.

3. Valenti S, A Scordamaglia: Transbronchial Lung Biopsy with Fiberoptik Bronchoscope. Scand J Resp Dis. 59:243. 1978.

4. Valenti S, P Crimi, A Ferrari, A Scordamaglia: Etude des fractions phospholipidiques et du surfactant dans le lavage broncho-alveolaire chez l'homme. Colloques de l'INSERM. 84:93. 1979.

5. Valenti S, Scordamaglia A, P Crimi, C Mereu: La fibrobroncoscopia e le sue applicazioni cliniche. Ed. Minerva Medica, Torino. 1980.

X.2.

1. Johnson AR: Human pulmonary endothelial cells in culture. J clin Invest. 65: (page not given. Ed). 1980.

2. Liebermann J: Elevation of serum ACE level in sarcoidosis. Am J Med. 59: (page not given. Ed). 1975.

3. Leuenberger PJ et al: Decrease in Angiotensin I Conversion by Acute Hypoxia in Dogs. Proc Soc exper Biol and Med. 158: (page not given. Ed). 1978.

4. Said SI: The lung as a metabolic organ. NEJM. 279:(page not given. Ed). 1968.

X.4.

1. Kronenberger H, K Morgenroth, S Tuengerthal, M Schneider, J Meier-Sydow, H Riemann, RF Kroidl, M Amthor: Pneumokoniosen bei einem Zahn-technikerkollektiv (w English abstract). Atemwegs- und Lungenkr. (In press).

2. Meier-Sydow J, M Amthor, H Hauk, H Kronenberger, S Tuengerthal: Die Diagnostik interstitieller Lungenkrankheiten. Internist. 21:65. 1980.

3. Morgenroth K: Elementaranalyse am histologische Schnitt (w English abstract). Prax Pneumol. 33:615. 1979.

X.8.

1. Nozawa Y, Y Kinoshita: Transbronchial lung biopsy for diffuse pulmonary diseases. Bronchoscopy. World Ass'n f Bronchology. Tokyo. 1978.

2. Matsui E, H Miyake, S Matsuura, S Shibayama, T iyashita: Trans-bronchial lung biopsy via Metras' catheter for diffuse pulmonary disease. Bronchoscopy. World Ass'n f Bronchology. Tokyo. 1978.

X.10.

1. Sherman AI, M Ter-Pogossian: Lymph-node concentration of radioactive colloidal gold following interstitial injection. Cancer. 6:1238. 1953.
2. Ege GN: Internal mammary lymphoscintigraphy. Radiology. 118:101. 1976.
3. Rouviére H: Anatomie de lymphatiques de l'homme. Masson et Cie. Paris. 1932.
4. Kubik I, Vizkeletz T, J Balint: Die Lokalisation der Lungensegmente in den regionalen Lymphknoten. Anat Anz. 104:104. 1957.
5. Kubik I, Tömböl T: Über die Abflussfolge der regionären Lympknoten der Lunge des Hundes. Acta anst. 33:116. 1958.

X.11.

1. Senno A, S Moallem, ER Quijano, A Adeyemo, RH Clauss: Thoracoscopy with the Fiberoptic Bronchoscope. Jou Thor Cardiovas Surg. 67:606. 1974.
2. Gwin E, F Pierce, M Boggan, G Kerby, WE Ruth: Pleuroscopy and Pleural Biopsy with the Flexible Fiberoptic Bronchoscope. Chest. 67:527. 1975.
3. Kerby GR, G Pierce, WE Ruth: Clinical Experience with Pleuroscopy Utilizing the Bronchofiberscope. Ann Otol Laryn. 84:602. 1975.
4. Borgeskov S, J Becker, AB Pederson: The Flexible Bronchofiberscope. Endoscopy. 5:177. 1973.
5. Ben-Issac FE, DH Simmons: Flexible Fiberoptic Pleuroscopy: Pleural and Lung Biopsy. Chest. 67:573. 1975.

XI. 4.

1. Ishikawa K, WJ Driskell, WJ Engelhardt: Magnesium in lung cancers of oat-cell type. Lancet. 8147:852. 1979.
2. Linder MC, JR Moor: Plasma ceruloplasmin and copper in pulmonary cancer: Studies on heavy smokers and patients with malignant and non-malignant pulmonary disease. In Prevention and Detection of Cancer, Part II, Vol I. Marcel Dekker, New York. 1978. (P. 191).
3. Pimentel JC, F Marques: Vineyard sprayers' disease. A new occupational disease. Thorax. 24:678. 1969.
4. Villar TG, R Avila, ADT Araújo: Pulmonary Granulomatosis due to inhaled Particles - Personal experience and some immunological considerations. Clin Allergy. 3:217. 1973.

5. Villar TG, R Avila, ADT Araújo: La pneumopathie des ouvriers exposés au ciment.- Comptes Renduse du XVII Congrés National de la Tuberculose et des Maladies Respiratoires. Clermont-Ferrand. Ed Masson, Paris. 1975.

XI. 7.

1. Levy MH, F Wheelock: The role of macrophages in defense against neoplastic disease. Adv Cancer Res. 20:131. 1974.

2. Reynolds HY, JP Atkinson, HH Newball, MM Frank: Receptors for immunoglobulin and complement on human alveolar macrophages. J immunol. 114: 1813. 1975.

3. Rhodes J: Altered expression of human monocyte Fc receptors in malignant disease. Nature. 265:253. 1977.

4. Reynolds HY, JD Fulmer, JA Kazmierowski, WC Roberts, MM Frank, RG Crystal: Analysis of cellular and protein content of broncho-alveolar lavage fluid from patients with idiopathic pulmonary fibrosis and chronic hypersensitivity pneumonitis. J Clin Invest. 59:165. 1977.

XI.10.

1. Sharma MP et al:(Titles not given. Ed) Cancer. 38:2457. 1976.

2. Kim YD et al: Immunol Commun. 5:619. 1976.

3. Vincent RG et al: Cancer. 36:2069. 1975.

4. Concanon JP et al: Cancer. 34:184.1974

5. Peter BD et al: Cancer. 42:1484. 1978.

XI.17.

1. Schönbein CF, comm by M Faraday. On some secondary physiological effects produced by atmospheric electricity. Med Chir Trans. 34:205. 1851.

2. Boatman ES et al: Acute effect of ozone on cat lungs. Am Rev Resp Dis 110:157. 1974.

3. Schwartz LW et al: Pulmonary responses of rats to ambient levels of ozone. Lob Invest. 34:565. 1976.

4. Martinez-Palomo A et al: The freeze-fracture technique: Application to the study of animal plasma membranes. 9th International Congress on Electron Microscopy. Toronto. Vol III. 1978.

5. Ailula NB, P Satir: The ciliary necklase, a ciliary membrane specializytion. J Cell Biol. 53:474. 1972.

XII.2.

1. Chopra SK, Taplin GV, Elam D, Carson SA, Golde D: Measurement of tracheal mucociliary transport velocity in humans - smokers versus nonsmokers (preliminary findings). Am Rev Resp Dis, 1979, 119 (Suppl.), 205.

2. Friedman M, Stott FD, Poole DO, Dougherty R, Chapman GH, Watson H, Sackner MA: A new roentgenographic method for estimating mucous velocity in airways. Am Rev Resp Dis, 1977, 115, 67-72.

3. Sackner MA, Rosen MJ, Wanner A: Estimation of tracheal mucous velocity by bronchofiberscopy. J Appl Physiol, 1973, 34, 495-499.

4. Santa Cruz R, Landa J, Hirsch J, Sackner MA: Tracheal mucous velocity in normal man and patients with obstructive lung disease; effects of terbutaline. Am Rev Resp Dis, 1974, 109, 458-463.

5. Spektor DM, Pitt BR, Yeates DB: Changes in regional mucociliary transport in the human lung resulting from systemic beta$_2$-adrenergic stimulation. Am Rev Resp Dis, 1979, 119 (Suppl.), 236.

6. Yeates DB, Aspin N, Levison H, Jones MT, Bryan AC: Mucociliary tracheal transport rates in man. J Appl Physiol, 1975, 39, 487-495.

XII.3.

1. Van As A: The Role of Selective Beta-2 Adrenoceptor Stimulants in the Control of Ciliary Activity. Respiration. 31:146. 1974.

2. Mossberg B, BA Afzelius, R Eliasson, P Camner: On the Pathogenesis of Obstructive Lung Disease. A Study on the Immotile Cilia Syndrome. Scand Rev Resp Dis. 59:55. 1978.

3. Sackner MA, GA Chapman, RD Dougherty: Effects of nebulized ipratropium bromide and atropine sulfate on tracheal mucous velocity and lung mechanics in anesthetized dogs. Respiration. 34:181. 1977.

4. Nakhosteen JA, G Wichtmann, W Petro, N Konietzko: Vergleich nuklearmedizinischer und röntgenologischer Methoden zur Bestimmung der Lungenklärfunktion. Atemwegs- u Lungendrankh (in Press).

XII.6.

1. Irivani J, GN Melville: Mucociliary function in the respiratory tract as influenced by physiochemical factors. Pharm Ther B. 2:471. 1976.

XII.8.

1. Geyer G: New histochemical techniques for the demonstration of carboxyl groups in mucosubstances. Histochem J. 3:241. 1971.

2. Hilding AC: Mucociliary insufficiency and its possible relation to chronic bronchitis and emphysema. Med Thor. 22:329. 1965.

3. Lamb D, L Reid: Histochemical and autoradiographic investigation of the serous cells of the human bronchial glands. J Pathol. 100:127. 1970.

4. Rambourg A: An improved silver–methenamine technique for the detection of periodic–acid–reactive complex carbohydrates with the electron microscope. J Histochem–Cytochem. 15:409. 1967.

5. Rhodin J: Ultrastructure and function of the human tracheal mucosa. Am Rev Resp Dis. 93.1. 1966.

XIII.3.

1. Marsh BR, JK Frost, YS Erozan et al: Flexible fiberoptic bronchoscopy. Its place in the search for lung cancer. Ann Otol. 82:757. 1973.

2. Sanderson DR, RS Fontana, LB Woolner et at:Bronchoscopic localization of radiographically occult lung cancer. Chest. 65:608. 1974.

3. Lundgren R, G Lundqvist, N Sternberg et al: Flexible fiberoptic bronchoscopy in the diagnosis of bronchial carcinoma. Scand J Respir Dis. 57:247. 1976.

4. Richardson RH, DC Zavala, PK Mukerjee et al: The use of fiberoptic bronchoscopy and brush biopsy in the diagnosis of suspected pulmonary malignancy. Amer Rev Respir Dis. 109:63. 1974.

XIV.5.

1. Jarisch R, I Sandor: Allergiediagnostik im Kindesalter. Wien klin Wschr. 89:455. 1977.

2. Kosenow W: Erkrankungen der Luftwege, der Lungen und der Ohren. In: Kinderheilkunde (Ed: von Harnack GA) 3d ed, Springer, Berlin-Heidelberg-NY. (P. 279 ff).

3. Mühlenberg R, D Glaubitt, K Siafarikas: Diagnostic efficiency of radioallergosorbent tests in children with respiratory diseases and simultaneous pollen allergy. 15 Int'le Jahrestagung der Ges f Nuclearmed, Groningen, 1977. In: Nuklearmedizin: Stand und Zukunft (Ed: Schmidt HAE, Woldring M). Schattauer, Stuttgart- NY. 1978. (P843).

4. Oprée W: Pathogenese atopischer Erkrankungen aus immunologischer Sicht. Chemie, Weinheim- NY. 1979. (P 38).

5. Siafarikas K, Glaubitt D, Mühlenberg R, Staude E: Klinische Bedeutung des RAST bei Kindern mit Schimmelpilzallergie. 2. Kölner RAST-Symposium. (in press).

XVI.1.

1. Slawson RG, RM Scott: Radiation Therapy in Bronchogenic Carcinoma. Radiology. 132:175. 1979.

2. Syed AMN, BH Feder, FW George. Afterloading Interstitial Implants in the Treatment of Oral Cavity and Oropharyngeal Cancers. Radiol Clin. 46:390. 1977.

3. Hilaris BS, N Martini, RK Luomanen: Endobronchial Interstitial Implantation. Clin Bull (Memorial Hospital). 9:17. 1976.

4. National Council on Radiation Protection and Measurements, Report No. 37: Precautions in the Management of Patients who have received Therapeutic Amounts of Radionuclides. NCRP Publications. 1970. Pp 24-35.

5. Albertini RE, JH Harrell II, N Kurihara, KM Moser: Arterial Hypoxemia induced by Fiberoptic Bronchoscopy. Jama. 230:1666. 1974.

6. Harrell II JH: Transnasal Approach for Fiberoptic Bronchoscopy. Chest. 735:704. 1978 (Supp).

XVI.3.

1. Marks C, M Marks: Bronchial adenoma. A clinicopathologic study. Chest. 71 (3):376. 1977.

2. Roenspies, U, E Pfenninger, R Otto, A Senning: Bronchial carcinoids. Thoraxchirurgie. 24 (3):154. 1976.

3. Attar S, JE Miller, J Hankins, JS McLaughkin: Bronchial adenoma. Benign or Malignant? South Med J. 71 (8):919. 1978.

4. Rui de Lima: Bronchial Adenoma. Chest. 77 (1):81. 1980.

5. Ikike N, PE Bernatz, LB Woolner: Carcinoid tumors of the lung. Ann Thorac Surg. 22 (3):270. 1976.

XVI.5.

1. Magnusson P, G Rotemark: Tracheobronchopathia osteochondroplastica. J Laryng. 88:159. 1974.

2. Martin CJ: Tracheopathia osteochondroplastica. Arch otolaryngol. 100: 290. 1974.

3. Ragaini L, P Piccoli: Rivista di anatomia et di oncologia. 13:188. 1957.
XVII.11.

1. Bartlett JG, J Alexander, J Maylen, N Sullivan-Sigler, SJ Gorbach: Should fiberoptic bronchoscopy aspirates be cultured? Am Rev Resp Dis. 114:73. 1976.

FIRST AUTHOR INDEX

Abe, R., M.D.
National Utano Hospital, Narutaki
Ondoyama-cho, Ukyo-ku
Kyoto, 616, Japan

Aizawa, Y., M.D.
Keio University Hospital
35, Shinanomachi, Shinjuku-ku
Tokyo, 160, Japan

Amemiya, R., M.D.
Tokyo Med. Coll.
6-7-1, Nishishinjuku, Shinjuku-ku
Tokyo, 160, Japan

Andersen, H.A., M.D., Prof.
Mayo Clinic
Rochester, Minn. 55901, U.S.A.

Anno, H., M.D.
2nd Clin. Dept., Research Inst. Hosp.
Japan Anti-Tuberculosis Ass.
3-1-24, Matsuyama, Kiyose-shi
Tokyo, 180-04, Japan

Antić, N., Prim. dr. sci.
Kliničko-bolnički centar,
Bežanijska Kosa
11000 Beograd, Yugoslavia

Aoki, M., M.D.
Department of Thoracic Surgery
Chest Disease Research Inst.
Kyoto University
53, Syogoin-Kawaramachi
Sakyo-ku, Kyoto-shi, 606, Japan

Arai, R., M.D.
Nakano National Chest Hospital
3-14-20, Ekoda, Nakano-ku
Tokyo, Japan

Arnoux, A., M.D.
Hôpital Laennec
42, rue de Sèvres, 75007 Paris, France

Atay, Z., M.D., Prof.
Pathologisches Institut der MHH
Karl-Wiechert-Allee 9
3000 Hannover 61, FRG

Atocha, J., M.D.
1435 Chapel Street
New Haven, Connecticut 06511, U.S.A.

Awataguchi, S., M.D.
Central Hosp. of Aomori, Prefecture,
Nagashima 1-2-24
Aomori, 030, Japan

Bánhidi, E., M.D.
Broncholog. Dept.
P.O.B. 107
Pécs, 7601, Hungary

Baumann, H.-R., M.D., P.D.   Pneumolog. Abt. Tiefenauspital
                                    CH-3004 Bern, Switzerland

Blaha, H., M.D., Prof.   Zentralkrankenhaus
                                    8035 Gauting, FRG

Borgeskov, S., M.D.   Rigshosp. afsn 3032
                                    Blegdamsvej
                                    Copenhagen, 2100 Ø, Denmark

Clarke, St. W., M.D.   The Brompton Hospital
                                    Fulham Road
                                    London, SW3 6HP, England

Couraud, L., M.D., Prof.   39 avenue Felix Faure
                                    33200 Bordeaux, France

Dedo, H., M.D., Prof.   University of California
                                    Room A-717
                                    400 Panassus Avenue
                                    San Francisco, CA 94143, U.S.A.

Dumon, J.-F., M.D.   Hôpital Salvator
                                    Service d'endoscopie thoracique
                                    Marseille cedex 2 BP51 - 13274,
                                    France

Eckert, R., M.D.   Zentralkrankenhaus
                                    8035 Gauting, FRG

Edens, E.Th., M.D.   University Medical Center
                                    P.O.Box 30.001
                                    9700 RB Groningen, Netherlands

Engel, J., M.D.   Reembroden 63
                                    2000 Hamburg 63, FRG

Fontana, R.S., M.D., Prof.   Mayo Clinic
                                    Rochester, Minn. 55901, U.S.A.

Freitas e Costa, M., M.D., Prof.   Department of Pneumonology
                                    Hospital Santa Maria
                                    University of Lisbon
                                    Lisboa, Portugal

Fukuoka, M., M.D.   Osaka Prefectural Habikino Hosp.
                                    3-7-1, Habikino, Habikino-shi
                                    Osaka, 583, Japan

Funatsu, T., M.D.   Kyoto-Katsura Hospital
                                    17, Yamadahirao-cho, Nishikyo-Ku
                                    Kyoto, 615, Japan

Gallinaro, A.E., M.D., Prof.

Via Alfani 40
Firenze, 50121, Italy

G. de Vega, J.M., M.D.

Avenida de Madrid, 8-11° D
Granada, Spain

Glaubitt, D., M.D., Prof.

Institut für Nuklearmedizin
Städt. Krankenanstalten
Lutherplatz 40
4150 Krefeld, FRG

Goeckenjan, G., M.D., P.D.

Medizinische Klinik B
Universität Düsseldorf
Moorenstr. 5
4000 Düsseldorf, FRG

Götz, R., M.D.

Mainzerstr. 1
8000 München 40, FRG

Greschuchna, D., M.D.

Ruhrlandklinik
4300 Essen 16, FRG

Haglund, S., M.D.

Department of Otolaryngology
Huddinge sjukhus
S 141 86 Huddinge, Sweden

Harrell II, J.H., M.D., Ass.Prof.

225 W. Dickinson
San Diego, CA 92103, U.S.A.

Hartmann, W., M.D.

Medizinische Hochschule Hannover
Podbielskistr. 380
3000 Hannover 51, FRG

Hata, E., M.D.

Department of Thoracic Surgery
Jichi Medical School
Minamikawachi-machi,
Tochigi-Ken, 329-04, Japan

Hayakawa, K., M.D.

Department of Surgery
Tokyo Med. Coll. Hosp.
6-7-1, Nishishinjuku
Shinjuku-ku
Tokyo, Japan

Hayashi, N., M.D.

Department of Surgery
Tokyo Med. Coll. Hosp.
6-7-1, Nishishinjuku
Shinjuku-ku
Tokyo, Japan

Heck, I., M.D.

Wilhelmstr. 35
5300 Bonn, FRG

Hershko, E., M.D.

Tel Hashomer Hospital
Chaim Sheba Medical Center
Tel-Hashomer, Israel

Hesse, H., M.D.

Camphausenstr. 10
4000 Düsseldorf 13, FRG

Hitomi, S., M.D.

Department of Chest Disease
Kansaidenryoku Hospital
Okutenzin 1-23-6,
Takatuki 569, Japan

Honda, J., M.D.

1-15-1, Kitasato
Sagamihara, Kanagawa Pref. 223
Japan

Honda, K., M.D.

148, Chozaichi-cho
Iwakura, Sakyo-ku
Kyoto, 606, Japan

Horie, S., M.D., Prof.

Dokkyo University School of Med.
Mibu, Tochigi 321-02, Japan

Hsieh, Y.-Ch., M.D.

Department of Medicine
Tri-Service General Hospital, N.D.M.C.
622, Ting-Chow Rd.
Taipei, Taiwan, China

Hsu, H.H., M.D.

53, Kawahara Machi Shogoin Sakyoku
Kyoto, 606, Japan

Hürzeler, D., M.D.

Klosbachstr. 107
CH-8032 Zürich, Switzerland

Hug, H., M.D.

Gellertstr. 45
CH-4052 Basel, Switzerland

Ishihara, T., M.D.

Dept. Surg., School of Medicine
Keio University
Tokyo, 160, Japan

Itoh, M., M.D.

Dept. Thorac. Surg.
Chest Disease Research Inst.
Kyoto University
53, Syogoin Kawaramachi, Sakyo
Kyoto, 606, Japan

Iwahashi, H., M.D.

Tokyo Metropolitan Cancer Detection
Center, Kanda Surugadai,
2-5, Chiyoda-ku
Tokyo, 101, Japan

Kahi, T., M.D.	Oita National Hospital 19, Minamikasugamachi Oita, 870, Japan
Kaneko, M., M.D.	Kitasato University, School of Med. 1-15-1, Kitasato Sagamihara, 228, Japan
Kasparek, R., M.D.	Ruhrlandklinik 4300 Essen 16, FRG
Kato, H., M.D.	Department of Surgery Tokyo Med. Coll. Hospital 6-7-1, Nishishinjuku, Shinjuku-ku Tokyo, Japan
Kawai, T., M.D.	Department of 2nd Surgery Boei Medical School 525, Tokorozawa Tokorozawa, 359, Japan
Kawauchi, T., M.D.	Tokyo Medical Coll. Hosp. Department of Surgery 6-7-1, Nishishinjuku, Shinjuku-ku Tokyo, Japan
Kertes, I., M.D.	1021 Budapest II. Pálos u. 1.VII.30. Hungary
Kimura, K., M.D.	The First Department of Medicine Faculty of Medicine North 14, West 5, Kitaku Sapporo, 060, Japan
Klippe, H.J., M.D.	Krankenhaus der LVA Hamburg Wöhrendamm 80 2070 Grosshansdorf, FRG
Klinke, F., M.D.	Chirurgische Klinik der Westf. Wilhelms-Universität Jungeblodtplatz 1 44 Münster/Westf., FRG
Ko, H.-C., M.D.	Taipei Municipal Jen-Ai Hospital 237, Yen-Pin North Road, Section 2 Taipei, 101, Taiwan, China
Kobayashi, T., M.D.	286, Yokota, Oaza, Matsumoto-City Nagano-Pref. 390, Japan

Kotake, Y., M.D.	Osaka Prefectural Habikino Hosp. 3-7-1, Habikino Habikino-City, Osaka, 583, Japan
Koyama, A., M.D.	Dept. of Thoracic Surgery Research Institute Hospital Japan Anti-Tuberculosis Ass. 3-1-24, Matsuyama, Kiyose-shi Tokyo 180-04, Japan
Kudo, H., M.D.	School of Medicine, c/o Juntendo Univ. 1-3, Hongo, 3 Chome Bunkyo-Ku, Tokyo 113, Japan
Kurasawa, T., M.D.	Chest Disease Research Institute Kyoto University Sakyo-ku, Kyoto, 606, Japan
Kurashima, A., M.D.	Department of Internal Medicine Tokyo National Chest Hospital No. 3-1-1, Takeoka, Kiyose-shi Tokyo 180-04, Japan
Kroidl, R., M.D.	2160 Stade, FRG
Kronenberger, H., M.D.	Universitätsklinik Frankfurt/Main 6000 Frankfurt/Main, FRG
Lindholm, C.-E., M.D., Prof.	Dept. of Otolaryngology 75014 Uppsala, Sweden
Loddenkemper, R., M.D.	Am Großen Wannsee 80 1000 Berlin 39, FRG
Lourenco, R.V., M.D., Prof.	Dept. of Medicine, Univ. of Illinois 840 S. Wood Street Chicago, Illinois, 60612, U.S.A.
Lundgren, R., M.D.	Gimoborgsv 4 S-902 40 Umeå, Sweden
Maeda, M., M.D.	Dept. Surgery, Osaka Univ. Med. School 1-1-50, Fukushima, Fukushima-ku Osaka-shi, Osaka, 553, Japan
Magnussen, H., M.D.	Medizinische Univ.-Poliklinik Wilhelmstr. 35-37 5300 Bonn 1
Matsui, E., M.D.	Department of Radiology Gifu University School of Medicine 40, Tsukasa-machi, Gifu-shi Gifu, 500, Japan

Matsui, K.,M.D.
Habikino Hospital, Surgery
3-7-1, Habikino, Habikino-shi
Osaka, 583, Japan

Mikami, H., M.D.
The First Depart. of Medicine
Faculty of Medicine
Hokkaido University
North 14, West 5, Kita-Ku
Sapporo, 060, Japan

Mitchell, D.M., M.D.
33 Countess Road
London N.W. 5, England

Mitchell, D.N., M.D.
MRC Tuberculosis & Chest Disease Unit
Brompton Hospital
Fulham Road
London, SW3 6HP, England

Molnár,B., M.D.
Kossuth st. 32
H-8900 Zalaegerszeg, Hungary

Mrckovcić, M., M.D.
Jordanovac 104
41000, Zagreb, Yugoslavia

Nagai, A., M.D.
1st Dept. of Internal Medicine
Tokyo Women's Medical School
10, Kawadacho, Shinjuku-ku
Tokyo, 162, Japan

Nagai, K., M.D.
Department of Surgery
Tokyo Med. Coll. Hospital
6-7-1, Nishishinjuku,
Shinjuku-ku, Tokyo, Japan

Nakamura, K., M.D.
National Kinki Central Hospital
Dept. of Surgery
1180, Nagasone-cho, Sakai-shi
Osaka, 591, Japan

Nakano, M., M.D.
Department of Internal Medicine
Nagasaki Municipal Hospital
6-39, Niichimachi, Nagasaki-City
Nagasaki-Pref. 850, Japan

Nakhosteen, J.A., M.D.
Ruhrlandklinik
4300 Essen 16, FRG

Naruke, T., M.D.
Department of Surgery
National Cancer Center Hospital
5-1-1, Tsukiji, Chuo-Ku
Tokyo, 104, Japan

Natsuizaka, T., M.D.

Internal Medicine (section3)
Sapporo Medical College
S.I., W.I. 6, Chuoku,
Sapporo, 060, Japan

Niederle, N., M.D.

Innere Universitätsklinik
Hufelandstr. 55
4300 Essen, FRG

Nordin, U., M.D., Prof.

Dept. of Otorhinolaryngology
University Hospital
S-75014 Uppsala, Sweden

Nerger, K., M.D.

Im Busch 3
6100 Darmstadt-Eberstadt, FRG

Ogihara, M., M.D.

Department of Internal Medicine
Tokyo Jikeikai University
8192, Fuchu-Cho, 20-Chome, Fuchu,
Tokyo, 183, Japan

Ohata, M., M.D.

The Thoracic Surgery Dept.
Nihon University Hospital
13-1, Oyaguchikami-cho, Itabashi-ku
Tokyo, 173, Japan

Oho, K., M.D.

Tokyo Med. Coll. Hosp.
6-7-1, Nishishinjuku
Shinjuku-ku,
Tokyo, 160, Japan

Ohsaki, Y., M.D.

The First Department of Medicine
Faculty of Medicine
Hokkaido Univ.
North 14, West 5,
Sapporo, 060, Japan

Ohtani, T., M.D.

Department of Surgery
6-7-1, Nishishinjuku,
Shinjuku-ku, Tokyo, 160, Japan

Okada, H., M.D.

Dept. of Thoracic Surgery
Kita no Hospital
13-3, Kamiyama-chyo, Kita-ku
Osaka, 530, Japan

Okayasu, M., M.D.

The First Dept. of Internal Med.
Nihon Univ., School of Medicine
No. 30-1, Oyaguchi-Kamimachi
Itabashi-ku,
Tokyo, 173, Japan

Ollman, B.G., M.D.   Ear, Nose & Throat Clinic
                                  Visby Hospital
                                  S-621 01 Visby, Sweden

Ono, R., M.D.   Division of Endoscopy (N.C.C.H.)
                                  7, Sakamachi, Shinjuku-ku
                                  Tokyo, 160, Japan

Osakabe, Y., M.D.   Showa University
                                  Fujigaoka
                                  Yokohama, Japan

Palojoki, A., M.D.   Vähä-Hämeenk 7 C 46
                                  20500 Turku 50, Finland

Paolini, A., M.D., Prof.   Via di Villa Massimo No. 1
                                  Roma, 00161, Italy

Parry, W.H., M.D., Ph. D.   Fitzsimons Army Medical Center
                                  Aurora, CO 30045, U.S.A.

Perng, R.-P., M. D.   Diagnostic Center of Chest Disease
                                  No. 128-5, Chin-Hwa St.
                                  Taipei, Taiwan, China

Petro, W., M.D.   Ruhrlandklinik
                                  4300 Essen 16, FRG

Piliś, I., M.D.   Institute of Lung Diseases & Tb
                                  Medical Faculty Novi Sad
                                  Stevana Musića ul. 10 a
                                  Novi Sad 21.000, Yugoslavia

Preussler, H., M.D.   Abteilung für Pathologie
                                  Am Großen Wannsee 80
                                  1000 Berlin 39, FRG

Reimann, B.G., M.D.   Raphaelsklinik
                                  Klosterstr. 75
                                  4400 Münster, FRG

Roglić, M., M.D.   Jordanovac 104
                                  41000 Zagreb, Yugoslavia

Roux, J., M.D.   Podbielskistr. 380
                                  Oststadtkrankenhaus
                                  3000 Hannover 51, FRG

Ruas da Silva, J., M.D.   Department of Chest Diseases
                                  Lisbon University
                                  Urbanisacão Portela Saccuòm
                                  Lote 112-1°. D^Rⁱ
                                  1885 Lisboa, Portugal

Saeed, A.H., M.D.	Sadar Bahadur Khan Sanatorium 1, Falak Numa Clinic Abdullah Haroon Road, Karachi, Pakistan
Sanderson, D.R., M.D., Prof.	Mayo Clinic Rochester, Minn. 55901, U.S.A.
Sato, A., M.D.	Hamamatsu University, School of Med. 3600, Handa-cho, Hamamatsu-shi Shizuoka-ken 431-31, Japan
Schaefer, M., M.D.	Johanniter-Krankenhaus 4200 Oberhausen, FRG
Schindl, R., M.D., Prim.	Elisabethinen Krankenhaus A 4020 Linz-Donau, Austria
Schlehe, H., M.D.	Klinik rechts der Isar Ismaninger Str. 22 8000 München 80, FRG
Schulz, V., M.D., Prof.	Universitätsklinikum Abt. Pneumonologie 6500 Mainz, FRG
Schuster, H., M.D.	Oewerweg 30 B 2800 Bremen 44, FRG
Sesterhenn,K., M.D.	HNO-Klinik, Universität Köln 5000 Köln, FRG
Shankar, P.S., M.D.	Deepti, Behind District Court Gulbarga 585 102, Karnataka State India
Shibayama, M., M.D.	Department of Radiology Gifu Medical College, 1-1, Yanagimachi, Gifu, 500, Japan
Shimada, H., M.D.	3rd Department of Internal Med. School of Medicine, Tokushima Univ. Kuramoto-chyo 3, Tokushima, 770 Japan
Šimeček, C., M.D.	Marxova 13, Plzeň, 305 99, ČSSR
Stjernberg, N., M.D.	Gimoborgsv 4 S-902 40 Umeå, Sweden
Suzuki, T., M.D.	Nakano National Chest Hospital 3-14-20, Ekoda, Nakano-ku Tokyo, 165, Japan

Suzuki, Y., M.D.

Josai Dental University
1-1, Keyakidai, Sakado,
Saitama, 350-02, Japan

Szüle, P., M.D.

XII. Diósárok-u.1.
Budapest, 1125, Hungary

Taguchi, H., M.D.

Division of Surgery, Tokyo Police
Hospital, 2-10-41, Fujimi Chiyoda-ku
Tokyo, 102, Japan

Takashima, T., M.D.

Hoshigaoka Koseinenkin Hospital
Dept. of Thoracic Surgery
4-8-1, Hoshigaoka
Hirakata, 573, Japan

Takayama, O., M.D.

Nihon Univ. Medical School
Broncho-esophagological Sec.
30-1, Oyaguchikami-cho, Itabashi-ku
Tokyo, 173, Japan

Takizawa, N., M.D.

Tokyo Med. Coll. Hosp.
6-7-1, Nishishinjuku, Shinjuku-ku
Tokyo, Japan

Tamada, J., M.D.

Dept. of Thoracic Surgery
Chest Disease Research Inst.
Kyoto University
53, Shogoinkawaramachi, Sakyo-ku
Kyoto, 606, Japan

Tan, T.D., M.D.

aalsterweg 259
5600 ML Eindhoven, Netherlands

Tanabe, H., M.D.

Habikino Hospital, Dept. of Surgery
3-7-1, Habikino, Habikino-shi
Osaka, 583, Japan

Teles de Araújo, A.D., M.D.

Department of Chest Diseases
Lisbon University Hospital
R. Victor Hugo, 18-4° ESQ
Lisbon, 1000, Portugal

Thal, W., M.D., Prof.

Kinderklinik der MAM
Halberstädter Str. 13
3014 Magdeburg, GDR

Thunell, M., M.D.

Department of Lung Diseases
University Hospital
S-901 85 Umeå, Sweden

Toomes, H., M.D.   Krankenhaus Rohrbach
                                    Amalienstr. 5
                                    6900 Heidelberg, FRG

Valenti, S., M.D., Prof.   Via Montallegro 2
                                    Genova, 16145, Italy

Watanabe, K., M.D.   Department of Internal Medicine
                                    Yokohama City Hospital
                                    56, Okazawa-cho, Hodogaya-ku
                                    Yokohama, 240, Japan

Weng, X.-Z., M.D., Prof.   Chao Yang Hospital
                                    Beijing, The People's Rep. of China

Wetzer, K., M.D.   Bezirkslungenklinik Lostau
                                    Friedrich-Engels-Str. 2
                                    327 Lostau, GDR

Wiman, L.-G., M.D.   Department of Lung Medicine
                                    Huddinge University Hospital
                                    14186 Huddinge, Sweden

Worch, R., M.D.   Kreiskrankenhaus
                                    Diekholzen, FRG

Wrabetz, W., M.D.   Med. Hochschule Hannover
                                    Karl-Wiechert-Alleee9
                                    3000 Hannover, FRG

Yasuoka, S., M.D.   3rd Dept. of Internal Medicine
                                    School of Medicine
                                    Tokushima University
                                    Kuramotochyo 2
                                    Tokushima, 770, Japan

Zavala, D.C., M.D., Prof.   1630 Derwen Drive
                                    Iowa City, Iowa 52240, U.S.A.

SUBJECT INDEX